MONITORING METABOLIC STATUS

Predicting Decrements in Physiological and Cognitive Performance

Committee on Metabolic Monitoring for Military Field Applications
Standing Committee on Military Nutrition Research
Food and Nutrition Board

INSTITUTE OF MEDICINE
OF THE NATIONAL ACADEMIES

THE NATIONAL ACADEMIES PRESS
Washington, D.C.
www.nap.edu

THE NATIONAL ACADEMIES PRESS 500 Fifth Street, N.W. Washington, DC 20001

NOTICE: The project that is the subject of this report was approved by the Governing Board of the National Research Council, whose members are drawn from the councils of the National Academy of Sciences, the National Academy of Engineering, and the Institute of Medicine. The members of the committee responsible for the report were chosen for their special competences and with regard for appropriate balance.

Support for this project was provided by U.S. Army Medical Research and Materiel Command through contract no. DAMD17-99-1-9478. The U.S. Army Medical Research Acquisition Activity, 820 Chandler Street, Fort Detrick, MD 21702-5014, is the awarding and administering acquisition office. The views presented in this report are those of the Institute of Medicine Committee on Metabolic Monitoring for Military Field Applications and are not necessarily those of the funding agency.

International Standard Book Number 0-309-09159-4 (Book)
International Standard Book Number 0-309-53052-0 (PDF)
Library of Congress Control Number: 2004108091

Additional copies of this report are available from the National Academies Press, 500 Fifth Street, N.W., Lockbox 285, Washington, DC 20055; (800) 624-6242 or (202) 334-3313 (in the Washington metropolitan area); Internet, http://www.nap.edu.

For more information about the Institute of Medicine, visit the IOM home page at: **www.iom.edu.**

Printed in the United States of America.

The serpent has been a symbol of long life, healing, and knowledge among almost all cultures and religions since the beginning of recorded history. The serpent adopted as a logotype by the Institute of Medicine is a relief carving from ancient Greece, now held by the Staatliche Museen in Berlin.

"Knowing is not enough; we must apply.
Willing is not enough; we must do."
—Goethe

INSTITUTE OF MEDICINE
OF THE NATIONAL ACADEMIES

Adviser to the Nation to Improve Health

THE NATIONAL ACADEMIES

Advisers to the Nation on Science, Engineering, and Medicine

The **National Academy of Sciences** is a private, nonprofit, self-perpetuating society of distinguished scholars engaged in scientific and engineering research, dedicated to the furtherance of science and technology and to their use for the general welfare. Upon the authority of the charter granted to it by the Congress in 1863, the Academy has a mandate that requires it to advise the federal government on scientific and technical matters. Dr. Bruce M. Alberts is president of the National Academy of Sciences.

The **National Academy of Engineering** was established in 1964, under the charter of the National Academy of Sciences, as a parallel organization of outstanding engineers. It is autonomous in its administration and in the selection of its members, sharing with the National Academy of Sciences the responsibility for advising the federal government. The National Academy of Engineering also sponsors engineering programs aimed at meeting national needs, encourages education and research, and recognizes the superior achievements of engineers. Dr. Wm. A. Wulf is president of the National Academy of Engineering.

The **Institute of Medicine** was established in 1970 by the National Academy of Sciences to secure the services of eminent members of appropriate professions in the examination of policy matters pertaining to the health of the public. The Institute acts under the responsibility given to the National Academy of Sciences by its congressional charter to be an adviser to the federal government and, upon its own initiative, to identify issues of medical care, research, and education. Dr. Harvey V. Fineberg is president of the Institute of Medicine.

The **National Research Council** was organized by the National Academy of Sciences in 1916 to associate the broad community of science and technology with the Academy's purposes of furthering knowledge and advising the federal government. Functioning in accordance with general policies determined by the Academy, the Council has become the principal operating agency of both the National Academy of Sciences and the National Academy of Engineering in providing services to the government, the public, and the scientific and engineering communities. The Council is administered jointly by both Academies and the Institute of Medicine. Dr. Bruce M. Alberts and Dr. Wm. A. Wulf are chair and vice chair, respectively, of the National Research Council

www.national-academies.org

COMMITTEE ON METABOLIC MONITORING FOR MILITARY FIELD APPLICATIONS

JOHN E. VANDERVEEN *(chair)*, San Antonio, Texas
BRUCE R. BISTRIAN, Clinical Nutrition, Beth Israel Deaconess Medical Center, Boston, Massachusetts
JOHN A. CALDWELL, Air Force Research Laboratory, Brooks City Air Force Base, San Antonio, Texas
JOHANNA T. DWYER, Office of Dietary Supplements, National Institutes of Health, Bethesda, Maryland, and Tufts University and New England Medical Center, Boston, Massachusetts
JOHN W. ERDMAN, Department of Food Science and Human Nutrition, University of Illinois at Urbana-Champaign
HELEN W. LANE, Habitability, Environmental Factors, and Bioastronautics Office, NASA Johnson Space Center, Houston, Texas
MELINDA M. MANORE, Department of Nutrition and Food Management, Oregon State University, Corvallis
WILLIAM P. MORGAN, Exercise Psychology Laboratory, University of Wisconsin, Madison
PATRICK M. O'NEIL, Weight Management Center, Medical University of South Carolina, Charleston
ESTHER M. STERNBERG, Section on Neuroendocrine Immunology and Behavior, National Institute of Mental Health, Bethesda, Maryland
BEVERLY J. TEPPER, Department of Food Science, Rutgers University, New Brunswick, New Jersey
JULIAN THAYER, Gerontology Research Center, National Institute on Aging, Baltimore, Maryland

Consultants
KIRA BACAL, Wyle Laboratories and Life Sciences, Houston, Texas
MARY I. POOS, Academic and Intellectual Partnerships, Food and Drug Administration, Rockville, Maryland (from November 2003)

Staff
MARIA ORIA, Study Director
MARY I. POOS, Study Director (through November 2003)
LESLIE J. VOGELSANG, Research Assistant
SANAIT B. TESFAGIORGIS, Senior Project Assistant
HARLEEN K. SETHI, Senior Project Assistant (through August 2003)

COMMITTEE ON MILITARY NUTRITION RESEARCH

JOHN W. ERDMAN *(chair)*, Department of Food Science and Human Nutrition, University of Illinois at Urbana-Champaign
BRUCE R. BISTRIAN, Clinical Nutrition, Beth Israel Deaconess Medical Center, Boston, Massachusetts
JOHANNA T. DWYER, Office of Dietary Supplements, National Institutes of Health, Bethesda, Maryland, and Tufts University and New England Medical Center, Boston, Massachusetts
HELEN W. LANE, Habitability, Environmental Factors, and Bioastronautics Office, NASA Johnson Space Center, Houston, Texas
MELINDA M. MANORE, Department of Nutrition and Food Management, Oregon State University, Corvallis
WILLIAM P. MORGAN, Exercise Psychology Laboratory, University of Wisconsin, Madison
PATRICK M. O'NEIL, Weight Management Center, Medical University of South Carolina, Charleston
ESTHER M. STERNBERG, Section on Neuroendocrine Immunology and Behavior, National Institute of Mental Health, Bethesda, Maryland
BEVERLY J. TEPPER, Department of Food Science, Rutgers University, New Brunswick, New Jersey

U.S. Army Grant Representative
COL KARL E. FRIEDL, Commander, U.S. Army Research Institute of Environmental Medicine, Natick, Massachusetts

Staff
MARIA ORIA, Project Director
MARY I. POOS, Project Director (through November 2003)
LESLIE J. VOGELSANG, Research Assistant
SANAIT TESFAGIORGIS, Senior Project Assistant
HARLEEN K. SETHI, Senior Project Assistant (through August 2003)

Reviewers

This report has been reviewed in draft form by individuals chosen for their diverse perspectives and technical expertise, in accordance with procedures approved by the NRC's Report Review Committee. The purpose of this independent review is to provide candid and critical comments that will assist the institution in making its published report as sound as possible and to ensure that the report meets institutional standards for objectivity, evidence, and responsiveness to the study charge. The review comments and draft manuscript remain confidential to protect the integrity of the deliberative process. We wish to thank the following individuals for their review of this report:

John Greenleaf, NASA, retired; J. Richard Jennings, University of Pittsburgh Medical Center; Gordon O. Matheson, Stanford University; Alan H. Morris, Intermountain Health Care; David C. Nieman, Appalachian State University; Clifford J. Rosen, St. Joseph Hospital, Bangor, Maine; Ronenn Roubenoff, Millennium Pharmaceuticals, Inc.; Stella L. Volpe, University of Pennsylvania.

Although the reviewers listed above have provided many constructive comments and suggestions, they were not asked to endorse the conclusions or recommendations nor did they see the final draft of the report before its release. The review of this report was overseen by Hugh Tilson, University of North Carolina at Chapel Hill. Appointed by the National Research Council and Institute of Medicine, he was responsible for making certain that an independent examination of this report was carried out in accordance with institutional procedures and that all review comments were carefully considered. Responsibility for the final content of this report rests entirely with the authoring committee and the institution.

Preface

This publication is the latest in a series of reports based on reviews of the scientific literature and workshops sponsored by the Standing Committee on Military Nutrition Research (CMNR) of the Food and Nutrition Board (FNB), the Institute of Medicine (IOM), and the National Academies. An ad hoc committee under the auspices of CMNR, the Committee on Metabolic Monitoring for Military Field Applications, was appointed to organize a workshop and prepare a report based on that workshop and a review of the relevant scientific literature. Other workshops or symposia conducted by CMNR have dealt with military weight management programs; caffeine for mental task performance; food components to enhance performance; nutritional needs in hot, cold, and high-altitude environments; nutrition and physical performance; cognitive testing methodology; fluid replacement and heat stress; and antioxidants and oxidative stress. These workshops form part of the response that the CMNR provides to the Commander of the U.S. Army Medical Research and Materiel Command regarding issues brought to the committee through the Military Operational Medicine Research Program at Fort Detrick, Maryland, and the U.S. Army Research Institute of Environmental Medicine at Natick, Massachusetts.

HISTORY OF THE COMMITTEE

The CMNR was established in October 1982 following a request by the Assistant Surgeon General of the Army that the Board on Military Supplies of the National Academy of Sciences set up a special committee to advise the U.S. Department of Defense (DOD) on the need for and conduct of nutrition research and related issues. This newly formed committee was transferred to the oversight of FNB in 1983. The committee's primary tasks are to identify factors that may critically influence the physical and mental performance of combat military personnel under all environmental extremes, to identify knowledge gaps, to recommend research that would remedy these deficiencies, to identify approaches for studying the relationship of diet to physical and mental performance, and to review and advise on military feeding standards.

As a standing committee of IOM, the membership of CMNR changes periodically, however the disciplines represented consistently have included human nutrition, nutritional biochemistry, performance physiology, food science, dietetics, psychology, and clinical medicine. For issues that require broader expertise than exists within the committee, CMNR has convened workshops, utilized consultants, or appointed subcommittees and ad hoc committees with expertise in the desired area to provide additional state-of-the art scientific knowledge and informed opinion to aid in the deliberations.

BACKGROUND

The U.S. military's concerns about the individual combat service member's ability to avoid performance degradation and the need to maintain both mental and physical capabilities in highly stressful situations have led to an interest in developing methods by which commanders could monitor the status of the combat service members in the field. This includes the ability to monitor physical and mental status of the combat service member, as well as monitoring his or her environment (e.g., ambient temperature, chemical exposure). This ability would allow commanders to determine when individuals needed to rest, eat, or consume fluids, or if their condition had deteriorated to the point that they needed to be replaced rather than risk combat injury.

Similarly, in the civilian sector, the ability to monitor physiological and cognitive status would also be crucial for individuals in situations such as sustained fire-fighting operations, chemical and other hazardous materials clean-up, industrial chemical plant work, and extended work shifts in emergency medicine. Metabolic monitoring techniques would also be valuable in the practice of telemedicine, and would enable health care workers to predict when an individual might need special attention or transport to a medical facility.

Technological advances in biological sensing of the past decade have not been accompanied by concomitant advances in the interpretation of biological signals to assess physiological status. A meaningful assessment calls for organization and interpretation of data and contextual information (e.g., ambient conditions, individual recent and historical reference points) from multiple sensors in a multidisciplinary effort between signal processing, mathematical modeling, and physiology. This is of special interest wherever physiological monitoring may predict problems in advance of a crisis.

For example, detection of high rates of bone and muscle turnover may be indicative of increased susceptibility to injury during an intensive physical training program and might provide an indication for optimal rest periods. Reduced cellular metabolism caused by glucose and insulin derangement may be signaled by early decrements in cognitive status, neurological functioning, or muscle action, allowing a combat service member operating in extreme conditions to take corrective actions. Dehydration may be marked by changes in skin turgidity, electrical impedance, heart rate, and/or skin temperature thus alerting an individual to impending risk of impaired performance and heat injury.

THE COMMITTEE'S TASK

Under the auspices of the Standing Committee on Military Nutrition Research, the Committee on Metabolic Monitoring for Military Field Applications was appointed to examine the state-of-the-science with respect to identification of biomarkers to predict individual health and performance outcomes related to regulation of water and substrate metabolism and cognitive function. This is a subset of a larger military effort in physiological monitoring. This study is focused on metabolic regulation during prolonged, exhaustive efforts where nutrition, hydration, and repair mechanisms may be mismatched to intakes and rest, or where specific metabolic derangements are present (e.g., following toxic chemical exposures or psychological threats). This report provides the Committee's response to the following questions posed by DOD:

(1) What are the most promising biomarkers for prediction of (a) excessive rates of bone and muscle turnover, (b) reduced glucose and energy metabolism (e.g., bioelectrical indicators of muscle and mental fatigue), (c) dehydration, and (d) decrements in cognitive function?

(2) What monitoring technologies would be required (that may not currently exist) to predict these intermediate targets in critical pathways?

(3) What tools currently exist for monitoring metabolic status that could be useful in the field?

(4) What algorithms are available that might provide useful predictions from combined sensor signals? What additional measurement would improve specificity of the predictions?

(5) What is the committee "blue sky" forecast for useful metabolic monitoring approaches (i.e., 10- to 20-year projection)? What are the current research investments that may lead to revolutionary advances?

ORGANIZATION OF THE REPORT

Chapter 1 of the report provides background information and the current status of military capabilities in monitoring and predicting physiological and cognitive status of individual combat service members. Chapter 2 provides a discussion of the importance of gathering individual data rather than group means and the need for individual baseline information. The role of physiological biomarkers and self-assessments in evaluating overall physical status are presented in Chapter 3. Potential biomarkers for monitoring bone and muscle turnover, hydration status and renal function, and stress and immune function are discussed in Chapter 4. Chapter 5 addresses monitoring of alertness and cognitive function and Chapter 6 presents the committee's conclusions and recommendations, including the committee's responses to the specific questions posed by the military in the Statement of Task. Appendix A presents a table that lists examples of physiological and cognitive markers of performance. Appendix B presents a discussion of metabolic monitoring strategies and algorithms under development at NASA that has implications for the military. Finally, the workshop agenda and workshop speaker manuscripts, as well as biographical sketches of workshop speakers and committee members are presented in Appendixes C through F.

ACKNOWLEDGMENTS

I wish to commend the workshop speakers for their excellent contributions to the workshop. Their manuscripts, presentations, participation in discussions, and willingness to take time from very busy schedules to prepare and deliver outstanding presentations made it possible for the committee to conduct a review of the area and prepare this report. Their thoughtful responses to questions posed by committee members and workshop participants also contributed immeasurably to the quality of the review. It would be neglectful not to mention the many experts who attended this open meeting at their own initiative and expense. Their questions and comments contributed in no small measure to broadening the exchange of scientific information.

Special thanks are extended to the U.S. Air Force personnel at Brooks City-Base in San Antonio, Texas, who hosted the committee's workshop. We thank COL Tom Travis, Commander of the School of Aerospace Medicine. COL Travis not only granted the committee permission to use the School's facilities, but took time from his busy schedule to address the workshop and share some of the history of the School of Aerospace Medicine with the committee and workshop attendees. Dr. Stefan Constable deserves special mention; he provided key assistance throughout the planning and execution of the workshop, including doing initial legwork on space availability, providing contact names and background information for catering needs, arranging transportation for committee members and speakers between the Base and the hotel each day, and providing names of San Antonio companies that could provide recording and transcription service. His assistance was truly invaluable. Thanks are also extended to SGT Monica Mandichak and Ms. Mary Bacerra for their assistance in setting up and demonstrating the microphones and audiovisual equipment in the Aerospace Medicine auditorium, and to Mr. Marvin Lee and SSGT Arnold Ashenbeck of the motor pool for providing transport buses and drivers who picked up and delivered workshop participants with punctuality and courtesy.

I express my deepest appreciation to the members of the committee who participated extensively during the workshop and in discussions and preparation of this report, and to Dr. Kira Bacal, who provided her considerable expertise in medical informatics and remote medical decision algorithms in her role as a consultant to the committee. Special thanks are also due to the FNB staff. In particular, I wish to acknowledge the skill and dedication of Dr. Mary I. Poos, the senior staff officer for CMNR, in organizing the workshop and preparing this report. She was instrumental in identifying and securing the expert panel of speakers, providing guidance to the committee members, and organizing and editing the report. I also want to recognize the efforts of Ms. Leslie J. Vogelsang, research assistant to CMNR, for providing outstanding expertise in recording committee deliberations, incorporating committee-drafted sections into the report, and checking all the references. The efforts of Ms. Harleen K. Sethi and Ms. Sanait Tesfagiorgis in providing excellent logistical support to committee members and workshop speakers are also recognized. Thanks are due to Dr. Maria Oria for integrating responses to reviewer comments and incorporating them into the final report. Thanks are also due to Ms. Gail Spears for copyediting the report. Finally, I wish to recognize Dr. Allison A. Yates, director emeritus of FNB during this study, for her continued interest and oversight of the CMNR during her tenure and Dr. Linda Meyers, who took the responsibilities as director of FNB in September 2003, for her role while completing the project.

JOHN E. VANDERVEEN, *Chair*
Committee on Metabolic
Monitoring for Military Field
Applications

Contents

Executive Summary

The U.S. military's concerns about the individual combat service member's ability to avoid performance degradation, in conjunction with the need to maintain both mental and physical capabilities in highly stressful situations, have led to an interest in developing methods by which commanders can monitor the status of combat service members in the field. This includes monitoring the physical and mental status of the combat service member, as well as monitoring the service member's environment (e.g., ambient temperature, geolocation, chemical exposure). Equally important are the development of methods for and the training of individual combat service members and unit commanders on self-monitoring (or monitoring of peers) of designated parameters predictive of performance. This ability would allow commanders to determine when individuals need to rest, eat, or consume fluids, or if their condition has deteriorated to the point that they need to be replaced rather than risk combat injury. Training service members in physiology and psychology then becomes an important aspect of their education.

Similarly, in the civilian sector, it is necessary to have the ability to monitor the physiological and cognitive status of individuals involved in situations such as sustained fire-fighting operations and chemical and other hazardous materials clean-ups, and for emergency medical personnel working extended shifts. Metabolic monitoring techniques would also be valuable in the practice of telemedicine and would enable healthcare workers to predict when an individual might need special attention or transport to a medical facility.

CHARGE TO COMMITTEE

This report examines appropriate biological markers, monitoring technologies currently available and in need of development, and appropriate algorithms to interpret the data obtained in order to provide information for command decisions relative to the physiological and psychological "readiness" of each combat service member. More specifically, this report also provides responses to questions posed by the military relative to monitoring the metabolic status of military personnel in training and operational situations, focusing on metabolic regulation during prolonged, exhaustive efforts (such as combat training or field operations), where nutrition/hydration and repair mechanisms may be mismatched to intakes and rest, or where specific metabolic derangements are present (e.g., following toxic chemical exposures or psychological threats). The committee was also asked to make a "blue sky" forecast for useful metabolic monitoring approaches and current research investments that may lead to revolutionary advances.

FINDINGS OF THE COMMITTEE

The Importance of Individual Differences

Biobehavioral research is among the most challenging of scientific endeavors as biological organisms display wide-ranging individual differences in physiology. A thorough exploration of biobehavioral responses requires the extensive study of individuals over time. In addition, the study of interactions between living systems and their environments has tested the limits of research methodologies and theoretical models. It is a truism in the biobehavioral sciences that no single measure or aspect of responding can adequately represent a complex latent construct; rather such constructs must be represented by an entire pattern of manifestations. In view of the prevalence and importance of rhythmicity in biological regulatory mechanisms, the inclusion of time-varying or temporal aspects of responding is crucial to accurately portray such activity. All recorded activity might be considered as relevant; functional relationships among ongoing physiological processes could then be extracted across observations.

In response to these various concerns, an alternative framework for research on monitoring the metabolic status of combat service members is suggested: a multivariate, systems perspective that emphasizes the study of individuals (combat service members). The three most important sources of variance (persons, occasions, and variables [or tests]) are present in nearly all experimental designs. Their relationship should be explicitly investigated, and the systematic variance associated with each should be accounted for before valid inferences can be drawn. The fact that such individualized, multivariate relationships have not been fully illuminated has seriously hampered the development of reliable monitoring strategies.

Biomarkers of Overall Physical Status

The overall physical status of service members in the field can be evaluated by analyzing either objective physiological measurements (e.g., energy expenditure, vital signs) or subjective measurements of self-assessments (or assessments by peers).

Monitoring core body temperature, skin temperature, and sweat losses would be invaluable in predicting if a service member was in danger of hypothermia, hyperthermia, heat stroke, or other environmentally induced overall physiological imbalance. Some technologies and algorithms currently exist that also consider environmental temperature, humidity, and wind speed.

There is evidence for the efficacy of using self-ratings of perceived and preferred levels of exertion to accurately predict physical performance in trained athletes. These methodologies need to be validated in military environments.

Biomarkers of Physiological Status

The specific metabolic systems of particular concern to the military are: bone and muscle metabolism, kidney function and hydration, and stress and immune function.

Maintaining a healthy bone is essential to minimize the incidence of fracture, which is predicted by measuring bone mineral density. However, the low level of precision of this method limits its use; therefore, for short-term changes, intermediate biological markers of bone remodeling may provide a better indication of potential fractures. Bone remodeling or the balance between resorption and formation dictates the risk of fracture. Because bone remodeling is a relatively slow process, it is more appropriate to monitor these changes during training rather than in actual combat situations. There are a variety of compounds that can be used as markers of bone resorption; however, for an accurate evaluation, biomarkers of bone formation also need to be monitored but, up to this time, their value is not clear. In addition to bone remodeling, stress is related to changes in bone health. Although cortisol appears to be a promising indicator of bone health, validation in the field is still needed.

Heavy physical exertion, inadequate energy intake, and psychological stress can all influence muscle metabolism, causing muscle damage and muscle protein breakdown. Single blood and urinary markers of these processes are difficult to interpret for a variety of reasons. For example, levels of cortisol as a measure of stress show diurnal patterns of variation. The urinary level of 3-methylhistidine, an ideal biomarker of protein catabolism because of its abundance in muscle, also may be misleading depending on the dietary consumption of muscle meats. More advanced technology for minimally invasive sampling of muscle tissue is needed before these methodologies are field-ready. Muscle soreness and ratings of self-assessment (or peer assessments) also can be good predictors of performance and indicate the need for rest.

Monitoring renal function is important because of the role of the kidneys in maintaining proper hydration, fluid homeostasis, and electrolyte balance, all of them critical to sustain both physical and cognitive functions; in addition, excretion of products of protein metabolism may also be an indicator of protein status. In the field, monitoring urinary output, color, odor, and specific gravity would all provide important information relative to hydration, electrolyte balance, muscle breakdown, and protein and energy status, as well as to the presence of infection. Changes in body weight, when coupled with knowledge of serum osmolality and/or serum sodium, would assist greatly in defining the presence and severity of disturbances in body volume status.

Stress can be defined as a constellation of events that begins with a stimulus called the stressor, which precipitates a reaction in the brain (stress perception) and subsequently activates physiological systems in the body, called the stress response. The stress response results in the release of neurotransmitters and hormones that serve as the brain's messengers for regulation of the immune and other systems and can be damaging when chronic. The rate of change of stress hormones in response to stressful stimuli is a critical variable in adaptive physiological responses. An important aspect of monitoring should include measurements (at baseline, during the stress exposure, and in the period of recovery) of indicators of stress and immune responses currently in use and in development, such as cortisol levels and heart rate variability. Self-report inventories could be adapted to offer valuable information about individual stress levels.

Biomarkers of Cognitive Status

Optimal performance in today's military is also increasingly dependent on a high level of cognitive fitness. The widespread use of computerized surveillance and reconnaissance systems, complex communications and targeting devices, highly interactive weapons systems, and even the technologically advanced diagnostic systems used in the maintenance of military equipment demands the highest level of cognitive readiness.

The efficiency of combatants in sustained operations can be significantly compromised by inadequate sleep, which can cause increased reaction time, mood declines, perceptual disturbances, motivational decrements, impaired attention, short-term memory loss, carelessness, reduced physical endurance, degraded verbal communication skills, and impaired judgment.

In all probability most technologies in development will be useful only in laboratory environments or in fixed-based operational facilities (such as posts in which radar and sonar equipment are monitored or stations from which remote-controlled vehicles are piloted) where complex equipment can be housed, lengthy recording procedures can be conducted, and rigid controls can be maintained. Only a small subset of the strategies is likely to be suitable for operational settings.

The most promising techniques for accomplishing real-time, continuous assessments of foot-soldier cognitive readiness in military field settings are: (1) actigraphy-based, or (2) electroencephalographic- (EEG) based, although neither technique is currently ready for widespread application. The most promising techniques for accomplishing real-time, continuous evaluations of the operators of military vehicles and monitoring equipment and those whose jobs consist of interfacing with computers and communications devices, are those suitable for stationary situations such as EEG based, or eye-movement based. Eye-movement parameters (i.e., PERCLOS) have already proven feasible for the detection of changes in truck-driver alertness, and efforts are underway to establish an automated PERCLOS that could be used in aviation settings.

Before implementing these methods, their feasibility in specific environments should be evaluated and a cost-benefit analysis should be performed. For example, the pilot of a B-2 bomber or other highly complex modern aircraft may be among the first to benefit from newly developed approaches because there are relatively few of these aircraft, and the cost of losing even one would be significant by any standard. On top of these considerations is the fact that aircrew fatigue is known to be an operational hazard in B-2s. Therefore, the costs associated with instrumentation of such a platform are easily justifiable.

A great deal of progress has been made toward helping the armed forces address fatigue-related cognitive decrements once they have been identified. However, highly reliable, efficient, and cost-effective technological means of initially detecting and predicting those decrements remain to be developed.

REPONSES TO THE MILITARY'S QUESTIONS

QUESTION 1

What are the most promising biomarkers for the prediction of: (a) excessive rates of bone loss and muscle turnover, (b) reduced glucose and energy metabolism (e.g., bioelectrical indicators of muscle and mental fatigue), (c) dehydration, and (d) decrements in cognitive function?

The committee recommends that, initially, simple protocol data of normal/abnormal ranges based on group averages may be used. However, these ranges may be sufficiently imprecise to make individual-based predictions dubious. Irrespective of the biological or cognitive markers selected, there is a need for baseline measurements of individual combat service members so that it can be determined, on an individual basis, if a marker is significantly altered under stress.

Biomarkers for Bone and Muscle Metabolism

Bone

Bone remodeling is a relatively slow biological process and thus not amenable to monitoring in field situations. Prediction of bone changes that increase fracture risk may be of greater importance in initial entry training, when individuals are transitioning to a greater state of fitness, than in combat.

There are no groups of intermediate markers of bone health that can provide a one-time identification of risk of fractures, including stress fracture. Markers should include bone density (as measured by dual-energy X-ray absorptiometry), sensation of bone pain, menstrual status, and mental state as related to cortisol responsiveness. The role of cortisol in bone health during military exercises, however, may be transient and may not have long-term effects on bone health.

Bone mineral density (BMD) is the most predictive measure of risk of fractures; this measure should be used in determining medical suitability for training and combat-related activities. Strategies should be developed to determine the BMD levels that are required to meet medical standards, and approaches should be identified to prevent significant loss of bone mass and fractures prior, during, and after intensive physical training.

Muscle

There are a number of biomarkers that may be indicative of muscle fatigue or increased catabolism, including protein turnover and 24-hour urinary 3-methylhistidine. However, there is insufficient evidence that can specifically correlate these biomarkers with actual decrements in muscle performance during activities such as weight lifting, timed running trials, and endurance running. In contrast, there is substantial evidence in the sports medicine literature that self- (or peer-) reported measures possess efficacy in predicting physical performance and, in fact, have often been found to be superior to other physiological measures.

Biomarkers for Reduced Glucose Metabolism

The potential biomarkers for anaerobic glucose metabolism are: Borg's 6–20 scale of perceived exertion (local, central, and overall); muscle soreness; tissue levels of lactate measured by near-infrared spectroscopy (NIRS); muscle biopsy for glycogen, cytokines, and enzymes; actigraphy; electroencephalography (EEC); heart-rate variability; profile of mood state; and visual analog scale. The use of these biomarkers for this purpose needs to be validated in the field.

Biomarkers of Dehydration and Renal Function

In the military setting, changes in water and osmotic balance are usually synergistic with increases in water loss. One of the most sensitive indicators of hydration status is short-term changes in body weight since most day-to-day variation in body weight is due to hydration status. The assessment of weight loss or loss of body mass, plasma sodium or plasma osmolality, urinary specific gravity, fluid balance, and the recovery of weight 24 hours after dehydration can be used for the identification of extent and type of dehydration. In the military setting, weight changes over a short period of time reflect fluid changes, and loss of body water coupled with measures of serum sodium or serum osmolality can define the degree of concomitant salt loss. Renal function is also a good indicator of hydration status.

Renal Function

There are a number of markers and technologies available that could be adapted for self- (or peer-) monitoring during training or field operations. The military should consider providing and training personnel in the use of simple urine dipstick-type test strips that would provide information on levels of urine protein (a marker for potential kidney damage), ketones and glucose (potential markers for energy metabolism), and leukocyte esterase and nitrates (indicators of urinary tract infections) as indicators of muscle damage and hydration status. These field measures should be taken at mid-day and after the day's exertion.

Biomarkers of Cognitive Function

The most promising techniques for accomplishing continuous assessments of ground combat service member cognitive readiness in field settings are actigraphy, EEG, and heart-rate variability. Actigraphy is useful because it offers a field-practical way of monitoring the sleep of combat service members, and insufficient sleep is the primary cause of cognitive degradations in operational environments. EEG is useful because it offers a relatively noninvasive assessment of the brain activity that underlies all types of performance, including vigilance and judgment. Heart-rate variability is a peripheral nervous system measure that also reflects the brain activity that underlies performance attention and mood. In vehicle operators or in radar or other fixed-based system operators, eye-movement monitoring is also promising. Saccadic velocity and percentage-of-eye-closure measures have been shown to reflect the status of the central nervous system. In all probability, most of these measures will be useful only in laboratory environments or in fixed-based operational facilities (such as posts in which radar or sonar equipment is monitored or stations from which remote-controlled vehicles are piloted) where complex equipment can be housed, lengthy recording procedures can be conducted, and rigid controls can be maintained. Only a small subset of these methods will likely be suitable for operational settings.

Besides these objective measures, subjective ratings of alertness and fatigue should be considered for use in the field since these have been shown to correlate with performance changes in some situations. However, it should be recognized that self-report data can be influenced by peer pressure (or supervisor pressure); also, there is evidence that self-reports may loose a degree of sensitivity when the stress or fatigue becomes so chronic that the individual has difficulty referencing his or her present feelings to more normal past experiences.

QUESTION 2

What monitoring technologies would be required (that may not currently exist) to predict these intermediate targets in critical metabolic pathways?

New biomarkers are likely to be identified in the future; still, the greater needs lie in: (1) the development of easier systems to measure and transmit data, and (2) the development of new mathematical models to provide enhanced data integration and analysis by using nonlinear discriminant algorithms. Future monitoring technologies should consist of an integrated system that incorporates noninvasive or minimally invasive sensor technology, communication interface and integration, data analysis tools, and local area networks. This infrastructure should be both redundant and noncentralized. A "black box" or "medical hub" is needed to gather data from multiple sensors or devices, standardize the outputs, and submit these data to a data reduction system or decision-making tool for the creation of both prioritized alarm signals and recommended interventions. Regarding development of models, the major obstacles to be overcome will be the selection of variables and the building of models that truly predict health performance status.

QUESTION 3

What tools currently exist for monitoring metabolic status that could be useful in the field?

Metabolic status can be defined in part by energy metabolism, intermediary fuels (glucose, fatty acids, and amino acids), acid/base and hydration status, and psychophysiological status. NIRS can examine many different biomarkers of metabolism, such as muscle function and hydration, and shows great promise in the field. Other tools to measure specific biomarkers are described below.

Muscle Fatigue

One measure that could be useful in the field, after validation in military settings, is self-perception. Predictors of fatigue at an earlier state have also been proposed. The challenge remains to differentiate diagnosis between acute damage from muscle injury, fatigue due to overuse or over conditioning, exercise until exhaustion, hydration, and nutritional status given the interactions of these factors in the subjective feeling of fatigue.

Renal Function and Hydration

Simple methods that measure renal function and hydration already exist. As mentioned previously, the military should train personnel in the field use of simple urine dipstick-type test strips that would provide information on levels of urine protein, ketones and glucose, and leukocyte esterase and nitrates as indicators of muscle damage and hydration status. Also, a practical method of monitoring weight changes in the field would be of value for monitoring hydration.

Energy Expenditure

Several field methods have been tested for predicting total daily energy expenditure, including heart-rate monitors, pedometers, and accelerometers. Accelerometer- and pedometer-based monitors provide valid indicators of overall physical activity, but they are less accurate at predicting energy expenditure. In addition, single-axis accelerometers or pedometers and most multidimensional accelerometers are not useful in detecting the increased energy costs of high-intensity exercise, upper-body exercise, carrying a load, or changes in surface or terrain.

The combination of doubly labeled water as a measure of total energy expenditure and hand-held indirect calorimetry to measure resting energy expenditure could be used to monitor metabolic status and assess energy metabolism over periods of up to 2 weeks. Self-selected pace, foot-strike devices, and activity monitors that integrate pulse, temperature, and movement could estimate activity and total energy expenditure and may be useful in the field.

If predicting total energy expenditure is the goal of monitoring the activity of the combat service member, then more sophisticated multidimensional devices must be developed.

Stress and Immune Function

The precise combination of measures chosen to monitor stress and immune function depends on the flexibility of the collection of the measures in the field setting. A full evaluation of the effects of activation of stress response systems on immune function requires measures of multiple functional and molecular biomarkers at multiple time points prior to, during, and after the stress exposure. Monitoring biomarkers of the stress response should include molecular and functional measures of the hypothalamic-pituitary-adrenal (HPA) axis, the adrenergic response systems, and the immune system at multiple levels. The HPA axis can be monitored by measuring levels of the corticotropin-releasing hormone, adrenocorticotropin, and cortisol in plasma, cerebrospinal fluid, urine, saliva, and sweat.

Measuring heart-rate variability should be considered as an accurate, sensitive, and noninvasive way to measure the relative activity of the sympathetic and parasympathetic nervous systems.

Indicators of stress and immune responses that are currently in use and in development include cortisol levels (measured from saliva, sweat, or urine), and heart-rate variability as measured with high-impedance electrocardiogram (ECG) electrodes that are currently available and are being further developed.

Sleep

Several companies currently offer wrist-worn actigraphs that are capable of estimating the quantity and quality of sleep in a variety of environments and for periods ranging from a few hours to several weeks. Associated software can present sleep/wake histories in a number of user-friendly formats.

Significant progress has already been made in developing and validating high-impedance sensors that could soon be mounted in helmets and clothing, a challenge when collecting electrophysiological measures (EEG and ECG) in field settings. The technology for field-portable, individual-worn systems for amplifying, recording, and to some extent analyzing these data already exist.

Assessment of eye movements and eye closures will only be possible in limited situations in which monitoring equipment can be mounted and aimed at the combat service member. A subset of oculomotor measures is sensitive to cognitive fatigue, but their utility needs to be validated.

Self-assessments, on the other hand, are quite easy to collect and many have been shown to be sensitive to operational stressors, such as mental and physical fatigue. However, readers are cautioned that self-assessments can be significantly confounded by motivational factors or peer pressure or in chronic-demand conditions (e.g., people who are very tired for several days at a time may lose their subjective ability to determine how tired they actually are).

QUESTION 4

What algorithms are available that might provide useful predictions from combined sensor signals? What additional measurements would improve specificity of the predictions?

Models, such as the Acute Physiologic and Chronic Health Evaluation Scores and Simplified Applied Physiological Score, that use physiological variables to predict health outcomes have worked quite well in the intensive care unit setting where pathological changes in physiological parameters are the rule, but there is little evidence that similar algorithms would be equally effective in the military setting where such parameters vary over a narrower range. The National Aeronautics and Space Administration also has undertaken a major research effort in this area, the design of which may be quite compatible with the military environment. Although it would be reasonable to explore whether new variables made possible by new field technologies would be predictive using simpler algorithms, a parallel initiative to explore presently available physiological measurements with more complex models seems appropriate.

The future development of algorithms must include the development of nonlinear models that allow discrimination of more complex decision surfaces (e.g., a graphical representation of a problem in space). More complex models, for example, involving artificial neural networks, are needed. In addition, as described in the response to question 2, the technology must evolve to permit the integration of data in multiple forms from different devices. Last, it is crucial to develop baseline data for each individual (combat service member) in order to implement effective field strategies for monitoring metabolic status.

QUESTION 5

What is the committee's "blue sky" forecast for useful metabolic monitoring approaches (i.e., 10- to 20-year projection)? What are the current research investments that may lead to revolutionary advances?

Evolution of New Cognitive Measurement Approaches

The prediction of cognitive responses to stress and fatigue needs to be improved. In addition to performing more research on the utility of traditional approaches using self-reported data, a significant focus should be placed on further developing and implementing new psychophysiological methods for monitoring brain activity, heart-rate variability, eye movements, and metabolites and validating these techniques as predictors of cognitive responses to stress and fatigue. New performance assessment methodologies may soon be available for computerized tasks in which cognitive probes can be unobtrusively introduced during the completion of primary operational demands. In addition, the use of hand-held computers to record ecological momentary assessments of cognitive function should be further developed.

In addition to developing new psychophysiological methods, more work needs to be undertaken on the mathematical integration of these data and the computer models that will synthesize numerous inputs into a field-useable status assessment.

Optimization of Markers to Monitor Stress and Immune Function

A limited battery of selected stress response and immune markers should be validated to monitor physiological adaptations to changes in the environment and to evaluate the readiness of individuals for impending deployment.

Odors as Biomarkers

Studies linking human perception of odors with emotion and cognitive states are currently in their infancy and need to be encouraged in order to ascertain the full range of information that human odors might convey. The military should promote innovative research in chemical signaling that will accelerate these advances. Also, research in the development of sensor technology is likely to yield smaller, more automated devices that reduce analysis time and increase reliability—two factors that are critical for field applications. These advances will go hand-in-hand with the development of sweat patches that can be uniquely designed to capture the substances of interest. It seems highly plausible that new insights from these diverse areas will converge in 5 to 10 years, making odor biomarkers a viable technology for military field applications.

Human Tears as Sources of Biomarkers

A number of disparate studies suggest that there may be merit in examining tears as a possible medium for monitoring relevant aspects of metabolic status. For example, it has been reported that tear glucose concentrations are related to blood glucose levels. This is an area where little research has been done, but one that may have significant potential as a noninvasive monitoring technology for a variety of physiological biomarkers.

New Algorithms to Integrate Complex Biological Information

The use of technology and "smart systems" are required to bridge the cognitive gap created by the lack of skilled clinicians in the field to provide individualized recommendations to support end users. Predictive medical algorithms can be utilized to generate specific recommendations and interventions from complex biological information gathered by metabolic monitoring systems. Further research is needed to develop and validate these models, with a particular emphasis on identifying prognostic factors in asymptomatic subjects.

The Impact of Biological and Chemical Hazards on Traditional Biomarkers of Health

It is largely unknown how hazards and toxins encountered during deployment will affect the biomarkers used by the military for monitoring. For example, low chronic exposure to a bacterial toxin or a heavy metal may alter serum electrolytes, glucose, or enzymes and confound usual interpretation of these values. In contrast, other biomarkers might serve as critical indicators for biological or chemical toxin exposure; for example, pulse rate alterations may be used as an indication of (sublethal) nerve toxin exposure.

Metabolomics/Nutrigenomics

The differential expression of genes creates individual differences or phenotypes. It is known, for instance, that single nucleotide polymorphisms can affect the way individuals respond to drugs, their vulnerability to microbiological infections, and their susceptibility to long-term degenerative diseases. Such knowledge is envisioned to enhance a combat service member's performance and lower the risk of life-threatening injury. Further, it is possible that such determinations would allow for prophylactic vaccinations, prescription of preventative pharmaceuticals, and the possible use of special monitoring sensors. Although it may be a number of years before it becomes possible, it would be ideal to be able to predict how a single combat service member will perform under a variety of different dietary and other environmental conditions based upon his or her phenotype. In this manner, the identification of differences between individuals by the use of genomic and metabolomic information collected on each combat servicemen are the ultimate "blue sky."

RESEARCH RECOMMENDATIONS

- To develop new algorithms that employ currently measurable biomarkers and nonlinear modeling techniques. In circumstances where average group data may not appropriately correlate with the performance of an individual, prediction models will need to be based on data from repeated measures from individuals.
- To develop patterns of rates of changes and resiliency. For example, research is needed to elucidate individual patterns of rates of change of stress hormones and to determine the resiliency of these stress responses in returning to baseline after the stressors have been removed.
- To conduct research to evaluate and validate available technology in the field. For example, technology related to self-assessment of perceived exertion, preferred exertion, and mood states that have been tested extensively in sports settings, but it needs to be evaluated and validated in military settings. Optimal combinations for use with physiological markers need to be determined.
- To further perform research activities in areas with the greatest long-range benefits, such as genomics/metabolomics, odors as biomarkers, tears as a new media for potential biomarkers, new cognitive measurements approaches, optimization of monitoring stress and immune function markers, the development of new algorithms to integrate complex biological information, and the impact of biological and chemical hazards on traditional biomarkers of health.
- To continue military activities in bone research. These should include studies of markers of bone loss, especially related to fracture risk and the prevention of lost duty time during initial entry training, advanced training, and combat operations.
- To continue to study cortisol levels during training and operations to ensure that its elevation is not a contributor to bone loss.
- To develop non- and minimally invasive technologies, particularly for the determination of muscle metabolism, hydration status, and cognitive function.
- To develop motion sensors that are inexpensive, but more convenient and reliable than current pedometers and accelerometers.

- To conduct research to validate the use of self- (and peer-) assessment tools in the field as indicators of fatigue and cognitive ability.
- To continue research on the use of NIRS to monitor muscle function and skin hydration status concurrently. This particular technology also has the potential for detecting the occurrence of inflammation.
- To develop simple field-friendly tests for urine specific gravity as an indicator of hydration status.
- To develop a practical method of monitoring body-weight change in the field.
- To conduct research to be able to mount or integrate high impedance EEG and ECG electrodes in helmets or into combat clothing. Although this technology will soon make it possible to continuously record brain activity, heart-rate data, and other electrophysiological parameters, some remaining challenges limit its use in the field.

1

Rationale for Military Interest and Current Capabilities in Monitoring Metabolism

Formidable monitoring capabilities exist for military hardware systems, but there is a lack of real-time information on the status of combat military personnel. Enhancing knowledge in this area would serve the U.S. Department of Defense (DOD) priority to assure the readiness of the Armed Forces (DOD, 2001). Based on the premise that metabolic processes are the bases of responses that allow organisms to survive in the face of environmental challenges and, thus, would be the earliest indicators of a change in physiological status, an understanding of regulatory mechanisms can suggest promising predictive markers of status and impending failure of adaptive response capabilities. Monitoring metabolic processes is needed to predict the readiness status of individuals in training and operational settings where human performance is important.

NEED FOR PHYSIOLOGICAL MONITORING

Monitoring combat service member status has become increasingly important as a result of new complex and lethal technologies that require high levels of cognitive readiness, such as computerized weapon systems; complicated communications and targeting devices; high-performance aircraft, tanks, and maritime vessels; and even the technologically advanced diagnostic systems used in the maintenance of military equipment. In addition, monitoring is necessary to ensure that operational personnel are as physically fit as possible because success on the battlefield is to a great extent dependent on the ability of combat service members to carry and operate weapons, to overcome physical obstacles, to traverse distances in harsh environments, and to endure a host of physical stresses and strains that could easily overwhelm unfit individuals. Also, battlefield tactics reduce line-of-sight contact with team members and increase the members' geographical distance and isolation.

Physiological monitoring is not just a nice-to-have technological replacement for common sense or for good leadership (which includes understanding the signs of an individual combat service member's limits). Combat service members may not be aware that they are reaching dangerous levels of overheating, dehydration, physical exertion, stress, fatigue, or sleep deprivation. They could develop performance-degrading problems unbeknownst to their team leaders, particularly if they are fully encapsulated in chemical protective suits, are flying aircraft, or are operating in a remote location. An alert or warning signal to the individual and to his or her squad leader could permit prompt intervention to alleviate the physiological danger and potentially save a mission.

The present-day U.S. military must be able to rapidly deploy around the globe on short notice and be capable of sustaining operations for long periods of time. In order to accomplish these objectives, a variety of occupational specialties are required. Ground combat military personnel have unique roles in combat operations and work in very different environments in order to achieve objectives in a coordinated fashion. Although a thorough discussion of the challenges faced by each group of combat service members is beyond the scope of this report, the reader can gain a small appreciation for the diversity by considering the problems faced by some Army ground personnel as opposed to those faced by some pilots.

The ground personnel's tasks often include a high level of physical energy expenditure in the face of constant and immediate threats from the environment, as well as from a wide range of enemy activities. Infantry personnel are constantly on the move, either walking, running, climbing, or at times, even swimming from one point to another. These activities are made more strenuous because of the need to carry heavy backpacks, weapons, and ammunition in all types of weather and across all types of terrain. Fatigue is a constant companion because of the physical workload, the environment, and the sleep deprivation that results from limited sleep opportunities and poor sleep environments. Air conditioning, hot water, and "normal" food are nonexistent for combat service members who often work long hours in the worst of circumstances.

The pilot's task is generally much less physically demanding than what is faced by infantry personnel, but his or her job presents challenges from other characteristics. Helicopter pilots must remain cognitively alert at all times if they are to successfully pilot their aircraft at speeds of 50 to 100 mph while maintaining altitudes of only 50 ft above terrain obstacles. Flying close combat support means that helicopter pilots are operating under conditions that are quite similar to those faced by combat military personnel on the ground: they are close to enemy threats, they are often hot or cold due to the lack of air conditioning, and they are required to live in the most austere and uncomfortable environments for days, weeks, or months at a time. Unlike their infantry comrades, they take off and land several times a day in stressful, low-visibility conditions and try to sleep during short intervals between flights, often in poor conditions. In addition, they are responsible for multimillion-dollar aircraft and the crews on board.

Air Force fighter pilots face different, but often equally challenging circumstances. For instance, F-117 pilots have been known to fly for 18 straight hours in a single-pilot aircraft, strapped into an ejection seat while wearing bulky, hot, protective gear. During this time, they must remain fully alert and fully prepared to engage or avoid enemy threats that arise from the air or ground while flying in a sterile, uncomfortable cockpit in a high-altitude, relatively featureless environment. Boredom and physical inactivity can decrease mental vigilance, and the fatigue from sleep deprivation and circadian disruptions are ever-present problems. Although their operational environment is generally more pleasant than the ones faced by infantry personnel, the continuous high-level cognitive demands of accomplishing the mission, combined with the responsibilities for an expensive aircraft that is fully-loaded with powerful weaponry, creates a high level of ongoing operational stress. Similar difficulties are faced by B-2 pilots who often fly missions that extend beyond 30 hours with only two pilots on board.

In addition, today's high-performance aircraft can easily exceed the limits of human physiological tolerances. One concept for physiological monitoring includes monitoring a pilot's approaching loss of consciousness in order to trigger an automatic take over of the plane's controls (Forster et al., 1994). On the other hand, for flights of extended duration, detection of alertness or deterioration in performance through self and distant monitoring becomes important. This calls for a highly responsive, rapid, and reliable system that identifies any major lapse in pilot capabilities.

Navy personnel would also benefit from physiological monitoring. The Navy is designing ships that require substantially fewer crew members for operation, which in turn calls for greater reliance on each individual. Monitoring the status of these crew members becomes especially important in case they become incapacitated in an isolated compartment during high-risk damage control operations, such as fighting fires or flooding. This monitoring is part of the concept of the Reduced Ships-Crew by Virtual Presence, which is designed for smart ships that continuously receive data on the status of the ship and on the crew within the ship (Street et al., 2002).

The military would also benefit from monitoring—during both training and operations—the factors that influence bone and muscle health, as well as other processes that underlie and optimize physical endurance and resistance to physical injury. It may be most useful for leaders to use monitoring to learn the physiological and cognitive limits of each individual under their command during the individual's training. Then, during an actual operational mission, the leaders could rely on specific warnings about real-time status. Monitoring during training may also prevent injuries. For example, if an individual is found to have reached a high state of bone and muscle remodeling during training, providing a day of rest might reduce a high probability of injury.

Physiological monitoring is also being explored for a wide variety of other military applications, including the forensic "black box" flight recorder-type of analysis (after a class A accident) of a pilot's mental state in order to prevent future accidents (Forster, 2002). There is also a need for overall "whole-body" health markers for easy assessment of global indices of service-members' health at regular intervals throughout their career. This could eventually include some combination of psychological and physiological health, monitoring brain metabolites through magnetic resonance spectroscopy (MRS) scans, whole-body oxidative stress load assessments, and mitochondrial redox potential of critical brain cells as common final pathways of health status.

RECENT EVOLUTION OF MONITORING RESEARCH

Physiological monitoring concepts are not new. Fifty years ago, the Office of Naval Research and the Army Surgeon General cooperatively studied infantrymen in combat to identify metabolic predictors of mental status (Davis et al., 1952). Using neuropsychological testing (including visual flicker fusion and auditory flutter fusion tests) and blood and urine testing, hydration status, adrenal stress markers, and corresponding changes in cognitive functioning were assessed. Studies by the Air Force explored the use of an electroencephalogram (EEG) to monitor pilot performance as early as the 1950s (Sem-Jacobsen, 1959). Current studies are examining many of the same factors and relationships that were tested in the studies conducted 50 years ago.

Although the current studies have some technological advantages, most notably electronic computing power, they have largely relied on available technologies instead of exploring the most suitable measurement targets and developing specifically needed monitoring technology. To date, efforts have focused on trying to find uses for new measurement technologies instead of pushing the development of technology to systematically test the current knowledge of physiology and predict the outcomes of greatest importance.

The greatest barrier to advances in performance monitoring has been the lack of suitably defined performance outcome measures. Until recently, aviator performance has been the most extensively studied model for physiological monitoring. Military aviators have been a logical focus because of need (i.e., the high costs associated with catastrophic performance failures) and because of experimental advantages. Performance outcome measures are better defined for aviator tasks, especially the ultimate outcome of successful landing versus disaster. Also, the cockpit provides an appropriate setting for prototype monitoring systems that are power hungry and tethered to heavy equipment. Aviator studies can provide early proof of concept for systems that are later reduced in size, weight, power, and invasiveness for untethered applications in combat military personnel. Nevertheless, the aviator monitoring studies cannot be generalized without further development of performance assessment methods and metrics.

Without suitable performance measures, results from laboratory-based studies cannot be translated into militarily relevant outcomes. These measures are also needed for field studies that are otherwise forced to rely on simple dichotomies of "no bad outcome" or catastrophic failure (e.g., heat stroke, serious injury, or mission failure). The Military Operational Medicine Research Program has invested heavily in the development and standardization of practical neuropsychological tests (e.g., the Automated Neuropsychological Assessment Metric) (Kane and Kay, 1992), and current field studies are attempting to link these test results with military performance. For example, simple reaction time remained impaired following sports concussions in military cadets even after they were cleared for return to duty by clinical criteria. The significance of this finding to other performance measures is being further investigated. Another study found that cold-water immersion affected performance tests (Vaughan, 1975); what this means to Navy diver performance capabilities is also being further investigated.

One eventual monitoring application may be to embed informative tests into common military tasks that could be monitored to obtain unobtrusive periodic assessments of an individual's performance status. DOD is currently reviewing methods and metrics for performance assessment in order to synthesize the current state of the knowledge on militarily relevant performance assessments and models (Ness et al., In preparation). A new research initiative is focused on the development of military performance assessment methods based on measures of neurological function (e.g., voice stress analysis and eye saccades).

In 1996 physiological monitoring became a central objective in the Army research program (Friedl, 2003). The goal of the Warfighter Physiological Status Monitoring (WPSM) initiative is to make real-time performance predictions that leaders can use to assess the readiness status of their forces. The concept is to develop a combat service member-acceptable, minimally invasive sensor set with on-the-combat service member analysis. The output (which can be queried for further information) will be a simple "green" (within normal limits), "amber" (physiological challenges are present), or "red" (systems have failed and the combat service member is a casualty). This system relies on environmental physiological and psychological data that have been collected and modeled in DOD research programs for many years. A key feature of the approach is that these systems must also learn the usual range of responses for each combat service member, thus accounting for individual variability (Friedl, 2003). Currently, WPSM is a research "tool kit" to learn more about normal and abnormal physiological signals encountered in real-combat service member environments; these include a range of responses that routinely exceed those that could be obtained in an ethically developed experimental laboratory setting. The ultimate goal of WPSM will be the minimal sensor set needed for highly reliable and important predictions.

The development of experimental signal acquisition, data handling systems, and data collection studies with combat military personnel in challenging training environments is underway (Hoyt et al., 1997a, 2001). The immediate goals for WPSM are to provide information on the individual's status for thermal strain, sleep history, energy expenditure, and live-dead detection for the Land Warrior system. More sophisticated monitoring capabilities and performance predictions are planned that will also include early casualty triage capabilities.

CURRENT RESEARCH EFFORTS

Several critical areas for metabolic monitoring have been chosen for review in this report: hydration and heat production, substrate utilization and energy metabolism, muscle and bone remodeling, and brain function. These traditionally separate research areas are interrelated through metabolic processes. For example, exertional rhabdomyolysis includes elements of hydration and heat exposure, energy flux, and muscle remodeling, with early effects on mental status (Gardner and Kark, 1994). These functions are closely interrelated through common measures that might signal changes in one or more of these physiological categories. For example, shivering may indicate a variety of threats that, when combined with one or two other measurements, can unambiguously distinguish conditions such as impending hypothermia risk, exposure to a neurotoxic chemical, or intense psychological fear. Brain function reflected in cognitive, mood, or psychomotor measures (e.g., speed of mental processing, irritability, and marksmanship) may be a common and sensitive marker of deficits of all the other stressors and functional deficits of interest, including carbohydrate metabolism in physical exhaustion (Frier, 2001), dehydration, or significant fluid shifts, such as those observed in the brain with acute mountain sickness (Singh et al., 1990), and perhaps even cytokine-mediated changes in brain function following intense muscular exertion (Febbraio and Pedersen, 2002). Thus brain function is both an early indicator of many stressors of concern and a direct reflection of specific performance capabilities.

Early metabolic changes to defend critical functions are likely to be more promising prognostic indicators than is awaiting change in the critical function itself (e.g., blood glucose, serum osmolality, or core body temperature). The critical function may be so well defended (e.g., serum osmolality and sodium concentration) that when a significant change is detected, homeostatic mechanisms have already failed and the individual is a casualty. Earlier changes in interstitial fluid or osmoregulatory hormones may signal a heroic defense against a threat to intravascular volume. There are also conditions under which a critical function measurement (e.g., body temperature) may have greater variation at performance extremes in healthy individuals, which may be appropriate compensation to sustain peak performance and defies the definitive classification of an impending performance failure. For example, core body temperature may be as low as 35°C at the circadian nadir in U.S. Army Ranger students who have lost most of their insulative fat and have metabolically adjusted to a reduced energy intake (Hoyt et al., 1997b), and it may be sustained at 40°C for several hours in marathoners while they are running (Maron et al., 1977). Monitoring the signs of compensation (e.g., changes in heat flux, activation of sweating or shivering mechanisms, cardiac response, and mental functioning) may predict a potential problem before unambiguous changes in core body temperature can be detected.

Bone and muscle turnover studies are important to the military to solve the near-term problem of high rates of injury during physical training—most importantly during the rapid train-up phase of the 8- to 12-week initial entry training course conducted in every service (half of all female combat service members incur musculoskeletal injury during initial entry training). A peak incidence of stress fractures by about the third week of training was hypothesized to be associated with high rates of bone remodeling stimulated by the training. This hypothesis was evaluated in an Army study that examined the benefits of a physical training rest period in the third week of training (Popovich et al., 2000). Unfortunately, the rest period did not modify the injury profile, suggesting a more complicated pathogenesis, including individual variability. The development of specific markers of susceptibility and impending injury in individuals is still urgently needed.

Table 1-1 suggests some of the outcomes that might be logical targets for monitoring within the next decade, along with some of the technologies that exist or could be developed for such monitoring. The boundary between current and near-term approaches is slightly blurred by the overlap of current technologies that require far more validation with projected near-term technologies that are just beginning to demonstrate promise. For example, fitness for duty based on various peripheral indicators of brain function is an important, but elusive, goal. In the past there was hope that performance could be predicted from recent sleep history measured by wrist-worn actigraphy (Redmond and Hegge, 1985). However, the current status of fatigue performance models is too immature and individual responses to this single measure are too variable to make actigraphy alone a useful measure. Potentially noninvasive methods that could be mounted in a helmet, such as measurement of pupil responses and saccadic eye movements, are being explored, but have so far not held up well compared with laboratory measures, such as the psychomotor vigilance task. A method that follows slow eye closure shows great promise, but will have to be proven in a helmet-type platform that keeps the monitor in line with the subject's eyes (Dinges et al., 1998). Another potential method, voice analysis, is specifically affected by emotional load, returning to normal with psychological adaptation even while general activation (e.g., accelerated heart rate) continues (Wittels et al., 2002). However, this measure has not yet been demonstrated to correspond to specific performance decrements. EEG analyses in fatigued individuals or in individuals involved in sustained vigilance tasks have been studied in military laboratories and show promise, but remain to be demonstrated as strong predictors of impending deficits (Caldwell et al., 2002).

Far-future technologies are concepts that might be achievable but have not been seriously explored and remain "marks on the wall." Mitochondrial redox state in specific brain tissues has been suggested a marker of brain function status based on the importance of neural cell bioenergetics (Ojaimi et al., 1999). Intracerebral monitoring of energy-related metabolites is currently being conducted with neurosurgical patients to follow acute conditions involving hypoxia and ischemia. As more is learned about what needs to be measured, the

TABLE 1-1 Technology Forecast for Practical Metabolic Assessment Measures (Measured Endpoints and Conceivable Technologies)

Past	Present[a]
Energy balance and fuel availability	
Blood and urine biochemistry	Activity-based predictions
Home test glucose monitors, laboratory tests	"Gluco-watch"
	Reverse iontophoresis, actigraphy
Ratings of perceived exertion	
Brain metabolic function	
Paper and pencil tests	Computerized neuropsychological testing
	EEG spectral analysis
	Palm-top test, dry electrodes in a hat band
Hydration and water balance	
Urine-specific gravity	Balance based on intake and predicted losses
	Instrumented canteen/camelbak, bioelectrical resistance
	Whole-body water estimates
Bone and muscle turnover	
"Hot spots"	Lab tests
Loss of strength and delayed onset muscle soreness	Specific blood and urinary markers (e.g., telopeptides, myoglobin, CPK, IGF-1)
Thermography	
Stress and Immune Function	
Psychological measures of: performance, stress, mood	Blood, urine, and saliva immune markers (e.g., ILs, NK cells, T-cells, IGs, neutrophils, macrophages)
Sleep patterns	
Stress hormones	Blood, urine, and saliva stress markers (cortisol, ACTH, catecholamines)
	Heart rate variability

[a] EEG = electroencephalogram, CPK = creatine phosphokinase, IGF-1 = insulin-like growth factor-1, IL = interleukin, NK = natural killer, IG = immunoglobulin, ACTH = adrenocorticotropic hormone.

technologists may be able to develop the noninvasive monitoring devices needed to monitor the identified biomarkers. For example, with higher-powered magnets, researchers are now able to detect glutamate peaks in MRS brain pixels. An elevated level of glutamate in the frontal lobe might signify a range of acute metabolic insults that would be very important to detect and countermand.

Current military research programs are leveraged with special Congressional appropriations that accelerate basic metabolic research in specific topic areas. The Bone Health and Military Medical Readiness research program (supported by the National Osteoporosis and Related Bone Disorders Coalition) is

Near Future[b]	Far Future[c]
Semi-invasive implantable sensors and "tattoos" Subdermal continuous glucose, lactate, pH, free fatty acids	Functional outcome (e.g., EMG, nerve conduction, changes in thermal flux) Noninvasive physiological sensors built into clothing
Saccades and pupil responses Voice analysis Task-embedded psychological tests Doppler, etc., in combat service member helmet/spectacles	Brain blood flow Chemical nose, respiratory sampling, personal intrahelmet brain imaging systems Sweat/exhaled cytokines Volatile compounds/pheromones
Intercellular fluid assessment Subdermal wicks, boot-sensor body weight tracking with electrolyte and BIA sensors Whole body water changes	Changes in skin properties Endocrine changes in defense of water volume Skin mechanical/electrical changes, semi-invasive sensing of osmoregulatory hormones
Altered biomechanics Sweat markers of calcium and protein metabolism Practical field test systems	Changes in redox status Deep muscle biochemical sensors Regional metabolism/blood flow changes
Field measures of: Blood, urine, or saliva immune markers (e.g., ILs, IGs) Blood, urine, or saliva stress markers (cortisol, ACTH, catecholamines) Sleep patterns	Human odors Sweat immune and stress biomarkers (e.g., neuropeptides, neurohormones, ILs, IGs)

[b] BIA = bioelectrical impedance analysis.
[c] EMG = electromyogram.
SOURCE: Friedl (2003).

focused on the improved understanding of bone remodeling processes and includes projects exploring markers of impending stress fracture injury. The Technologies for Metabolic Monitoring research program (supported by the Juvenile Diabetes Research Foundation) is testing novel approaches to measure functional outcomes related to biochemical status and energy metabolism, notably glucose regulation, but including the development of lactate sensors and the exploration of other physiological indicators of metabolic status. Projects supported by the Force Health Protection research program are examining methods to monitor global health status in combat service members, including the use of breath condensates to measure cytokines and other markers of lung function following blast or toxic inhalation exposures. Two large projects are currently in progress to assess the association of brain MRS measures and symptom reporting in chronic, multisymptom illnesses in order to determine objective markers of well-being. Finally, the Neurotoxin Exposure Treatment Research Program (sponsored by the Parkinson's Action Network) includes the exploration of voice analysis and neuropsychological testing methods for the early detection of neurological changes.

CURRENT STATUS OF FIELD APPLICATIONS OF PHYSIOLOGICAL MONITORING

The dismounted combat service member's workplace is fairly unique within the variety of occupational challenges encountered by the American population. Modern infantry combat service members commonly engage in intense, mentally and physically demanding, 3- to 10-day missions, often in rugged terrain or complex urban settings. These individuals carry heavy loads (35–65 kg) and are often food- and sleep-restricted. Environmental conditions—ambient temperature, humidity, wind speed, solar load, and barometric pressure—can vary widely. Recent examples of operational environments include the desert heat conditions of the Persian Gulf; cold, wet weather in Bosnia; and cold and high altitude challenges in the mountains of Afghanistan.

The WPSM concept includes wearable metabolic and physiological status monitors to help improve combat service members' performance. This monitoring plays important roles in: (a) sustaining physical and mental performance; (b) reducing the likelihood of nonbattle injuries, such as heat stroke, frostbite, and acute mountain sickness; and (c) improving casualty management in remote situations.

Ambulatory WPSM technologies are being developed to provide useful performance and health status indicators for combat service members, medics, commanders, and logisticians. The WPSM program uses a novel research "tool kit" to collect ambulatory physiological data from military personnel operating in stressful field environments. Analyses of the data sets are providing a better understanding of the physiological strains associated with operations in a multi-stressor environment.

Sensor hardware is important in ambulatory metabolic and physiological monitoring. However, sensor development is only one of a series of steps needed to reliably generate a useful flow of health status information in a harsh and highly constrained wearable environment. Other steps include: reliable sensor data collection, data cleaning, data reduction and interpretation, and the communication, synthesis, interpretation, and presentation of the data. Key technologies that support this process, including post-hoc, time-series data management and the medical Personal Area Network, are reviewed elsewhere (Hoyt et al., 2002).

Power, weight, and volume constraints and the need for truly "wear-and-forget" comfort limit the functionality of wearable sensors. For example, estimating sleep by monitoring activity is possible, but it is not currently practical to do so by EEG in the field. An intelligent sensor network that reliably generates useful information from a number of disparate sources is needed to provide a holistic, rather than a "keyhole," view of the physiological status of individuals.

THE PHYSIOLOGICAL STATUS MONITOR

A prototype WPSM user interface (display) for the medic or field commander (Figure 1-1) illustrates the relevant types of contextual and physiological information that are available. This heuristic display shows: (1) thermal/work strain as the Physiological Strain Index (PSI) (Moran et al., 1998), (2) hydration state or water balance, (3) metabolic rate, (4) environmental conditions, (5) cognitive/sleep status (hours of sleep, etc.), and (6) clinical status and location information. The knowledge display includes a baseline characterization of the individual, real-time combat service member and environmental sensor input, and historical and group mean data. Some of the measurements provided by the WPSM and their potential uses are described in the following sections.

Combat Service Member Characteristics

Combat service member characteristics, along with clothing, diet, load, geolocation, and meteorological conditions (air temperature, solar load, wind speed, and humidity), are important determinants of an individual's physiological and pathophysiological responses to environmental stresses and trauma. Relevant combat service member characteristics include job type (military occupational specialty), gender, ethnicity, age, height, body weight, percent body fat, thermal and altitude acclimation history, and aerobic fitness. These factors change slowly, if at all, and can be recorded well before any training or combat mission begins. Percent body fat can be estimated easily from weight and waist circumference (Wright and Wilmore, 1974), but simple field techniques for characterizing thermal and altitude acclimation states are currently not well defined. Aerobic fitness can be estimated from the Army Physical Fitness Test 2-mile-run-for-time score (Mello et al., 1988) or from foot-ground contact time and heart rate using the method of Weyand and colleagues (2001).

Heat Strain

Understanding why hot weather injuries occur and developing ways to prevent heat injuries are important concerns given the approximately 1,800 heat injuries that occurred in active-duty combat service members in the Army in 2002 (USACHPPM, 2003). The graphic display in Figure 1-2 shows core temperature, measured by an ingested radio telemetry pill (O'Brien et al., 1998), and heart rate, typically derived from an electrocardiogram. The PSI (lumped core temperature) and heart rate index that reflects thermal and work strain on a scale

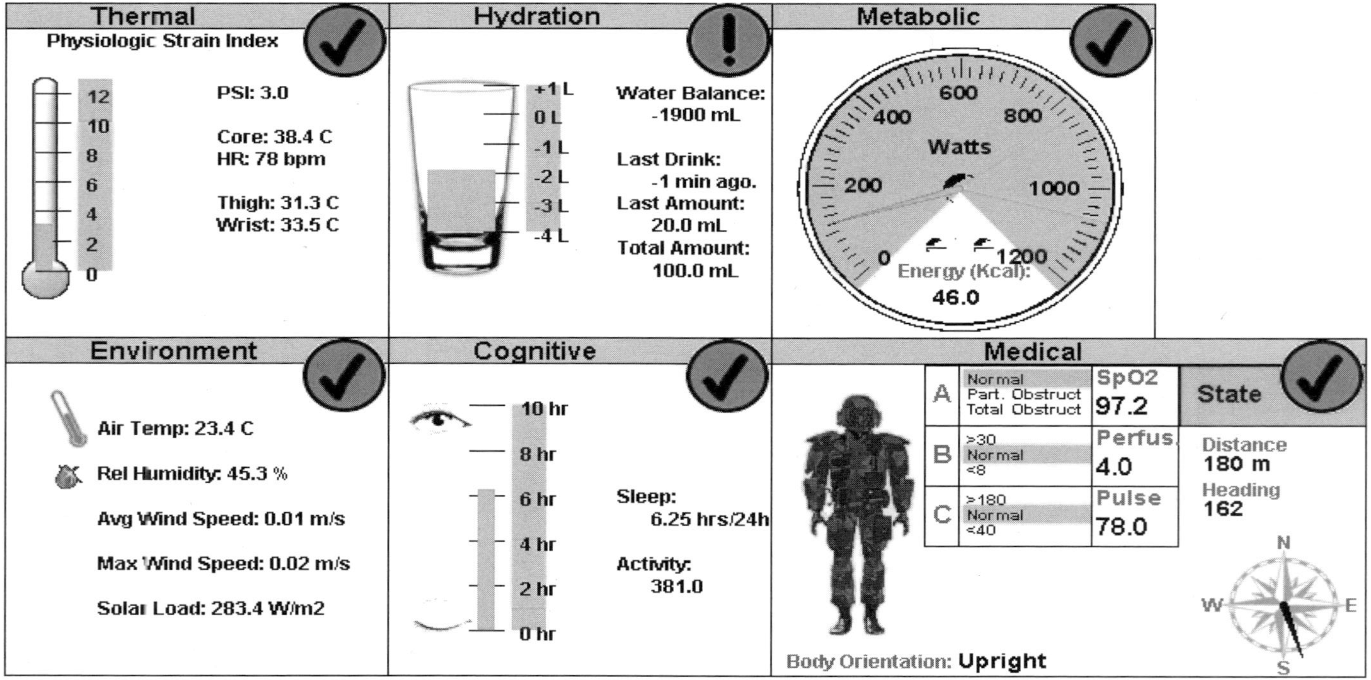

FIGURE 1-1 Prototype combat service member physiological status monitoring user interface (display) for the medic or field commander illustrating contextual and physiological information. This heuristic display shows (1) thermal/work strain as physiological strain index (PSI), (2) hydration state or water balance, (3) metabolic rate, (4) environmental conditions, (5) cognitive/sleep status (hours of sleep, etc.), and (6) clinical status and location information.
SOURCE: Hoyt and Friedl (2003).

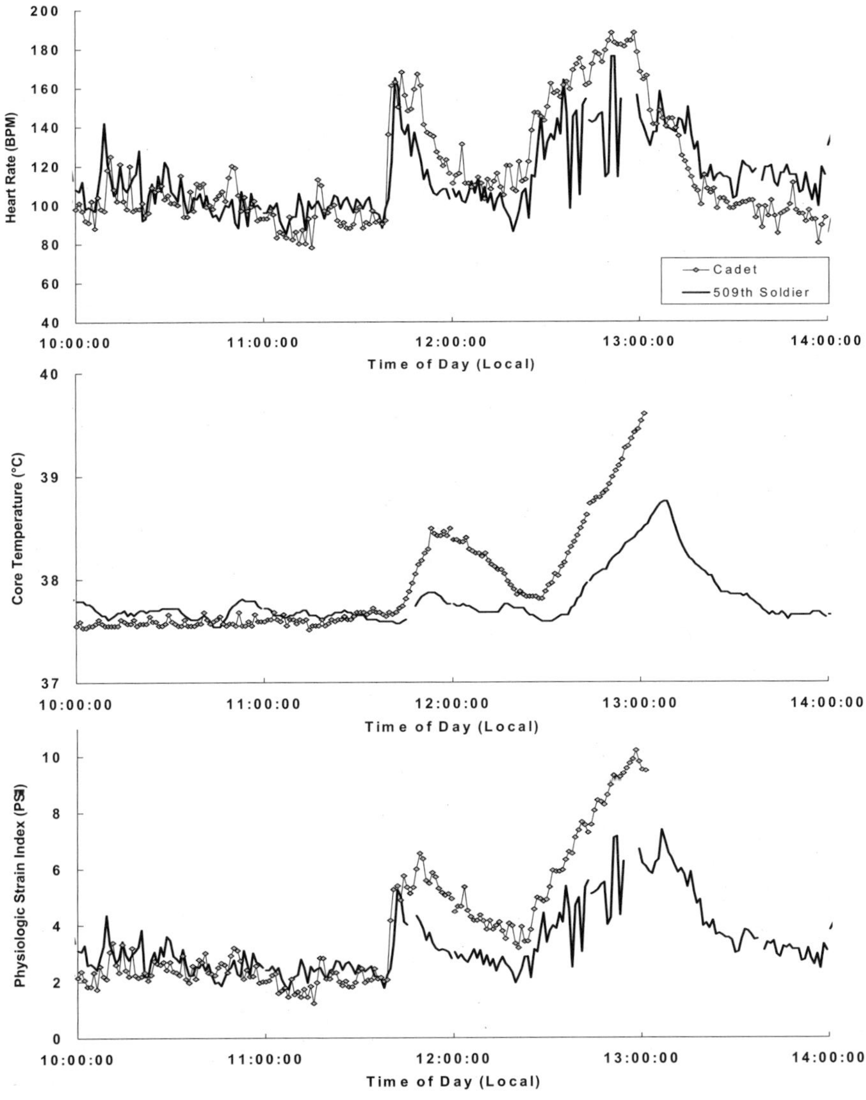

FIGURE 1-2 Heart rate, core temperature, and physiological strain index in two combat service members engaged in similar training activities during a hot-weather field exercise at the Joint Readiness Training Center, Ft. Polk, Louisiana. The thermal/work strain levels associated with two bouts of marching (1145–1200 h and 1230–1300 h) were more pronounced in the heat-exhaustion casualty (cadet) than in the less-affected 509th combat service member. The heat casualty had a higher body fat percent, carried a heavier load, was less physically fit, and was not heat acclimated as compared with his 509th cohort. SOURCE: Hoyt and Friedl (2003).

of 0 to 10 (Moran et al., 1998) is currently used to generate green, amber, or red alerts as thresholds are passed. PSI values may prove useful in assessing acclimation status, guiding heat acclimation routines, and setting the timing and duration of work/rest cycles. A prototype thermal strain model, SCENARIO, estimates core temperature from work rate, clothing characteristics, and ambient meteorological conditions (Kraning and Gonzalez, 1997). This and other surrogate measures of core temperature may be appropriate when risk of hypo- or hyperthermia is moderate and more precise core temperature measurements, such as those provided by the ingested radio telemetry pill, are not needed. The core temperature requirement is likely to be replaced by improvements in heat flux modeling from measures of cutaneous responses and temperatures. Combined with other sensor measurements, cutaneous responses and temperature may provide strong inferences not only about thermal status, but also about shock and hemorrhage.

Cold Strain

Cold injuries, that is, hypothermia and peripheral cold injuries are also a major concern for combat service members (USACHPPM, 2001). Temperature radio telemetry pills can be used to monitor for hypothermia (O'Brien et al., 1998). Peripheral temperature and heat flux sensors can be used to assess the risk of peripheral cold injury and to guide improvements in clothing, boots, and gloves. The Cold Strain Index (Moran et al., 1999) uses core and peripheral temperatures to track cold strain. However, this algorithm needs to be modified to account for altered thermoregulation during underfeeding and sleep. (For a discussion of physiological adjustment of humans to the cold, see Toner and McArdle, 1988.)

Hydration

Under- or overhydration can lead to decrements in physical and cognitive performance, increased risk of heat injury, hyponatremia, and death (Montain et al., 2001; Sawka, 1988). Mission water requirements, largely driven by basal water needs and sweat losses, can be predicted based on the anticipated weather, clothing, load weight, and metabolic rate during the mission (Kraning and Gonzalez, 1997). Technologies to monitor water intake from bladder-type canteens, the "drink-o-meter" concept, can help ensure adequate water intake (water discipline). However, practical field methods to assess overall body tissue hydration or to monitor hydration through urine output have yet to be developed. Tests of the use of body resistance measurements have consistently failed to demonstrate accurate tracking of water changes, perhaps in part because of the inability to control for variability in electrolyte concentrations during various types of dehydration (Berneis and Keller, 2000; Koulmann et al., 2000). It may be possible in the future to improve electrical resistance-derived estimates of hydration with minimally invasive subdermal electrolyte sensors. Alternatively, future automatic monitoring of urinary excretion rates and solute concentrations may provide valuable insight into hydration status and other aspects of acute combat service member health.

Metabolic Status and Energy Reserve: Modeling Metabolic Fuel Requirements

Field rations may not always meet the nutritional needs of combat service members (Friedl and Hoyt, 1997). Negative energy balance, commonly associated with undereating in the field, can usually be managed with little consequence by drawing on substantial body fat reserves. Body energy reserves can be calculated from percent body fat (estimated from waist circumference) less the 5 percent absolute minimum body fat levels attainable in underfed, healthy male combat service members (Friedl et al., 1994). However, negative carbohydrate balance, which is common in the field and is associated with decreased endurance capacity and loss of lean mass, is more difficult to manage due to the body's limited carbohydrate reserves.

Carbohydrate requirements can be estimated from aerobic fitness, daily activity patterns, and the metabolic cost of locomotion (Hoyt and Weyand, 1997). Maximum aerobic capacity can be derived from the Army's Annual Physical Fitness Test 2-mile-run-for-time results (Mello et al., 1988), and daily activity patterns can be derived from heart rate or actigraphy (Redmond and Hegge, 1985). The metabolic cost of locomotion can be derived from total weight and foot-ground contact times (pedometry) (Hoyt and Weyand, 1997; Kram and Taylor, 1990) or from the Pandolf equation, which includes body weight, load weight, and geolocation (including velocity of movement, grade, and footing) (Pandolf et al., 1977). Knowing metabolic rate and the maximum aerobic capacity for each individual, an exercise intensity profile can be generated (i.e., percent of maximum aerobic capacity over time). Oxygen consumption can be partitioned into carbohydrate and fat combustion by assuming a given relationship between resting or exercise intensity and nonprotein respiratory exchange ratio (carbon dioxide production/oxygen consumption) and using standard conversion factors. The exercise intensity-respiratory exchange ratio relationship chosen might be more fat-predominant than that of fully fed individuals (Åstrand and Rodahl, 1986) due to practical limits on the amount of food that can be carried.

Remote Trauma Triage

Combat service members are expected to be widely dispersed on the battlefield and often minimal medical care is available to combat casualties. To help improve remote casualty management, a remote trauma triage system is being developed. This system, part of the WPSM, will contain sensors and algorithms that allow medics to remotely detect ballistic wounding events and to determine casualty life signs and the need for a major surgical life-saving intervention (Holcomb et al., In press). Parameters important in life-sign detection after wounding include responsiveness to radio contact, motion, body position, cardiac activity, and systolic blood pressure. Distilled health status information will foster the effective use of medical resources (e.g., time, equipment, and supplies).

Altitude Acclimatization

Combat service members deploying to elevations above 2,800 m (~ 8,000 ft) may experience Acute Mountain Sickness (Pandolf et al., 1988), which is characterized by headache, nausea, fatigue, decreased appetite, and poor sleep, often with signs of poor balance and mild swelling of the face, hands, and feet. Without special preparation, a large proportion of a military unit rapidly inserted at high altitude is likely to develop acutely debilitating symptoms. Normally, Acute Mountain Sickness is either absent or resolves within 3 to 7 days following ascent. However, maladaptation can lead to life-threatening high-altitude pulmonary or cerebral edema. An individual's acclimatization state can be assessed by comparing blood-oxygen saturation for a given ascent profile (i.e., S_aO_2 for the reported or measured exposure to hypobaric hypoxia) with that expected in normal acclimatization. An ability to monitor and model acclimatization status will make it easier to plan high-altitude missions and minimize altitude illnesses.

EXAMPLE APPLICATION: CHARACTERISTICS OF A HEAT CASUALTY

Heat strain provides a demonstration of nascent capabilities for physiological monitoring. Progressive heat strain moves on a continuum from impaired cognitive function to actual casualty status and presents one of the first opportunities to provide commanders with useful predictions of failing performance before a combat service member becomes an environmental stress casualty. Collection of field data that includes clear medical outcomes makes it possible to backtrack to earlier indicators of the impending health risk and to develop more precise predictive thresholds of individual risk.

Hoyt and Friedl (2003) discussed a recent example that studied individual responses to heat stress. A pair of combat service members were engaged in similar training activities during a hot-weather field exercise at the Joint Readiness Training Center, Ft. Polk, Louisiana. Although the two combat service members performed similar activities from about 1130 to 1400 h (ambient temperature = 32°–34°C; relative humidity = 46–55 percent; solar load = 800–875

TABLE 1-2 Age, Physical Characteristics, Total Load Carried, and Maximal Aerobic Capacity of Two Combat Service Members—A Heat Exhaustion Casualty (Cadet) and an Unaffected 509th Combat Service Member from the 1/509th Infantry Brigade (Airborne)

Combat Service Member	Age (y)	Height (cm)	Weight (kg)	Body Fat (%)	Load (kg)	VO_{2max} (ml O_2/kg^1 min^{-1})
Cadet	21	175	79.3	18	45.3	47
509th combat service member	22	170	68	13.3	35.3	53

NOTE: These combat service members were engaged in similar hot-weather training activities at the Joint Readiness Training Center, Ft. Polk, Louisiana. During a road march, the nonheat-acclimated, less-lean, more-burdened, less physically fit cadet became a heat casualty, while the heat-acclimated, leaner, less-burdened, more fit combat service member from the 1/509th Infantry Brigade (Airborne) tolerated the thermal/work stress.
SOURCE: Hoyt and Friedl (2003).

W/m^2; wind speed = 1–2 ms^{-1}), and both were fed and hydrated, only one became a heat casualty. Combat service member characteristics (Table 1-2), including analysis showed that the combat service members' differences in response to the heat stress were due to a number of factors. The heat casualty had a higher percent body fat, carried a heavier load, was less physically fit, and was not heat acclimated (by interview) as compared with his unaffected cohort. These results illustrate the importance of integrating multiple data streams in the process of understanding multistressor physiological events.

As illustrated in the paragraph above, individuals respond differently to similar work loads in hot environments. In the example, the differences in body size, level of fitness, and acclimation to the heat appeared to be the primary factors contributing to one combat service member being overcome by the heat while the other was fine. Based on the extensive research literature, it is known that a number of factors determine how a particular individual responds to exercise in a hot environment. These factors include the environment (temperature, altitude, wind chill index, humidity), physical factors associated with the individual (body temperature, level of acclimation, fluid intake, level of fitness, level of exercise intensity required to do the work), and the individual's overall health and well-being. Those who are well fed and hydrated, are fit and adapted to the environment, and are wearing appropriate clothing will typically fair better than those who are not. Understanding how individuals respond to specific environmental challenges will aid in training individuals to monitor their own well-being and make appropriate change so that heat stress does not occur.

REFERENCES

Åstrand PO, Rodahl K. 1986. *Textbook of Work Physiology. Physiological Bases of Exercise.* 3rd ed. New York: McGraw-Hill Book Co.

Berneis K, Keller U. 2000. Bioelectrical impedance analysis during acute changes of extracellular osmolality in man. *Clin Nutr* 19:361–366.

Caldwell JA, Hall KK, Erickson BS. 2002. EEG data collected from helicopter pilots in flight are sufficiently sensitive to detect increased fatigue from sleep deprivation. *Int J Aviat Psychol* 12:19–32.

Davis SW, Elmadjian F, Hanson LF, Liddell HS, Zilinsky AA, Johnston ME, Killbuck JH, Pace N, Schaffer FL, Walker EL, Minard D, Kolovos ER, Longley GH. 1952. *A Study of Combat Stress, Korea 1952.* Technical Memorandum ORO-T-41(FEC). Chevy Chase, MD: Operations Research Office, The Johns Hopkins University.

Dinges DF, Mallis MM, Maislin G, Powell JW. 1998. *Evaluation of Techniques for Ocular Measurement as an Index of Fatigue and as the Basis for Alertness Management.* DOT-HS-808-762. Washington, DC: National Highway Traffic Safety Administration.

DOD (U.S. Department of Defense). 2001. *Annual Report to the President and the Congress.* Washington, DC: U.S. Government Printing Office.

Febbraio MA, Pedersen BK. 2002. Muscle-derived interleukin-6: Mechanisms for activation and possible biological roles. *FASEB J* 16:1335–1347.

Forster EM. 2002. *Safety of Flight: The Physiologic Aspect of the Weapon System.* Patuxent River, MD: Naval Air Warfare Center Aircraft Division.

Forster EM, Morrison JG, Hitchcock EM, Scerbo MW. 1994. *Physiologic Instrumentation in the Naval Air Warfare Center Human-Use Centrifuge to Determine the Effects of Cumulative +Gz on Cognitive Performance.* NAWCADWAR-95006-4-6. Warminster, PA: Naval Air Warfare Center Aircraft Division.

Friedl KE. 2003. *Predicting and Protecting Performance using Metabolic Monitoring Strategies: It's All Wet Stuff Anyway, Isn't It?* Presented at the Institute of Medicine, Committee on Metabolic Monitoring Technologies for Military Field Applications Workshop on Metabolic Monitoring Technologies for Military Field Applications, San Antonio, Texas, January 8–9.

Friedl KE, Hoyt RW. 1997. Development and biomedical testing of military operational rations. *Annu Rev Nutr* 17:51–75.

Friedl KE, Moore RJ, Martinez-Lopez LE, Vogel JA, Askew EW, Marchitelli LJ, Hoyt RW, Gordon CC. 1994. Lower limit of body fat in healthy active men. *J Appl Physiol* 77:933–940.

Frier BM. 2001. Hypoglycaemia and cognitive function in diabetes. *Int J Clin Pract* 123:30–37.

Gardner JW, Kark JA. 1994. Fatal rhabdomyolysis presenting as mild heat illness in military training. *Mil Med* 159:160–163.

Holcomb JB, Niles SE, Hinds D, Aoki N, Salinas J, Flannigan TJ, Macaitis JM, Duke JH, Moore FA. In press. Prehospital physiologic data and life saving interventions in trauma patients. *J Trauma.*

Hoyt RW, Friedl KE. 2003. *Current Status of Field Applications of Physiological Monitoring for the Dismounted Soldier.* Presented at the Institute of Medicine, Committee on Metabolic Monitoring Technologies for Military Field Applications Workshop on Metabolic Monitoring Technologies for Military Field Applications, San Antonio, Texas, January 8–9.

Hoyt RW, Weyand PG. 1997. Advances in ambulatory monitoring: Using foot contact time to estimate the metabolic cost of locomotion. In: Carlson-Newberry SJ, Costello RB, eds. *Emerging Technologies for Nutrition Research.* Washington, DC: National Academy Press. Pp. 315–343.

Hoyt RW, Buller M, Redin MS, Poor RD, Oliver SR. 1997a. *Soldier Physiological Monitoring—Results of Dismounted Battlespace Battle Lab Concept Experimentation Program Field Study.* Natick, MA: U.S. Army Research Institute of Environmental Medicine.

Hoyt RW, Young AJ, Matthew WT, Kain JE, Buller M. 1997b. *Warfighter Physiological Status Monitoring (WPSM): Body Core Temperatures during 96 H of Swamp Phase Ranger Training.* Technical Report T97-4. Natick, MA: U.S. Army Research Institute of Environmental Medicine.

Hoyt RW, Buller MJ, DeLany JP, Stultz D, Warren K. 2001. *Warfighter Physiological Status Monitoring (WPSM): Energy Balance and Thermal Status during a 10-day Cold Weather U.S. Marine Corps Infantry Officer Course Field Exercise.* Natick, MA: U.S. Army Research Institute of Environmental Medicine.

Hoyt RW, Reifman J, Coster TS, Buller MJ. 2002. Combat medical informatics: Present and future. In: Kohane IS, ed. *Biomedical Informatics: One Discipline.* Proceedings of the 2002 AMIA Annual Symposium, November 9–13, 2002, San Antonio, Texas. Bethesda, MD: American Medical Informatics Association. Pp. 2335–2339.

Kane RL, Kay GG. 1992. Computerized assessment in neuropsychology: A review of tests and test batteries. *Neuropsychol Rev* 3:1–117.

Koulmann N, Jimenez C, Regal D, Bolliet P, Launay JC, Savourey G, Melin B. 2000. Use of bioelectrical impedance analysis to estimate body fluid compartments after acute variations of the body hydration level. *Med Sci Sports Exerc* 32:857–864.

Kram R, Taylor CR. 1990. Energetics of running: A new perspective. *Nature* 346:265–267.

Kraning KK, Gonzalez RR. 1997. A mechanistic computer simulation of human work in heat that accounts for physical and physiological effects of clothing, aerobic fitness, and progressive dehydration. *J Therm Biol* 22:331–342.

Maron MB, Wagner JA, Horvath SM. 1977. Thermoregulatory responses during competitive marathon running. *J Appl Physiol* 42:909–914.

Mello RP, Murphy MM, Vogel JA. 1988. Relationship between a two mile run for time and maximal oxygen uptake. *J Appl Sport Sci Res* 2:9–12.

Montain SJ, Sawka MN, Wenger CB. 2001. Hyponatremia associated with exercise: Risk factors and pathogenesis. *Exerc Sports Sci Rev* 29:113–117.

Moran DS, Shitzer A, Pandolf KB. 1998. A physiological strain index to evaluate heat stress. *Am J Physiol* 275:R129–R134.

Moran DS, Castellani JW, O'Brien C, Young AJ, Pandolf KB. 1999. Evaluating physiological strain during cold exposure using a new cold strain index. *Am J Physiol* 277:R556–R564.

O'Brien C, Hoyt RW, Buller MJ, Castellani JW, Young AJ. 1998. Telemetry pill measurement of core temperature in humans during active heating and cooling. *Med Sci Sports Exerc* 30:468–472.

Ojaimi J, Masters CL, Opeskin K, McKelvie P, Byrne E. 1999. Mitochondrial respiratory chain activity in the human brain as a function of age. *Mech Ageing Dev* 111:39–47.

Pandolf KB, Givoni B, Goldman RF. 1977. Predicting energy expenditure with loads while standing or walking very slowly. *J Appl Physiol* 43:577–581.

Pandolf KB, Sawka MN, Gonzalez RR, eds. 1988. *Human Performance Physiology and Environmental Medicine at Terrestrial Extremes*. Indianapolis, IN: Benchmark Press.

Popovich RM, Gardner JW, Potter R, Knapik JJ, Jones BH. 2000. Effect of rest from running on overuse injuries in army basic training. *Am J Prev Med* 18:147–155.

Redmond DP, Hegge FW. 1985. Observations on the design and specification of a wrist-worn human activity monitoring system. *Behav Res Methods Instrum Comp* 17:659–669.

Sawka MN. 1988. Body fluid responses and hypohydration during exercise-heat stress. In: Pandolf KB, Sawka MN, Gonzalez RR, eds. *Human Performance Physiology and Environmental Medicine at Terrestrial Extremes*. Indianapolis, IN: Benchmark Press. Pp. 227–266.

Sem-Jacobsen CW. 1959. Electroencephalographic study of pilot stresses in flight. *J Aviat Med* 30:797–801.

Singh MV, Rawal SB, Tyagi AK. 1990. Body fluid status on induction, reinduction and prolonged stay at high altitude of human volunteers. *Int J Biometerol* 34:93–97.

Street TT, Nguyen X, Williams FW. 2002. *Wireless Communication Technologies on Ex-USS Shadwell*. NRL-MR-6180-02-8631. Washington, DC: Naval Research Laboratory.

Toner MM, McArdle WD. 1988. Physiological adjustments of man to the cold. In: Pandolf KB, Sawka MN, Gonzalez RR, eds. *Human Performance Physiology and Environmental Medicine at Terrestrial Extremes*. Indianapolis, IN: Benchmark Press. Pp. 361–399.

USACHPPM (U.S. Army Center for Health Promotion and Preventive Medicine). 2001. Cold weather injuries among active duty soldiers, U.S. Army, 1997–2001. *Med Surveill Month Rep* 7:2–5.

USACHPPM. 2003. Heat-related injuries, U.S. Army, 2002. *Med Surveill Month Rep* 9:2–4.

Vaughan WS Jr. 1975. Diver temperature and performance changes during long-duration, cold water exposure. *Undersea Biomed Res* 2:75–88

Weyand PG, Kelly M, Blackadar T, Darley JC, Oliver SR, Ohlenbusch NE, Joffe SW, Hoyt RW. 2001. Ambulatory estimates of maximal aerobic power from foot-ground contact times and heart rates in running humans. *J Appl Physiol* 91:451–458.

Wittels P, Johannes B, Enne R, Kirsch K, Gunga HC. 2002. Voice monitoring to measure emotional load during short-term stress. *Eur J Appl Physiol* 87:278–282.

Wright HF, Wilmore JH. 1974. Estimation of relative body fat and lean body weight in a United States Marine Corps population. *Aerospace Med* 45:301–306.

2

The Study of Individual Differences: Statistical Approaches to Inter- and Intraindividual Variability

This chapter outlines some basic issues in research design and analysis. It is included to inform the reader about the manner in which researchers have typically explored relationships among environmental, task, or psychological stressors and specific biomarkers or performance outcomes. Although this standard approach has been invaluable up to the present, continued reliance on this approach to the exclusion of more complex, nonlinear methods may impede progress toward developing predictors that are reliable across unique individuals, times, and circumstances. To start, a discussion of the research hypothesis and its relationship to the partitioning of variance is presented. Attention is then shifted to the elements of a statistical test, followed by an examination of the selection perspective on research design and the distinction between inter- and intraindividual variability. A rationale for the use of multivariate, replicated, repeated-measures, single-subject designs in research with combat service members is offered. It is imperative to keep in mind that the most important aspect of any statistical test is the informed judgment of the researcher. As such, a clear understanding of these basic issues contributes greatly toward the appropriate design and analysis of experiments.

OVERVIEW

Biobehavioral research is among the most challenging of scientific endeavors. The study of interactions between living systems and their environment has tested the limits of research methodologies and theoretical models. The typical research design oversimplifies the complexity of these relationships and thus does not unambiguously allow for inferences about organism-environment interactions. Rather, these designs tend to obscure underlying processes by shrouding rich individual data with group data aggregation procedures (Glass and Mackey, 1988; O'Connor, 1990).

It is a truism in the biobehavioral sciences that no single measure or aspect of responding can adequately represent a complex latent construct (Nesselroade and

Ford, 1987; Schwartz, 1986). Rather, such constructs must be represented by an entire pattern of manifestations (Cattell, 1966). In studying the behavior of living systems, a description and elucidation of the nature of underlying regulatory processes should precede any premature hypothesis testing with group means of individual variables (Barton, 1994). In view of the prevalence and importance of rhythmicity in biological regulatory mechanisms, inclusion of time-varying or temporal aspects of responding is crucial to accurately portray such activity (Glass and Mackey, 1988; Goldbeter and Decroly, 1983; Hrushesky, 1994).

Unfortunately, the analysis of variance (ANOVA) design, a staple of psychophysiological research, confuses temporal information by splitting physiological events into discrete epochs, thereby disrupting the continuity of responding (O'Connor, 1992). Furthermore, precise mapping of physiological activity from these distinct periods onto experimental manipulations is fraught with hazards, such as delayed physiological responses and compensatory homeostatic processes (Levenson, 1988). Alternatively, all recorded activity might be considered as relevant; functional relationships among ongoing physiological processes could then be extracted across observations (O'Connor, 1990).

In response to these various concerns, an alternative framework for research with combat service members is suggested: a multivariate, systems perspective that emphasizes the study of individuals. A distinctive feature of this approach is its focus on intraindividual variability in the behavioral and physiological processes of an organism. Moreover, within-group variance (typically treated as error in traditional experimental psychology) is also investigated since it contains a wealth of relevant information (Cronbach, 1957). Thus it is appropriate first to address these basic methodological issues in design and analysis for research involving combat service members.

SEX AND GENDER

Sex and gender factors, including genetic, hormonal, and behavioral factors, are important variables that contribute to differences in biological responses in all species. Sex and gender should therefore always be considered and taken into account when designing and analyzing studies at all levels of biomedical- and health-related research (IOM, 2001b). Data related to sex and gender variables in health and disease have been recently summarized in an Institute of Medicine report (IOM, 2001b). This report pointed out that incidence and severity of diseases vary between the sexes and may be related to differences in genetic, hormonal, cellular, or behavioral responses, as well as to differences in exposures, routes of entry, or the processing of a foreign agent. The report also underscored the importance of performing studies at different stages of the life span to determine how sex and developmental differences influence health, illness, and longevity.

Several examples of sexually dimorphic biomarkers are relevant to this report. For example, in the context of a military setting, it is known that the incidence of stress fractures during military training is significantly higher in females than in males (Shaffer, 1997; Stoneman, 1997). Furthermore, recent research indicates that stress responses differ in males and females, and that the hormonal stress response (hypothalamic-pituitary-adrenal axis) is modulated by sex hormones. Conversely, stress hormones modulate the sex hormone axis (hypothalamic-pituitary-gonadal axis) (Castagnetta et al., 2003; Cutolo et al., 2003). Clinically relevant conditions related to this interplay between these axes that could apply to a military setting include amenorrhea in female athletes. Pain responses also differ in males and females (Sternberg et al., 2001), as do cognitive and behavioral differences in response to sleep deprivation (IOM, 2001a). The committee therefore emphasizes that sex- and gender-related differences at the biological level will impact outcome measures of all the biomarkers considered in this report; therefore when designing and analyzing relevant studies, consideration should be always be given to these differences.

RESEARCH: WHAT ARE WE REALLY TRYING TO DO?

Variance Partitioning and Hypothesis Testing

The research enterprise is primarily concerned with the detection of systematic relationships amidst the morass of variability in biobehavioral responses. This task calls for the partitioning of observed variability into systematic and random components, which in turn will reveal patterns of associations such that events can be described, predicted, controlled, and ultimately understood. In the simplest case, a research question or hypothesis is tested by an investigation of the existence, direction, and magnitude of a relationship between an independent or predictor variable (IV) and a dependent or criterion variable (DV).

It is a basic and often implicit assumption of most scientific research that the whole is equal to the sum of its parts. It then follows that the partitioning of observed variability will lead to an explicit set of relationships between IVs and DVs. This premise is the basis of all common statistical procedures and is the foundation of the general linear model, that is, the presumption of linearity allows for unambiguous partitioning of variability. As such, small causes lead to small effects and large causes lead to large effects. This concept of proportionality is a cornerstone of the general linear model (West, 1990). However, linearity, and thus this ability to neatly partition variance, often does not hold in nature, and so arose the impetus for contemporary work on nonlinear dynamics: the science of complexity, also called chaos theory (Gleick, 1987). In spite of the notoriety that has been attained by this field, most research methodologies are based on the presumption of linearity.

Variance Partitioning in a Linear World

When trying to assess the relative importance of a particular association, one typically asks if the systematic relationship is large relative to random fluctuations. In a simple t-test or one-way, between-subjects ANOVA, this question becomes a test of the ratio of two variances: one representing systematic variability (between-subject variance) and the other representing unsystematic variability (within-subject variance). In the one-way, between-subjects ANOVA, this ratio is expressed as:

$$F = \text{between-subject variance/within-subject variance}$$

When this ratio is much greater than one, with the appropriate degrees of freedom (df), there is evidence for a statistically significant association between the IV and DV. However, in numerous situations there are many possible systematic relationships, only some of which will be of interest. Thus it is preferable to think of a statistical test as the ratio of the variance of interest to the variance of noninterest:

$$F = \text{variance of interest/variance of noninterest}$$

Another important consideration is the magnitude or size of the effect. Since one is not only attempting to estimate the probability, but also the direction and magnitude of relationships, a direct index of the latter is very useful. Unfortunately, the tradition of null-hypothesis testing has tended to divert the focus of research away from the dimension of magnitude. In fact, any significance test represents the confluence of four mathematical components: (1) the size of the study, which refers to the number of subjects under investigation and is often represented in the significance test by the df associated with the denominator of the ratio of variances; (2) the size of the effect, which refers to the magnitude of the relationship between the IV and DV, a quantity that represents the amount of variability in the DV that is due to variation in each IV; (3) the Type I error; and (4) the power and Type II errors.

The Alpha Level or Type I Error Rate

The Type I error rate is the probability of falsely rejecting the null hypothesis, that is, the chance of concluding that a systematic relationship exists in the population when in fact it does not. This possibility tends to dominate the consciousness of investigators, so many post hoc techniques (e.g., the Bonferoni inequality, the Newman-Keuls test) have been developed to control it. By convention, the level of alpha is usually set at 0.05, but this figure is arbitrary.

The Power and Type II Error Rate (Beta)

Power refers to the probability that a relationship in the population will be detected when one in fact exists. Power and its related Type II error rate (failure to reject a false null hypothesis) are probably the most neglected aspects of a statistical test. Power might reflect what Fisher (1966) called the "sensitivity" of an experiment. Importantly, the power of an obtained statistical test reflects the probability that such a result can be replicated (Goodman, 1992). The effects of low statistical power on the reproducibility of research findings have been well documented (Abelson, 1997; Goodman, 1992; Harris, 1997; Hunter, 1997; Scarr, 1997; Shrout, 1997). The Type II error occurs when one fails to reject a false null hypothesis. This error is inversely related to the power of a test:

$$\text{Power} = 1 - \text{beta}$$

One factor that leads to low power or inflated Type II error risk is an inadequate sample size.

As a convention, Type I error rates of 0.05 and implicit Type II error rates of 0.20 (power of 0.80) are adopted. However, in practice in many areas of investigation, one rarely has adequate power (that is, power ≥ 0.80), and therefore the Type II error rate is much higher (Cohen, 1992).

The following equation reveals the relationship between the statistical test value on the one hand, and the effect size and size of the study on the other:

$$\text{Statistical (i.e., significance) test} = \text{effect size} \times \text{size of the study}$$

or more concretely for a two-group test:

$$F = \text{mean square error of interest} \div \text{mean square error of noninterest} \times df_{\text{denominator}}$$

with the appropriate F distribution based on the numerator and denominator *df*s and the mean squares representing the variability per *df*. Thus the numerator is an estimate of the variability of interest and the denominator is an estimate of the variability of noninterest (Rosenthal and Rosnow, 1984).

What is clear from the equation of the experiment is that statistical significance is a function not only of the magnitude of the relationship (the effect size), but also of the size of the study. Thus one way to achieve a statistically significant result is to increase the size of the study. A consequence of this fact is that any nonzero association between IVs and DVs can be statistically significant if one runs enough subjects (Meehl, 1978). In fact, the probability that the so-called "null" hypothesis, if taken literally, is truly false is essentially zero. Perhaps the best information derived from a significant statistical test result is that a lot of subjects were run, which one knows without having do to any mathematical calculations.

Moreover, all other things being equal, the probability of a Type I error is inversely related to the probability of a Type II error. Thus as the risk of a Type I error is decreased, for example by decreasing the alpha level considered acceptable, the risk of a Type II error increases. The appropriate balancing of Type I and Type II errors is very much content-area specific (Rosenthal and Rosnow, 1984). However, using the conventional values for Type I and Type II errors (0.05 and 0.20, respectively), a Type I error is deemed to be four times more egregious than a Type II error. In areas such as those involving monitoring metabolic status of combat service members, where the cost per datum tends to be relatively high, this level of balance in which we are more apt to accept a Type II error and thus conclude that no relationship exists when in fact one does, may not be cost effective.

Though an extended discussion of the relative merits of statistical hypothesis testing is beyond the scope of this chapter (for a recent debate, see Ableson, 1997; Harris, 1997; Hunter, 1997; Scarr, 1997; Shrout, 1997), knowledge of the nature of these tests is crucial for the design of the experiment. At the very least, this awareness can help to determine the number of subjects necessary to have a good chance of detecting an effect of a certain size while balancing the risk of Type I and Type II errors. Moreover, reasoned consideration of the effect size can greatly enhance the ability to determine the practical significance—and not just the statistical significance—of the results of an experiment.

Choosing What to Measure

On the IV side, Cattell (1988) presented a system of relationships based on three dimensions (persons, occasions, and variables [or tests]), termed the data box. Common to both data theory and the data box is the notion that the researcher, explicitly or more often, implicitly, selects from a broad range of possible dimensions or modes of interest. This critical decision involves selection from a universe of possible scores those that will be the subject of investigation. That this choice often occurs without full knowledge of the various selection effects threatens not only the validity of the inferences drawn from such experiments, but also ultimately the quality of research that serves as the collective database of the field.

Nesselroade and Jones (1991) have provided a cogent exposition on the nature of these selection effects. They noted that a single datum can be characterized as a "...'draw' of one piece of information from a universe of information" (P. 21). Minimally, this hypothesized universe represents the scores for every conceivable person and variable on all possible measurement occasions. Thus the three dimensions of persons, variables, and occasions represent a minimum universe from which data are selected. Since each possible score is not likely to be available due to constraints such as time, money, and population base rates, most of the data will remain unrealized. Therefore, in attempting to make generalizations from the results, the necessity of selecting a representative subset of scores to comprise the data cannot be overestimated.

A thornier situation exists in biobehavioral research, in which there are a myriad of possible dimensions to select from. Cattell (1988) mentioned ten such dimensions, and innumerable others are possible. Thus this decision is a complex, multimodal selection operation (Nesselroade and Jones, 1991). For example, if an investigator attends exclusively to the persons mode, which is often the case, even appropriate sampling methods do not protect against selection effects on the variables or occasions modes.

Known Systematic Sources of Variability

The three sources of variance (persons, occasions, and variables) are present in nearly all experimental designs. Their relationship with a set of scores should be explicitly investigated and the systematic variance associated with each accounted for before valid inferences can be drawn (Cattell, 1988). The most familiar source is that of persons; the effects of inadequate selection on this dimension are widely known. However, the exclusive emphasis on this mode has tended to distract investigators from selection effects on the variables and occasions dimensions, inadvertently providing a false sense of security to experimenters who have accounted for bias on person selection while neglecting these other equally important dimensions.

Multivariate techniques are required to assess multiple sources of variance. Yet there has generally been a paucity of multivariate studies in experimental psychology and in experimental research in general (Harris, 1992). In addition, the occasions dimension holds particular significance for biobehavioral research since most studies involve repeated measurements to some degree (Vasey and Thayer, 1987).

The dynamics of a system cannot be investigated unless the organism is observed repeatedly over time. Organismic theory views the human being as a unified entity whose component parts function according to laws that direct the whole organism (Goldstein, 1939). These principles guide which aspects of the environment the organism attends and reacts to. Goldstein asserted that in-depth investigations of single individuals, over a wide range of observation conditions, are necessary to comprehend the operation of these superordinate functions in naturalistic environments.

Indeed, a full description of human responses requires an observation on some measure in a certain individual at a particular time and place (occasion) (Nesselroade and Ford, 1987). Thus three known sources of variability must be taken into account in the design and analysis of studies involving combat service members. First, experiments should be designed to highlight the particular variability of interest. For example, if one is interested in individual differences, persons should be observed over many different occasions to estimate the variance in scores that is relatively unchanging. Moreover, one may want to use "raw" rather than "change" scores, since partial ipsatization (from subtraction of base values; see Cattell, 1988) tends to minimize the variance due to persons. Second, the focus should be on indices of the magnitude of the association; less reliance should be placed on tests of statistical significance. Third, a program of research studies should be examined in aggregate, that is, the results of several studies should be combined to produce estimates of the magnitude of associations. Meta-analytical procedures for this purpose can produce more stable estimates of the importance of various factors and can aid in the accumulation of knowledge that lies at the heart of any scientific enterprise (Guzzo et al., 1987). However, for meta-analysis to be meaningful, scientific and explicit protocols that ensure comparability of randomized, controlled clinical trials should be followed. Furthermore, a significant *p* value found in any one study yields essentially no useful information regarding the probability of replicating that finding (Goodman, 1992; Guttman, 1985).

Inter- Versus Intraindividual Variability

An important and often overlooked distinction that has led to confusion in the literature is the difference between inter- and intraindividual variability. Relationships that exist *among* individuals may not be the same as those relationships that exist *within* individuals. From a research design perspective, it is important to be clear which of these associations is being investigated. A common mistake is to formulate a hypothesis concerning an intraindividual association, say, on the effects of different treatments on an individual's blood pressure, but to then conduct an experiment in which each person receives a different treatment or manipulation.

Another relevant example is that few studies have truly tested the James (1884) model of emotion, which suggests that the physiological responses and the subjective experience of a given emotion are highly related (an intraindividual hypothesis). Instead, most studies have involved an emotional response elicited from a group of individuals exposed to several manipulations, such as viewing pictures of facial expressions (for a review, see Ellsworth, 1994). Subjects may have various physiological measures taken, such as the facial electromyogram (EMG) from the brow and the cheek, and then are asked to rate their subjective emotional state after viewing each picture. The data are then analyzed by correlating physiological and self-reported responses aggregated across all individuals. In this case, inter- and intraindividual differences are confounded. A more appropriate test of the Jamesian hypothesis (James, 1884) would be to correlate the physiological and subjective responses within individuals and then combine the results of these within-person correlations. Using this within-person approach with a multivariate measure of association (redundancy analysis; Lambert et al., 1988), responses aggregated across subjects revealed little relationship (shared variance on the order of magnitude of 10 percent) between EMG and subjective responses (Uijtdehaage and Thayer, 1988). When the same data were analyzed using within-subject measures of association, the shared variance increased to approximately 80 percent.

Clearly, different data aggregation procedures lead to vastly different inferences about the Jamesian hypothesis (James, 1884). In a related study, it was reported that the physiological measures that best discriminated the group emotion profiles were not those that best discriminated among any individual's emotion profiles (Thayer and Faith, 1994). These findings suggest that the effects of confounding inter- and intraindividual variability can have enormous consequences for the generalizations and conclusions reached in any particular study.

Multivariate, Replicated, Repeated-Measures, Single-Subject Designs

In any one study, it is generally not feasible to represent all possible modes of data classification in a completely satisfactory manner. Therefore, it behooves investigators to make informed choices on these dimensions rather than let chance and expediency dictate research design. Preparation for conducting large group studies may involve prior intensive study of individuals with multiple measures on numerous occasions in order to discern information on sampling of variables and occasions (Nesselroade and Jones, 1991). Indeed, the history of biobehavioral research is replete with prominent examples in which principles of broad applicability emerged from the intensive study of individuals (for a review, see Barlow and Hersen, 1984). Importantly, it is only through intensive studies of individuals that behavior patterns can be examined as they unfold over time, a critical feature in the study of nonlinear dynamics. Finally, the individual has long been recognized as the ultimate entity in biobehavioral research, for it is there that processes occur and applications are made (Rosenzweig, 1958). This point is especially salient to research on combat service members.

In summary, multivariate, replicated, repeated-measures, single-subject designs are highly compatible with the aims of research on combat service members. Central to these aims is the desire to develop applications that are relevant to specific individuals as they carry out complex, multivariate behaviors that evolve over time. Repeated-measures designs and the collection of multiple interrelated measures are common in biobehavioral research, and so the considered application of this research paradigm can enhance the quality of research that is already being conducted. Thus no radical change in experimental procedures is required; only a more reasoned data extraction from the rich corpus of already available information is necessary.

Furthermore, recent statistical advances have expanded the repertoire of tools with which to analyze data from these designs. For example, hierarchical linear models (Schwartz et al., 1994), random regression models (Jacob et al., 1999), and pooled cross-sectional time series (Dielman, 1983) allow for the partitioning of inter- and intraindividual variability from a number of different sources. Complemented by *set* analytical techniques that allow for the examination of multiple DVs (Cohen, 1982), these methods offer many data analytical strategies for multivariate, replicated, repeated-measures, single-subject designs.

An Example Using Multilevel Models

Recent advances in statistical software have brought the use of hierarchical linear models and stochastic regression models into easy reach. PROC MIXED in the SAS software package (SAS Institute Inc.) and BMDP 5V in the Biomedical software package (SPSS Inc.) can be used to estimate these types of models. There are numerous advantages to these approaches compared with previous methods. First, inter- and intraindividual variability can be simultaneously estimated. Second, the use of random coefficients allows for the generalizability of these estimates beyond the particular data sample. Third, differing numbers of observations per participant can be accommodated. Finally, missing data can be easily handled in these models.

Ambulatory monitoring of physiological responses has the potential to greatly impact research on combat service members. Researchers are no longer confined to the laboratory; subjects can now be monitored during actual work situations. Several versions of these multilevel models have been applied to study the effects of various factors, such as mood, location, and postural effects on ambulatory heart rate and blood pressure (Jacob et al., 1999; Schwartz et al., 1994). Schwartz and colleagues (1994) present a simple illustration of the model; for a single, within-person factor, such as location (work versus home), the model is:

$$Y_{ij(k)} = (\mu + \alpha_i) + (\beta_k + \delta_{ik}) + \varepsilon_{ij(k)}$$

where $Y_{ij(k)}$ is the jth blood pressure reading for person i, taken in the kth location; μ is the weighted grand mean of an individual's average awake blood pressures, weighted by the number of readings per person; α_i is the deviation of person i's average awake blood pressure (from the grand mean μ); β_k is the average intra-individual (main) effect of being in location k (the weighted average of the βs equals zero); δ_{ik} is the deviation of the effect for person i of being in location k from β_k, the person by location interaction effect (the weighted average of the δs equals zero for each person); $\varepsilon_{ij(k)}$ is the deviation of person i's j^{th} observation from its predicted value, based upon the preceding parameters (the mean of these deviations for all observations of person i taken in the kth location equals zero); the first term on the right side of the equation ($\mu + \alpha_i$) is the interindividual variance; and the second term on the right side ($\beta_k + \delta_{ik}$) is the intraindividual variance. (Full details for estimation of the model are given in Schwartz et al., 1994.)

Application of this model to multiple-parameter estimation is illustrated by Schwartz and colleagues (1994); a similar model and estimation procedure has been applied to longitudinal regression (Jacob et al., 1999). These models allow for the estimation of multiple influences on a DV in a nonarbitrary metric. For example, Schwartz and colleagues (1994) found that the average intraindividual effect of being at work versus at home on systolic blood pressure was 2 to 4 mm Hg. Thus the implications of this result are easy to comprehend, whereas traditional ANOVA-type models may state results in standard deviation units or other derived indices, the practical significance of which is often difficult to gauge.

SYSTEMS THEORY AND THE STUDY OF INDIVIDUALS

Systems theory seeks principles that are widely applicable across diverse complex systems (Miller, 1978; Schwartz, 1982). The ideal venue for modeling such organismic systems may be the single-subject paradigm (Denenberg, 1982; Goldstein, 1939; Nesselroade and Ford, 1987). A basic advantage of such designs is their sensitivity to temporal patterns in biobehavioral processes. Multivariate, multioccasion, single-subject paradigms have the resolving power necessary to portray patterns of stability and change that characterize organism-environment interactions (Nesselroade, 1991). The replication of these patterns across individuals in turn can bridge specific and general applicability. This spiraling process is therefore congruent with the quest for principles that are relevant at multiple levels of analysis.

It is fundamental to systems theory that basic processes operating at the level of the individual will also be manifested at both lower and higher levels of analysis (Schwartz, 1982). In nonlinear dynamics terminology, these similarities are referred to as fractals and occur frequently in nature (Barton, 1994; Bassingthwaighte, 1988; Goldberger, 1992; Nonnenmacher et al., 1994; West, 1990). In general, systems approaches have revealed the utility of seeking correspondences across multiple layers of biobehavioral inquiry (Friedman and Thayer, 1998a, 1998b; Kandel, 1983; Mandell et al., 1981). For example, perception of the relationship between individual and population disease-prevention strategies has been underscored in epidemiological research (Rose, 1992). Clearly, studies of individuals are integral components in the scientific quest for general laws of behavior; they are complementary parts of a whole (Rosenzweig, 1958).

Another aspect of this area that is of great concern to research on combat service members is the study of individual differences. Biological organisms display wide-ranging individual differences in physiology (Fahrenberg, 1986; Sargent and Weinman, 1966; Woodhead et al., 1985). The importance of individual differences for research on combat service members can be illustrated by the effects of differences in visual acuity on cardiovascular responses to a computer display (Tyrrell et al., 2000).

A thorough exploration of biobehavioral responding requires the extensive study of individuals over time, a highly problematic enterprise in large *N* designs. Beyond pragmatic concerns, these designs constrain individual response patterns into group molds. To take advantage of the emerging field of dynamic systems, experiments must be designed in such a way as to mine the rich inter-

and intraindividual variability inherent in living systems. In this context, time-series analysis is a useful adjunct to traditional data analysis strategies. Time-series analysis has been used extensively in many fields, from econometrics to physiology, and it allows for the examination of the temporal structure of a set of sequentially collected data points. Time series from individual subjects can be examined and parameters extracted that can be used in data aggregation procedures. For example, the time series of heart periods (the time between successive heart beats) has been used to extract indices of autonomic nervous system control that can be used to characterize the physiological, emotional, and cognitive state of an individual (Friedman et al., 1996; Thayer and Lane, 2000).

Moreover, the parameters extracted from time-series analyses can be combined and the pattern of these parameters examined using pattern classification and neural network techniques. These techniques allow for the investigation of nonlinear patterns in data that might usefully distinguish subjects or conditions into meaningful classes or categories at the level of the individual (see Tyrrell et al., 1995).

SUMMARY

In this chapter we have attempted to expose assumptions that are often deceptively implicit in the design and analysis of experiments. Research on combat service members, with its focus on person-environment interactions, has a pressing need to elucidate those factors that contribute to interindividual differences *and* distinguish them from sources of intraindividual variability. The search for associations among IVs and DVs can be expressed as the partitioning of system variability into factors that contribute to this observed variation. Furthermore, although the assumption of linearity has been useful in promoting well-controlled studies of biobehavioral variables, it also represents a limiting influence on the burgeoning study of complexity and dynamic systems. However, designs that can be used to partition data into linear estimates of variance can also be used to investigate the dynamics of person-environment transactions. It is hoped that researchers will not only take advantage of contemporary analytical techniques for the study of dynamic systems, but also pursue research that will aid in the understanding and appropriate use of extant data analytical tools.

REFERENCES

Abelson RP. 1997. On the surprising longevity of flogged horses: Why there is a case for the significance test. *Psychol Sci* 8:12–15.

Barlow DH, Hersen M. 1984. *Single Case Experimental Designs. Strategies for Studying Behavior Change.* New York: Pergamon Press.

Barton S. 1994. Chaos, self-organization, and psychology. *Am Psychol* 49:5–14.

Bassingthwaighte JB. 1988. Physiological heterogeneity: Fractals link determinism and randomness in structures and functions. *News Physiol Sci* 3:5–9.

Castagnetta LA, Carruba G, Granata OM, Stefano R, Miele M, Schmidt M, Cutolo M, Straub RH. 2003. Increased estrogen formation and estrogen to androgen ratio in the synovial fluid of patients with rheumatoid arthritis. *J Rheumatol* 30:2597–2605.

Cattell RB. 1966. Multivariate behavioral research and the integrative challenge. *Multivariate Behav Res* 1:4–23.

Cattell RB. 1988. The data box. Its ordering of total resources in terms of possible relational systems. In: Nesselroade JR, Cattell RB, eds. *Handbook of Multivariate Experimental Psychology*. 2nd ed. New York: Plenum Press. Pp. 69–130.

Cohen J. 1982. Set correlation as a general multivariate data-analytic method. *Multivariate Behav Res* 17:301–341.

Cohen J. 1992. A power primer. *Psychol Bull* 112:155–159.

Cronbach LJ. 1957. The two disciplines of scientific psychology. *Am Psychol* 12:671–684.

Cutolo M, Capellino S, Montagna P, Villaggio B, Sulli A, Seriolo B, Straub RH. 2003. New roles for estrogens in rheumatoid arthritis. *Clin Exp Rheumatol* 21:687–690.

Denenberg VH. 1982. Comparative psychology and single-subject research. In: Fiske DW, ed. *New Directions for Methodology of Social and Behavioral Science*. Vol. 13. San Francisco: Jossey-Bass. Pp. 19–31.

Dielman TE. 1983. Pooled cross-sectional and time series data: A survey of current statistical methodology. *Am Statist* 37:111–122.

Ellsworth PC. 1994. William James and emotion: Is a century of fame worth a century of misunderstanding? *Psychol Rev* 101:222–229.

Fahrenberg J. 1986. Psychophysiological individuality: A pattern analytic approach to personality research and psychosomatic medicine. *Adv Behav Res Ther* 8:43–100.

Fisher RA. 1966. *The Design of Experiments*. 8th ed. New York: Hafner Publishing.

Friedman BH, Thayer JF. 1998a. Anxiety and autonomic flexibility: A cardiovascular approach. *Biol Psychol* 49:303–323.

Friedman BH, Thayer JF. 1998b. Autonomic balance revisited: Panic anxiety and heart rate variability. *J Psychosom Res* 44:133–151.

Friedman BH, Thayer JF, Tyrrell RA. 1996. Spectral characteristics of heart period variability during cold face stress and shock avoidance in normal subjects. *Clin Auton Res* 6:147–152.

Glass L, Mackey MC. 1988. *From Clocks to Chaos*. Princeton, NJ: Princeton University Press.

Gleick J. 1987. *Chaos. Making a New Science*. New York: Viking Penguin.

Goldberger AL. 1992. Applications of chaos to physiology and medicine. In: Kim JH, Stringer J, eds. *Applied Chaos*. New York: John Wiley & Sons. Pp. 321–331.

Goldbeter A, Decroly O. 1983. Temporal self-organization in biochemical systems: Periodic behavior vs. chaos. *Am J Physiol* 245:R478–R483.

Goldstein K. 1939. *The Organism. A Holistic Approach to Biology Derived from Pathological Data in Men*. New York: American Book.

Goodman SN. 1992. A comment on replication, *p*-values and evidence. *Stat Med* 11:875–879.

Guttman L. 1985. The illogic of statistical inference for cumulative science. *Appl Stochastic Models Data Anal* 1:3–10.

Guzzo RA, Jackson SE, Katzell RA. 1987. Meta-analysis analysis. In: Cummings LL, Staw BM, eds. *Research in Organizational Behavior*. Vol. 9. Greenwich, CT: JAI Press. Pp. 407–442.

Harris RJ. 1992. Multivariate statistics. When will experimental psychology catch up? In: Koch S, Leary DE, eds. *A Century of Psychology as Science*. Washington, DC: American Psychological Association. Pp. 678–697.

Harris RJ. 1997. Significance tests have their place. *Psychol Sci* 8:8–11.

Hrushesky WJM. 1994. Timing is everything. *Sciences* 34:32–37.

Hunter JE. 1997. Needed: A ban on the significance test. *Psychol Sci* 8:3–7.

IOM (Institute of Medicine). 2001a. *Caffeine for the Sustainment of Mental Task Performance. Formulations for Military Operations*. Washington, DC: National Academy Press.

IOM (Institute of Medicine). 2001b. *Exploring the Biological Contributions to Human Health: Does Sex Matter?* Washington, DC: National Academy Press.

Jacob RG, Thayer JF, Manuck SB, Muldoon MF, Tamres LK, Williams DM, Ding Y, Gatsonis C. 1999. Ambulatory blood pressure responses and the circumplex model of mood: A 4-day study. *Psychosom Med* 61:319–333.

James W. 1884. What is an emotion? *Mind* 9:188–205.

Kandel ER. 1983. From metapsychology to molecular biology: Explorations into the nature of anxiety. *Am J Psychiat* 140:1277–1293.

Lambert ZV, Wildt AR, Durand RM. 1988. Redundancy analysis: An alternative to canonical correlation and multivariate multiple regression in exploring interset associations. *Psychol Bull* 104:282–289.

Levenson RW. 1988. Emotion and the autonomic nervous system: A prospectus for research on autonomic specificity. In: Wagner HL, ed. *Social Psychophysiology and Emotion Theory and Clinical Applications*. Chichester, Eng: John Wiley & Sons. Pp. 17–42.

Mandell AJ, Stewart KD, Russo PV. 1981. The Sunday syndrome: From kinetics to altered consciousness. *Fed Proc* 40:2693–2698.

Meehl PE. 1978. Theoretical risks and tabular asterisks: Sir Karl, Sir Ronald, and the slow progress of soft psychology. *J Consult Clin Psychol* 46:806–834.

Miller JG. 1978. *Living Systems*. New York: McGraw-Hill.

Nesselroade JR. 1991. Interindividual differences in intraindividual change. In: Collins LM, Horn JL, eds. *Best Methods for the Analysis of Change. Recent*

Advances. Unanswered Questions, Future Directions. Washington, DC: American Psychological Association. Pp. 92–105.

Nesselroade JR, Ford DH. 1987. Methodological considerations in modeling living systems. In: Ford ME, Ford DH, eds. *Humans as Self-Constructing Living Systems. Putting the Framework to Work*. Hillsdale, NJ: Lawrence Erlbaum Associates. Pp. 47–79.

Nesselroade JR, Jones CJ. 1991. Multi-modal selection effects in the study of adult development: A perspective on multivariate, replicated, single-subject, repeated measures designs. *Exp Aging Res* 17:21–27.

Nonnenmacher TF, Losa GA, Weibel ER, eds. 1994. *Fractals in Biology and Medicine*. Basel: Birkhauser Verlag.

O'Connor K. 1990. Towards a process paradigm in psychophysiology. *Int J Psychophysiol* 9:209–223.

O'Connor K. 1992. Design and analysis in individual difference research. In: Gale A, Eysenck MW, eds. *Handbook of Individual Differences: Biological Perspectives*. New York: John Wiley & Sons. Pp. 45–79.

Rose G. 1992. Strategies of prevention: The individual and the population. In: Marmot M, Elliott P, eds. *Coronary Heart Disease Epidemiology. From Aetiology to Public Health*. New York: Oxford University Press. Pp. 311–324.

Rosenthal R, Rosnow RL. 1984. *Essentials of Behavioral Research. Methods and Data Analysis*. New York: McGraw-Hill.

Rosenzweig S. 1958. The place of the individual and of idiodynamics in psychology: A dialogue. *J Indiv Psychol* 14:3–21.

Sargent F, Weinman KP. 1966. Physiological individuality. *Ann NY Acad Sci* 134:696–719.

Scarr S. 1997. Rules of evidence: A larger context for the statistical debate. *Psychol Sci* 8:16–20.

Schwartz GE. 1982. Cardiovascular psychophysiology: A systems perspective. In: Cacioppo JT, Petty RE, eds. *Perspectives in Cardiovascular Psychophysiology*. New York: Guilford Press. Pp. 347–372.

Schwartz GE. 1986. Emotion and psychophysiological organization: A systems approach. In: Coles MGH, Donchin E, Porges SW, eds. *Psychophysiology. Systems, Processes, and Applications*. New York: Guilford Press. Pp. 354–377.

Schwartz JE, Warren K, Pickering TG. 1994. Mood, location and physical position as predictors of ambulatory blood pressure and heart rate: Application of a multi-level random effects model. *Ann Behav Med* 16:210–220.

Shaffer RA. 1997. *Physical Training Interventions to Reduce Stress Fracture Incidence in Navy and Marine Corps Recruit Training*. Presented at the Institute of Medicine, Subcommittee on Body Composition, Nutrition, and Health of Military Women Workshop on Reducing Stress Fracture in Physically Active Young Servicemembers, Washington, DC, December 10.

Shrout PE. 1997. Should significance tests be banned? Introduction to a special section exploring the pros and cons. *Psychol Sci* 8:1–2.

Sternberg WF, Bokat C, Kass L, Alboyadjian A, Gracely RH. 2001. Sex-dependent components of the analgesia produced by athletic competition. *J Pain* 2:65–74.

Stoneman P. 1997. *Stress Fracture Experience at Fort Jackson.* Presented at the Institute of Medicine, Subcommittee on Body Composition, Nutrition, and Health of Military Women Workshop on Reducing Stress Fracture in Physically Active Young Servicemembers, Washington, DC, December 10.

Thayer JF, Faith ML. 1994. Idiographic nonlinear pattern classification of autonomic and self-report measures of emotion. *Psychosom Med* 56:178.

Thayer JF, Lane RD. 2000. A model of neurovisceral integration in emotion regulation and dysregulation. *J Affect Disord* 61:201–216.

Tyrrell RA, Thayer JF, Friedman BH, Leibowitz HW, Francis EL. 1995. A behavioural link between the oculomotor and cardiovascular systems. *Integr Physiol Behav Sci* 30:46–67.

Tyrrell RA, Pearson MA, Thayer JF. 2000. Behavioral links between the oculomotor and cardiovascular system. In: Franzén O, Richter H, Lawrence S, eds. *Accommodation and Vergence Mechanisms in the Visual System.* Basel: Birkhäuser Verlag. Pp. 151–160.

Uijtdehaage SHJ, Thayer JF. 1988. Pattern classification of emotions: Autonomic, somatic, and self-report measures. *Psychophysiology* 25:486.

Vasey MW, Thayer JF. 1987. The continuing problem of false positives in repeated measures ANOVA in psychophysiology: A multivariate solution. *Psychophysiology* 24:479–486.

West BJ. 1990. *Fractal Physiology and Chaos in Medicine.* Teaneck, NJ: World Scientific.

Woodhead AD, Blackett AD, Hollaender A, eds. 1985. *Molecular Biology of Aging.* New York: Plenum Press.

3

Monitoring Overall Physical Status to Predict Performance

There is an extensive body of literature dealing with the prediction of maximal physical performance in a variety of settings, including both the prediction of optimal performance and the prediction of performance deterioration. Most of this literature is based on research carried out with healthy men and women performing various physical tasks, such as prolonged endurance efforts in exercise and sports settings, but some has involved combat service members performing military tasks under controlled laboratory and field conditions. There are two main types of measures used to predict physical performance: physiological measures and self-assessment measures.

The usual predictor variables employed in the research have consisted of physiological markers, such as heart rate; core temperature; blood and muscle lactate; plasma levels of epinephrine, norepinephrine, and beta-endorphin; plasma and salivary levels of cortisol; circulating glucose; ventilatory minute volume and related metabolic measures; plasma creatine phosphokinase; glycogen stores as determined by serial muscle biopsy; and regional cerebral blood flow. This chapter describes some of the physiological measures used to indicate overall physical status, such as vital signs and temperature, while more specific surrogate measures for muscle fatigue, bone health, and renal and immune function are described in Chapter 4.

Although measuring overall physical status in the field presents a challenge, the importance of measuring total daily energy expenditure as an indication of energy intake needs cannot be overemphasized. Limitations of the direct and indirect measurements of energy expenditure are described in this chapter, along with potential technological advances for the future.

There is evidence that self-assessment measures also possess efficacy in predicting both optimal physical performance and deterioration in performance. Self-assessment measures include perceived exertion, muscle soreness, muscle pain, ratings of sleep quality, and mood states. A number of investigations suggest that a single measure of effort sense or mood state may be superior to each of the above-mentioned physiological measures when used singly or in combination. This chapter describes some of the research, along with some of the advantages and limitations, of self-assessment.

GENERAL CONSIDERATIONS WHEN MONITORING PHYSICAL STATUS

The ultimate goal of collecting data on biomarkers that measure or predict the status of physiological and cognitive function of military personnel is to assess any change in these functions that could compromise an individual's health and ability to perform mission tasks. The usual approach to the interpretation of these data is to compare them with the range of values determined to support normal physiological and cognitive function. If the data are outside this range, then there is a risk that the health of the individual and/or the mission success will be compromised. Corrective actions should be available to bring the physiological or cognitive function back to the normal range or to save the individual and accomplish the mission objective.

To implement such a system, several steps must be accomplished. First, there must be devices for continuously or intermittingly monitoring the biomarkers. Second, there must be some system for transmitting the data to a command and control unit or to the individual so that corrective action can be taken. Third, there must be baseline or reference data (normal range) that can be used to interpret the data. (The development of devices for measuring biomarkers and the system for transmission of data is beyond the scope of this report.)

For practical reasons it is likely that the data-monitoring system will be able to calculate and screen the incoming data so only those data that require action will be brought to the attention of the individual and/or the command and control unit. This means that the standard used in the analysis (the baseline data) becomes important. It is widely recognized that many individuals have biomarker values that may fall outside the normal range for some physiological or cognitive functions (Sargent and Weinman, 1966). Although the normal range is useful in the practice of clinical medicine because there are other opportunities to make judgments about a patient's condition, a more rigorous approach may be needed for a system monitoring the vital functions of a combat service member.

A biomarker is a surrogate marker for an important outcome and therefore the choice of biomarkers will have a significant impact on the types and design of the devices and systems that will be needed. Major issues that must be considered are related to the validation of the biomarker, such as reliability and the potential for false positive or false negative results. Therefore, prior to implementing performance testing to assess "readiness to perform," careful planning is necessary. Test development and validation can be a rather daunting and complex problem. For instance, even when a given measure has good reliability and validity under laboratory conditions, the efficacy of the procedure may not generalize to field settings. At the most basic level, it is first necessary to develop an idea about the model that underlies the performance of interest and how specific tests relate to this model (paradigm development). Next, evidence must be gathered that proves the validity of specific individual tests for measuring what they purport to measure (e.g., does a psychomotor tracking task really predict flying ability?). Finally, if several cognitive tests are going to be combined into a generalized assessment battery, the entire battery (as opposed to the individual tests) should be validated. It should be noted that the validation results generally will apply only to a set of standardized testing conditions that must be maintained in the actual assessment context (this may be a significant obstacle to the implementation of test batteries for use in field environments).

Once an assessment battery is formulated and validated, personnel must be trained to the point at which no more learning effects would be expected to occur on the tests to be used. Then, during operational use of the battery, specific test outcome measures (e.g., reaction time, percent correct, accuracy) will need to be subjected to standard statistical treatments, and scores from individual test sessions will need to be compared with the individual's baseline performance (defined as the average of his or her passing scores over numerous past sessions). Based on past results (or on unique validation studies, if desired) "cut" scores can be determined using traditional psychometric approaches. These cut scores can be used to determine whether or not the individual is within his or her normal performance envelope. Some test batteries use a cut score of 1.5 standard deviations from a person's running average of numerous past sessions to indicate an alerting (nonsafety-critical) change, and a cut score of 2.0 standard deviations to indicate a safety-critical change. However, these values could be different for different criterion groups, which is another issue that must be addressed (Robert O'Donnell, NTI, Inc., Dayton, OH, personal communication, January 2004). In summary, the introduction of any type of fitness-for-duty test (whether for medical health, psychological well-being, or cognitive performance) will require a great deal of "up-front" work prior to implementation if valid and useful results are to be expected.

PHYSIOLOGICAL MEASUREMENTS

There are two general categories of physiological parameters that are used to monitor physical changes in humans: conventional and surrogate. These parameters have been used in a variety of settings (e.g., hospitals, military operations, clinical trials). When disease is present, measures of conventional physiological parameters, such as vital signs (e.g., pulse, temperature, blood pressure, and respiratory rate), are sensitive and specific for predicting the potential for adverse outcomes. More specifically, the level of blood glucose of diabetics or the level of blood urea nitrogen or creatine in those with chronic renal failure has considerable value for prognostic and treatment purposes. In addition to using vital signs and other conventional parameters to monitor physiological status, surrogate measures (e.g., hormones, metabolic substrates) have also been used. The difficulty with using these conventional or surrogate physiological measures in normal humans under extreme conditions is their general lack of predictability for the individual, which is generally due to their poor sensitivity in asymptomatic healthy individuals.

In the critically ill, physiological measurements have been used in the Acute Physiologic and Chronic Health Evaluation Score (APACHE II and APACHE III). The APACHE II and III use conventional parameters to determine the risk of death of acutely ill patients (Knaus et al., 1985). These scores have been validated (Knaus et al., 1985; Rivera-Fernandez et al., 1998; Rosenberg, 2002) and have universal acceptance in defining the risk of mortality. As a result, APACHE has become the benchmark for comparing outcomes of care and for the evaluation of the efficacy of new therapies. There is also a simpler version of these scores, the Simplified Applied Physiology Score, which also primarily uses physiological variables (Le Gall et al., 1984).

Surrogate measures, on the other hand, use hormonal levels, such as cortisol, insulin-like growth factor-1, growth hormone, or metabolic substrates (e.g., glucose, lactate, ketone bodies, or amino acids). Unlike some conventional parameters, surrogate measures do not have validated scores or available algorithms to assess overall health status and predict the performance of individual combat service members in hostile situations.

Another significant limitation with many physiological measures is that they are based upon average group data, referred to as nomothetic data, which are frequently ineffective in predicting the performance of an individual. In circumstances where average group data may not appropriately correlate with the performance of an individual, prediction models will need to be based on the unique characteristics of the individual (see also Chapter 2). One approach is to monitor each combat service member during rigorous training to determine the values of the critical biomarkers that are "normal" for that individual under a variety of situations. For example, the concentration of electrolytes in sweat varies widely among individuals in very hot, humid conditions, and an estimate of normal electrolyte loss based on water loss may underestimate the actual loss by a large margin. If the individual has a major disconformity (in this example, either a very high or a very low electrolyte concentration in sweat), then that data can be inserted in the personal profile used to monitor his or her condition. Similarly, it may be found that some individuals are capable of optimum performance outside of the "normal range" for some biomarker of a physiological or cognitive function. If such observations are verifiable, then the profiles of those individuals could be modified to take advantage of those observations.

Despite the limitations mentioned above, some conventional measures are valuable for monitoring the physical status of combat service members in field operations; however, more research is needed to validate these measures. The following sections review current physiological monitoring methods and suggest potential uses of these conventional measures for monitoring in the field.

Energy Expenditure

Accurate measurement of total daily energy expenditure provides an estimate of total energy needs if weight is to be maintained. An individual is said to be in energy balance if energy input (calories consumed) matches energy expenditure. When energy expenditure is larger than energy intake, balance is not maintained, weight is lost and the energy available for physical activity is decreased. Severe weight loss can dramatically impair performance and cognitive ability in high physical and mental stress situations.

The components of total daily energy expenditure are generally divided into three main categories: (1) basal metabolic rate, also known as resting metabolic rate (RMR), or resting energy expenditure; (2) the thermic effect of food (TEF); and (3) energy expended in physical activity or, as it is frequently called, the thermic effect of activity (TEA).

RMR is the energy required to maintain the systems of the body and to regulate body temperature at rest. It is measured by indirect calorimetry in the morning after an overnight fast (12 hours) and while the individual is resting in a bed. The individual must be comfortable and free from stress, medications, or any other stimulation that could increase metabolic activity (Manore and Thompson, 2000). In addition, the room where RMR is measured needs to be quiet, temperature controlled, and free of distractions. In most sedentary, healthy adults, RMR accounts for approximately 60 to 80 percent of total daily energy expenditure (Poehlman, 1989; Ravussin and Bogardus, 1989). However, this percentage varies greatly in active individuals. It is not unusual for some active individuals to expend 1,000 to 2,000 kcals/day in exercise activities. Thompson and colleagues (1993) determined energy balance in 24 elite, male endurance athletes over a 3- to 7-day period and found that their RMR represented only about 35 percent of total daily energy expenditure. Similar results have been reported in active females (Beidleman et al., 1995). During days of repetitive heavy competition, such as ultramarathons, RMR may represent less than 20 percent of total energy expenditure (Rontoyannis et al., 1989).

TEF is the increase in energy expenditure above RMR that results from the consumption of food throughout the day and includes the energy cost of food digestion, absorption, transport, metabolism, and storage. It usually accounts for approximately 7 to 10 percent of total daily energy expenditure, with women sometimes having a lower value (Poehlman, 1989; Ravussin et al., 1986). However, this value varies depending on the total number of kilocalories in the meal, the types of foods consumed, and the degree of obesity.

TEA is the most variable component of energy expenditure in humans. It includes the energy cost of daily activities above RMR and TEF, such as purposeful activities of daily living (e.g., making dinner, dressing, cleaning house) or planned exercise events (e.g., running, weight training, walking). It also includes the energy cost of involuntary muscular activity, such as shivering and fidgeting (also called spontaneous physical activity). TEA may account for only 15 percent of total daily energy expenditure in sedentary individuals, but it may be as high as 30 percent in active individuals (Poehlman, 1989). The addition of RMR, TEF, and TEA should account for 100 percent of total energy expenditure. However, there are a variety of factors that may increase energy expenditure above normal, such as cold, fear, stress, and various medications or drugs. The thermic effect of these factors is frequently referred to as adaptive thermogenesis, which represents a temporary increase in thermogenesis that may last for hours or even days, depending on the duration and magnitude of the stimulus. For example, a serious physical injury, the stress associated with an upcoming event, or going to a higher altitude may all increase RMR above normal levels.

The measurement of total daily energy expenditure or its components can be conducted in the laboratory using direct measures, such as calorimetry, doubly labeled water (DLW), motion sensors, or observation. In general, field methods of measuring or predicting energy expenditure use indirect methods (e.g., self-report questionnaires, surveys, fitness measures) or devices (e.g., movement devices, heart-rate monitors) that have been validated against more precise laboratory methods. Energy expenditure prediction equations have also been developed and are typically based on age, gender, and body size.

Laboratory Methods

Calorimetry. Energy expenditure in humans can be assessed by either direct or indirect calorimetry. Direct calorimetry measures the amount of heat given off by the body through radiation, convection, and evaporation and must be conducted in an airtight calorimetric chamber in which the amount of heat produced by the body warms the water surrounding the chamber. The change in water temperature is recorded, and the amount of energy expended is calculated. This method is very expensive and is not currently used to any extent. However, some field devices are based on the direct calorimetry principle and use changes in body heat to predict total energy expenditure. Under basal conditions, both direct and indirect calorimetry give identical results, but due to the cyclical changes in body temperature throughout the day, direct calorimetry cannot be used to assess heat production for periods of less that 24 hours (Jequier and Schutz, 1983).

Indirect calorimetry uses a much less expensive method for assessing energy expenditure and is frequently the method of choice for many researchers. A metabolic chamber is used, and a mask, hood, or mouthpiece is used to collect gases. This method assumes that metabolic rate can be estimated by measuring the rate of transformation of chemical energy into heat. The amount of oxygen and carbon dioxide exchanged in the lungs closely represents the use and release of these substances by the body tissues, so the amount of oxygen consumed and the amount of carbon dioxide produced are measured during various activities to estimate the amount of energy being expended. The ratio between the volume of carbon dioxide produced (VCO_2) and the volume of oxygen consumed (VO_2)

can be calculated (VCO_2/VO_2). This ratio is termed the "nonprotein respiratory quotient" and represents the ratio between the oxidation of carbohydrate and lipid. By knowing the amount of each energy substrate oxidized, the amount of oxygen consumed, and the amount of carbon dioxide produced, total energy expenditure (in kilocalories) can be estimated using various published formulas (Manore and Thompson, 2000). In general, consuming 1 L of oxygen results in the expenditure of approximately 4.81 kcals if the fuels oxidized represent a mixture of protein, fat, and carbohydrate.

Doubly Labeled Water. Recently, the DLW technique has been validated and accepted as a gold standard method for determining free-living total daily energy expenditure. This method was first developed for use in animals and was eventually applied to humans (Schoeller et al., 1986). The DLW method is a form of indirect calorimetry based on the differential elimination of deuterium ($^2H_2$) and ^{18}oxygen (^{18}O) from body water following a load dose of water labeled with these two stable isotopes. The $^2H_2$ is eliminated as water, while the ^{18}O is eliminated as both water and carbon dioxide. The difference between the two elimination rates is a measure of carbon dioxide production (Coward and Cole, 1991; Prentice et al., 1991). This method differs from traditional indirect calorimetry in that it only measures carbon dioxide production, not oxygen consumption. The major disadvantages of this technique are that it requires frequent urine collection and it is very expensive, thus making it prohibitive for use in field situations. This method has become a valuable tool for the validation of other less-expensive field methods of measuring energy expenditure, such as the use of accelerometers (Schoeller and Racette, 1990).

Field Methods

Because measurements of calorimetry require that an individual be confined to a laboratory setting or a metabolic chamber, it is difficult to measure an individual's free-living or habitual activity. However, there is a new hand-held indirect calorimetry instrument (BodyGem, HealtheTech, Inc., Golden, Colorado) available that could be used in the field. This instrument measures RMR in 12 minutes and has been validated against oxygen consumption measured with a metabolic cart or a Douglas bag. These studies (Melanson et al., 2003; Nieman et al., 2003) showed high correlations (r = 0.81–0.97) between the BodyGem and the laboratory methods used for validation. Unfortunately, this instrument measures resting energy expenditure. Total daily energy expenditure still needs to be estimated from the methods outlined below or from prediction equations. Thus the usefulness of this instrument in the field is still limited.

Subjective Measures. These measures include the direct observation of physical activity by a trained observer or the recording of daily physical activity by the subject. Use of direct observation is limited because it requires a trained individual for each participant being measured. Recording daily physical activity using activity logs is time consuming and requires training of the individual since each activity needs to be quantified as to time, intensity, and type. Both of these methods require that the input of the data and the calculation of total energy expenditure be conducted by trained researchers (Chen, 2003). These two methods are impractical for large military field operations.

Objective Measures. These measures use some type of mechanical or electronic device (e.g., pedometers, heel- or foot-strike monitors, accelerometers, heart-rate monitors, heat-flow sensors) that measures changes in body movement, heart rate, or body temperature. The data acquired from these devices are generally integrated with personal data (e.g., age, weight, stride length, gender) and then converted into a mathematical formula that predicts total physical activity or energy expenditure. The advantages of these devices are that they can generally be worn either on the wrist, waist, arm, or ankle; they require little manipulation once they are attached; and they can measure free-living movement over an extended period of time. Recorded data are either directly integrated into a formula that predicts energy expenditure or are downloaded to a computer for further analysis.

Validation of these devices is typically conducted by using whole-room indirect calorimetry or DLW (Chen, 2003) for total energy expenditure and by using treadmills or measured distances for physical activity. Many of these devices incorporate a number of methods for assessing body movement, motion, and heat production. Below are the methods used by three different sensors currently being sold:

- The SenseWear Armband (BodyMedia, Inc., Pittsburgh, Pennsylvania) utilizes a two-axis accelerometer, a heat-flux sensor, a galvanic skin-response sensor, a skin-temperature sensor, and a near-body ambient temperature sensor to gather the data used to calculate energy expenditure from an algorithm (Liden et al., 2002).
- The IDEEA (Intelligent Device for Energy Expenditure and Activity) (MiniSun, Fresno, California) measures body and limb motions constantly through five sensors attached to the chest, thighs, and feet, and can correctly provide identification of 98.9 percent of posture and limb movements and 98.5 percent of gait movements (Zhang et al., 2003).
- The Actical Activity Monitor (Mini Mitter Co., Inc., Bend, Oregon) utilizes a motion sensor known as a piezoelectric accelerometer to monitor motion. This type of sensor integrates the degree and intensity of motion and produces a voltage output signal with varying magnitudes and durations that are dependent on the amount of motion. Based on recent validation studies using whole-room calorimetry, this monitor is a good predictor of total energy expenditure in children (Puyau et al., 2002). Validation studies using portable SensorMedics (Yorba Linda, California) systems performed with adolescents, teens, and adults to predict activity energy expenditure are still being conducted and algorithms are being refined (Heil and Klippel, 2003; Klippel and Heil, 2003).

Preliminary data show reasonably accurate predictions using the Actical Activity Monitor in these populations, depending on the sites chosen for monitor placement.

These second-generation devices may be much better at predicting energy expenditure than devices that only use one method for determining motion (e.g., vertical acceleration). Extensive research has examined the validity and usefulness of pedometers and accelerometers for the measurement of physical activity or energy expenditure (Hendelman et al., 2000; Jakicic et al., 1999; Tudor-Locke et al., 2002). In general, accelerometer- and pedometer-based monitors provide valid indicators of overall physical activity, but they are less accurate at predicting energy expenditure (Bassett and Strath, 2002; Welk, 2002). If pedometers are used to predict levels of physical activity, then the correlation is stronger (average r = 0.82) than if they are used to predict total daily energy expenditure (average r = 0.68; range = 0.46–0.88) (Tudor-Locke et al., 2002). The same appears to be true for accelerometers that use only one dimension to measure physical activity. Single-method motion detectors appear to underestimate energy expenditure by 42 to 67 percent in field conditions where a variety of exercises are used (Welk et al., 2000) and during cycling as work intensities are increased (Iltis and Givens, 2000). In addition, single-axis accelerometers or pedometers and most multidimensional accelerometers are not useful in detecting increased energy cost of high-intensity exercise, upper-body exercise, carrying a load, or changes in surface or terrain (Bassett et al., 2000; Hendelman et al., 2000; Iltis and Givens, 2000; Jakicic et al., 1999). However, single-axis accelerometers may work well when estimating energy expenditure during low-intensity single activities, such as walking, and they may be useful in assessing daily activity patterns of individuals (Schutz et al., 2002) unless the subjects are the frail elderly with very slow gaits (Le Masurier and Tudor-Locke, 2003).

If predicting total energy expenditure is the goal of monitoring the activity of the combat service members, then more sophisticated devices must be used (multidimensional devices that include multiple types of metabolic measurements) since they are better at predicting energy expenditure (Chen, 2003; Hoyt et al., 1994; Schutz et al., 2001). Based on a review by Schutz and colleagues (2001), measuring the total daily energy expenditure of combat service members at the accuracy required by the military will require the development of a motion sensor that is inexpensive and is more convenient and reliable than current pedometers or accelerometers. When this instrument becomes available, researchers, those responsible for monitoring the combat service members, or the combat service members themselves will be able to accurately monitor their daily free-living energy expenditure.

Summary

There are a number of methods for assessing total daily energy expenditure in an individual in an objective manner. In a more subjective manner, however, combat service members (or their peers) can easily tell whether they are maintaining energy balance by changes in their total body weight. If their weight does not change, then their energy intake matches their energy expenditure.

Vital Signs

There are three conventional measurements discussed below that may have success in monitoring the physiological status of combat service members under field conditions. These measures are: pulse rate, a combination of respiratory rate and pulse rate, and a combination of all the major vital measures. This section also includes measurements of core temperature because it is the most common method for assessing the impact of environmental conditions and exercise on the body, in addition to being an indicator of physical status (e.g., inflammation).

Pulse Rate

Pulse rate, which is easy to measure noninvasively and is amenable to telemetry, can be used to estimate the degree and duration of aerobic workload. It might also be used to assess periods of rest and sleep.

Respiratory Rate and Pulse Rate

In the present environment of potential exposure to chemical and biological agents, other parameters, such as respiratory rate and pulse rate, might be patterned. For instance, wearing chemical biological weapon suits and breathing apparatus is likely to alter respiratory rate and pulse rate, both at rest and in response to activity. How these parameters are affected would be important to determine under experimental conditions, both in the laboratory setting and in the field, to gather baseline data for the individual combat service member.

Overall Vital Signs

With the measurement of pulse rate, respiratory rate, and core body temperature, one could potentially design algorithms to distinguish the following conditions: moderate activity, more intense activity, cold exposure affecting performance, sleep, and systemic inflammatory response (usually due to infection under battlefield conditions if the soldier is otherwise unaware of injury) (see Table 3-1).

TABLE 3-1 Summary of Vital Signs Under Specific Activity and Environmental Conditions

Condition	Pulse Rate	Respiratory Rate	Core Body Temperature
Moderate activity	Moderately high (> 120)	Increased	Normal
Intense activity	High (> 160)	Elevated for a prolonged period	Prolonged elevated respiratory rate may lead to increased core body temperature
Cold exposure	Normal to low	Normal to low	Low
Sleep	Lower than awake pulse rate	Lower than awake pulse rate	Slightly lower to normal
Systemic inflammatory responses	> 90, but usually < 120	Elevated, but less than intense activity	Higher

Ambient Temperature

Although ambient temperature is not a vital sign, it is included here because environmental temperature can have a dramatic effect on the body's ability to maintain physiological stability, especially during exercise (Cheung et al., 2000). If extreme environmental conditions are combined with fluid losses and the development of dehydration or the wearing of protective clothing (Kulka and Kenney, 2002), a significant decrease in mental function and exercise performance can occur. As temperature and humidity increase, exercising becomes harder and the risk of heat-related problems increases. Hydration can also be a problem for individuals who exercise in cold environments because fluid is being lost while the desire to drink may be reduced. As temperature decreases, the ability to maintain body heat and normal body temperature may decline depending on the severity of the cold stress (e.g., temperature, altitude, wind chill index, humidity), the intensity of the exercise being performed, the level of sleep deprivation, the negative energy balance, and the insulating effect of the clothing worn. In addition, the body tries to minimize heat loss through vasoconstriction and to increase heat production through shivering. Thus cold can dramatically increase metabolic demands on the body.

Table 3-2 outlines recommendations and precautions that should be taken by individuals who exercise under conditions of varying air temperature, relative humidity, and solar radiation. As shown in the table, when the wet bulb globe temperature (WBGT) rises, the health risks associated with exercising also rise. The WBGT is comprised of three measurements. First is the wet bulb, an index of relative humidity. Second is the black bulb, an index of radiation of heat from the environment (e.g., from the sun). The third measurement is the dry bulb, an index of ambient temperature (the actual air temperature measured on a thermometer). If the wet bulb and the dry bulb temperatures are the same, then the

TABLE 3-2 Various Wet Bulb Globe Temperatures (WBGT) and Exercise Recommendations and Precautions That Need to Be Taken

WBGT	Exercise Recommendations	Comments
Less than 80°F (< ~27°C)	All can exercise	Most individuals without a risk of heat problems can perform activities
80° to 85°F (~ 27° to 29°C)	Exercise with caution	All individuals should drink frequently; look for signs of heat illness (dizziness, rapid heart rate, nausea, chilling, headache, and decreased coordination) Distances greater than 10 km should not be done or conducted with caution when the WBGT is greater than 82°F (28°C)
85° to 88°F (~ 29° to 31°C)	Limited exercise	Physical activity for unconditioned or unacclimatized individuals should be suspended Frequent water breaks should be taken by exercising individuals
Greater than 88°F (> ~31°C)	Suspend exercise	All activities should be suspended or moved indoors to a cooler environment

NOTE: WBGT = 0.7 (wet bulb temperature) + 0.2 (black bulb temperature) + 0.1 (dry bulb temperature). Wet bulb temperature measures the temperature when the bulb is moist (relative humidity); black bulb temperature measures radiated heat (this bulb absorbs the radiated heat); and dry bulb temperature measures the ambient room temperature.
SOURCE: Adapted from Pivarnik and Palmer (1994).

air has a humidity of 100 percent and evaporation is impossible. The following method is used to calculate the WBGT:

$$\text{WBGT} = 0.7\ (\text{wet bulb temperature}) + 0.2\ (\text{black bulb temperature}) + 0.1\ (\text{dry bulb temperature})$$

The greatest contributor to WBGT is the humidity (wet bulb), while the ambient temperature (dry bulb) contributes the least. Thus it is easier and safer to exercise in a hot environment with a low humidity than in a hot environment with a high humidity. As the humidity rises, it is harder for the body to cool itself through evaporation of sweat from the skin. By measuring WGBT before exercising in hot environments, proper precautions can be taken to reduce the risk of heat exhaustion.

Environmental conditions that predispose an active individual to heat exhaustion or stroke are hot, humid, windless conditions or unseasonably hot conditions where an individual is not acclimatized to the environment. Sunstroke, heat cramps, or heat exhaustion are likely, and heatstroke is possible with prolonged exposure or physical activity in temperatures ranging from 105° to 130°F (41°–54°C). If the temperature rises to 130°F (54°C) or more, heat stroke and sunstroke are highly likely with continued exposure (NWS, 2003). Individuals who are unfit, overweight, dehydrated, unacclimatized to the heat, or ill are more susceptible to heat stroke. Finally, the young and the old are more susceptible to heat-related injury due to less sensitive homeostatic mechanisms for fluid balance (Sutton, 1990). Studies that examined exertional heat illness in military recruits showed that risk was greatest when temperatures rose above 65°F (18°C), when strenuous exercise was performed (e.g., running), or when recruits had heat-stress exposure on previous days (Kark et al., 1996). For new recruits, a body mass index (kg/m^2) over 22 and a 1.5-mile run time over 12 minutes also increased the risk of heat illness (Gardner et al., 1996).

Less has been written on the body's response to cold weather exercise; however, when exercise is performed in cold environments, the body's thermoregulation mechanisms are stressed (O'Brien et al., 1998b; Young et al., 1998). If exercise in the cold is combined with high altitude, the metabolic stresses on the body are extremely high, which increases the demand for adequate energy and fluid intake. Like in hot environments, fluid balance can be compromised while exercising in cold environments (Murray, 1995). First, cold can increase urinary fluid losses, while fluid intake is reduced. Individuals generally have less desire to drink in the cold, the need to drink is less obvious, fluids may be less available, and fluid intake may be reduced to avoid having to urinate. Active women may be more likely to restrict fluid intake in cold environments to avoid removing layers of clothing in order to urinate or to avoid traveling some distance to a restroom. Fluid losses are increased through respiration and sweat losses, especially if heavily insulated clothing is worn.

Body Temperature

A number of factors can influence body temperature. Therefore, a number of physiological parameters may need to be measured to assess thermal strain on the combat service member.

Core Body Temperature. Measuring core body temperature is the most commonly used method for assessing the impact of environmental conditions (either hot or cold) and exercise on the body. The most common places for measuring core body temperature are the esophagus, rectum, mouth, tympanum, and auditory meatus (Young et al., 2003), but most thermal physiologists consider the esophagus to be the best site (Moran and Mendal, 2002; Young et al., 2003). Measurement of esophageal temperature is best for research settings, but it is problematic in clinical or field assessments because the sensor causes irritation to the nasal passages and general subject discomfort (Moran and Mendal, 2002), and it is difficult to insert. Overall, these probes are impractical to use

TABLE 3-3 Definitions of Various Temperature Measurements Used in Wearable Body Activity Monitors

Measurement	Definition
Heat flux	Measurement of the heat being dissipated by the body; sensors in the wearable devices use very low thermally resistant materials and sensitive thermocouple arrays to determine this measurement
Skin temperature	Sensors placed in the device are in contact with the skin and measure changes in skin temperature
Near-body ambient temperature	Sensors measure air temperature immediately around the wearable device and are designed to directly reflect the change in environmental conditions; an example is walking into an air-conditioned building from outside on a hot day
Galvanic skin response	This measurement represents the electrical conductivity between two points on the wearer's arm or leg, depending on where the device is worn; skin conductivity is affected by the sweat from physical activity and by emotional stimuli; it can also be used as an indicator of evaporative heat loss by identifying the onset, peak, and recovery of maximal sweat rates

SOURCE: Liden et al. (2002).

in a field setting where individuals are participating in strenuous physical activity.

Skin Temperature Sensors. These sensors measure skin temperature at a particular body site and may not correlate well with core body temperature. In order to use skin sensors, multiple sites may need to be measured, and the information gained from the sensors may need to be integrated with other temperature and thermal stress-related data (e.g., heart rate, ambient temperature, exercise intensity, level of hydration, wind speed, and perceived effort or exertion). As discussed previously, new, wearable body-activity monitors (typically worn on the arm, wrist, or ankle) are being used to assess total energy expenditure or physical activity. They also measure a variety of temperature-related variables, such as heat flux, skin temperature, near-body ambient temperature, and galvanic skin response (see Table 3-3). One device, the Mini-Logger (Mini-Metter Co., Inc., Bend, Oregon), has four temperature channels that can measure skin, rectal, and ear canal temperature. Only the assessment of skin temperature would be practical for military personnel in the field. Many of these devices can be worn continuously for 4 to 5 days without recharging their batteries, and they may have the capability for remote transmission of data.

Oral Temperature Thermometer. The measurement of oral temperature can readily track changes in core body temperature. Unfortunately, oral temperature measurements are not always possible, because of equipment being worn over the face, or accurate, because the head and face can be easily influenced by the environment. Hot and cold drinks, smoking, or irregular breathing patterns can also alter oral temperature measures (Moran and Mendal, 2002).

Temperature Pill Telemetry System. The ingestible temperature pill provides a valid measure of core temperature during rest, exercise, and changes in environmental conditions (e.g., hot, cold) (Kolka et al., 1993; O'Brien et al., 1998a). The temperature pill has been validated by comparison with rectal and esophageal temperature. The pill contains a sensor that transmits a continuous, low-frequency radio wave that varies with temperature. This signal can be received and stored by a data logger and later downloaded to a computer (Castellani et al., 2002; O'Brien et al., 1998a). The pill moves through the gastrointestinal tract and most accurately measures core temperature when it reaches the small intestine. Because it is eventually eliminated, a new pill needs to be consumed if temperature monitoring is to continue over long periods of time. The use of this technology in the field is possible; however, a mechanism for data transmission over long distances to a collection site is required, as is a way of displaying the data so it can be easily observed by the soldier.

Summary. Currently there is no accurate and easy method to measure core body temperature in a field setting. The development of a simple, noninvasive, universally used device that can measure core body temperature in individuals exercising or working in extreme environments would be quite useful (Moran and Mendal, 2002). Such an instrument would help prevent many of the heat-related illnesses that occur in field settings.

Physiological Strain Index

The U.S. Army and the Israeli military have been working together to develop and test a physiological strain index (PSI) based on rectal temperature and heart rate—two physiological parameters that adequately depict the combined strain reflected by the cardiovascular and thermoregulatory systems (Moran et al., 1998b). The PSI is based on a scale of 1 to 10, with a high value indicating a high risk of heat stress. It was developed using individuals performing exercise in the heat under a variety of conditions (e.g., in different heat-related environments, with protective clothing, and with varying hydration levels) (Moran et al., 1998a, 1998b). Comparisons of the PSI based on gender, age, and level of exercise training and intensity have also been conducted (Moran et al., 1999b, 2002). Overall, the PSI may be a simple method for examining the impact of environmental temperatures and exercise stress on individuals in order to predict who might be at risk for heat stress (Moran, 2000). Once a field method for assessing core body temperature is developed, the PSI could be a useful tool for the prevention of heat illnesses.

Cold Strain Index

Similar to the PSI, the U.S. Army and the Israeli military have developed a cold strain index (CSI) based on rectal temperature and mean skin temperature measured at multiple sites (Moran et al., 1999a). The CSI is also based on a rating scale of 1 to 10, where high numbers indicate risk of hypothermia. As with the PSI, the CSI's usefulness in the field will depend on the development of a reliable method for measuring core body temperature.

SELF-ASSESSMENT MEASUREMENTS

As discussed in the previous section, it might be possible to employ some physiological markers in field settings, although some still need validation in the field and others encounter practical limitations. In addition to conventional measures, self-assessments have the potential for use as indicators of physical status in the field. Self-assessment measures include: perceived exertion, muscle soreness, muscle pain, ratings of sleep quality, and mood states. There is evidence that self-assessment measures possess efficacy in predicting both optimal physical performance and deterioration in performance.

In a number of investigations a single measure of effort sense or mood state has been found to be superior to specific physiological measures used singly or in combination. Relying on self-assessments to evaluate physical status, however, is not without limitations. For example, it is an established fact that sleep-deprived individuals lose their ability to accurately assess their own levels of sleepiness and impairment after the first day or two of sleep reduction. Also, it is well known that inexperienced individuals are often unable to pace themselves as well as people who have been frequently exposed to a given situation. In addition, peer and supervisory pressures continue to present major confounds to the validity of self-assessments in circumstances involving team relationships. For these reasons, more objective assessments that are immune to such judgment and social confounds, such as direct physiological measurements, are generally more desirable.

If these limitations to self-assessment can be overcome, then the advantages to this measurement method can be realized. First, the continued use of this approach does not require the development and application of sophisticated instrumentation; that is, "perceptual" models can be taught and used now. Second, the data based on the unique characteristics of the individual are not confounded by other individuals' responses within a group. As discussed in Chapter 2, research on combat service members, with its focus on person-environment interactions, has a pressing need to elucidate those factors that contribute to interindividual differences *and* to distinguish them from sources of intraindividual variability. The educated athlete (combat service member) can learn how to monitor sensations provided by the working muscle, as well as other physiological systems, and he or she can titrate the pace (e.g., increase, decrease, maintain) without experiencing performance decay or the morbidity and mortality often associated with performance of prolonged efforts under extreme conditions (Morgan, 1981, 2000; Morgan and Pollock, 1977). If educated athletes (combat service members) and coaches (commanders) learn how to train hard without overtraining, when they are placed in a situation (competition or combat) where maximal or supramaximal efforts are required their output can be titrated and optimized (Morgan et al., 1988; Verde et al., 1992). The body of scientific literature relevant to this hypothesis emphasizes the importance of considering the individual in efforts designed to prevent morbidity, as well as to predict maximal physical performance.

Perceived Exertion

Perceived exertion involves the individual's sensation of effort, and the rating of perceived exertion (RPE) obtained during prolonged physical efforts can reliably predict performance. Physiological variables (e.g., heart rate, blood pressure, and cortisol, epinephrine, norepinephrine, muscle and blood lactate, glycogen, oxygen uptake, and ventilatory minute volume) and individual variables (e.g., gender, training state, personality structure, and mood state) contribute to RPE. According to Borg (1973, 1998), RPE can be viewed as the gestalt or whole (i.e., configuration of all sensory inputs responsible for the formation of the percept), while variables such as heart rate or lactate should be regarded as parts of the whole. Hence, perceptual ratings such as RPE could be more accurate in predicting or monitoring exertion than any part of the whole.

The literature dealing with self-assessment has been summarized in volumes by Borg (1998) and Noble and Robertson (1996). These comprehensive reviews of self-assessment demonstrate the efficacy of perceptual models in quantifying stress responses associated with exercise and, in some circumstances, their superiority to selected physiological models.

Borg (1998) developed a number of rating scales for use in quantifying the distress or strain associated with exercise, but the one most frequently employed has been his 6–20 category scale. This scale has verbal anchors associated with the odd-numbered ratings (7 = very, very light, 9 = very light, 11 = fairly light, 13 = somewhat hard, 15 = hard, 17 = very hard, 19 = very, very hard) (Borg, 1973). The terms "easy," "heavy," and "moderate" are sometimes used in place of light, hard, and somewhat hard, respectively. The 6–20 category scale is employed in most exercise laboratories around the world and has been shown to possess good construct validity when employed with English-speaking individuals and across cultures.

In his early formulations, Borg (1973) asserted that RPE correlated very well with physiological measures (e.g., heart rate), and it was proposed that heart rate was equal to RPE × 10. While this proposal may have been overly simplistic, it actually worked reasonably well in the case of healthy young men and women evaluated on maximal bicycle ergometer or treadmill tests. However, as the scale became more widely applied with younger and older age groups, elite distance runners, and selected patient groups, it became apparent that RPE and heart rate were often uncoupled. In the case of healthy men and women performing selected types of exercise (e.g., isometric, concentric), as well as exercise in extreme environments (e.g., hot, cold, hyperbaric, hypobaric), the RPE-heart rate relationship is not strong. However, RPE works effectively in such settings because it includes other inputs that possess greater primacy.

In summary, perceptual ratings of effort, sense, fatigue, pain, and mood are often regarded as *subjective*, whereas physiological measures are regarded as *objective.* However, since perceptual ratings have some advantages and some studies have showed that they may be more accurate than some physiological measures in predicting performance, a case can be made for developing and employing perceptual models in efforts to monitor distress during training and special operations.

Perceived Exertion as a Predictor of Physical Strain and Physical Endurance

Although heart rate may be easy to measure, the case has been made that ratings of perceived exertion may be a better measure of the whole physiological situation of an individual. As a result, there are studies that compare the physiological measure of heart rate with RPE. These studies evaluate any possible correlations of these two measures, specifically through physical strain and physical endurance studies.

Patton and colleagues (1977) evaluated ratings of perceived exertion and heart rate in two groups of 60 male military personnel who differed in level of fitness (Group I untrained, Group II trained), measured by maximal oxygen uptake (VO_{2max}). Group II scored significantly higher than Group I on VO_{2max} at the outset of the study, as anticipated. When the two groups performed submaximal runs on the treadmill, Group I (untrained) had a significantly higher heart rate than Group II (trained) at each minute of exercise, as expected; however, the RPE for the two groups did not differ. While this finding is surprising, a similar observation was later reported by Dishman and colleagues (1994). These results represent examples of the uncoupling of heart rate and perceived exertion, and they suggest that heart rate may not be an adequate measure of strain during physical exertion. When both groups were retested following 6 months of training, they experienced a significant decrease in perceived exertion and heart rate during submaximal exercise (Patton et al., 1977). Furthermore, the RPE and heart-rate values were identical for the two groups following the training. This finding indicates that although a valuable measure of strain, effectiveness of the RPE model is dependent in part on habituation or familiarization; this phenomenon needs to be addressed during educational and training programs. In addition to these issues, it is important to support the honest reporting of RPE despite encouragement to report overly positive results. Individuals may feel that it runs counter to military expectations of stoicism and toughness to admit to high levels of perceived exertion. Both habituation and overly positive reporting have to be monitored during actual field situations.

The efficacy of perceptual versus heart-rate monitoring in the development of physical endurance was evaluated by Koltyn and Morgan (1992) in a study involving two groups of college women engaged in aerobic dance classes. The two groups used either heart rate or perceived exertion to regulate exercise intensity. The outcome measure used in this study was endurance performance as measured by the amount of distance that could be covered during a 15-minute run. This test was administered at the beginning and the conclusion of the 14-week course. Both groups experienced an increase in endurance, but the gain for the perceived exertion group was 11 percent compared with 6 percent for the heart-rate group. This led to the conclusion that regulation of exercise intensity with the use of perceived-exertion monitoring is superior to heart-rate monitoring for improvement in endurance performance.

In a case study conducted with one of the participants in the above study (Morgan, 1981), a volunteer attempted to complete a simulated marathon (26.2 miles, 385 yards) on the treadmill at a pace of 7.5 mph and 0 percent grade. Heart rate, rectal temperature, state anxiety, and RPE were obtained throughout the simulation. There was a gradual increase in heart rate and rectal temperature during this simulation, but extrapolation from values obtained at 5, 10, and 15 miles into the run suggested that the individual would complete the planned run without difficulty. Ratings of state anxiety and RPE obtained at the same points in time predicted otherwise. The individual was unable to continue beyond the 23-mile point—the precise point predicted by the RPE data. This case study supports the theoretical views advanced by Borg (1973, 1998) that ratings of perceived exertion are more accurate in predicting endurance performance than measures of heart rate and rectal temperature.

In conclusion, it has been shown that heart rate is not an adequate measure of physical strain during exertion or during the development of physical endurance.

RPE as a Predictor of Maximal Physical Performance

A test of maximal physical performance involving progressive increments in workload on a bicycle ergometer was performed by Morgan and Borg (1976) using 30 trained male cyclists with a mean age of 23 years. Heart rates measured at submaximal levels of work (50, 100, and 150 W) were employed to predict the actual maximum and compared with a prediction based upon ratings of RPE. The actual maximal performance capacity was 14,316 kpm. The predicted maximal performance capacity using heart-rate values was 16,500 kpm, whereas the prediction using RPE was 14,250 kpm. This observation demonstrates that RPE values obtained at submaximal exercise intensities are superior to heart-rate values in predicting maximal performance capacity. This is important since the most frequent measure employed to predict maximum capacity is submaximal heart rate (Åstrand and Rodahl, 1986).

RPE as a Predictor of Total Exhaustion Time

In research carried out at the U.S. Army Research Institute of Environmental Medicine by Horstman and colleagues (1979), the perception of effort was studied in healthy combat service members during constant work to self-imposed exhaustion. In the first experiment, 26 healthy male volunteers completed a test of VO_{2max} on one day, and were retested at 80 percent of VO_{2max} on two subsequent days in the walking and running modes. Heart rate, VO_2, V_{CO2}, minute ventilation, end tidal CO_2, and RPE were obtained throughout the exercise. Plasma lactate, epinephrine, and norepinephrine concentrations were obtained following exercise. These values did not differ between the walking and running conditions. At the time of exhaustion, the test subjects reported less respiratory distress for the walk compared with the run, but perception of effort for the legs did not differ in the two conditions. Values of RPE were identical for the walking and running conditions, and these ratings increased in a linear fashion from a value of 12.9 at 25 percent of total exhaustion time to 18.9 at exhaustion. The results from this experiment were replicated in the walking mode with an independent sample involving another 28 combat service members. It was found that changes in perception of effort occurring early during work were sensitive predictors of exhaustion time in this study.

RPE as a Predictor of Coronary Heart Disease

There is recent evidence that RPE obtained from individuals for customary or usual exercise is predictive of coronary heart disease (CHD). Lee and colleagues (2003) reported that an inverse relationship exists between an individual's RPE and the risk of CHD. These investigators studied 7,337 men who were free of CHD at the outset of the study; 551 of these men developed CHD at follow-up. The men who reported RPE as "moderate" to "strong" had a lower risk of CHD compared with those who reported RPE in the "weak" or "less intense" range. This study suggests that the efficacy of RPE could be extended from the performance domain to include morbidity and mortality due to CHD.

Other Potential Uses of Self-Assessment Measurements

Optimal Pace

Prolonged endurance efforts lasting several hours, as well as repeated efforts of shorter duration, are more likely to be optimal if a steady-state pace is employed (Wilmore and Costill, 1994). Use of a steady-state pace results in the more economical use of energy with conservation of energy stores, whereas accelerating and decelerating during a given endurance effort results in uneven energy expenditure with a more rapid depletion of energy stores. In fact, it has been recognized for many years that athletes, industrial workers, military personnel, and individuals who engage in various forms of exercise for health, fitness, and recreational purposes (e.g., cycling, jogging, swimming, gardening, dancing, walking) do so at a self-regulated pace. In the case of the athlete performing vigorous exercise at a high intensity for prolonged periods, the concept of pace represents a very important principle in terms of both optimal performance and prevention of injury (Morgan, 2000; Morgan and Pollock, 1977). Indeed, the ability to maintain optimal pace in endurance events is not only a principal focus in the training programs of many athletes, but steady state-expenditure of energy is often developed in an exquisite manner. Runners and swimmers, for example, often repeat segments of a given distance within a second or fraction of a second throughout an event.

While most of this research has been carried out with trained athletes, there is no reason to believe that combat service members cannot be trained to perform prolonged efforts in a steady state. There is research evidence that perception of effort, the key component of steady-state energy expenditure, can be an effective tool in applications with military personnel engaged in physical efforts (Horstman et al., 1979; Morgan, 1977, 1981; Morgan et al., 1983; Patton et al., 1977; Soule and Goldman, 1973).

Some of the earliest research dealing with the subject of pace was performed by Ralph Goldman and his colleagues at the U.S. Army Research Institute of Environmental Medicine. It was reported by Hughes and Goldman (1970), for example, that an energy expenditure of 425 kcal/hr (±10 percent) is voluntarily adopted by healthy, physically fit young men engaged in hard physical work. As a matter of fact, this research group demonstrated that self regulated pace is not only very consistent, but inclusion of terrain and load coefficients in mathematical models enables one to accurately predict the time requirement to traverse a given distance (Givoni and Goldman, 1971; Goldman and Iampietro, 1962; Hughes and Goldman, 1970; Soule and Goldman, 1969, 1972). This work has potential military applications as it has involved multiple terrains, and the resulting prediction models included load coefficients based on energy expenditure associated with loads positioned on the head, back, and legs.

Preferred Exertion

One of the most innovative lines of research carried out by Goldman's group involved a study dealing with the pacing of intermittent work during a 31-hour period without sleep (Soule and Goldman, 1973), designed to examine what has come to be known as "preferred exertion." This concept represents a distinct construct from RPE, but it is related since it represents the exertional level the individual chooses to adopt (Morgan, 2001).

In the study described by Soule and Goldman (1973), 10 men with a mean age of 21 years walked on a motor-driven treadmill at a self-selected pace. The individuals in this study walked for 1 hour or until completion of 4.8 km, whichever occurred first, on six occasions at 5-hour intervals during a 31-hour period without sleep. This task was completed on one day while wearing a 15-kg pack, and on a second day while wearing a 30-kg pack. The speed of walking was self-regulated by means of a servo-controlled treadmill. The time required to walk each 400 m was recorded, as well as the distance covered during each 5-minute epoch. An RPE was obtained near the end of each 1-hour exercise bout, and heart rate was measured at the conclusion of each walk. Times for the 15-kg condition were faster than those for the 30-kg condition as expected, but walk times were not impaired significantly by sleep deprivation. The investigators suggested that the improved performance at 31 hours of sleep deprivation was due to what has traditionally been termed "end spurt" in human performance research, that is, the participants walked faster since they knew this was the last work bout.

Additional research dealing with the concept of preferred exertion has been conducted with civilian samples, and the findings have generally supported the earlier work by Goldman and his associates involving young combat service members. Furthermore, preferred exertion has been found to be consistent when exercise is performed in the early morning, at noon, and in the late afternoon, and the stability of this phenomenon has been shown to hold for both men and women (Trine and Morgan, 1997). A summary of additional research involving preferred exertion has been described by Morgan (2001).

Preferred Intensity

Indirect support for the use of perceptual monitoring is offered by Pollock and colleagues (1972). These investigators evaluated the influence of aerobic training in 22 men ranging in age from 30 to 45 years who were randomly assigned to one group that trained at 90 percent of maximum heart rate or a second group that trained at 80 percent of maximum heart rate. Both groups experienced significant increases in aerobic power, but they did not differ in the amount of improvement. The investigators had hypothesized that the group training at 90 percent of maximum heart rate would have the greatest gain in aerobic power, and the unexpected finding was explained on the basis of preferred exertion. The investigators reported that it was necessary throughout the study to encourage the 90-percent group to go faster and maintain the desired intensity, while at the same time it was necessary to urge the 80-percent group to slow their pace. It was found that both groups "preferred" an intensity of ~85 percent of maximum heart rate, and there was a regression toward this intensity. Hence the finding that training at 90 percent of maximum heart rate was no more effective than training at 80 percent was due to the fact that both groups were actually training at 85 percent of maximum heart rate most of the time.

There is additional evidence that healthy men and women tend to have a comfort zone based on preferred intensity. It has been reported by Morgan (1973) that male college students tested at five work loads (i.e., 50, 100, 150, 200, and 250 W) on a bicycle ergometer had a preferred intensity of 120 W for a 30-minute exercise bout. However, there was considerable individual variability in preferred intensity. The preferred exercise intensity in any given setting is undoubtedly due to many factors. In this particular study it was found that values of RPE were correlated with extroversion. This finding supports Borg's view that perception of effort is a configuration of numerous physiological, psychological, and demographic factors (Borg, 1973, 1998).

Perception of effort was assessed in six well-trained endurance athletes by Farrell and colleagues (1982) on a treadmill test involving 30-minute runs at 60 percent and 80 percent of VO_{2max} performed on separate days. These runners were assessed on a third occasion with instructions to select the pace they would prefer to use for a 30-minute run. The preferred intensity was found to be 75 percent of VO_{2max}, and the mean ratings of perceived exertion for this intensity were below those observed at 80 percent and above those observed at 60 percent of VO_{2max}. In this case there was considerable individual variability that further demonstrates the limitation of nomothetic guidelines.

Overtraining

There is also a great deal of research demonstrating that physical training, when carried to excess, usually results in performance decrements (see also Chapter 4). The reduced performance in such cases has been associated with a number of undesirable physiological and psychological changes. Examples of the physiological changes associated with overtraining include:

- elevated heart rate and blood pressure;
- elevated cortisol, creatine kinase, epinephrine, and norepinephrine at rest, along with greater increases in these values following a standard exercise stimulus; and
- decreased glycogen stores (Costill et al., 1988; Kirwan et al., 1988; Morgan et al., 1987, 1988; O'Connor et al., 1989, 1991; Wilmore and Costill, 1994).

There is also evidence that mood disturbance occurs with overtraining, and common changes include increases in:

- tension and state anxiety,
- depression,
- anger,
- fatigue,
- confusion, and

- decreased vigor as measured by the Profile of Mood States (POMS) (Morgan et al., 1987, 1988; O'Connor et al., 1989, 1991; Verde et al., 1992).

In the early phases of overtraining, performance is not affected, but this is followed by a decrease in performance as the overtraining continues (Costill et al., 1988; Morgan et al., 1987, 1988). The decreased performance resulting from excessive physical training has consistently been shown to be associated with mood disturbance, and this relationship can be viewed as causal for the following reasons: (a) the strength of association is strong, (b) there is a temporal sequence, (c) there is consistency for the observed relationship, (d) there is an association independent of other factors, (e) there is a dose-response gradient between increased training volume and mood disturbance, (f) there is biological plausibility for the association (e.g., hypercortisolism), and (g) there is experimental confirmation showing a causal link. There is also evidence that titration of training volume in a systematic manner is effective in preventing the onset of mood disturbance and performance decline. The resulting syndrome is sometimes termed "staleness" in the sports medicine literature, and this breakdown is also associated with reports of muscle soreness, decrements in physical performance, loss of appetite, sleep disturbance, and reduced libido (Costill et al., 1988; Morgan et al., 1987, 1988; O'Connor et al., 1989, 1991).

One of the overtraining studies cited above included a sudden increase in training volume from 4,000 to 9,000 m/day at 94 percent of VO_{2max} in 12 male competitive swimmers. Measures of perceived intensity of exercise, muscle soreness, and mood disturbance (total POMS score) progressively increased through training until midway, at which point self-reports of perceived exertion reached a plateau. Four of the twelve individuals were unable to adapt, and these individuals experienced performance decrements. The self-report (total POMS score [Morgan et al., 1988]) and physiological data (Costill et al., 1988; Kirwan et al., 1988) were in agreement on predicting the negative impact of the sudden increase in training volume for three of the four swimmers, but the psychological data identified all of the impaired swimmers. In a subsequent study by Verde and colleagues (1992) involving heavy training in highly trained distance runners, it was reported that the self-report measure of mood state as measured by POMS was superior to a battery of physiological variables in the prediction and identification of disturbed function.

SUMMARY

The overall physical status of service members in the field can be evaluated by analyzing either objective physiological measurements or subjective measurements of self-assessments (or assessments by peers). For many of the physiological measurements (e.g., energy expenditure), technological advances need to be achieved before the parameters are practical for field situations. Even with this limitation, objective measurements of physiological factors, such as heart rate or temperature, are generally preferable to more subjective methods of measurement for a variety of reasons. For example, individuals that self-report their status tend to overestimate endurance and performance due to peer and commander pressure. The validity of self-assessments is also compromised when, as is often the case, the service members are tired or sleep deprived. Last, unfamiliarity with a given situation may alter pace and therefore also may confound the results of a test. However, when measuring overall physical status, the subjectivity of self-assessments may offer an advantage over other more objective measurements. In fact, self-assessments often include the influence of psychological factors, which are not accounted for when physiological measurements are used. This may be one of the reasons why studies have shown that self-assessment measurements, such as rating of perceived exertion, are better indicators of physical performance than a single physiological measurement.

Whether physiological measurements or self-assessments are used to measure performance, it is critical that before implementation in the field, the biomarker is validated not only in the laboratory, but also in the field. This validation is a complex problem that requires a great deal of planning and research.

REFERENCES

Åstrand PO, Rodahl K. 1986. *Textbook of Work Physiology. Physiological Bases of Exercise*. 3rd ed. New York: McGraw-Hill.

Bassett DR, Strath SJ. 2002. Use of pedometers to assess physical activity. In: Welk GJ, ed. *Physical Activity Assessments for Health-Related Research*. Champaign, IL: Human Kinetics. Pp. 163–177.

Bassett DR, Ainsworth BE, Swartz AM, Strath SJ, O'Brien WL, King GA. 2000. Validity of four motion sensors in measuring moderate intensity physical activity. *Med Sci Sports Exerc* 32:S471–S480.

Beidleman BA, Puhl JL, De Souza MJ. 1995. Energy balance in female distance runners. *Am J Clin Nutr* 61:303–311.

Borg GAV. 1973. Perceived exertion: A note on 'history' and methods. *Med Sci Sports* 5:90–93.

Borg G. 1998. *Borg's Perceived Exertion and Pain Scales*. Champaign, IL: Human Kinetics.

Castellani JW, O'Brien C, Stulz DA, Blanchard LA, DeGroot DW, Bovill ME, Francis TJ, Young AJ. 2002. Physiological responses to cold exposure in men: A disabled submarine study. *Undersea Hyperb Med* 29:189–203.

Chen KY. 2003. *The Use of Portable Accelerometers in Predicting Activity Energy Expenditure*. Presented at the Institute of Medicine, Committee on Metabolic Monitoring Technologies for Military Field Applications Workshop on Metabolic Monitoring Technologies for Military Field Applications, San Antonio, Texas, January 8–9.

Cheung SS, McLellan TM, Tenaglia S. 2000. The thermophysiology of uncompensable heat stress. Physiological manipulations and individual characteristics. *Sports Med* 29:329–359.

Costill DL, Flynn MG, Kirwan JP, Houmard JA, Mitchell JB, Thomas R, Park SH. 1988. Effects of repeated days of intensified training on muscle glycogen and swimming performance. *Med Sci Sports Exerc* 20:249–254.

Coward WA, Cole TJ. 1991. The doubly labeled water method for the measurement of energy expenditure in humans: Risks and benefits. In: Whitehead RG, Prentice A, eds. *New Techniques in Nutrition Research.* San Diego: Academic Press. Pp. 139–176.

Dishman RK, Farquhar RP, Cureton KJ. 1994. Responses to preferred intensities of exertion in men differing in activity levels. *Med Sci Sports Exerc* 26:783–790.

Farrell PA, Gates WK, Maksud MG, Morgan WP. 1982. Increases in plasma beta-endorphin/beta-lipotropin immunoreactivity after treadmill running in humans. *J Appl Physiol* 52:1245–1249.

Gardner JW, Kark JA, Karnei K, Sanborn JS, Gastaldo E, Burr P, Wenger CB. 1996. Risk factors predicting exertional heat illness in male Marine Corps recruits. *Med Sci Sports Exerc* 28:939–944.

Givoni B, Goldman RF. 1971. Predicting metabolic energy cost. *J Appl Physiol* 30:429–433.

Goldman RF, Iampietro PF. 1962. Energy cost of load carriage. *J Appl Physiol* 17:675–676.

Heil DP, Klippel NJ. 2003. Validation of energy expenditure prediction algorithms in adolescents and teens using the actical activity monitor. *Med Sci Sports Exerc* 35:S285.

Hendelman D, Miller K, Baggett C, Debold E, Freedson P. 2000. Validity of accelerometry for the assessment of moderate intensity physical activity in the field. *Med Sci Sports Exerc* 32:S442–S449.

Horstman DH, Morgan WP, Cymerman A, Stokes J. 1979. Perception of effort during constant work to self-imposed exhaustion. *Percept Motor Skill* 48:1111–1126.

Hoyt RW, Knapik JJ, Lanza JF, Jones BH, Staab JS. 1994. Ambulatory foot contact monitor to estimate metabolic cost of human locomotion. *J Appl Physiol* 76:1818–1822.

Hughes AL, Goldman RF. 1970. Energy cost of "hard work." *J Appl Physiol* 29:570–572.

Iltis PW, Givens MW. 2000. Validation of the CALTRAC accelerometer during simulated multi-geared cycling at different work rates. *J Exerc Physiol* 3:21–27.

Jakicic JM, Winters C, Lagally K, Ho J, Robertson RJ, Wing RR. 1999. The accuracy of the tritrac-R3d accelerometer to estimate energy expenditure. *Med Sci Sports Exerc* 31:747–754.

Jequier E, Schutz Y. 1983. Long-term measurements of energy expenditure in humans using a respiration chamber. *Am J Clin Nutr* 38:989–998.

Kark JA, Burr PQ, Wenger CB, Gastaldo E, Gardner JW. 1996. Exertional heat illness in Marine Corps recruit training. *Aviat Space Environ Med* 67:354–360.

Kirwan JP, Costill DL, Flynn MG, Mitchell JB, Fink WJ, Neufer PD, Houmard JA. 1988. Physiological responses to successive days of intense training in competitive swimmers. *Med Sci Sports Exerc* 20:255–259.

Klippel JN, Heil DP. 2003. Validation of energy expenditure prediction algorithms in adults using the Actical Electronic Activity Monitor. *Med Sci Sports Exerc* 35:S284.

Knaus WA, Draper EA, Wagner DP, Zimmerman JE. 1985. APACHE II: A severity of disease classification system. *Crit Care Med* 13:818–829.

Kolka MA, Quigley MD, Blanchard LA, Toyota DA, Stephenson LA. 1993. Validation of a temperature telemetry system during moderate and strenuous exercise. *J Therm Biol* 18:203–210.

Koltyn KF, Morgan WP. 1992. Efficacy of perceptual versus heart rate monitoring in the development of endurance. *Br J Sports Med* 26:132–134.

Kulka TJ, Kenney WL. 2002. Heat balance limits in football uniforms. *Physician Sportsmed* 30:29–35.

Le Gall JR, Loirat P, Alperovitch A, Glaser P, Granthil C, Mathieu D, Mercier P, Thomas R, Villers D. 1984. A simplified acute physiology score for ICU patients. *Crit Care Med* 12:975–977.

Le Masurier GC, Tudor-Locke C. 2003. Comparison of pedometer and accelerometer accuracy under controlled conditions. *Med Sci Sports Exerc* 35:867–871.

Lee IM, Sesso HD, Oguma Y, Paffenbarger PF Jr. 2003. Relative intensity of physical activity and risk of coronary heart disease. *Circulation* 107:1110–1116.

Liden CB, Wolowicz M, Stivoric J, Teller A, Vishunubhatla S, Pelletier R, Farringdon J. 2002. *Accuracy and Reliability of the SenseWear™ Armband as an Energy Expenditure Assessment Device*. Online. BodyMedia. Available at http://www.bodymedia.com/pdf/Accuracy.pdf. Accessed September 23, 2003.

Manore M, Thompson J. 2000. *Sport Nutrition for Health and Performance*. Champaign, IL: Human Kinetics. Pp. 136–137, 148–149, 219–220, 224, 225, 228.

Melanson EL, Coelho LB, Tran ZV, Haugen HA, Kearney JT, Hill JO. 2003. Validation of the BodyGem™ hand-held indirect calorimeter. Abstract presented at the Nutrition Week Conference, San Antonio, Texas, January 18–22.

Moran DS. 2000. Stress evaluation by the physiological strain index (PSI). *J Basic Clin Physiol Pharmacol* 11:403–423.

Moran DS, Mendal L. 2002. Core temperature measurement: Methods and current insights. *Sports Med* 32:879–885.

Moran DS, Montain SJ, Pandolf KB. 1998a. Evaluation of different levels of hydration using a new physiological strain index. *Am J Physiol* 275:R854–R860.

Moran DS, Shitzer A, Pandolf KB. 1998b. A physiological strain index to evaluate heat stress. *Am J Physiol* 275:R129–R134.

Moran DS, Castellani JW, O'Brien C, Young AJ, Pandolf KB. 1999a. Evaluating physiological strain during cold exposure using a new cold strain index. *Am J Physiol* 277:R556–R564.

Moran DS, Shapiro Y, Laor A, Izraeli S, Pandolf KB. 1999b. Can gender differences during exercise-heat stress be assessed by the physiological strain index? *Am J Physiol* 276:R1798–R1804.

Moran DS, Kenney WL, Pierzga JM, Pandolf KB. 2002. Aging and assessment of physiological strain during exercise-heat stress. *Am J Physiol Regul Integr Comp Physiol* 282:R1063–R1069.

Morgan WP. 1973. Psychological factors influencing perceived exertion. *Med Sci Sport* 5:97–103.

Morgan WP. 1977. Perception of effort in selected samples of Olympic athletes and soldiers. In: Borg G, ed. *Physical Work and Effort*. Oxford: Pergamon Press. Pp. 267–277.

Morgan WP. 1981. The 1980 C.H. McCloy Research Lecture. Psychophysiology of self-awareness during vigorous physical activity. *Res Q Exerc Sport* 52:385–427.

Morgan W. 2000. Psychological factors associated with distance running and the marathon. In: Pedoe DT, ed. *Marathon Medicine*. London, UK: Royal Society of Medicine Press Limited. Pp. 293–310.

Morgan WP. 2001. Prescription of physical activity: A paradigm shift. *Quest: The Academy Papers* 53:137–161.

Morgan WP, Borg GAV. 1976. Perception of effort in the prescription of physical activity. In: Craig TT, ed. *The Humanistic and Mental Health Aspects of Sports, Exercise and Recreation*. Chicago, IL: American Medical Association. Pp. 126–129.

Morgan WP, Pollock ML. 1977. Psychologic characterization of the elite distance runner. *Ann NY Acad Sci* 301:382–403.

Morgan WP, Horstman DH, Cymerman A, Stokes J. 1983. Facilitation of physical performance by means of a cognitive strategy. *Cogn Ther Res* 7:251–264.

Morgan WP, Brown DR, Raglin JS, O'Connor PJ, Ellickson KA. 1987. Psychological monitoring of overtraining and staleness. *Br J Sports Med* 21:107 114.

Morgan WP, Costill DL, Flynn MG, Raglin JS, O'Connor PJ. 1988. Mood disturbance following increased training in swimmers. *Med Sci Sports Exerc* 20:408–414.

Murray R. 1995. Fluid needs in hot and cold environments. *Int J Sport Nutr* 5:S62–S73.

Nieman DC, Trone GA, Austin MD. 2003. A new handheld device for measuring resting metabolic rate and oxygen consumption. *J Am Diet Assoc* 103:588–592.

Noble BJ, Robertson RJ. 1996. *Perceived Exertion*. Champaign, IL: Human Kinetics.

NWS (National Weather Service). 2003. *Heat Index*. Online. National Oceanic and Atmospheric Administration. Available at http://www.crh.noaa.gov/pub/heat.htm. Accessed September 24, 2003.

O'Brien C, Hoyt RW, Buller MJ, Castellani JW, Young AJ. 1998a. Telemetry pill measurement of core temperature in humans during active heating and cooling. *Med Sci Sports Exerc* 30:468–472.

O'Brien C, Young AJ, Sawka MN. 1998b. Hypohydration and thermoregulation in cold air. *J Appl Physiol* 84:185–189.

O'Connor PJ, Morgan WP, Raglin JS, Barksdale CM, Kalin NH. 1989. Mood state and salivary cortisol levels following overtraining in female swimmers. *Psychoneuroendocrinol* 14:303–310.

O'Connor PJ, Morgan WP, Raglin JS. 1991. Psychobiologic effects of 3 d of increased training in female and male swimmers. *Med Sci Sports Exerc* 23:1055–1061.

Patton JF, Morgan WP, Vogel JA. 1977. Perceived exertion of absolute work during a military physical training program. *Eur J Appl Physiol* 36:107–114.

Pivarnik JM, Palmer RA. 1994. Water and electrolyte balance during rest and exercise. In: Wolinsky I, Hickson JF, eds. *Nutrition in Exercise and Sport*. 2nd ed. Boca Raton, FL: CRC Press. Pp. 245–262.

Poehlman ET. 1989. A review: Exercise and its influence on resting energy metabolism in man. *Med Sci Sports Exerc* 21:515–525.

Pollock ML, Broida J, Kendrick Z, Miller HS, Janeway R, Linnerud AC. 1972. Effects of training two days per week at different intensities on middle-aged men. *Med Sci Sports* 4:192–197.

Prentice AM, Diaz EO, Murgatroyd PR, Goldberg GR, Sonko BJ, Black AE, Coward WA. 1991. Doubly labeled water measurements and calorimetry in practice. In: Whitehead RG, Prentice A, eds. *New Techniques in Nutrition Research*. San Diego: Academic Press. Pp. 177–206.

Puyau MR, Adolph AL, Vohra FA, Butte NF. 2002. Validation and calibration of physical activity monitors in children. *Obes Res* 10:150–157.

Ravussin E, Bogardus C. 1989. Relationship of genetics, age, and physical fitness to daily energy expenditure and fuel utilization. *Am J Clin Nutr* 49:968–975.

Ravussin E, Lillioja S, Anderson TE, Christin L, Bogardus C. 1986. Determinants of 24-hour energy expenditure in man. Methods and results using a respiratory chamber. *J Clin Invest* 78:1568–1578.

Rivera-Fernandez R, Vazquez-Mata G, Bravo M, Aguayo-Hoyos E, Zimmerman J, Wagner D, Knaus W. 1998. The Apache III prognostic system: Customized mortality predictions for Spanish ICU patients. *Intensive Care Med* 24:574–581.

Rontoyannis GP, Skoulis T, Pavlou KN. 1989. Energy balance in ultramarathon running. *Am J Clin Nutr* 49:976–979.

Rosenberg AL. 2002. Recent innovations in intensive care unit risk-prediction models. *Curr Opin Crit Care* 8:321–330.

Sargent F, Weinman KP. 1966. Physiological individuality. *Ann NY Acad Sci* 134:696–719.

Schoeller DA, Racette SB. 1990. A review of field techniques for the assessment of energy expenditure. *J Nutr* 120:1492–1495.

Schoeller DA, Ravussin E, Schutz Y, Acheson KJ, Baertschi P, Jequier E. 1986. Energy expenditure by doubly labeled water: Validation in humans and proposed calculation. *Am J Physiol* 250:R823–R830.

Schutz Y, Weinsier RL, Hunter GR. 2001. Assessment of free-living physical activity in humans: An overview of currently available and proposed new measures. *Obes Res* 9:368–379.

Schutz Y, Weinsier S, Terrier P, Durrer D. 2002. A new accelerometric method to assess the daily walking practice. *Int J Obes Relat Metab Disord* 26:111–118.

Soule RG, Goldman RF. 1969. Energy cost of loads carried on the head, hands, or feet. *J Appl Physiol* 27:687–690.

Soule RG, Goldman RF. 1972. Terrain coefficients for energy cost prediction. *J Appl Physiol* 32:706–708.

Soule RG, Goldman RF. 1973. Pacing of intermittent work during 31 hours. *Med Sci Sports* 5:128–131.

Sutton JR. 1990. Clinical implications of fluid imbalance. In: Lamb DR, Gisolfi CV, eds. *Perspectives in Exercise Science and Sports Medicine. Fluid Homeostasis During Exercise.* Vol 3. Carmel, IN: Benchmark Press. Pp. 425–455.

Thompson J, Manore MM, Skinner JS. 1993. Resting metabolic rate and thermic effect of a meal in low- and adequate-energy intake male endurance athletes. *Int J Sport Nutr* 3:194–206.

Trine MR, Morgan WP. 1997. Influence of time of day on the anxiolytic effects of exercise. *Int J Sports Med* 18:161–168.

Tudor-Locke C, Williams JE, Reis JP, Pluto D. 2002. Utility of pedometers for assessing physical activity: Convergent validity. *Sports Med* 32:795–808.

Verde T, Thomas S, Shephard RJ. 1992. Potential markers of heavy training in highly trained distance runners. *Br J Sports Med* 26:167–175.

Welk GJ. 2002. Use of accelerometry-based activity monitors to assess physical activity. In: Welk GJ, ed. *Physical Activity Assessments for Health-Related Research*. Champaign, IL: Human Kinetics. Pp. 125–141.

Welk GJ, Blair SN, Wood K, Jones S, Thompson RW. 2000. A comparative evaluation of three accelerometry-based physical activity monitors. *Med Sci Sports Exerc* 32:S489–S497.

Wilmore JH, Costill DL. 1994. *Physiology of Sport and Exercise*. Champaign, IL: Human Kinetics Publishers.

Young AJ, Castellani JW, O'Brien C, Shippee RL, Tikuisis P, Meyer LG, Blanchard LA, Kain JE, Cadarette BS, Sawka MN. 1998. Exertional fatigue, sleep loss, and negative energy balance increase susceptibility to hypothermia. *J Appl Physiol* 85:1210–1217.

Young AJ, Sawka MN, Pandolf KB. 2003. *Biomarkers of Physiological Strain during Exposure to Hot and Cold Environments*. Presented at the Institute of Medicine, Committee on Metabolic Monitoring Technologies for Military Field Applications Workshop on Metabolic Monitoring Technologies for Military Field Applications, San Antonio, Texas, January 8–9.

Zhang K, Werner P, Sun M, Pi-Sunyer FX, Boozer CN. 2003. Measurement of human daily physical activity. *Obes Res* 11:33–40.

4

Physiological Biomarkers for Predicting Performance

This chapter provides scientific background on biomarkers that could be useful in monitoring metabolic status in the field. It includes a discussion of the most promising biomarkers for the prediction of: (a) excessive rates of bone and muscle turnover, (b) renal function and hydration, and (c) stress and immune function. Intermediate biomarkers that might be predictive of outcome function, performance, or injury of these systems are addressed, as are factors that influence the validity of each marker as a predictor of performance (e.g., individual variability, gender differences, and environmental exposures). The sensitivity of these biomarkers as surrogates for predicting performance outcomes under a variety of conditions is also explored. In addition, other potential markers of physiological status that have not yet been thoroughly researched are discussed. The measures presented in this chapter are meant as a comprehensive list from which selected measures can be chosen as appropriate, depending on circumstance and feasibility for measurement in the field. Therefore, appropriate groupings of biomarkers can be selected from this list, depending on specific conditions and goals.

BIOMARKERS OF BONE HEALTH

Healthy bone is essential to minimize fracture incidence, including stress fractures that decrease the availability of combat military personnel for training and combat action (Burr, 1997; IOM, 1998). The most accepted predictor of fractures is bone mineral density (BMD) (Black et al., 1992; Chailurkit et al., 2001; Cummings et al., 1993; Gluer et al., 1996; Kelly and Eisman, 1992; Kelsey et al., 1992; Marshall et al., 1996; Melton et al., 1993; Watts, 1999). BMD is measured by dual-energy X-ray absorptiometry, ultrasound, or quantitative computed tomography (Bass and Myburgh, 2000; Bennell et al., 1998; Ingle et al., 1999; IOM, 1998; Ravn et al., 1999).

Bone remodeling is a continuous process of breakdown (bone resorption by osteoclasts) and resynthesis (bone formation by osteoblasts) (Kleerekoper, 2003) of bone that begins after puberty and continues throughout life. Homeostatic processes involve both the cortical and trabecular bone, with remodeling of mature bone occurring more rapidly in trabecular regions. Net bone growth is seen primarily at the growth plate during longitudinal growth. Once the growth plate is closed, bone remodeling occurs at both the trabecular and cortical sites, but it is much slower in cortical bone. Bone health is related to both adult peak bone mass and the rate of bone loss after peak bone mass (Recker et al., 1992). Peak bone mass occurs in individuals between 20 and 30 years of age (Bass and Myburgh, 2000). Since fracture risk is related to bone density, BMD is the primary predictor of risk regardless of age or health status of an individual (Black et al., 1992; Chailurkit et al., 2001; Cummings et al., 1993; Gluer et al., 1996; Kelly and Eisman, 1992; Kelsey et al., 1992; Marshall et al., 1996; Melton et al., 1993; Watts, 1999).

As a sole measure, BMD provides a good indication of the state of bone health over the lifetime of the individual. Currently available instrumentation for measuring BMD has a level of precision from 1 to 3 percent of BMD, depending on the machine, the site of measurement, and the operator (Chailurkit et al., 2001; LeBlanc et al., 1986; Nguyen et al., 1997). This limits the use of BMD for determining short-term changes because it generally takes months to years for a significant change to be detected (Nguyen et al., 1997). Consequently, intermediate biochemical markers of bone resorption and formation may provide earlier indications of potential fractures. (See Appendix A for the available biochemical markers for bone health.)

Biochemical Markers of Bone Resorption

Intermediate markers of bone resorption are used as early indicators of changes in bone homeostasis. Historically, urinary hydroxyproline, a bone breakdown product, was the marker for resorption (Latner, 1975; Lueken et al., 1993). However, this marker was not specific for bone changes and is affected by diet. Currently the most commonly used markers of bone loss are the collagen breakdown products N-telepeptide, carboxy-terminal telopeptide, and the pyridinium cross-links pyridinoline and deoxypridinoline (Chailurkit et al., 2001; Fukuoka et al., 1994; Ladlow et al., 2002; LeBlanc et al., 2002; Lueken et al., 1993; Nishimura et al., 1994; Ravn et al., 1999; Smith et al., 1998). Calcium balance and increases in urinary (24-h) calcium excretion levels are also used to indicate changes in bone resorption (LeBlanc et al., 1995; Matkovic and Heaney, 1992; Weaver et al., 2000), as is tartrate-resistant acid phosphatase, a specific gene product of the osteoclast related to bone resorption (Ingle et al., 1999; Nishimura et al., 1994). These intermediate biochemical markers track well with the elevated bone resorption that is found in individuals during space flight, suggesting that they are good indicators. (These compounds increased immediately upon entrance into microgravity [Smith et al., 1998] and correlated with changes in BMD.)

There is great intraindividual variability in the urinary products of collagen breakdown, making these products difficult to use as a one-time measure to predict bone health (Ingle et al., 1999; Ladlow et al., 2002; Smith et al., 1998). These products, like other measures of bone metabolism, have circadian rhythms, with their highest excretion point at waking and their lowest point 12 hours later (Ladlow et al., 2002). Smith and colleagues (1998) reported on the variability of these markers: an average baseline level for eight individuals was determined over 5 or 10 weeks of 24-hour urinary collections. The longer period of collections reduced error from daily variation and circadian rhythms. The urinary excretion of N-telepeptide varied from 375 ± 66 nmol/day to 1,065 ± 118 nmol/day. This threefold difference reflects the interindividual variability (i.e., the between-subject variation).

When these same individuals participated in a bed-rest study for 1 week, their levels of N-telepeptide increased. The increases ranged from 63 percent for the individual with the lowest baseline level to 7 percent for the individual with the highest baseline level. In fact, with the exception of very elevated bone resorption due to space flight or diseases such as Paget's disease, these urinary products of collagen breakdown are only helpful in indicating a change from an individual's baseline (Kleerekoper, 2003; Ladlow et al., 2002). As a measure of change in bone resorption status, these early markers could be used in clinical assessment of decreases in bone resorption after therapy or after a return to health.

Endocrine markers of bone resorption are important for understanding the balance between bone loss and bone formation. Hormonal measures of bone resorption include 1,25-dihydroxyvitamin D, osteocalcin, and parathyroid hormone (PTH) (LeBlanc et al., 1995). These markers were determined in spaceflight studies and in bed-rest studies—periods known to increase bone resorption (LeBlanc et al., 1995; Lueken et al., 1993; Smith et al., 1999; Weaver et al., 2000). In spaceflight-induced bone resorption, PTH and osteocalcin increased, compared with 17 weeks of bed rest where PTH and osteocalcin were unchanged. In both the spaceflight and bed-rest studies, 1,25-dihydroxyvitamin D decreased (LeBlanc et al., 1995; Smith et al., 1999). The loss of bone density was similar between these two studies, but the endocrine changes were somewhat different, making it difficult to draw conclusions about the best endocrine markers.

Both chronic and acute exercise affects endocrine makers for bone metabolism. For instance, Chilibeck (2000) summarized several studies showing that with acute exercise, PTH increased bone resorption when continuously released, but increased bone formation when intermittently released. In contrast, extreme training decreased calcitonin (which decreased bone resorption) and increased vitamin D (which increased calcium absorption). Extreme training also impacts the reproductive hormones estrogen and testosterone, thyroid hormones, and growth hormone, all of which affect bone health (Chilibeck, 2000).

Biochemical Markers of Bone Formation

Bone remodeling combines resorption with formation (Kohrt and Jankowski, 2003). When bone resorption is high, bone formation is often also high, and it is the balance of these two that produce healthy bones. Intermediate markers of bone formation are also important to ensure a correct clinical evaluation of the balance between resorption and formation before changes in BMD can be detected.

Markers of bone formation have been difficult to elucidate (Ingle et al., 1999; Ladlow et al., 2002; LeBlanc et al., 2002; Lueken et al., 1993; Smith et al., 1999). In one study, total alkaline phosphatase and bone-specific alkaline phosphatase were measured to evaluate the efficacy of bisphosphonates to reduce bone resorption. These two enzymes decreased with reduction of resorption (LeBlanc et al., 2002). In another study of bone healing after fractures, osteocalcin, procollagen type I, N-terminal propeptide, and bone-specific alkaline phosphatase increased; however, the variability was two- to threefold (Ingle et al., 1999). It is unclear if these are good markers for a one-time determination of bone formation status.

Biomarkers of Stress and Bone Metabolism

Other indicators of changes in bone health are related to markers of stress. The cytokines interleukin (IL-1 and IL-6), tumor necrosis factor, transforming growth factor, and insulin-like growth factor-1 (IGF-1) have been studied (Conover, 1996; Margolis et al., 1996). Increases in stress indicators have been shown to correlate with increases in bone resorption. However, a clinical prediction of bone health using these stress markers cannot yet be made because often stress indicators appear over a limited time and may not result in significant bone loss and an increase in fracture risk.

Since there is still a need for intermediate markers of bone metabolism, research is on-going with other markers, such as specific IGF-1 markers. Recent work (Rosen et al., 2003; Zhang et al., 2002; Zhao et al., 2000) suggests that the determination of IGF-1 may relate directly to signaling in the bone matrix. Other studies of specific genes may lead to a better marker for bone health (Simon et al., 2002).

Cortisol as a Biomarker of Bone Health

Glucocorticoid excess directly affects bone resorption and formation (Ziegler and Kasperk, 1998) (Figure 4-1). Chronic elevated corticoid levels stimulate the loss of BMD through decreased formation and increased resorption. The chronic nature of corticoid-induced bone loss is of particular concern as this may cause the fracture rate to increase, causing reduced mobility and general health. Possible glucocorticoid-induced osteoporosis is documented in patients with endocrine-related diseases, such as Cushing's syndrome (Ziegler

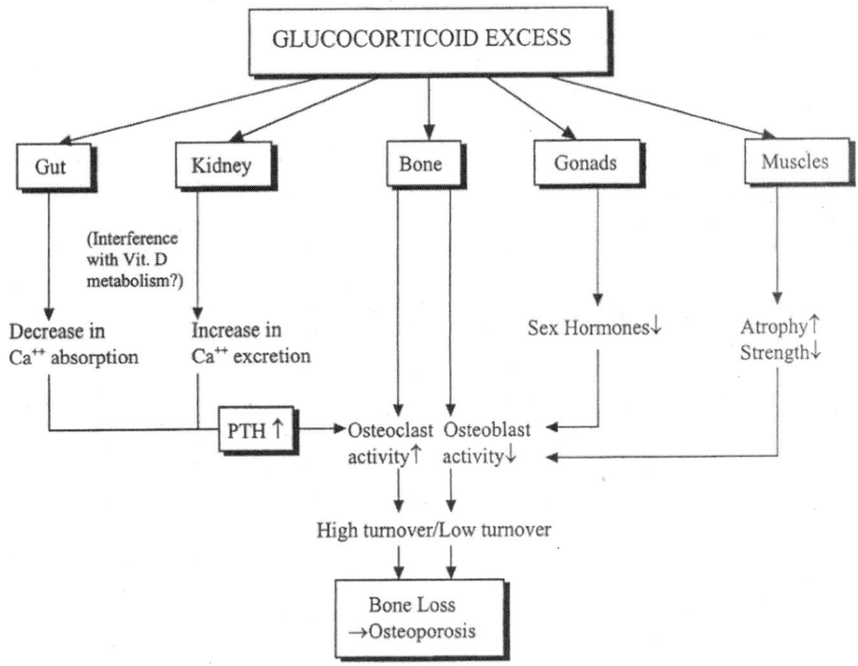

FIGURE 4-1 Mechanisms of bone loss due to glucocorticoid excess.
SOURCE: Reprinted from Ziegler and Kasperk (1998), with permission from Elsevier.

and Kasperk, 1998), patients with depression (Cizza et al., 2001; Robbins et al., 2001; Wong et al., 2000), and transplant patients.

Cortisol, measured in U.S. Army Rangers during 8 weeks of training (Friedl et al., 2000), did not significantly increase until the Rangers' fourth week of training and remained elevated, albeit within normally accepted levels (Figure 4-2). During training, the Rangers experienced sleep deprivation, heavy exercise, and inadequate food intake. Yet these service members' cortisol levels did not change until their body fat was significantly reduced; their muscle and hepatic glycogen were probably also depleted. The authors concluded that the Rangers' cortisol response was related to their increased need to catabolize alternate body-energy sources, similar to that found in research with starvation. In contrast to the cortisol response, the Rangers' IGF-1 levels decreased by week 2 (Figure 4-3), showing earlier adjustments to the physical activity of training. In comparison, astronauts (Smith et al., 1997) had increased plasma cortisol levels immediately upon entry into space. These levels remained above baseline during space flight, but all levels were within their normal ranges with considerable variation between crew members.

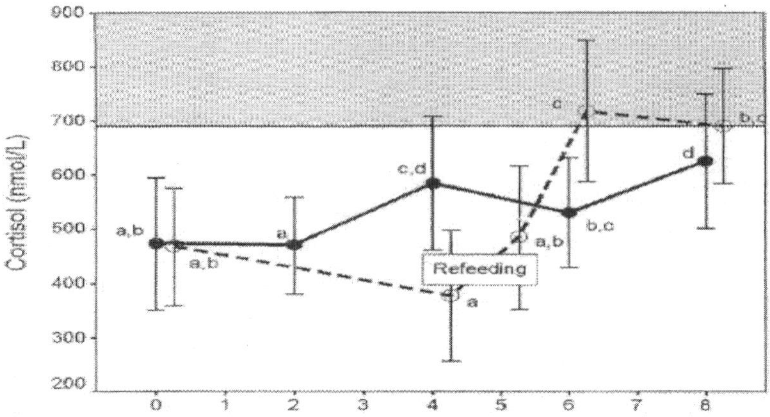

FIGURE 4-2 Serum cortisol for group 1 (solid lines) and group 2 (dashed lines) over an 8-week Ranger training course. Values are means ± standard deviation. Letters indicate means that are not significantly different (Scheffé's test); shaded regions represent areas outside of normal range for morning serum concentrations in normal young men. There were differences between group means at all of the common measurement points for cortisol.
SOURCE: Reprinted, with permission from *JAP* 88:1820 by Friedl et al. (2000).

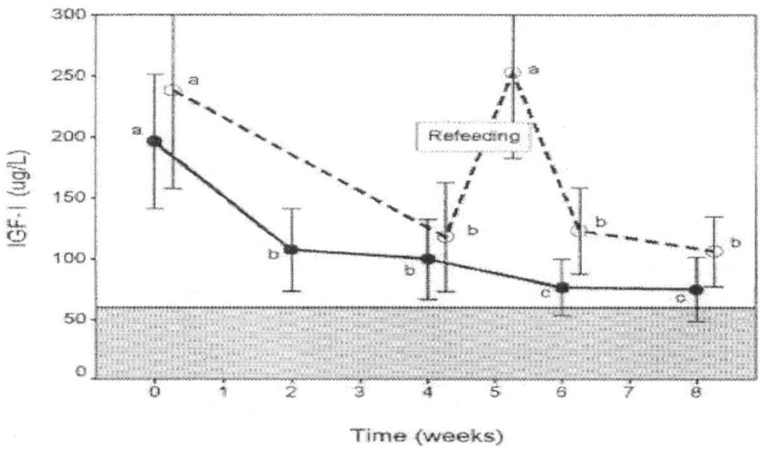

FIGURE 4-3 Serum insulin-like growth factor-1 (IGF-1) for group 1 (solid lines) and group 2 (dashed lines) over an 8-week Ranger training course. Values are means ± standard deviation. Letters indicate means that are not significantly different (Scheffé's test); shaded regions represent areas outside of normal range for morning serum concentrations in normal young men. There were differences between group means at all of the common measurement points for IGF-1.
SOURCE: Reprinted, with permission from *JAP* 88:1820 by Friedl et al. (2000).

Although cortisol is a marker of physical and emotional stress (Hackney and Viru, 1999; Obminski et al., 1997), its circadian rhythms make it difficult to obtain reliable measures during field operations. Circadian rhythms are also disrupted during operations (especially with sleep deprivation), further exacerbating reliable measures of change. When the cortisol elevations are not chronic, there may be no long-lasting effect on bone health. Finally, the levels of cortisol found in healthy individuals performing Ranger-like activities and in astronauts were within normal ranges.

Although the relationship of cortisol and bone turnover is well known, this relationship has not been verified under actual operational experiences, such as during Ranger training. Astronauts did have elevated urinary excretion of collagen cross-links within the first week of space flight (Smith et al., 1998), but the relationship between the urinary excretion of collagen cross-links and cortisol levels has not been studied. However, there is evidence that cortisol decreases BMD in the healthy population when cortisol levels are chronically elevated. Because increased cortisol levels did not occur in Rangers until their fourth week of training, it may be expected that after training, cortisol levels would return to pretraining levels and, similar to astronauts, their bone formation would increase.

BIOMARKERS OF MUSCLE METABOLISM AND FATIGUE

Skeletal muscle structure is highly adaptable in that the individual muscle cells (myocytes) comprising the complex muscle system have the ability to change their mass, metabolic capacity, and contractile properties in accordance with the level of demand placed on them (Baldwin et al., 2003).

In the context of this report, skeletal muscle function is defined as the composite of muscle activities needed for strength, endurance, and rapid-burst, quick movements like short sprints. Each component is essential for military training and combat activities; however, endurance is probably most critical (IOM, 1998). Reduction in any of these muscle capabilities may lead to decrements in overall performance (Behm et al., 2001; Budgett, 1998; Clarkson et al., 1992; Davis, 1995). Chronic muscle fatigue is a generalized problem caused by inadequate recovery from multiple acute bouts of muscle activity. Lack of adequate rest, hydration, and nutritional support (Ardawi et al., 1989; Barac-Nieto et al., 1980; Fitts, 1994) increase the time needed for recovery from muscle fatigue.

Skeletal muscle activity, which can involve either single muscles or muscle groups (for review, see Wilmore and Costill, 1994), includes fine intricate movements, heavy lifting, long-duration traveling, or very fast (rapid-burst) movements. Muscle contraction is initiated through the nervous system by a combination of biochemical and electrochemical reactions that cause shortening of the fibers (Fitts, 1994; Saltin and Gollnick, 1983). Muscle capabilities can be improved or lost through training, overuse that produces fatigue, and disuse that produces atrophy (ACSM, 2002; Ferrando et al., 1996; LeBlanc et al., 1992).

The muscle contractible unit (sarcomere) contains myofibrils, composed of actin and myosin filaments (Fitts, 1994). Through neurological activation, the membrane potential of the muscle cell changes, which in turn causes the filaments to slide together (interdigitate), producing a contraction. All the muscle fibers innervated by a single motor neuron (anterior horn cell of the spinal cord) by contact with its axon are termed a motor unit (Fitts, 1994).

Muscle Fatigue

A common definition of muscle fatigue is "failure to maintain the required or expected force" (Edwards, 1981; Fitts, 1994). Muscle fatigue limits physical activity. The etiology can be of either local or central origin. Local fatigue originates within the muscle, whereas central fatigue is secondary to alterations within the brain. Several neurological and biochemical changes may cause local muscle fatigue, including the following (Fitts, 1994):

- inability of the sodium-potassium pump to maintain the membrane excitability necessary for contraction,
- inability of the muscle fiber to maintain normal contractility because calcium ions are not efficiently removed from the intermyofibrillar space into the sarcoplasmic reticulum,
- inability to provide oxygen to the muscle cell for energy metabolism (oxidative phosphorylation),
- lack of available energy substrates, such as glucose and phosphocreatine, to provide sufficient adenosine triphosphate (ATP), and
- increased lactic acid that reduces intracellular muscle fiber pH, thereby inhibiting further contractions.

It is postulated that in central mechanisms, exercising muscle releases factors that act systemically and impact the central nervous system. In the context of military performance, systemic effects are likely to be of greater significance because of their potential to impact both physical and mental performance.

Muscle fatigue is not the same as muscle soreness. Muscle soreness is the pain that occurs about a day after exercise and peaks 2 to 3 days postexercise (Clarkson et al., 1992). The underlying mechanisms for delayed-onset muscle fatigue and soreness are different. Soreness is believed to be due to a localized inflammatory response (Smith, 1991), and so the appropriate markers are markers for an inflammatory response. The onset of pain is also not considered to be a marker for muscle fatigue. Pain by itself is performance limiting and therefore is not a "predictor."

The majority of studies of muscle fatigue have assumed that the fatigue is the result of events localized within skeletal muscle (Davies and White, 1981;

Edwards, 1981). Prior studies of muscle fatigue have focused on the relationship of a putative marker to the underlying biochemical or histological changes (Banister et al., 1985). For a marker to be of practical use, certain conditions must be met. The marker must apply to all subjects; a statistical relationship is inadequate when applied to the individual (Barron et al., 1985). In addition, the measurement must be technically feasible on a large number of subjects. These criteria currently limit assays to "spot" blood and urine measurements. In-line sensors in a selected muscle are not likely to be of much use because an isolated muscle may not reflect the whole musculoskeletal system, and the muscle selected may not be one of the muscles that is becoming fatigued.

Fatigue may occur with the inability of the sodium-potassium pump to maintain the muscle membrane excitability necessary for contraction (Evans and Cannon, 1991; Fitts, 1994). Determined by electrophysiological measurement, this fatigue is transient and probably not related to the phenomenon of chronic muscle fatigue (Fitts, 1994).

The muscle cell membrane (sarcolemma) is electrically excitable due to selective permeability to potassium and sodium (Fitts, 1994). The electrical potential across the resting muscle cell membrane is due to the ion concentration gradients maintained by the ATPase-dependent sodium-potassium pump that transports sodium ions out of the cell in exchange for potassium ions back into the cell. The neurological excitation is through the release of acetylcholine at the neural membrane; this neurotransmitter causes conformational changes that open channels for the movement of calcium, sodium, and potassium ions. Initially, more sodium ions flow through these channels, resulting in a negative potential on the muscle membrane, which produces a contraction. With the metabolism of acetylcholine, the potassium ions move across the cell membrane to reduce the negative potential. Generally, this fast reaction is not primarily related to fatigue, but research with artificial electrical stimulation demonstrates that there is a point where the rate of destruction of acetylcholine is limited. At that point, the cell membrane cannot recover the resting potential for a subsequent contraction.

Muscle contraction requires movement of calcium ions into the intermyofibrillar fluid (intermyofibrillar space) (Fitts, 1994; Westerblad et al., 1991). Muscle fatigue may relate to the process by which free calcium ions are removed from the intermyofibrillar space back into the sarcoplasmic reticulum (Westerblad et al., 1991). Essentially, if calcium ions are not efficiently removed (increased sarcoplasmic free calcium), then the muscle fiber will not be able to maintain normal contractility. Also, chronic increases of sarcoplasmic calcium ions are associated with the activation of calcium-dependent proteases, which in turn can lead to destruction of the contractile proteins and muscle atrophy.

Myofibrils are surrounded by the transverse tubule-sarcoplasmic reticulum system. These tubules transverse the entire cell and, by branching, form planes of T tubules that interlace the myofibrils (Fitts, 1994). In the resting state, the troponin-tropomyosin complex blocks the action-filaments binding sites, which maintains the muscle in a relaxed state. An action potential at the muscle fiber membrane spreads along these T tubules to the interior of the myofibril, and this causes the increase in calcium ions in the intermyofibrillar fluid. Calcium ions diffuse through the intermyofibrillar space and cause conformational changes in the fiber proteins (troponin-tropomyosin complex), which results in the availability of actin binding sites for the globular heads of the myosin filaments. Muscle contraction will continue as long as the calcium concentration is high in the sarcoplasmic tubules. Calcium-ATPase pumps the calcium into the sarcoplasmic reticulum, leaving few free calcium ions, so muscle relaxation occurs. This reaction time is extremely fast, 1/20 of a second, and continued repetitive contractions may prevent the reestablishment of calcium equilibrium prior to the next stimulus.

Muscle fatigue is also related to decreases in the availability of oxygen to the muscle cell (Barac-Nieto et al., 1980; Fitts, 1994; Gollnick et al., 1972). This may be due to decreases in cardiovascular function, hemoglobin concentrations, and respiratory exchange rates. Dehydration, or decreased plasma volume (Nose et al., 1983), can also reduce the availability of oxygen to the cell. Even with very highly trained athletes, there are limits in the ability to perfuse the muscle cell with oxygen, and fatigue occurs. Obviously combat service members must maintain hydration, high levels of cardiovascular/pulmonary fitness, and good hemoglobin status (no iron or other nutrient deficiency).

ATP provides energy for muscle contraction (Meyer and Foley, 1996). ATP is generated through several different pathways, including glycolysis and oxidative phosphorylation. The instantaneous source of energy, phosphocreatine, produces ATP immediately. When this ATP is used, the adenosine diphosphate is regenerated through the phosphocreatine shuttle to resynthesize ATP. With high resistance and/or fast repetitions of contractions, the source of phosphorus for ATP synthesis (phosphocreatine) is depleted and fatigue occurs. Replenishment of the phosphocreatine from glucose may take minutes before contractions can continue.

Muscle fibers store energy as glycogen. It is estimated that 2,000 muscle fiber contractions may be required to deplete muscle glycogen stores, suggesting that this is a good source of energy for muscle contractions, particularly during quick-burst activities. Muscle glycogen depletion may occur with endurance types of muscle activity, such as marathon running, when no dietary glucose is available. Since muscle glycogen metabolism does not require oxygen (anaerobic metabolism), it is not dependent upon an immediate blood supply of oxygen. Under anaerobic conditions, for each glucose-6-phosphate molecule released from glycogen stores, three ATP molecules are generated with two molecules of lactic acid. Thus glycogen metabolism in the absence of oxygen leads to a buildup of lactic acid, which can be measured in the blood. Lactic acid levels become a problem when the intracellular muscle fiber pH changes, (an increase in H^+ ions) producing muscle fatigue (Fitts, 1994; Westerblad et al., 1991).

Accumulating lactic acid reduces intracellular muscle fiber pH, which inhibits further contraction and results in fatigue. Nuclear magnetic resonance spectroscopy has shown that prolonged strong muscle contraction can reduce the intracellular pH from normal resting values near 7.02 to as low as 6.34 (de Kerviler et al., 1991). Adenosine monophosphate (AMP) accumulation also activates the enzyme myoadenylate deaminase (localized particularly in type II fibers), which hydrolyzes AMP to inosine monophosphate with the release of ammonia. This ammonia partially neutralizes lactic acid, modulating the drop in intracellular pH. Ultimately, muscle fatigue is accompanied by cessation of contraction, which restores capillary blood flow with the consequent removal of lactic acid and the recovery of normal intracellular pH. Regeneration of AMP is then possible from inosine monophosphate through a guanosine-triphosphate-mediated reaction (Meyer and Foley, 1996).

Fiber Types and Muscle Performance

The ability of the muscle tissue to perform burst versus endurance activities is due to the percentage of the two fiber types found in the muscles: types I and II, and two subtypes: types IIA and IIB; these are defined by their morphological, physiological, and biochemical characteristics (Pette and Staron, 1990; Saltin and Gollnick, 1983). Genetically predetermined, human muscles are a mosaic of these various fiber types. An individual with more type I (slow twitch) muscle cells excels at endurance activities, while an individual with more type II (fast twitch) excels at quickness and strength activities. Different muscles have different proportions of the fiber types. The leg muscles provide an example. The gastrocnemius has more than 50 percent fast-fiber types, while the solcus muscle may have less than 40 percent fast types. There is a great deal of interindividual variation in the percentage of fiber types found in muscles.

Type 1 fiber types have low glycogen content, high resting levels of phosphocreatine (with ample mitochondria), a rich capillary network, and high blood flow—all indicative of reliance on aerobic metabolism. In general, these fiber types are considered to be resistant to fatigue due to their slower contraction speed and their postural and prolonged sustained contracile functions. Type 1 fibers rely on a continuous delivery of glucose and oxygen for energy production. As long as oxygen and glucose are available, these muscles will continue to function. With reduced oxygen availability due to altered cardiovascular-pulmonary function, dehydration (reduction of plasma volume), or low hemoglobin levels, glucose metabolism is limited to nonmitochondrial metabolism, resulting in increased lactic acid concentrations. Maintaining blood glucose through feeding during endurance exercise delays the onset of this fatigue by providing necessary energy. During long-duration exercise, both intracellular and plasma fatty acids can be used for energy metabolism by type I muscle fibers. A noteworthy sex difference is that women have higher muscle lipid levels, which are related to the estrogenic influences that enhance aerobic endurance activities.

Type II muscle fibers produce rapid, strong contractions of short duration (quick burst), but these fibers are sensitive to fatigue (Saltin and Gollnick, 1983). They are dependent largely on glycogen metabolism and do not require oxygen for contraction because they are not highly dependant on oxidative phosphorylation. They contain ample glycogen stores, few mitochondria, a sparse capillary network, and low intracellular resting levels of phosphocreatine, all of which are indicative of the fibers' reliance on anaerobic glycolysis for the production of energy. In fact, they can contract in the absence of oxygen until their stored glycogen supply is exhausted. When phosphocreatine is completely metabolized and there is inadequate time for regeneration (Westerblad et al., 1991), the muscle does not have available energy and fatigue occurs. Usually a rest period of several hours is required to regenerate enough phosphocreatine and ATP from blood glucose for another fast-exercise activity. If muscle glycogen is depleted, it may take several days for regeneration.

In summary, individuals experience fatigue when muscle energy sources are inadequate or when faced with inadequate energy substrates when oxygen delivery falls below the point for lactate accumulation (a decrease in intracellular pH) (Westerblad et al., 1991). One subjective measure of muscle fatigue is self perception, as described previously in Chapter 3; however, predictors of fatigue at an earlier state have been proposed (see following sections).

Measures of Muscle Performance and Indicators of Fatigue

A differential diagnosis between acute damage from muscle injury, fatigue due to overuse or overconditioning, exercise until exhaustion, hydration, and nutritional status is difficult given the interactions of these factors in the subjective feeling of fatigue. For heavy lifts and sprint activities, highly available energy sources are essential, and energy depletion results in fatigue. Aerobic endurance depends on glucose and fat for energy and on the adequate delivery of oxygen to tissues. The level of these energy nutrients depends on the nutritional status of the individual. Undernutrition contributes to fatigue and makes biochemical diagnosis difficult (Barac-Nieto et al., 1980; Lieberman et al., 2002).

For this report, it is assumed that military training requires high standards for high muscle performance and teaches the importance of muscle conditioning, including maximized hydration, nutrition, and rest. Tools have been developed to evaluate the physical fitness of military personnel, including running distances in a certain time, lifting weights, and calisthenics (IOM, 1998).

The most common measure of muscle strength (besides functional performance) is muscle diameter, which relates to muscle volume or mass (Evans, 2001; Roth et al., 2001). Muscle mass is measured by circumference (tape measure) (Takahashi et al., 2003) or magnetic resonance imaging (LeBlanc et al., 1992), and by dual-energy X-ray absorptiometry (Ferrando et al., 1996) for lean mass in specific regions (Suzuki et al., 1994). Muscle responses to nervous stimuli are measured by electromyography (Evans and Cannon, 1991). Decreases in muscle performance and muscle volume as determined by magnetic resonance imaging (LeBlanc et al., 1992) are related, although a direct linear correlation has not been found. Muscle strength is not just due to mass, but is also related to neurological and cardiovascular factors, with decrements found with deconditioning.

Heavy muscle performance causes muscle damage with the release of creatine kinase, lactic acid dehydrogenases, and glutamic oxaloacetic transaminase into the blood (Evans and Cannon, 1991; Manfredi et al., 1991). Circulating creatine kinase, as a marker of acute damage, is different for trained and untrained individuals and does not always correlate with muscle damage (Heymsfield et al., 1983; Manfredi et al., 1991). While this parameter may indicate acute muscle damage, it is not a reliable measure of chronic fatigue. Muscle soreness may accompany these biochemical changes and is actually a good indicator of the need to rest (see Chapter 3).

Cortisol

Stress causes increased muscle protein breakdown that results in loss of muscle mass and potentially in muscle atrophy (Wolfe and Børsheim, 2003). The most common stress indicator is increased blood or urinary cortisol levels (IOM, 1999). Short-term heavy exercise increases plasma cortisol levels, but over-training decreases this cortisol response (Wittert, 2000). Physiological increases in plasma cortisol initiate protein breakdown (Darmaun et al., 1988; Gelfand et al., 1984). Hypercortisolemia increases whole-body protein turnover without the offsetting increase in protein synthesis (Wolfe and Børsheim, 2003). Under experimental conditions, 6 days of hypercortisolemia produced a 15 percent decrease in rat soleus muscle mass (Jaspers and Tischler, 1986). This stress-induced proteolysis may increase the incidence of chronic fatigue in military personnel under conditions of continuous stress (Wolfe and Børsheim, 2003). However, blood and urinary cortisol have diurnal rhythms, making the use of a single measurement difficult to interpret (Braunwald et al., 2001).

3-Methyl Histidine

Other indicators of protein catabolism in muscle are urinary 3-methyl histidine (Stein, 2003; Young et al., 1973) and urinary creatinine levels (Afting et al., 1981). Urinary creatinine provides a marker for long-term change in lean body mass, while increases in urinary 3-methyl histidine levels indicate muscle tissue catabolism. Three-methyl histidine is released during muscle protein breakdown and is not reutilized for synthesis, but is excreted in the urine. Since muscle contains the largest level of 3-methyl histidine in the body, urinary levels relate directly to muscle breakdown. However, 3-methyl histidine urinary levels are not always good predictors of muscle performance levels since they are also affected by the dietary consumption of muscle meats.

Protein Turnover

Protein turnover in muscles may indicate changes in muscle capabilities. In general, protein synthesis equals protein breakdown in normally maintained muscles. Under stress or chronic fatigue, protein turnover is increased, but catabolism increases more than synthesis (Wolfe and Børsheim, 2003). In general, markers that indicate protein breakdown may overemphasize the changes in muscle. Markers of synthesis are also needed to provide insight into the overall changes in muscle protein metabolism that relate to changes in muscle performance. The only methods available to determine the rates of breakdown versus synthesis are invasive measures (infusion technologies and muscle biopsies) of incorporation and release of labeled amino acids from muscles. These studies are important, however, because they provide insight into understanding the conditions of muscle metabolism during different forms and levels of metabolic stresses (Ferrando et al., 1995, 1996).

Blood amino acids are incorporated into the muscle and are used for synthesis. Conversely, during breakdown, some amino acids (e.g., branched-chain amino acids [BCAAs]) are released from the muscle into the blood. The rate of these changes can be measured. Protein synthesis increases during the postprandial period and decreases during the fasting period. However, even with an imbalance of protein breakdown to synthesis, a 15-percent loss in muscle mass can occur without significant effect on muscle performance (Wolfe and Børsheim, 2003). Studies by Wolfe and Børsheim (2003) demonstrate that changes in blood essential amino acids, including plasma alanine and glutamine levels, do not always indicate changes in muscle protein turnover. Plasma alanine and glutamine levels are related to stress and exercise. Alanine is released after exercise and is probably related to the stimulation of gluconeogenesis (Darmaun et al., 1988). Plasma glutamine levels appear to be maintained even when the intramuscular glutamine pool is depleted. Therefore, blood amino acids are not considered good markers of muscle changes (Wolfe and Børsheim, 2003).

Neutrophil Infiltration and Cytokines

Other markers of muscle damage include neutrophil infiltration into the muscle cells and increased concentrations of the cytokines IL-1 and tumor necrosis factor. These become elevated with muscle-damaging exercises. For instance, after endurance downhill skiing at 70 percent of maximum heart rate (HR), IL-1β in vastus lateralis biopsy increased 135 percent after 45 minutes and 250 percent after 5 days. This correlated to accumulation of neutrophils in muscles (Fielding et al., 1993).

IGF-1 has an anabolic effect on skeletal muscle cells (Adams and Haddad, 1996; Adams et al., 1999; Eliakim et al., 2000; Evans, 2001), and due to the significant positive correlation between increased muscle overloading and IGF-1 level, it is a potential marker for muscle overuse. IGF-1 is an insulin-like peptide that is primarily secreted in the liver and is stimulated by growth hormone. There are paracrine and autocrine forms that are only partially regulated through growth hormone. Most of the circulating IGF-1 is bound to proteins, and as many as six forms have been identified. In rodent studies, muscle IGF-1 increased after muscle overloading. Adams and Haddad (1996) suggested that this muscle-produced IGF-1 might mediate muscle hypertrophy. Additional research is needed to determine if IGF-1 (especially the muscle-produced form of the peptide) can be a specific biomarker for muscle damage. There is evidence that IGF-1 levels are stable during the day (i.e., no diurnal variation) (Eliakim et al., 2000). However, IGF-1 levels are decreased with malnutrition and change depending on an individual's level of fitness (training effect) and length and duration of exercise.

Some genetic markers, such as myosin heavy chain (Baldwin et al., 2003; Giger et al., 2002; Ohira et al., 1992), have been studied. Although these studies are important to understand the expression of proteins under different nutritional and stress conditions, they have not been useful in predicting changes in the functional muscle capacity.

Near-Infrared Spectroscopy

Near-infrared spectroscopy (NIRS) and surface electromyography studies indicate muscle ischemia and fatigue during isometric contractions (Alfonsi et al., 1999). NIRS is a potential tool to determine fatigue (Neary et al., 2002; van Beekvelt et al., 2002; Wariar et al., 2000). The military should study the use of NIRS to concurrently monitor muscle oxygenation/deoxygenation, intramuscular pH, and skin hydrations status. With NIRS, muscle function and hydrations status can be measured under field conditions with telemetry units.

Near-infrared light (700–1,000 nm) has the ability to deeply penetrate tissue and be bound to oxygenated or deoxygenated hemoglobin that allows the measurement of tissue oxygen and blood flow (Quaresima et al., 2003). It is a relatively low-cost and noninvasive way to measure muscle oxidative metabolism that has found wide application in sports medicine (Puente-Maestu et al., 2003; Xu et al., 2003). Among the other important variables that would be valuable to assess noninvasively would be tissue pH, redox potential, hydration, extracellular sodium and glucose concentration, osmolality, and evidence of inflammation. This technology has already been shown to be feasible for measuring tissue pH (Soller et al., 2002), blood pH (Rosen et al., 2002), glucose (Cohen et al., 2003), blood flow (Kell and Bhambhani, 2003), and hemoglobin (Rendell et al., 2003) or hematocrit (Soller et al., 2002) levels. When used with fluorescent labels, tissue imaging is possible (Sevick-Muraca et al., 2002). This technology could also potentially be used for assessing inflammation since superoxide, one of the more potent reactive oxygen substances that develop with inflammation, reacts with nitric oxide to produce peroxynitrite. Peroxynitrite interacts with tyrosine to produce nitrotyrosine, which can be measured by NIRS (Massip et al., 2002). Recently it has been shown that the measurement of nitrotyrosine levels is a very sensitive measure of inflammation (Shishehbor et al., 2003). There is a possibility as well that states of hydration could be assessed (Zhou et al., 2003). Finally, in combination with deuterium oxide, NIRS can be used to measure total body water to determine body composition (Macías et al., 2002). Argon lasers with a shorter wave length might also be useful (Massip et al., 2002) for a number of these purposes.

Central Fatigue and the Tryptophan Hypothesis

The neurotransmitter serotonin (5-hydroxytryptamine [5-HT]) is a critical central modulator of sleep, arousal, mood, and cognitive function (Graeff, 1997). Plasma free tryptophan (TRP) is the precursor for brain 5-HT. The rate-limiting step in the synthesis of 5-HT is the transport of free TRP across the blood-brain barrier as it competes for a barrier carrier system with other large neutral amino acids, especially BCAAs. Thus an increase in free TRP and a reduction in BCAAs favors uptake of TRP across the blood-brain barrier and increased 5-HT synthesis. Both exercise and diet can influence the ratio of TRP:BCAA, thus altering serotonergic pathways (Blomstrand et al., 1988; Fernstrom, 1990).

Newsholme and colleagues (1987) first proposed that prolonged exercise increased brain serotonergic activity leading to a loss of physical and mental efficiency in athletes, known as "central fatigue." At rest, the majority of plasma TRP is bound to albumin and unavailable for transport across the blood-brain barrier. During exercise, free fatty acids displace TRP from albumin leading to an increased availability of free TRP in plasma. Concurrently, BCAAs are taken up by muscle for oxidative metabolism. The net effect is that the TRP:BCAA ratio increases several-fold, and more TRP is taken up into the brain and available for conversion to 5-HT (Blomstrand et al., 1988). Although considerable evidence suggests that endurance exercise alters serotonergic activity, links between the neuroendocrine changes and alterations in performance and perceived exertion have been more difficult to demonstrate. The administration of 5-HT reuptake inhibitors (which alter central serotonin transmission) has been shown to reliably modify human mental and physical performance (Strüder et al., 1998; Wilson and Maughan, 1992). However, a recent review of more than 20 human studies concluded that nutritional manipulation of the brain 5-HT system has variable effects on reducing fatigue and enhancing performance outcomes (see Strüder and Weicker, 2001). Specifically, oral supplementation with 5-HT precursor, BCAAs, or carbohydrate, either alone or in combination, has generally led to contradictory results.

There is some evidence that down-regulation of 5-HT receptors or other counter-regulatory mechanisms might protect the well-conditioned athlete from excessive neurotransmission of 5-HT (Jakeman et al., 1994; Strachan and Maughan, 1999). Strüder and Weicker (2001) speculate that prolonged, exhaustive exercise disturbs this physiological balance leading to 5-HT dysregulation and the syndrome known as over training. As described earlier in this chapter, over training has been related to reduced physical performance, prolonged fatigue, altered mood states, loss of appetite, and sleep disturbances even in highly conditioned athletes (Morgan et al., 1988; O'Connor et al., 1991). Thus the search for potential markers for the prediction of the onset of fatigue might include plasma levels of free TRP, BCAAs, albumin, and free fatty acids. However, it seems unlikely that these parameters would be sufficiently informative to predict cognitive state or physical performance of *individuals* because "normal" values were derived using group data. Moreover, there would be difficult technical challenges to measuring free amino acids in saliva or by sweat patch, which would severely limit the practical application of this strategy for military field use.

In summary, increased TRP uptake into the brain and the subsequent increase in 5-HT biosynthesis does not induce excessive neural transmission of 5-HT or central fatigue. A high TRP:BCAA ratio during exercise would be considered normal, except when accompanied by evidence of fatigue and exhaustion. Thus, the TRP:BCAA ratio does not appear to be a useful marker since it cannot reliably predict performance decrements. Various feedback controls regulate central serotonergic transmission. Oral administration of TRP before or during exercise has been suggested but not proven as a possible strategy to "down regulate" 5-HT receptors and avoid this 5-HT dysregulation. Insufficient evidence exists at this time to support this approach.

BIOMARKERS OF HYDRATION AND RENAL FUNCTION

Water comprises an average 60 percent (range 45–70 percent) of total body weight, depending on an individual's body composition (Sawka and Pandolf, 1990). Individuals with more muscle mass have a higher percentage of body water than individuals with more body fat since water comprises about 72 percent of muscle and organ weight, but only about 20 to 30 percent of fat weight. In general, men have a higher percentage of lean body mass and thus a higher percentage of their total body weight is comprised of water. For example, the average adult man's body weight is comprised of about 65 percent water, while the average adult woman's body weight is comprised of about 55 percent water (Kleinman and Lorenz, 1996).

As defined by Manore and Thompson (2000), dehydration is a decrease in total body water (TBW) that occurs anytime that fluid intake does not keep up with fluid loss. During exercise, involuntary dehydration occurs since most active individuals do not voluntarily consume enough water or other fluids to offset the water losses that occur from sweating. This means that even if an active individual drinks to satisfy thirst, the amount of water or fluid consumed does not usually suffice to return this individual to a state of euhydration (normal hydration). Thus most individuals end a session of extensive physical exertion (e.g., exercise) in a state of dehydration that must be corrected by eating and drinking during the postexercise period. Hyponatremia (abnormally low plasma sodium concentrations) generally occurs when water intake is high, but sodium intake is low. This will occur if the fluid being consumed during exercise does not have adequate sodium to replace losses.

Effects of Dehydration

The effects of dehydration on exercise performance and physiological functions within the body are well documented. For example, even small levels of dehydration (1 percent) can cause obvious signs of heat exhaustion if strenuous exercise occurs in hot (41°C or 105°F) environments (Casa and Armstrong, 2001; Sawka and Montain, 2000) and can lead to decrements in physical work capacity and cognitive function (Epstein and Armstrong, 1999; Montain and Coyle, 1992). When dehydration exceeds 2 to 2.5 percent of body weight, physical work capacity can decrease as much as 35 to 48 percent (Casa et al., 2000; Shirreffs and Maughan, 2000). Dehydration of greater than 3 percent of body weight increases the risk of developing exertional heat illness and of producing significant reductions in cardiac output since the reduction in stroke volume can be greater than the increase in heart rate (ACSM, 1996; Casa et al., 2000). Table 4-1 provides a general overview of the effect that continued dehydration has on thirst, on the ability to perform work, and on physiological functions. It is important to remember that the impact of a particular degree of dehydration and heat on exercise performance is highly variable within and among individuals.

Dehydration increases hemoconcentration, blood viscosity and osmolality, core body temperature, and HR, while causing a decrease in stroke volume (Montain and Coyle, 1992; Murray, 1995). It promotes the onset of fatigue and makes any given exercise intensity seem harder than it would if the individual was well hydrated (Gonzalez-Alonso et al., 1999; Maughan, 1992; Murray, 1995). In addition, dehydration increases carbohydrate oxidation (Gonzalez-Alonso et al., 1999), thus increasing the amount of carbohydrate utilized during exercise. However, the most serious effect of progressive dehydration is that the body decreases its ability to sweat because of decreased blood flow to the skin.

TABLE 4-1 Adverse Effects of Dehydration on Work Capacity

Body Weight Lost (%)	Symptoms
0	Well hydrated; no dehydration
1	Thirst threshold and threshold for impaired exercise thermoregulation leading to decrement in physical work capacity; core body temperature can begin to rise and increased cardiovascular strain; dehydration at this level can cause serious problems if moderate-to-strenuous exercise occurs in very hot environments
2	Stronger thirst, vague discomfort, sense of oppression, loss of appetite
3	Dry mouth, increasing hemoconcentration, reduction in urinary output; exercise at high intensity is difficult; decrease in aerobic power
4	Decrements of 20–30% in physical work capacity, more depending on individual
5	Difficulty in concentrating, headache, impatience, sleepiness
6	Severe impairment in exercise temperature regulation and increased respiratory rate lead to tingling and numbness of extremities
7	Likely to collapse if combined with heat and exercise; individuals can experience dizziness, fatigue, dyspnea, tingling, indistinct speech, headache, and spasticity

SOURCE: Adapted from Casa and Armstrong (2001) and Greenleaf (1992).

This in turn decreases the body's ability to cool itself, which leads to an increased core body temperature and the risk of heat illness and collapse and, in rare situations, life-threatening heat stroke (Sutton, 1990). Various types of heat-related disorders and factors that increase risk for heat illness are outlined in Table 4-2.

Water is lost first from the extracellular space. Next, a proportionately greater percentage of water comes from the intracellular spaces. Costill and colleagues (1976) found that when subjects lost 6 percent of their body weight due to dehydration, approximately 50 percent of the water lost came from intracellular water. Thus muscle cells, which are 70 percent water, are depleted of the water necessary to maintain metabolic functions. This is one reason why dehydration negatively impacts exercise performance. One study showed that moderate exercise (50 percent of maximum oxygen uptake) in cool environmental temperatures (14.4°C or 60°F) without prior dehydration resulted in most of the fluid losses coming from the extracellular interstitial fluid (Maw et al., 1998). However, when subjects repeated the same protocol in a hot environment (36.2°C or 97°F), 23 percent of the fluid losses came from the intracellular environment. Thus progressive dehydration in well-hydrated individuals performing moderate exercise primarily depletes extracellular fluid. However, when the stress of heat is added, fluid is drawn from the intracellular spaces.

TABLE 4-2 Signs and Symptoms of Exertional Heat Illnesses

Heat Illness	Signs and Symptoms	Reference
Heat syncope	Occurs when unacclimatized people stand for a long period of time and the blood pools in the vasodilated periphery. Dehydration does not need to be a prerequisite for this disorder. It generally occurs when individuals stand for long periods of time in the heat, stop suddenly after a race, or stand suddenly from a lying position. Symptoms may include dehydration, fatigue, tunnel vision, pale or sweaty skin, decreased pulse rate, dizziness, lightheadedness, or fainting.	Binkley et al., 2002; Sutton, 1990
Heat cramps	Painful cramps involving abdominal and skeletal muscles that occur after strenuous exercise where sweat losses and fluid intakes were high, urine volume low, sodium intake was inadequate to replace losses, and there was neuromuscular fatigue. Sunstroke, heat cramps, and heat exhaustion are possible with prolonged exposure and/or physical activity in temperatures between 90°–105°F (~32°–41°C). Symptoms include dehydration, thirst, sweating, transient muscle cramps, and fatigue.	Binkley et al., 2002; NWS, 2003
Heat exhaustion	During exercise, plasma volume decreases, causing decreased blood flow from the muscles to the skin and decreases the body's ability to dissipate the heat generated during exercise. This results in the body's heat production to exceed the body's ability to dissipate heat and core body temperature rises to ≥ 104°F (≥ 40°C). Dehydration exacerbates these physiological changes and contributes to heat-related problems. The causes of heat exhaustion may be associated with a combination of heavy sweating, dehydration, sodium losses, and energy depletion. Symptoms include elevated or normal core body temperature, dizziness, lightheadedness, headache, syncope, nausea, decreased urine output, persistent muscle cramps, pallor, profuse sweating, chills, intestinal cramps, weakness, and hyperventilation.	Binkley et al., 2002

continued

TABLE 4-2 Continued

Heat Illness	Signs and Symptoms	Reference
Heat stroke	Heat exhaustion can lead to heat stroke, which can lead to loss of consciousness and even death. Early symptoms of heat injury are excessive sweating, headache, nausea, dizziness, and a gradual impairment of consciousness and the ability to concentrate. Along with an increased core body temperature (≥ 104°F or 40°C) and hot, dry skin, altered mental status is the universally accepted sign that distinguishes exertional heat stroke from heat exhaustion. The central nervous system neurological changes are typically the first signs of heat stroke and can include dizziness, drowsiness, irrational behavior, confusion, irritability, emotional instability, hysteria, apathy, aggressiveness, seizures, loss of consciousness, and coma. Other symptoms include dehydration, weakness, hot and wet or dry skin, tachycardia, vomiting, hyperventilation, hypotension, and diarrhea.	Binkley et al., 2002; Shapiro and Seidman, 1990

NOTE: Symptoms for each of the above conditions were adapted from Binkley et al. (2002). Not all combat service members will present with all the signs and symptoms for the suspected condition.

Electrolyte Losses

Electrolytes are also lost in the sweat, but the quantity lost appears to be highly variable and dependent on when the sweat sample is taken, on the individual's state of acclimation, and on the physiological differences between individuals (Manore and Thompson, 2000; Sawka and Montain, 2000). Because the methods for collecting sweat and estimating total electrolyte losses are crude and cumbersome, values for sweat electrolyte concentrations in the research literature vary dramatically. Although a number of minerals are lost in sweat, including sodium, chloride, potassium, magnesium, calcium, and iron, the electrolytes lost are primarily sodium and potassium. Typical values for sodium concentrations in sweat range from 20 to 80 mmol/L, while potassium values range from 4 to 8 mmol/L (Maughan and Shirreffs, 1997). The amount of electrolytes lost in sweat for any one individual depends on many variables, such as exercise intensity and duration, acclimation, environmental conditions, and clothing. Because direct sweat electrolyte loss is difficult to measure, electrolyte losses are generally estimated based on data collected under various laboratory environmental conditions in individuals performing a wide range of exercises.

As mentioned above, it is now known that sweat electrolyte losses vary widely among individuals, and research aimed at identifying who is a risk for these losses is underway. For example, football players in the National Football

League had sweat losses of 1.3 to 5.2 L/h and sodium losses of 22 to 101 mmol/L (Stofan et al., 2002). These data indicate that sodium loses for some individuals can be much higher than the normal range. The players who have higher sweat and sodium losses may be at a greater risk of dehydration and of adverse health effects due to these losses. This was demonstrated in a study conducted with NCAA Division 1 football players. The sports medicine staff identified those football players with a history of whole-body muscle cramp during practices and competition. During two 2.5-hour training practices, sodium and fluid intakes and losses were measured. Sodium losses were twice as high (55 vs. 26 mmol/L or 5.2 vs. 2.4 g/2 practice sessions) in players who frequently had muscle cramps compared with those players who were classified as non-crampers. The crampers also had significantly higher sweat losses (0.5 L more/hr) and significantly higher dehydration rates at the end of practice than noncrampers (Stofan et al., 2003), even though both groups consumed the same amount and types of fluids. These preliminary research data suggest that there is a great deal of variation in sweat and sodium losses among individuals. Thus some individuals have a great need to replace sodium and fluids during physical activity. Efforts are needed to identify these individuals and train them on the importance of increasing fluid and sodium intakes before, during, and after physical activity, especially in hot environments.

Hyponatremia

Hyponatremia is the development of abnormally low plasma sodium concentrations (< 130 mmol/L). This condition usually occurs when excess water accumulates, relative to sodium, in the extracellular water compartments of the body. The general symptoms of hyponatremia are fatigue and nausea (Armstrong et al., 1993), but severe cases can result in grand mal seizures, respiratory arrest, acute respiratory distress syndrome, and coma (Armstrong et al., 1993; Noakes et al., 1990). The cause of hyponatremia in healthy individuals is not known, but it is generally attributed to prolonged endurance exercise in a warm environment while drinking excessive amounts of low-sodium fluids. In these individuals, the fluid-electrolyte control mechanisms are either defective or are overwhelmed by the environmental conditions and the intense exercise (Armstrong et al., 1993). When hyponatremia develops in the presence of a modest fluid load, the cause may be due to an impaired renal capacity and the inability to excrete a fluid load (Speedy et al., 2001).

Hyponatremia has been document in recreational and endurance runners. Noakes and colleagues (1990) reported that in the 1986 and 1987 Comrades Marathon in South Africa, 9 percent of collapsed runners had hyponatremia. Another case of hyponatremia was reported in an individual hiking all day in the heat in the Grand Canyon in Arizona (Richards, 1996). Finally, Flinn and Sherer (2000) reported a case study of a 20-year-old male military recruit who suffered a generalized tonic-clonic seizure following 9 hours of moderate activity in a hot, humid environment. He consumed at least 5.8 L of plain water before the seizure, and his blood sodium level dropped to 113 mmol/L. Although there are a number of research papers reporting hyponatremia in individual athletes (Armstrong et al., 1993), overall the incidence of hyponatremia in active individuals is low. As illustrated in the case study by Flinn and Sherer (2000), combat service members exercising in hot environments need to be aware of the importance of replacing the fluids and electrolytes lost in sweat in order to prevent the development of hyponatremia. Under these conditions, consumption of plain or bottled water may not provide enough electrolytes to maintain good fluid and electrolyte balance.

Measurement of Total Body Water

In general, assessment of TBW requires a laboratory setting and uses the dilution principle, which states that the volume of the compartment is equal to the amount of the tracer added to the compartment divided by the concentration of the tracer in the compartment (Schoeller, 1996). Using this principle and some basic assumptions about the tracer selected (tritium, deuterium oxygen-18), a tracer is administered to an individual and urine samples collected over time to determine TBW.

Deuterium Dilution

The most common property-based method of measuring TBW is deuterium dilution. This method measures the dilution in the body of a known dose of deuterium isotope using a body fluid sample.

Bioelectrical Impedance

Bioelectrical impedance analysis (BIA) is based on the relationship among a conductor's volume (the body), length (height), and impedance (which reflects the resistance to the flow of an electric current). Impedance measurements are made with an individual lying flat on a nonconducting surface with electrodes attached to specific sites on the wrist and ankle of the right side of the body. A low-dose (800 μA), single-frequency (50 KHz) current is passed through the individual and the value for resistance is measured. A prediction equation that includes the resistance value from the measured impedance plus height-squared is then used to estimate fat-free mass. Validity of BIA measurements are significantly affected if measurements are not made using standard measurement techniques and appropriate prediction equations (Houtkooper et al., 1996). Standard techniques include having the individual recline on a nonconducting surface, restriction of the individual's food intake 3 to 4 hours prior to measurement, and the standard placement of electrodes. The accuracy of prediction equations derived from BIA is improved when population-specific equations that have been validated and crossvalidated using multicomponent criterion methods are used (Houtkooper et al., 1996; Lohman, 1992).

Biomarkers of Renal Function

Identifying potential markers of renal function (see Figure 4-4) deserves attention because of the role of the kidney in maintaining protein status, electrolyte balance, and hydration status. Acute renal failure may occur within hours, and without proper kidney functioning, death ensues within a few weeks to a month (Kopple, 1999).

Large amounts of protein are not usual constituents of the urine and when they are present, they indicate pathology. Perhaps the most common pathological state associated with proteinuria is rhambdomyosis, secondary to the breakdown of muscle; but other possible causes, such as fever, infection, and unidentified renal damage from other causes (e.g., diabetes and renal disease), may also be involved. It is important to eliminate the possibility of contamination from feces (or in females, menstrual blood) in the urine sample. This is often done by discarding the early portion of the void. Urinary tract infections may be signaled by the presence of leukocyte esterase or nitrites in the urine (Beers and Berkow, 1999), and although urinary tract infections may not be debilitating, they may cause later renal damage (Beers and Berkow, 1999).

Dipstick strips that test for blood, protein, urobilinogen, glucose, ketones, pH, leukocyte esterase, and nitrites are now available on a single-purpose strip in 1-oz dispensers that are color coded, permitting the individual to read them easily. If a digital camera were available, it could be used to record the calorimetric information as well. Readings are usually on a scale (e.g., protein 1, 2, 3, 4, etc.) for each indicator; values above 3 or 4 signify significant abnormality. A reading of blood hemoglobin or myoglobin greater than 3 or 4 and a high urine protein greater than 3 or 4 might signal that the risk of kidney damage is elevated. If this is combined with a high specific gravity, there is even greater cause for concern. Abnormal nitrates and leukocyte esterase values suggest that urinary tract infection may be present. If core temperature is above 38°C (~100°F) or below 36°C (~97°F) and/or pulse is over 70 beats/min, the index of suspicion for urinary tract infection rises further.

Protein

One of the kidney's functions is to eliminate the products of protein metabolism, and when this does not occur, as in renal failure, metabolism is severely deranged. As mentioned above, having relatively large amounts of protein in the urine is abnormal and is likely to signal renal damage. Other pathological conditions can lead to losses of protein in the urine; these include nephrolithiasis (major losses), early renal failure, and glomerulosclerosis (Walser, 1999). However, under field conditions among individuals who have

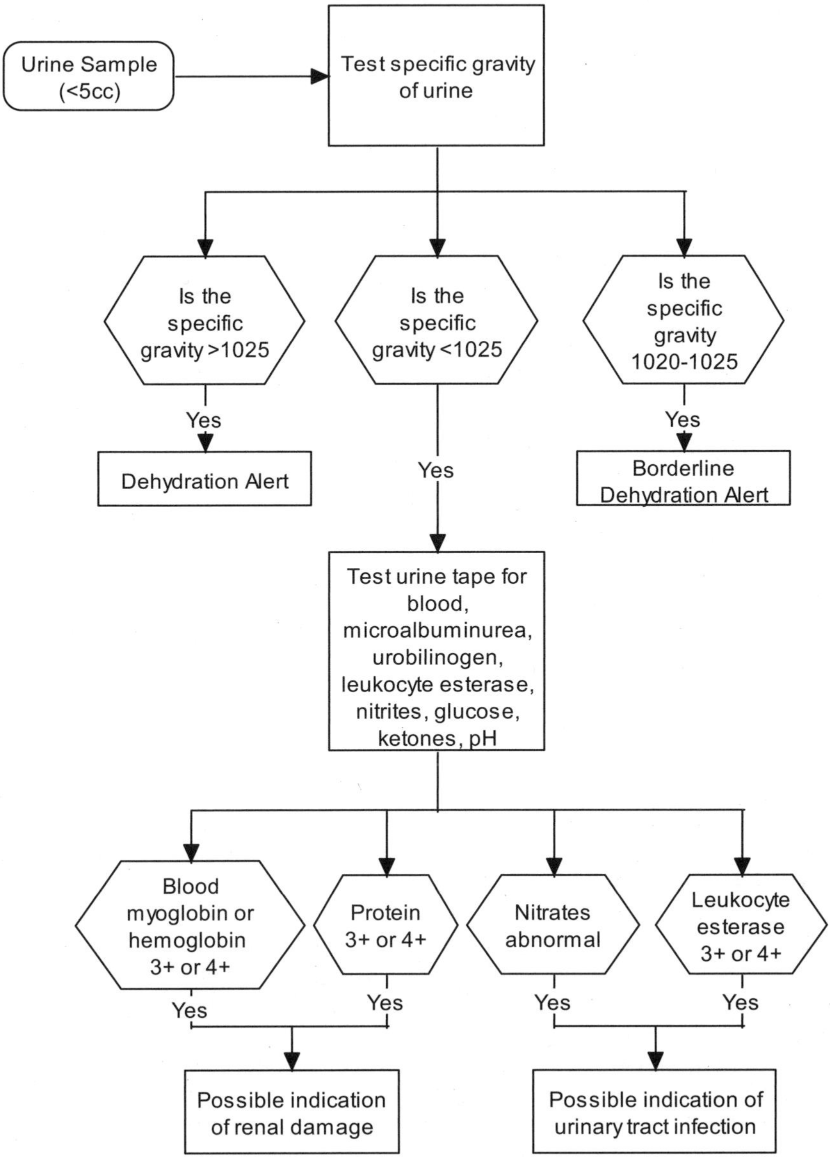

FIGURE 4-4 Procedure for renal function assessment.

TABLE 4-3 Various Types of Dehydration and Their Effects on Body Fluid Spaces

Status	Extracellular Volume	Intracellular Volume
Normal	Normal	Normal
Isotonic dehydration	Decreased	Normal
Hypertonic dehydration	Decreased	Decreased
Hypotonic dehydration	Decreased	Increased

engaged in heavy exertion and exercise, protein in the urine often signals muscle damage. If it is extensive, it can lead to acute renal failure.

Several biochemical indicators, including blood urea nitrogen and serum creatinine, have some associations with protein status. However, concentrations of these indicators will also be influenced by hydration status. High blood urea nitrogen or high serum creatinine suggests that protein intake is very high, protein catabolism is very high, the individual is very dehydrated, or kidney function is abnormal. The problem with these measures is that multiple processes and factors, not simply hydration status, influence all of them. There are no simple method to measure these markers.

Possible urine measures of protein status might include urinary nitrogen, urinary creatinine, and 3-methylhistidine. These might signal changes in protein status, but they do not appear to be useful under field conditions.

Electrolytes

The kidneys also play a vital role in electrolyte homeostasis. Fluid intake regulation is influenced by plasma osmolality and volume, both of which are affected by kidney function, as well as by other factors (Nose et al., 1994). Exertion and other stresses during field operations affect not only water metabolism, but also electrolytes. Water shifts between the intracellular and extracellular compartments cause shifts in sodium, potassium, magnesium, and chloride ions. Sweating also causes electrolyte loss. In hot environments, "...individuals routinely have sweat rates of 1 liter per hour. Dehydration from sweat loss increases plasma tonicity and decreases blood volume, both of which reduce heat loss and result in elevated core temperature levels during exercise heat stress. Additionally, during exercise-heat stress, competing metabolic and thermoregulatory demands for blood flow make it difficult to maintain adequate cardiac output" (IOM, 1993, P. 71), and with continued stress, may result in renal failure. Prolonged moderate- to high-intensity activity, especially in hot environments, will lead to a significant loss of electrolytes (sodium, potassium, and magnesium), especially in individuals who are not adapted to hot environments.

The relative amounts of electrolytes versus water that are lost will determine whether the dehydration is isotonic (net salt and water loss equal), hypertonic (water alone is lost or water in excess of electrolytes is lost) or hypotonic (electrolyte loss exceeds water loss; see Table 4-3) (Oh and Uribarri, 1999).

Urinary water excretion varies greatly depending on the total amount of solute that is excreted, the urine osmolality, and the presence of fever or sweating.

Isotonic dehydration under field conditions might occur due to gastrointestinal fluid loses, with salt lost with an equal or larger quantity of water lost, and depletion of the extracellular volume. The osmolality of the body fluids can be adjusted to isotonicity either by urinary excretion of water or by oral salt intake.

Hypertonic dehydration is due to water deficit that in turn may be due to either inadequacy of water intake or excessive water loss. Under field conditions, inadequate water intake might be due to defective thirst signals, the lack of water, or an inability to drink water. Increased water loss due to sweating, osmotic diarrheas, vomiting, and hyperventilation may also occur. The end result of hypertonic dehydration is depletion in both the extracellular volume and the intracellular volume.

The various forms of dehydration (isotonic, hypotonic, and hypertonic) could theoretically be distinguished from each other by the use of "point of care" electrolyte kits that are relatively compact (egg size) and assess sodium, potassium, carbon dioxide, and chloride. However, from the standpoint of field conditions, all forms of dehydration are of concern. Water replacement is important for all forms. Although hypotonic salt replacement is most important in hypotonic dehydration, isotonic dehydration will not be harmed by the provision of modest salt replacement in addition to water, whereas in hypertonic dehydration salt replacement should be dilute (< 40 mEq/L water replacement).

Hydration Status Measures

The maintenance of proper hydration status is a critical issue facing combat military personnel in the field, especially in hot environments (IOM, 1994). Fluid deprivation may be due to extracellular volume deficiency, pure water deficiency (dehydration), or both (see Table 4-4) (Hoffer, 1999). Both water loss and a combination of water and sodium loss may deplete the extracellular fluid volume. Changes in weight over a short time (hours) are indicators of hydration status. At present, changes in hydration status cannot easily be measured by strain gauges or by other techniques in the field. Similarly, hyper- or hyponatremic dehydration cannot accurately be measured in the field. In the future, if miniaturized and field-usable forms of NIRS become available to measure serum sodium, and measures of weight are feasible in the field, it will be possible to refine these measurements (see earlier section, "Biomarkers of Muscle Metabolism and Fatigue"). Carter and colleagues (2003) described various methods for measuring hydration (see Appendix A), but only some of these are promising at present for use in the field.

TABLE 4-4 Various Types of Fluid Deprivation

Condition	Symptoms
Volume deficiency: combination of sodium and water loss deplete extracellular fluid volume	Anorexia Nausea Thirst either present or absent
Dehydration (water deficiency)	Anorexia with continued deprivation of water and hyperosmolality, confusion, weakness, lethargy, obtundation, coma Dry mouth Fatigue Headache, but a late symptom that develops slowly Thirst
Combinations of these	

Urine Specific Gravity

The most straightforward method for measuring hydration status is to assess urine specific gravity. If this were done at mid-day and at the end of the day, it might be most helpful since it would assess hydration status during or afterstress experiences that might perturb it. Miniaturized (pen-size) instruments with eyepieces are available—a drop of urine is all that is needed—and can be read in the field. When available, methods based on measurement of osmolality should also be used.

Although the measurement of first-morning urine specific gravity in the field may be feasible, individuals could also be trained to associate a urine specific gravity that represents dehydration with their urine color (urine color charts are available) (Casa et al., 2000). They could then use either color or odor to monitor their own level of hydration.

Clinical Signs	Biochemical Signs
Diminished sweat Dry mucous membranes Poor skin turgor Postural hypotension Weight loss	Hyponatremia (variable) Increased serum urea concentration due to decreased renal glomerular filtration and urea clearance
Diminished sweat Dry mucous membranes For each 1% loss in body weight, there is approximately an increase of 0.4°–0.5°C in rectal temperature, a 2.5% decrease in plasma volume, and a 1% decline in muscle water Poor skin turgor Postural hypotension Renal failure with extreme dehydration There is increased strain on the cardiovascular and thermoregulatory systems with as little as 2% body-weight loss; at 4% body-weight loss, muscle strength declines Weight loss	Hypernatremia Increased plasma viscosity with lesser increases in serum sodium, albumin, and hematocrit; with continuing water deprivation, rising serum sodium and hyperosmolality and increased blood urea and hemoconcentration

Urine Color and Odor

Urine color and odor are more subjective methods and therefore are not ideal for determining dehydration, but a deep color or strong odor is corroborative. If the urine has a dark color or strong odor, then the individual is dehydrated. Urine color may be a better field indicator of dehydration than urine volume (Armstrong et al., 1998). Individuals should drink until their urine color is either a "very pale yellow" or "pale yellow." However, this may not be the best measure of hydration status within 6 hours of physical activity-caused dehydration (Kovacs et al., 1999).

Urine Volume

Urine volume is difficult and impractical to track, but it may corroborate other measures of dehydration. If urine color cannot be measured, then urine volume may be the only field indicator of hydration level available. Active individuals should drink enough fluids to produce 1 to 2 L of urine per day.

Voids per Day

Voids per day are also difficult to track under field situations, but few or no voids are corroborative of dehydration.

Calculation of Sweat Rate Using Changes in Body Weight

A decrease in body weight by 1 percent can cause a decrease in exercise performance. In order to measure changes in body mass due to physical activity, body weight needs to be measured before and after exercise. Sweat rate is calculated as follows:

Sweat rate = preexercise body weight – postexercise body weight + fluid intake – urine volume/exercise time in hours

Although the measurement of sweat rate and changes in body weight may be easy in a sport setting where locker rooms are available, this becomes more difficult in a field setting. It might be easier to determine an individual's sweat rate in a controlled setting and then use this rate to estimate sweat losses in the field. For example, an individual's sweat rate could be determined by measuring weight loss after a 1-hour, intense training period under environmental conditions that mimic what is expected to occur in the field. The amount of fluid lost in this hour would then represent the amount an individual would need to drink in the field for every hour of physical activity. The development of a way for combat service members to monitor short-term changes in body weight in the field would be a useful method for measuring fluid balance. These same measurements, over a longer period, could be used to determine if adequate energy is being provided to cover total energy expenditure.

Thirst

By the time an individual is thirsty, some level of dehydration has already occurred (~1 percent). Individuals can be trained to drink frequently in hot environments even when they are not thirsty, thus reducing their risk of dehydration. Teaching military personnel how to drink frequently for adequate hydration can be easily done through training and by providing military personnel with quantitative camel packs or insulated sport bottles for carrying fluids.

BIOMARKERS OF STRESS AND IMMUNE FUNCTION

Evidence revealing bidirectional communications between the neuroendocrine and immune systems has been derived from neuroendocrine, behavioral, and immunological studies using animals and humans (Ader et al., 1995; Cohen and Kinney, 2001; Maier et al., 1994; Sternberg et al., 1992; Webster et al., 2002). Other studies have shown that a variety of physical and psychosocial stressors can alter immune responsiveness (Biondi, 1991; Esterling et al., 1996; Kiecolt-Glaser et al., 1993; Kusnecov et al., 2001). While previous studies assumed that all stress was generally immunosuppressive, recent evidence indicates that different types of stress and different components of the physiological stress response have specific effects on different components of the immune response. In addition, the duration and timing of the stressor in relation to immune exposures also affect how stress influences immunity and immune-mediated processes.

Stress can be defined as a constellation of events that begins with a stimulus, called the stressor, that precipitates a reaction in the brain (stress perception) and subsequently activates physiological systems in the body, called the stress response (Dhabhar and McEwen, 2001). The stress response results in the release of neurotransmitters and hormones that serve as the brain's messengers for regulation of the immune and other systems. The consequences of this response are generally adaptative in the short run, but can be damaging when stress is chronic (Dhabhar and McEwen, 2001).

Conversely, the immune system produces chemical messengers (cytokines) that play a crucial role in mediating inflammatory and immune responses and that also serve as mediators between the immune system and the central nervous system (Kronfol and Remick, 2000).

Considering the interactions between these systems, monitoring of biomarkers of stress and immune function should ideally include monitoring the immune system and the neuronal and hormonal arms of the stress response at multiple levels. This includes monitoring the expression of immune and nervous system genes, receptors, and maturation or activation markers in accessible cells and tissues (Wei et al., 2003). Thus categories of molecules that could be monitored include: immune mediators (cytokines including ILs) (Kang et al., 1997; Rothermundt et al., 2001; Song et al., 1999), immune-cell activation markers, and neuropeptides and neurohormones secreted in bodily fluids, including blood, saliva, or sweat (Ahmed et al., 1996; Murphy, 1995; Niess et al., 2002; Scott and Dinan 1998; Strickland et al., 1998).

Intermediate functional measures of neuronal and neuroendocrine responsiveness, which should also be monitored, include measures of heart rate variability (HRV) as an indicator of relative sympathetic and parasympathetic responsiveness (Brook and Julius, 2000), and hormonal measures of adrenergic and hypothalamic-pituitary-adrenal (HPA) axis responsiveness, such as cortisol (Biondi et al., 1994; Moynihan, 2003; Niess et al., 2002) and neuropeptide Y (Zukowska et al., 2003) secretion, respectively. Functional measures of immune responsiveness that can be measured include the production of antibodies to vaccine and measures of cellular and innate immunity (Glaser et al., 1992; Vedhara et al., 1999). Functional integrity at the organ and system levels may include outcome measures of the central nervous system, cognitive function and mood, immune outcome measures of susceptibility to infection (Kasl et al.,

1979; Totman et al., 1980), and speed of wound healing (Kiecolt-Glaser et al., 1995; Marucha et al., 2001).

The measures selected to monitor stress and immune function will depend on the setting in which the monitoring is performed. While a full battery of biomarkers and functional measures can be assessed in the clinical laboratory setting (see Appendix A), a more limited battery may be applied in ambulatory or field settings. For example, a minimum battery of cytokine measures that is currently used include IL-10 and IL-4 as markers of T helper type 1 (Th1) response, and interferon-gamma (IFNγ) and IL-6 as markers of Th2 response and innate immunity response. In addition, cortisol and HRV are currently used as markers of neuroendocrine and neuronal responsiveness, respectively

The rate of change of stress hormones away from and back to baseline in response to stressful stimuli is a critical variable in adaptive physiological responses. An important aspect of monitoring should include measurements at baseline (prior to exposure to the stressor), during the stress exposure, and during the period of recovery (postexposure to the stressor) (Ader et al., 1995; Biondi, 2001). The first two measurement periods, baseline and stress exposure, provide insights into individual degrees of stress responsiveness that cannot be detected by baseline measures alone. The latter period, poststress exposure, is important to gain insight into the pattern and resiliency of the individual's stress responsiveness and the speed and completeness with which the responses return to baseline.

In ambulatory settings, the less invasive the method for obtaining samples, the less the measurement itself will perturb the system. It is thus important to develop methods to measure and validate intermediate neural and immune markers in tissues other than blood. Any electronic monitoring should be relatively noninvasive, and any psychological instruments to measure cognition and mood should be relatively noninvasive.

The Stress Response

The HPA axis and the sympathetic adrenomedullary system are the primary neuroendocrine components of the stress response (Chrousos, 1998; Eskandari and Sternberg, 2002; Goldstein, 1995; Sternberg, 1998) and are further described below. Release of cortisol from the adrenal cortex, catecholamine from the adrenal medulla, and norepinephrine from nerve terminals prepare the individual to cope with the demands of metabolic, physical, and psychological stressors. These two systems interact in a dynamic fashion in response to challenge. The stress response must be tightly controlled because an exaggerated response can by itself be a source of illness to the individual (Dhabhar and McEwen, 2001; Webster et al., 2002)

After exposure to any stressor, the neuronal response is first activated and then elicits the hormonal stress response (Guyton and Hall, 1997). Contrary to previous belief, it is now known that the stress response is not nonspecific, but shows specificity in patterns of response depending on the nature of the stimulus. Thus different stressors (physiological, psychological, inflammatory, or infectious) differentially activate components of the stress response and activate different brain regions (Goldstein, 1995; Sawchenko and Arias, 1995; Sawchenko et al., 2000).

Autonomic Nervous System

There is growing evidence for a role of the autonomic nervous system (ANS) in a wide range of diseases. The ANS is generally conceived to have two major branches: the sympathetic system, associated with energy mobilization, and the parasympathetic system, associated with vegetative and restorative functions. Normally the activity of these branches is in dynamic balance. For example, there is a well-documented circadian rhythm such that sympathetic activity is higher during daytime hours and parasympathetic activity increases at night. There are other periodicities present, and the activity of the two branches can be rapidly modulated in response to changing environmental demands.

More modern conceptions of organism function that are based on complexity theory hold that organism stability, adaptability, and health are maintained through variability in the dynamic relationship among system elements (Friedman and Thayer, 1998a, 1998b; Thayer and Friedman, 1997; Thayer and Lane, 2000). Thus patterns of organized variability, rather than static levels, are preserved in the face of constantly changing environmental demands. This conception, in contrast to homeostasis, posits that the system has multiple points of stability, which necessitates a dynamic organization of resources to match specific situational demands. These demands can be conceived in terms of energy regulation such that the points of relative stability represent local energy minima required by the situation. For example, in healthy individuals average HR is greater during the day than during the night because energy demands are greater during the day. Thus the system has a local energy minimum, or attractor, for daytime and another for nighttime. Because the system operates "far-from-equilibrium," it is always searching for local energy minima to minimize the energy requirements of the organism. Consequentially, optimal system functioning is achieved via lability and variability in its component processes, and rigid regularity is associated with mortality, morbidity, and ill health (Lipsitz and Goldberger, 1992; Peng et al., 1994).

Another corollary of this view is that autonomic imbalance, in which one branch of the ANS dominates over the other, is associated with a lack of dynamic flexibility and health. Empirically, there is a large body of evidence to suggest that autonomic imbalance, in which typically the sympathetic system is hyperactive and the parasympathetic system is hypoactive, is associated with various pathological conditions (Malliani et al., 1994). In particular, when the sympathetic branch dominates for long periods of time, the energy demands on the system becomes excessive and ultimately cannot be met, eventually causing death. The prolonged state of alarm associated with negative emotions likewise places an excessive energy demand on the system. On the way to death, however, premature aging and disease characterize a system dominated by negative effect and autonomic imbalance.

Like many organs in the body, the heart is dually innervated. Although a wide range of physiologic factors determines HR, the ANS is the most prominent. Importantly, when both cardiac vagal (the primary parasympathetic nerve) and sympathetic inputs are blocked pharmacologically (for example, with atropine plus propranolol, the so-called double blockade), intrinsic HR is higher than normal resting HR (Jose and Collison, 1970). This fact supports the idea that the heart is under tonic inhibitory control by parasympathetic influences. Thus, resting cardiac autonomic balance favors energy conservation by way of parasympathetic dominance over sympathetic influences. In addition, the HR time series is characterized by beat-to-beat variability over a wide range, which also implicates vagal dominance. Lowered HRV is associated with increased risk of mortality, and HRV has been proposed as a marker for disease (Task Force of the European Society of Cardiology the North American Society of Pacing Electrophysiology, 1996).

Resting HR can be used as a rough indicator of autonomic balance, and several large studies have shown a largely linear, positive dose-response relationship between resting HR and all-cause mortality (see Habib, 1999). This association was independent of gender and ethnicity and showed a threefold increase in mortality in persons with HR over 90 beats/min compared with those persons with HRs less than 60 beats/min. It was suggested that this relationship is due to the role of HR as a major determinant of myocardial oxygen demand and the direct link of HR to the rate of myocardial energy use.

Brook and Julius (2000) have recently detailed how autonomic imbalance in the sympathetic direction is associated with a range of metabolic, hemodynamic, trophic, and rheologic abnormalities that contribute to elevated cardiac morbidity and mortality. Although the relationship between HR and cardiovascular morbidity and mortality may be assumed, the fact that autonomic imbalance and HR are related to other diseases may not be as obvious. However, links do exist. For example, HRV has been shown to be associated with diabetes mellitus, and decreased HRV has been shown to precede evidence of disease provided by standard clinical tests (Ziegler et al., 2001). In addition, immune dysfunction and inflammation have been implicated in a wide range of conditions associated with aging, including cardiovascular disease, diabetes, osteoporosis, arthritis, Alzheimer's disease, periodontal disease, and certain types of cancers, as well as with declines in muscle strength and increased frailty and disability (Ershler and Keller, 2000; Kiecolt-Glaser et al., 2002). The common mechanism seems to involve excess proinflammatory cytokines, such as IL-1, IL-6, and tumor necrosis factor. Importantly, increased parasympathetic tone and acetylcholine (the primary parasympathetic neurotransmitter) have been shown to attenuate release of these proinflammatory cytokines, and sympathetic hyperactivity is associated with their increased production (Das, 2000). Thus autonomic imbalance may be a final common pathway to increased morbidity and mortality from a host of conditions and diseases.

Although the idea is not new (Sternberg, 1997), several recent reviews have provided strong evidence linking negative affective states and dispositions to disease and ill health (Friedman and Thayer, 1998a; Kiecolt-Glaser et al., 2002; Krantz and McCeney, 2002; Musselman et al., 1998; Rozanski et al., 1999; Verrier and Mittleman, 2000). All of these reviews implicate altered ANS function and decreased parasympathetic activity as a possible mediator in this link.

An additional pathway between psychosocial stressors and ill health is an indirect one in which psychosocial factors lead to poor lifestyle choices, including a lack of physical activity and the abuse of tobacco, alcohol, and drugs. Both sedentary lifestyle and substance abuse are associated with autonomic imbalance and decreased parasympathetic tone (Nabors-Oberg et al., 2002; Reed et al., 1999; Rossy and Thayer, 1998; Weise et al., 1986). In fact, the therapeutic effectiveness of smoking cessation, reduced alcohol consumption, and increased physical activity rest in part on their ability to restore autonomic balance and increase parasympathetic tone.

In sum, autonomic imbalance, and decreased parasympathetic tone in particular, may be the final common pathway linking negative effective states and dispositions, including the indirect effects of poor lifestyle, to numerous diseases and conditions associated with aging and increased morbidity and mortality.

Several lines of research point to the significance of HRV in emotions and health. Decreased HRV is linked with a number of disease states (e.g., cardiovascular disease, diabetes, and obesity), and a lack of physical exercise (Stein and Kleiger, 1999). Reduced vagally-mediated HRV is also associated with a number of psychological disease states (e.g., anxiety, depression, and hostility). For example, low HRV is consistent with the cardiac symptoms of panic anxiety, as well as with its psychological expressions in poor attentional control, poor emotion regulation, and behavioral inflexibility (Friedman and Thayer, 1998a, 1998b). Similar reductions in HRV have been found in depression (Thayer et al., 1998), generalized anxiety disorder (Thayer et al., 1996), and post-traumatic stress disorder (Cohen et al., 1999). Low levels of vagal cardiovascular influence serve to disinhibit sympathoexcitatory influences. Due to differences in the temporal kinetics of the autonomic neuroeffectors, sympathetic effects on cardiac control are relatively slow (an order of magnitude of seconds) compared with vagal effects (an order of magnitude of milliseconds; see Saul, 1990). Thus when this rapid vagal cardiac control is low, HR cannot change as quickly in response to environmental changes. In this view, the prefrontal cortex modulates subcortical motivational circuits to serve goal-directed behavior. When the prefrontal cortex is taken "off-line" for whatever reason, a relative sympathetic dominance associated with disinhibited defensive circuits is released.

The Hypothalamic-Pituitary-Adrenal Axis

The hormones of the hormonal stress response, which together constitute the HPA axis, include corticotropin-releasing hormone (CRH), which is released from the hypothalamus; adrenocorticotropin (ACTH), which is released from the pituitary gland; and cortisol, which is released from the adrenal glands (Webster et al., 2002). CRH, released into the median eminence through the portal circulation from neuronal cells of the paraventricular nucleus in the hypothalamus, acts on the anterior pituitary in conjunction with arginine vasopressin to release ACTH. Secretion of ACTH signals the adrenal glands to increase the production and secretion of cortisol (Chrousos and Gold, 1992; Scott and Dinan, 1998).

Negative feedback by cortisol is the principal mechanism of regulatory control of the HPA axis, specifically on the pituitary-adrenal component. In addition, cortisol may modulate some of the physiological effects of catecholamines (Eskandari and Sternberg, 2002; Ligier and Sternberg, 2001). CRH is also negatively regulated by ACTH and itself, as well as by other neuropeptides, such as γ-aminobutyric acid/benzodiazepines and opioid peptide systems (Calogero et al., 1988b, 1988d).

The HPA axis is also positively regulated by neurotransmitters, such as serotonin (Bagdy et al., 1989; Calogero et al., 1989, 1990), acetylcholine (Calogero et al., 1988c), and catecholamines (Calogero et al., 1988a).

Almost immediately after an activation of the HPA axis (e.g., a stressful event), the levels of the regulatory hormones ACTH and CRH increase, causing a rise in cortisol levels. Once released into the circulation, a primary function of cortisol is to make energy stores available for use throughout the body by increasing protein catabolism and gluconeogenesis (Gold et al., 1988).

Recent studies show that depending on dose or preparation, cortisol may enhance or suppress immunological and other physiological parameters. Low levels of glucocorticoids are generally stimulatory for a physiological process, whereas higher levels are inhibitory (Dhabhar and McEwen, 2001). Also, most of the adaptive changes conferred by cortisol are limited to its acute, rather than chronic, release (Gold and Chrousos, 2002). Chronic cortisol release is almost always deleterious and results in a variety of physical and emotional effects, including insulin resistance, visceral fat deposition and its many proatherogenic sequelae, osteopenia/osteoporosis, and excessive fear (Gold and Chrousos, 2002).

When cortisol is secreted it causes a breakdown of muscle protein, leading to release of amino acids into the bloodstream. These amino acids are then used by the liver for gluconeogenesis. This process raises the blood sugar level so that the brain will have more glucose for energy. At the same time, the other tissues of the body decrease their use of glucose as fuel. Cortisol also causes the release of fatty acids from adipose tissue for use by the muscles. Taken together, these energy-directing processes prepare the individual to deal with stressors and ensure that the brain receives adequate energy sources (Gold and Chrousos, 2002).

Glucocorticoids regulate a wide variety of immune cell expressions and function, including production of cytokines, adhesion molecular expression, immune cell trafficking, immune cell maturation and differentiation, expression of chemoattractants and cell migration, and production of inflammatory mediators and other inflammatory molecules (Webster et al., 2002). Exposure to physiological concentrations of stress hormones exerts biphasic effects on immune function, that is, they are immunomodulatory rather than simply immunosuppressive. Some important factors that determine the nature of the effects that glucocorticoids have on a given immune response include the source (natural vs. synthetic), concentration (physiological vs. pharmacological), the effects that other factors have (hormone, cytokines, and neurotransmitters), and the state of activation of an immune parameter (naive vs. activated leukocyte vs. late activated) (Dhabhar, 2002).

Acute administration of physiological doses of endogenous cortisol can significantly enhance some immune responses (Dhabhar and McEwen, 1999), whereas chronic and acute administration of high doses of endogenous cortisol are immunosuppressive (Dhabhar and McEwen, 1999). This dose-response relationship has been described for the biphasic effects of cortisol on several immunological parameters, including the skin delayed-type hypersensitivity response in vivo (Dhabhar, 1998; Dhabhar and McEwen, 1999), synthesis and secretion of immunoglobulin (Levo et al., 1985), T-cell mitogenesis (Stanulis et al., 1997; Wiegers et al., 1994), and macrophage phagocytosis (Forner et al., 1995). The immunomodulatory actions of glucocorticoids may be related to a shift of cytokine production from a primarily proinflammatory to an anti-inflammatory pattern (Elenkov et al., 2000; Sternberg, 2001), also categorized as Th1 or Th2. A Th1 pattern of cytokines is characterized by production of largely proinflammatory IL-2 and IFNγ and generally mediates cellular immune reactions. A Th2 pattern of immunity is characterized by production of IL-4 and IL-10 and is associated with a primarily humoral or antibody response (Sternberg, 2001). At physiological concentrations, glucocorticoids inhibit Th1 and enhance Th2 cytokine production, thus causing a shift in immune responses from a cellular immune to a humoral pattern of response. Such glucocorticoid-induced shifts may protect against some forms of autoimmune disease (Sternberg, 2001), but exacerbate others (Elenkov et al., 2000).

Psychological Stress and Immunity

Psychological stimuli exert profound effects on the HPA axis, generally causing cortisol elevations. However, in some circumstances, the stimuli cause the suppression of cortisol (Biondi, 2001).

Some important parameters that should be considered in determining the HPA responses to a stress situation and these HPA response effects on immune responses include stress characteristics (magnitude, psychological, physical, and avoidable or not), immunological outcome measure (cellular or humoral), biological characteristics of the individual under study, and the individual's perception, interpretation, and evaluation of the stress situation and specific stress-coping strategies (Ader et al., 1995; Olff, 1999).

Thus to assess the consequences of stress on immune responses, it is important to first identify the specific characteristics of the stress and to quantify its magnitude, which can be regarded as a combination of its intensity, duration, and frequency (Dhabhar and McEwen, 2001). The intensity of a stress can be measured by peak levels of stress hormones and neurotransmitters, and by physiological changes, such as increases in HR and blood pressure. The duration of stress can be classified as acute (for a period of minutes to hours), or chronic (for a period of several hours to a number of months) (Dhabhar and McEwen, 2001).

Another important point to address in such studies is the individual's perception of the stressful situation and the availability and effectiveness of the individual's ways of coping with the situation. A situation may be perceived as threatening if the individual does not have control and appraises his or her resources as less than effective in dealing with the situation. In general, distressing situations (e.g., those characterized by threat, lack of control, uncertainty, novelty, and anticipation of aversive events) are associated with an increase in cortisol release (Olff, 1999). In addition to these psychological measures, changes in cortisol secretion can be used as a measure of the reactivity of the stress response system. Chronic hypersecretion of cortisol has been associated with the melancholic form of depression, while hyposecretion of cortisol has been associated with atypical depression, emotional numbing, withdrawal, and avoidance in post-traumatic stress disorder and in normal populations (Holsboer et al., 1984; Yehuda et al., 1996, 2000).

Immunological Alterations After Acute and Chronic Psychological Stress

Under normal conditions, acute stress may serve a protective role by enhancing immune responses directed toward a wound, infection, or cancer. However, such immune enhancement can be deleterious for autoimmune and inflammatory disorders (Dhabhar and McEwen, 2001). Immunological changes that have been reported in association with acute psychological stress include enhanced delayed-type hypersensitivity and immune cell trafficking into tissues (Dhabhar and McEwen, 1999), transient increases in the number and activity of natural killer (NK) cells (van der Pompe et al., 1998), and transient increases in leukocyte count (Mills et al., 1995).

During chronic stress, high levels of glucocorticoids suppress most aspects of the immune responses, including humoral, cellular, and innate immunity; immune cell trafficking out of the blood and into tissues (Dhabhar and McEwen, 1997); and the ability to fight infection and mount an antibody response (Dhabhar, 2002). Thus chronic or subacute stress is consistently associated with decreased immune cell function and maturation, decreased mitogen responses (Weiss et al., 1996), reduced numbers of NK cells and NK-cell activity (Irwin et al., 1988), reduced antibody production in response to vaccine (Kiecolt-Glaser et al., 1988, 1993), suppressed delayed-type hypersensitivity response (Dhabhar and McEwen, 1997), and suppressed and prolonged wound healing (Kiecolt-Glaser et al., 1995). Also during stress, patterns of immune responses are shifted from a Th1 (mainly cellular) to a Th2 (mainly humoral) pattern of response. Thus levels of proinflammatory cytokines are suppressed by glucocorticoids, and anti-inflammatory cytokines are increased, leading to overall immunosuppression.

Both the sympathetic and neuroendocrine arms of the stress response are involved in these effects of stress on immunity, as evidenced by the fact that in animal models pharmacological interruption with both beta adrenergic and glucocorticoid antagonists is required to completely abrogate these effects (Webster et al., 2002).

Interruption of the neuroendocrine stress response (HPA axis) is associated with enhanced mortality and incidence of septic shock in rodent animal models. Thus interruption of the HPA axis at the level of the pituitary with hypophysectomy, at the level of the adrenal with adrenalectomy, and through pharmacological interruption at the level of the glucocorticoid receptor, have all been shown to be associated with increased mortality from septic shock after exposure to salmonella, streptococcal bacterial cell walls, bacterial lipopolysaccharide (Webster et al., 2002), murine cytomegalovirus (Ruzek et al., 1999), and toxicity related to Shiga toxin (Gomez et al., 2003). Furthermore, a blunted HPA-axis hormone response has been associated with susceptibility to a variety of autoimmune and inflammatory diseases across species and in chicken, mice, rats, and humans (Bonneau et al., 1993; Mason et al., 1990; Sternberg et al., 1992; Wick et al., 1987).

Thus systemically, an over-reactive immune response, through activation of the stress system, stimulates an important negative feedback mechanism that protects the organism from "overshoot" of proinflammatory cytokines and other products of activated macrophages with tissue damaging potential. Conversely, a blunted hormonal stress response may enhance immune responses and susceptibility to autoimmune disease as a consequence of inadequate responsiveness of this negative feedback loop.

Immunological Alterations After Physical Stress: Overtraining Syndrome and Excessive Exercise

Immunological alterations can also appear in the Overtraining Syndrome (OTS). This is a condition that occurs when an athlete is training intensely but, instead of showing improvement, shows deterioration in performance, even after an appropriate rest period (MacKinnon, 2000).

Classic symptoms of overtraining include profound mood changes (feelings of depression and emotional instability), extreme fatigue (apathy), and frequent illnesses (flu-like illness, bacterial infection, allergies). Others symptoms, such as deficits in concentration, fear of competition, prolonged recovery, decreased muscular strength, loss of coordination, insomnia, and loss of appetite, may also occur. Biochemical alterations, such as negative nitrogen balance, depressed muscle glycogen concentration, elevated cortisol, and a low level of free testosterone, are also seen (Fry et al., 1991). The condition should be distinguished from overreaching, which is a temporary deterioration in athletic performance with recovery and improvement after sufficient rest (Fry and Kraemer, 1997).

Evidence in a few empirical studies of OTS and in excessive exercise showed immune alterations manifested as increased susceptibility to infectious illnesses, such as upper respiratory tract infections, usually with a viral etiology (MacKinnon, 2000; Nieman, 2000; Sevier, 1994; Shephard and Shek, 2001). Other infections may occur in the ear and skin (Sevier, 1994). Intestinal upset, slow wound healing, and increased sensitivity to environmental and food allergens have also been reported (Sevier, 1994). Laboratory measures show suppressed neutrophil function, suppressed lymphocyte count and proliferation, suppressed NK cell count and activity, changes in polymorphonuclear cell priming potential, and decreased serum, nasal, and salivary immunoglobulins (MacKinnon, 2000; Müns, 1994; Pedersen et al., 1999; Suzuki et al., 2000). Alterations in others measures, such as cytokine levels and stress hormones, were found in some studies (Müns, 1994; Suzuki et al., 2000).

Some theories have attempted to explain the relationship among immune suppression, OTS, and excessive exercise. Some studies have found lower serum glutamine levels in athletes during seasonal periods of intense training, which may interfere with optimal immune function (MacKinnon, 2000; Newsholme, 1994). Other theories focus on the "open window" model, which is a similar situation where immunosuppression is seen after exhaustive aerobic exercise, such as marathon running. Pedersen and colleagues (1999) have suggested that the time period between 3 and 72 hours after exercise represents an open window that is associated with an increased risk of developing subclinical and clinical infections. Some researchers have proposed that the athlete who trains excessively without sufficient recovery time shows a cumulative effect of the vulnerable open window period, which leads to a more chronic form of immunosuppression (Lakier Smith, 2003).

It has also been proposed that in OTS, excessive exercise, and marathon running, athletes may develop trauma in muscle and connective tissues, which activates local cells to produce cytokines that stimulate a Th2 humoral profile (Lakier Smith, 2003). As described above, when Th2 responses are up-regulated (humoral immunity), there is a suppression of Th1 responses (cellular immunity) (Abbas et al., 2000). Evidence for this hypothesis has been shown in studies of athletes after a marathon, where higher levels of tumor necrosis factor-α and Th2 cytokines, including IL-6 and IL-10 (Lakier Smith, 2003; Suzuki et al.,

2000), and lower levels of IL-12 and IFNγ (Lakier Smith, 2003) are seen. This pattern of immune responses—an up-regulation of the Th2 humoral response and suppressed Th1 cellular responses—would be consistent with reported higher levels of stress hormones (cortisol and catecholamine) in athletes postexercise (Steensberg et al., 2001) and in OTS (MacKinnon, 2000). It should be pointed out that higher levels of stress hormones also occur in response to psychological stress. Thus in OTS and excessive exercise, the stress of high-intensity training may be superimposed with psychological stressors, leading to further increases in an athlete's susceptibility to infection (Lakier Smith, 2003). For studies in this field, it may be important to measure immunological parameters in the open window period, as it seems to be a particularly vulnerable period (Nieman, 2000; Smith, 2000).

Monitoring Stress and Immune Function

This section outlines general categories of biomarkers that are currently used to measure both physiological stress responses and immune responses, but they are neither comprehensive nor exhaustive. Monitoring biomarkers of the stress response should include molecular and functional measures of the HPA axis, the adrenergic response systems, and the immune system at multiple levels. The HPA axis can be monitored by measuring CRH, ACTH, and cortisol in plasma, cerebral-spinal fluid, urine, saliva, or sweat. HRV is an accurate, sensitive, and noninvasive way to measure the relative activity of the sympathetic and parasympathetic nervous systems. Monitoring the parasympathetic system (which generally acts as a brake to oppose sympathetic nervous system responses) also provides insights for the action of the ANS. Acetylcholine (the main neurotransmitter of the parasympathetic nervous system) and other neurotransmitters and neurohormones can be measured in the serum, urine, saliva, or sweat.

Immunological evaluation may include measures of the numbers, maturity, activation, and function of immune cells, including such measures as macrophage phagocytosis, lymphocyte proliferation in stimulation test, NK activity, cytokine production patterns, expression of genes and receptors, antibody production, skin delayed-type hypersensitivity, antibody response to vaccine, wound healing, and infection rate. The precise combination of measures chosen will depend on the flexibility of the collection of these measures in the laboratory or field setting.

A full evaluation of the effects of activation of stress response systems on immune function requires measures of multiple functional and molecular biomarkers at multiple time points prior to, during, and after the stress exposure. The precise measures selected should be determined by the specific conditions and setting of the study. In the field setting, a minimum battery of biomarkers may be selected as compared with a more extensive battery applied in the laboratory setting.

HUMAN ODORS AS BIOMARKERS

Chemical signals that are present in body odors provide information about many characteristics of an organism and are involved in the coordination and regulation of all aspects of behavior and physiology. Also known as pheromones, these chemical signals elicit a broad range of behavioral and physiological responses within members of a species. Several classes of pheromones have been defined (McClintock, 2000; Wysocki and Preti, 2000):

- Releaser pheromones generate immediate behavioral responses, such as aggression, sexual attraction, and copulation.
- Primer pheromones elicit slower physiological, endocrine, and neuroendocrine responses, such as estrus synchrony and sexual maturation.
- Signaler pheromones include chemical signals that convey information such as individual identity, age, or health status. No obvious primer or releaser effect has been established for this class.
- Recently, an additional group, modulator pheromones, has been introduced. This group has the potential to affect the psychological state or mood of the receiver (Jacob and McClintock, 2000).

Body odors have a number of inherent characteristics that should make them particularly useful for monitoring organic states of individual humans. First, many body odors evolved to communicate messages between individuals. As a consequence, these messages ought to be relatively unambiguous and difficult to falsify. Second, as mentioned above, body odors often directly reflect physiological processes. For example, odors associated with stress have been suggested to arise from the action of stress hormones (e.g., cortisol) on odor-producing body structures (e.g., underarm axillae). Third, odors can be detected from a distance, hence they can be monitored noninvasively. Finally, in principle, it should be possible to identify the odorous materials in human emanations with the long-range goals of developing sensors that could recognize individuals by their characteristic body odors and of developing devices that could detect and recognize specific chemical signatures indicative of particular physiological states. In practice, however, this has remained a challenge, as described below.

Messages in Body Odor

Individual Identity

Many species rely on chemical signals to recognize the individual identity of other members of the same species. The individual identity of a mouse, for example, is coded in part by the genes of the major histocompatability complex (MHC), the same genes involved in activation of immunological defenses and self/nonself recognition (Penn and Potts, 1998a; Yamazaki et al., 1999). MHC genes are highly polymorphic. Conservation of this extreme allelic variation may help the organism recognize and evade a greater array of pathogens, leading to increased resistance to infection and parasites (Apanius et al., 1997). In one study, congenic mice strains were coinfected with *Salmonella enterica* and a murine encephalomyelitis virus where one haplotype was resistant to *Salmonella* and the other was resistant to the encephalomyelitis virus. MHC heterozygotes had lower susceptibility profiles to the two pathogens than did homozygotes (McClelland et al., 2003). This finding provides evidence that MHC diversity provides superior protection against multiple pathogens and might explain the persistence of alleles conferring lower susceptibility to disease.

This protection extends to subsequent generations as well. In a study in which male and female mice were randomly infected with mouse hepatitis virus prior to mating, virus-infected mice produced more heterozygous embryos than sham-infected mice. Thus the presence of a viral infection during fertilization could influence the MHC-genotype of the progeny (Rülicke et al., 1998).

MHC genes also influence characteristic body odors and mating preferences. Female mice prefer to mate with male mice expressing MHC genes different from their own (Penn and Potts, 1998b). Thus preference for MHC-dissimilar mates may have evolved as a strategy to increase genetic diversity of the individual's offspring in order to preserve immunocompetence and enhance survival fitness.

Female mice can be trained to distinguish the odor of mice that vary genetically from themselves (Yamaguchi et al., 1981; Yamazaki et al., 1979). This discrimination has also been demonstrated in untrained MHC-mutant mouse strains differing in only five amino acids (Carroll et al., 2002).

In humans the influence of MHC odor types on odor preferences and mate selection is controversial (Hedrick and Black, 1997; Ober et al., 1997; Wedekind et al., 1995). Ober and colleagues (1997) studied 411 couples from the Hutterites, an isolated community that expresses a limited number of MHC-derived, human leucocyte antigen (HLA) alleles. Fewer matches in HLA genotypes were found between spouses than expected by chance. Among couples that did match, the matched genotype was more often inherited from the father. These results are consistent with the hypothesis that mate choice is influenced by HLA genes, with an avoidance of spouses with genotypes that are the same as one's own. Hedrick and Black (1997), on the other hand, found no mate choice effect in 194 couples from 11 South Amerindian tribes who were characterized by two HLA variants.

McClintock's group (Jacob et al., 2002) recently studied the odor preferences of females exposed to male axillary odors. Forty-nine women were recruited from an isolated community in which a limited number of HLA types were expressed. Six males from diverse ethnic backgrounds were selected as odor donors. The men carried HLA alleles that were common in the women's community, as well as completely foreign alleles. Each man wore a T-shirt for two consecutive nights to capture body odors. In a double-blind study design, the women sniffed and rated each T-shirt for familiarity, intensity, pleasantness, and spiciness. Each woman's most-preferred odors were from male donors whose number of HLA matches differed on average by 1 allele from her own HLA alleles. The least-preferred odors were from donors with few matches (0 or 1 HLA matches) or more matches (up to 7 HLA matches were possible). None of the odor donors in this study shared identical or near-identical MHC with the women, thus avoidance of haplotypes identical to one's own was not an option. Nevertheless, the findings of this study are consistent with a small, intermediate number of matches being preferred over either zero matches or identical MHC as suggested by previous studies (Ober et al., 1997; Wedekind et al., 1995).

Jacob and colleagues (2002) also showed that a woman's odor choices were strongly associated with matches to the alleles inherited from her father, but not her mother, similar to the earlier finding of Ober and colleagues (1997) for mate choices. Preferred odor donors had an average of 1.4 allele matches, and the least-preferred odor donors had an average of 0.6 allele matches to a woman's paternally inherited haplotype. These provocative findings suggest that paternally inherited HLA-associated odors influence women's odor preferences and may serve as social cues.

Disease Recognition

Throughout history physicians have used body odor to diagnose metabolic diseases (e.g., diabetes, scurvy, and gout) and infectious diseases (e.g., smallpox, typhoid, and yellow fever) (see Penn and Potts, 1998a). There are also anecdotal accounts of dogs' abilities to detect human skin cancers before overt symptoms of the disease were present (Church and Williams, 2001). These observations need to be confirmed with rigorous experimental study.

Nevertheless, female mice could discriminate between parasitized males and healthy males (Kavaliers and Colwell, 1992) and showed less attraction to the odor of male mice infected with intestinal parasites than they did to healthy controls (Kavaliers and Colwell, 1995). In another experiment, female mice were less attracted to male mice infected with a respiratory virus than they were either before or after the infection (Penn et al., 1998).

Yamazaki and colleagues (2002) studied the ability of mice to discriminate the urine odors of other mice experimentally infected with mouse mammary tumor virus (MMTV), a B-type retrovirus that is tightly linked to immune responses. MMTV can be acquired either through infection (when newborn pups suckle on infected mothers that shed the virus into milk) or genetically (when the virus is transmitted as an endogenous provirus). Trained mice discriminated male and female mice or their urine odors based on the presence or absence of MMTV, regardless of how the virus was acquired. These odor differences were observed in the absence of overt symptoms of infection. These findings may have relevance for human disease since MMTV-like genes may play a role in human breast cancers (Etkind et al., 2000). There is also a wide variety of other viruses (e.g., human immunodeficiency virus) for which obvious symptoms are slow to develop and could give rise to unique odor profiles. Further investigation of the volatile profiles that give rise to these odor differences could be important for the early diagnosis of human disease.

Psychological State

There has been very little empirical research on the ability of humans to communicate emotions such as fear, anger, and happiness through body odors. Nevertheless, a large body of work has shown that stressed animals communicate fear and alarm through changes in body odor (Agosta, 1992). For example, in one study rats distinguished the odor from stressed and unstressed rats (Valenta and Rigby, 1968). Odors from stressed rats lowered the immune responses of unstressed rats (Cocke et al., 1993), and they induced avoidance behavior (Rottman and Snowdon, 1972).

Only two studies have investigated the ability of humans to communicate emotions through body odor. Chen and Haviland-Jones (2000) collected underarm odors from young men and women under two different conditions: when viewing a "scary" movie or viewing a "funny" movie. A panel of 40 women and 37 men were asked to sniff bottles containing odor pads collected from odor donors during the two viewing conditions. When asked to select which bottles contained the odors of people who were happy (or frightened), women chose the correct bottle more often than chance would suggest. Interestingly, neither men nor women correctly identified fearful odors from women donors. This negative finding could reflect the fact that odor donors reported their fear to be only moderate, and that underarm odors are generally less intense and more pleasant in young women than in young men (Chen and Haviland-Jones, 1999; Doty et al., 1978).

A similar study was conducted by Ackerl and colleagues (2002) in which female donors wore odor pads during a "fear" film or a "neutral" film. Salivary cortisol was measured before and after the films as a measure of stress. Female observers were able to discriminate between fear and nonfear odor pads in a forced-choice test significantly better than chance. However, cortisol levels were unrelated to the level of induced fear or to the odor ratings. These findings implied that cortisol was not the inducer of these odors, and that other mechanisms need to be investigated.

Although the results of these studies should be interpreted cautiously, they suggest that there may be information in human body odors that communicate emotional state. These experiments need to be repeated with stimuli that arouse more intense emotions, although ethical considerations may limit the conduct of some extreme study designs.

Recognition and Detection of Human Odor Profiles

Studies reviewed here suggest there is a rich potential for monitoring human physical and psychological states using body odors. For this potential to be realized, however, three critical issues need to be addressed: (1) ascertainment of what specific information human body odors convey, (2) identification of which compounds of the odor profile to measure, and (3) development of convenient and reliable devices to monitor odor profiles in individuals under various physical and psychological states. Currently there is a lack of definitive studies in all three areas, but future work is likely to fill many gaps in our understanding of these issues. It is encouraging that the Defense Advanced Research Projects Agency has an interest in funding studies to identify individuals based on their body odors.

Information Conveyed in Human Body Odors

Current evidence suggests that genetically based odor profiles play a role in individual identity and immune and stress responses and may be useful for monitoring a variety of physical and emotional states in humans. These signals may be mediated by MHC genes, whereas others may not (Beauchamp and Yamazaki, 2003).

Whether these signals can be reliably discriminated against background variation in such factors as diet, perfume use, and odors associated with home and work place remains a major question. Apparently dogs can discern the individual signature of a person in spite of these potential distracters indicating that, at least in principle, it should be possible for a device to do this as well.

Studies should be encouraged to investigate further how odors reflect emotional states. Based on animal studies, it is highly likely that human stress induces specific odor changes, but this must be rigorously demonstrated before programs that try to identify specific odorants and that try to develop sensors are instituted. No studies have examined odor profiles that might be associated with fatigue; this remains a novel area for future investigation.

It is also important to recognize that for volatile signals indicative of emotional states to be useful for monitoring emotion, it is not necessary that human noses be able to detect these substances. More discriminative devices, be they other biological ones, such as rats or dogs, or specialized nonbiological sensors (see below), may be able to detect these volatile signals and thereby serve as monitors, even if humans find these discriminations difficult or impossible.

A major problem with using human odors as biomarkers is identifying which odorants to monitor. The olfactory system is exquisitely sensitive to a large repertoire of molecules. Recently much progress has been made in our understanding of this system, although many mysteries remain. Briefly, it is now thought that mammals have about 1,000 different genes that express receptors for odorants (in humans, however, two-thirds of these are not functional). Each receptor (located on an individual receptor cell that is actually a primary sensory neuron) is responsive to a variety of structurally similar odorants (Zhang and Firestein, 2002). It is thus the pattern of receptor activity that is monitored and that determines odor quality and intensity. Processing and fine-tuning this pattern begins at the first synapse in the olfactory bulbs, but how further central nervous system processing occurs remains mostly unknown.

It is clear that the olfactory system is capable of decoding MHC-derived body odors (Schaefer et al., 2001). How MHC genes alter odors is largely unknown, although recent studies have shown that they influence the concentration of volatile acids that serve as sexual attractants (Singer et al., 1997). It has also been proposed that MHC odor types may result from a linkage between MHC loci and olfactory receptor genes (Amadou et al., 1999; Fan et al., 1996). MHC-specific odors may be soluble MHC proteins, odor molecules selectively bound to MHC proteins, or by-products of MHC-specific bacteria localized to skin or axillae (Pearse-Pratt et al., 1999; Yamazaki et al., 1999). Further identification of MHC-derived and non-MHC-derived odors is an important prerequisite for developing a viable monitoring system based on odor profiles.

Odor Sensors

One strategy to designing odor sensors is to develop devices that mimic or even use biological principles to detect specific body odors. Particularly attractive is the idea that one might be able to express olfactory receptors in a device that monitors receptor activity using, for example, fluorescence to express overall patterned activity. This is a promising approach, but its development is clearly quite far in the future.

A very active research area involves using a variety of nonbiological sensors (called electronic noses, or e-noses) as artificial odor-sensing devices. In principle, an e-nose consists of an array of chemophysical detectors that change frequency or conductivity in a characteristic pattern upon binding of an odorant. The e-nose does not identify the specific chemical structure of the odorant, rather it detects differences in the molecular composition of odors by comparing signal patterns among samples (Gardner and Bartlett, 1999; Persaud and Travers, 1996). Such devices have been employed in the food industry to distinguish among different types of olive oils, tomatoes, and cheeses (Concepción Cerrato Oliverosa et al., 2002; Maul et al., 2000; Pillonel et al., 2003).

Recently Montag and colleagues (2001) utilized e-nose technology in a comprehensive study of MHC-derived individual odor types of mice and humans. The output from the sensors was analyzed using principal component analysis, an algorithm used to find the optimum representation of a given data set in n-dimensional space. In this case, the data were visualized in two-dimensional spaces where each odor type was represented by a primary and secondary component. The e-nose reliably distinguished urine and serum odor types among MHC congenic and mutant mice strains and also detected the difference between male and female mouse urine. Human serum from eight HLA-homozygous males was also distinguished by the e-nose. The human serum was also represented by two odor components: one influenced by MHC genes and the other by non-MHC genes. The authors speculated that differences in food intake might have influenced the non-MHC odor component. Other environmental variables, such as perfumes and soaps, could have contributed to these differences as well.

Gas chromatography/mass spectrometry headspace analysis was also used to detect and identify individual volatile odors from mouse urine. Preliminary evidence suggested that the ratio of some common volatile compounds varied with HLA expression. For example, the peaks for 3-methylbutanal and 2-pentanone occurred in markedly different ratios in H-2 congenic mouse strains. Moreover, one partially identified substance was present in HLA-A2 transgenic mice, but was absent from their nontransgenic counterparts, suggesting that the presence of this substance depended on the expression of a single gene (Montag et al., 2001). Compounds of low volatility, such as organic acids, also contribute to the odor profile (Singer et al., 1997) and need to be considered as well. Further identification of these odor substances—both in absolute as well as relative quantity—may eventually lead to objective, on-line detection of individual odor profiles.

E-nose technology has also been used in clinical applications. Mohamed and colleagues (2002) used an e-nose to qualitatively classify urine samples from type 2 diabetic patients and healthy controls. Data were analyzed by principal component analysis, artificial neural network, and logistic regression. Correct clinical classification ranged from 88 to 96 percent across methods and was highest with principal component analysis. Others (Hay et al., 2003; Lai et al., 2002; Pavlou et al., 2002) have used the e-nose to diagnose urogenital and upper respiratory infections, with different degrees of success. As e-nose technology continues to develop (Harper, 2001), it represents a promising technology for the early detection of a variety of medical conditions.

Over the next 5 to 10 years, major strides are likely to be made in understanding the molecular mechanisms of olfaction and the relationship between gene expression and individual odor profiles and their links with emotion and cognitive states. Development of sensor technology are ongoing and are likely to yield smaller, more automated devices that reduce analysis time and increase reliability—two factors critical for field applications. These advances will go hand-in-hand with the development of sweat patches that can be uniquely designed to capture the substances of interest (Cizza et al., 2003). The military is encouraged to promote innovative research in chemical signaling that will accelerate these advances.

Two final caveats need to be mentioned. First, to be truly valuable as a monitoring technology, odor profiling must be reproducible at the individual level. That is, an individual's odor profile during rest must be easily distinguished from that same individual's odor profile during stress. Furthermore, information contained in an individual's odor profile must be capable of predicting decrements in cognitive performance or changes in health status under different environmental and physiological conditions. Future study of these parameters will determine if odor profiles possess these performance characteristics.

HUMAN TEARS AS BIOMARKERS

Bodily excretions and secretions that are noninvasively accessible and that reflect the current internal concentrations of substances within physiologically relevant systems represent possible targets of metabolic monitoring technology. Saliva and sweat have been discussed elsewhere. An often overlooked external secretion is lachrymal fluid, or tears.

Although there appears to be little currently accepted clinical analytic use of tears as indicants of nonophthalmic internal status, a number of disparate studies suggest that there may be merit in examining tears as a possible medium for monitoring relevant aspects of metabolic status.

It has been reported that tear glucose concentrations are related to blood glucose levels (Das et al., 1995). Also, insulin concentrations in tears of subjects who were fasted for 12 hours were lower than those in tears of fed subjects (Rocha et al., 2002).

Among marginally nourished Thai children, tear levels of retinol increased 2 months after a single dose of vitamin A supplementation, whereas they were unchanged among an unsupplemented group (van Agtmaal et al., 1988). In adults administered varying doses of aspirin, salicylic acid levels in tears were dose-dependent and proportional to plasma levels (Valentic et al., 1980). Fluoride concentrations in tears have been found to be in constant proportion to plasma concentrations in the face of twofold increases in plasma levels induced by acute fluoride ingestion (Chan et al., 1990).

Several studies have shown that tear concentrations of certain anticonvulsant drugs are closely related to both plasma and cerebrospinal fluid drug levels. Tear concentrations of valproic acid were directly correlated to cerebrospinal fluid concentrations as strongly as were plasma concentrations, and more so than were salivary concentrations (Monaco et al., 1982). Further, tear concentrations of valproic acid were correlated with plasma concentrations among adults and among children under 3 years of age (Nakajima et al., 2000; Monaco et al., 1982, 1984). Tear levels of diphenylhydantoin, phenobarbital, and carbamazepine correlated more strongly than salivary levels with their respective plasma and cerebrospinal fluid concentrations (Monaco et al., 1979, 1981).

Research is needed to determine which physiological and pharmacological variables may be reliably assessed from tear concentrations. It may be possible to identify potential exogenously administered tracers that in their tear concentrations indicate the status of certain physiological variables. It will also be necessary to delineate the conditions that affect the validity of tear levels as indicants. For example, it has been suggested that the tear:plasma ratio of levels of certain drugs is affected by the pH of the tears and plasma and by the drug's lipid solubility and degree of ionization (van Haeringen, 1985). Environmental agents may also influence the tear concentrations of certain analytes that might have physiological significance. Among subjects with indoor air complaints, exposures to two concentrations of a mixture of organic gases and vapors associated with new homes led, in a dose- and time-dependent manner, to dilution of tear levels of serum albumin, sodium, and potassium (Thygesen et al., 1987). While this may limit the extent to which tear concentrations of some substances accurately represent internal levels, it also suggests that analysis of tears may indicate exposure to some environmental toxins in subperceptible concentrations. Thus tears may also provide a medium for obtaining early indications of exposure to toxins.

SUMMARY

This chapter presents the current monitoring methods for specific metabolic systems of particular concern to the military, which are bone and muscle metabolism, kidney function and hydration, and stress and immune function. The development of sensors and applicability in the field remains at different stages; some of them, such as the monitoring of renal function by dipstick strips, are ready for field use, while others, such monitoring methods for bone health or muscle fatigue, still need validation in the field.

Maintaining a healthy bone to minimize the incidence of fracture is predicted by measuring bone mineral density. However, the low level of precision of this method limits its use; therefore, for short-term changes, intermediate biological markers of bone remodeling (i.e., the balance between resorption and formation) may be better indicators of potential fractures. There are a variety of compounds that can be used as markers of bone resorption, including collagen break-down products, specific gene products, and hormonal markers. For an accurate evaluation, however, biomarkers of bone formation also need to be monitored, but they have been difficult to elucidate. In addition to bone remodeling, stress is related to changes in bone health. Although cortisol appears to be a promising indicator of bone health, validation in the field is still needed.

Heavy physical exertion, inadequate energy intake, and psychological stress can all influence muscle metabolism, causing muscle damage and muscle protein breakdown. Single blood and urinary markers of these processes are difficult to interpret because their levels may be confounded by diurnal patterns or dietary consumption of muscle meats; also, other markers of turnover exist but their measure involves invasive procedures unsuitable for field monitoring. More advanced technology for minimally invasive sampling of muscle tissue is needed before this monitoring application is field-ready. Subjective measures, such as muscle soreness and ratings of self-assessment, may be of great value as predictors of performance and indicators of the need for rest.

Monitoring renal function is important because of the role of the kidneys in maintaining proper hydration, fluid homeostasis, and electrolyte balance, all of which are critical to sustain both physical and cognitive functions. In the field, monitoring urinary output, color, odor, and specific gravity would all provide important information relative to hydration, electrolyte balance, muscle breakdown, and protein and energy status, as well as to the presence of infection. Being able to field-monitor fluctuations in body weight would also be an excellent indicator of hydration status, since short-term changes in body weight are directly attributable to changes in body water volume. Changes in body weight, when coupled with knowledge of serum osmolality and/or serum sodium, would assist greatly in defining the presence and severity of disturbances in body volume status.

In addition to muscle, bone, and renal function, stress and immune responses need to be monitored because they affect both physical and cognitive performance through a variety of mechanisms. The stress response to an stressor results in the release of neurotransmitters and hormones that serve as the brain's messengers for regulation of the immune and other systems. The consequences of this response are generally adaptive in the short run, but can be damaging when stress is chronic. Indicators of stress and immune responses that are currently in use or development include cortisol levels and heart-rate variability. Self-report (and peer-report) inventories could be adapted to offer valuable information about individual stress levels.

Over the next several years, major strides are likely to be made in understanding the molecular mechanisms of olfaction and the relationship between individual odor profiles and emotion and cognitive states. Development of sensor technology suitable for field applications, along with the development of sweat patches designed to capture substances of interest, are ongoing. Future studies on their reproducibility and the ability to predict decrements in performance under different environmental and physiological conditions will be critical.

A number of studies suggest the possibility of using tears as a possible medium for monitoring relevant aspects of metabolic status. For example, the analysis of tears may indicate exposure to some environmental toxins in subperceptible concentrations and its use merits future research.

REFERENCES

Abbas AK, Lichtman AH, Pober JS. 2000. *Cellular and Molecular Immunology*. 4th ed. Philadelphia: WB Saunders. P. 307.

Ackerl K, Atzmueller M, Grammer K. 2002. The scent of fear. *Neuroendocrinol Lett* 23:79–84.

ACSM (American College of Sports Medicine). 1996. Exercise and fluid replacement. *Med Sci Sports Exerc* 28:i–vii.

ACSM. 2002. Progression models in resistance training for healthy adults. *Med Sci Sports Exerc* 34:364–380.

Adams GR, Haddad F. 1996. The relationships among IGF-1, DNA content, and protein accumulation during skeletal muscle hypertrophy. *J Appl Physiol* 81:2509–2516.

Adams GR, Haddad F, Baldwin KM. 1999. Time course of changes in markers of myogenesis in overloaded rat skeletal muscles. *J Appl Physiol* 87:1705–1712.

Ader R, Cohen N, Felten D. 1995. Psychoneuroimmunology: Interactions between the nervous system and the immune system. *Lancet* 345:99–103.

Afting EG, Bernhardt W, Janzen RW, Rothig HJ. 1981. Quantitative importance of non-skeletal-muscle N^{τ}-methylhistidine and creatine in human urine. *Biochem J* 200:449–452.

Agosta WC. 1992. *Chemical Communication: The Language of Pheromones*. New York: Scientific American Library.

Ahmed AA, Nordlind K, Schultzberg M, Liden S. 1996. Proinflammatory cytokines and their corresponding receptor proteins in eccrine sweat glands in normal and cutaneous leishmaniasis human skin. An immunohistochemical study. *Exp Dermatol* 5:230–235.

Alfonsi E, Pavesi R, Merlo IM, Gelmetti A, Zambarbieri D, Lago P, Arrigo A, Reggiani C, Moglia A. 1999. Hemoglobin near-infrared spectroscopy and surface EMG study in muscle ischaemia and fatiguing isometric contraction. *J Sports Med Phys Fitness* 39:83–92.

Amadou C, Kumánovics A, Jones EP, Lambracht-Washington D, Yoshino M, Lindahl KF. 1999. The mouse major histocompatibility complex: Some assembly required. *Immunol Rev* 167:211–221.

Apanius V, Penn D, Slev PR, Ruff LR, Potts WK. 1997. The nature of selection on the major histocompatibility complex. *Crit Rev Immunol* 17:179–224.

Ardawi MS, Majzoub MF, Masoud IM, Newsholme EA. 1989. Enzymic and metabolic adaptations in the gastrocnemius, plantaris and soleus muscles of hypocaloric rats. *Biochem J* 261:219–225.

Armstrong LE, Curtis WC, Hubbard RW, Francesconi RP, Moore R, Askew EW. 1993. Symptomatic hyponatremia during prolonged exercise in heat. *Med Sci Sports Exerc* 25:543–549.

Armstrong LE, Herrera Soto JA, Hacker FT, Casa DJ, Kavouras SA, Maresh CM. 1998. Urinary indices during dehydration, exercise, and rehydration. *Int J Sport Nutr* 8:345–355.

Bagdy G, Calogero AE, Murphy DL, Szemeredi K. 1989. Serotonin agonists cause parallel activation of the sympathoadrenomedullary system and the hypothalamo-pituitary-adrenocortical axis in conscious rats. *Endocrinology* 125:2664–2669.

Baldwin KM, Haddad F, Adams GR. 2003. *Molecular Markers of Mechanical Activity/Inactivity Induced Anabolic and Catabolic States in Striated Muscle*. Presented at the Institute of Medicine, Committee on Metabolic Monitoring Technologies for Military Field Applications Workshop on Metabolic Monitoring Technologies for Military Field Applications, San Antonio, Texas, January 8–9.

Banister EW, Rajendra W, Mutch BJ. 1985. Ammonia as an indicator of exercise stress: Implications of recent findings to sports medicine. *Sports Med* 2:34–46.

Barac-Nieto M, Spurr GB, Dahners HW, Maksud MG. 1980. Aerobic work capacity and endurance during nutritional repletion of severely undernourished men. *Am J Clin Nutr* 33:2268–2275.

Barron JL, Noakes TD, Levy W, Smith C, Millar RP. 1985. Hypothalamic dysfunction in overtrained athletes. *J Clin Endocrinol Metab* 60:803–806.

Bass SL, Myburgh KH. 2000. The role of exercise in the attainment of peak bone mass and bone strength. In: Warren MP, Constantini NW, eds. *Sports Endocrinology*. Totowa, NJ: Humana Press. Pp. 253–280.

Beauchamp GK, Yamazaki K. 2003. Chemical signalling in mice. *Biochem Soc Trans* 31:147–151.

Beers MH, Berkow R, eds. 1999. *The Merck Manual of Diagnosis and Therapy*. 17th ed. Whitehouse Station, NJ: Merck Research Laboratories.

Behm DG, Baker KM, Kelland R, Lomond J. 2001. The effect of muscle damage on strength and fatigue deficits. *J Strength Cond Res* 15:255–263.

Bennell KL, Malcolm SA, Brukner PD, Green RM, Hopper JL, Wark JD, Ebeling PR. 1998. A 12-month prospective study of the relationship between stress fractures and bone turnover in athletes. *Calcif Tissue Int* 63:80–85.

Binkley HM, Beckett J, Casa DJ, Leiner DM, Plummer PE. 2002. National Athletic Trainers' Association position statement: Exertional heat illnesses. *J Athlet Train* 37:329–343.

Biondi M. 1991. The application of the human stress model to psychoneuroimmunology. *Acta Neurologica* 13:328–334.

Biondi M. 2001. Effect of stress on immune functions: An overview. In: Adler RF, Felten DL, Cohen N, eds. *Psychoneuroimmunology*. Vol 2, 3rd ed. San Diego: Academic Press. Pp. 189–226.

Biondi M, Peronti M, Pacitti F, Pancheri P, Pacifici R, Altieri I, Paris L, Zuccaro P. 1994. Personality, endocrine and immune changes after eight months in healthy individuals under normal daily stress. *Psychother Psychosom* 62:176–184.

Black DM, Cummings SR, Genant HK, Nevitt MC, Palermo L, Browner W. 1992. Axial and appendicular bone density predict fractures in older women. *J Bone Miner Res* 7:633–638.

Blomstrand E, Celsing F, Newsholme EA. 1988. Changes in plasma concentrations of aromatic and branched-chain amino acids during sustained exercise in man and their possible role in fatigue. *Acta Physiol Scand* 133:115–121.

Bonneau RH, Sheridan JF, Feng N, Glaser R. 1993. Stress-induced modulation of the primary cellular immune response to herpes simplex virus infection is mediated by both adrenal-dependent and independent mechanisms. *J Neuroimmunol* 42:167–176.

Braunwald E, Fauci AS, Kasper DL, Hauser SL, Longo DL, Jameson JL, eds. 2001. *Harrison's Principles of Internal Medicine*. 15th ed. New York: McGraw-Hill.

Brook RD, Julius S. 2000. Autonomic imbalance, hypertension, and cardiovascular risk. *Am J Hyperten* 13:S112–S122.

Budgett R. 1998. Fatigue and underperformance in athletes: The overtraining syndrome. *Br J Sports Med* 32:107–110.

Burr DB. 1997. Bone, exercise, and stress fractures. *Exerc Sport Sci Rev* 25:171–194.

Calogero AE, Gallucci WT, Bernardini R, Saoutis C, Gold PW, Chrousos GP. 1988a. Effect of cholinergic agnonists and antagonists on rat hypothalamic coricotropin-releasing hormone secretion in vitro. *Neuroendocrinology* 47:303–308.

Calogero AE, Gallucci WT, Chrousos GP, Gold PW. 1988b. Catecholamine effects upon rat hypothalamic corticotropin-releasing hormone secretion in vitro. *J Clin Invest* 82:839–846.

Calogero AE, Gallucci WT, Chrousos GP, Gold PW. 1988c. Interaction between GABAergic neurotransmission and rat hypothalamic corticotropin-releasing hormone secretion in vitro. *Brain Res* 463:28–36.

Calogero AE, Gallucci WT, Gold PW, Chrousos GP. 1988d. Multiple feedback regulatory loops upon rat hypothalamic corticotropin-releasing hormone secretion. Potential clinical implications. *J Clin Invest* 82:767–774.

Calogero AE, Bernardini R, Margioris AN, Bagdy G, Gallucci WT, Munson PJ, Tamarkin L, Tomai TP, Brady L, Gold PW, Chrousos GP. 1989. Effects of serotonergic agonists and antagonists on corticotropin-releasing hormone secretion by explanted rat hypothalami. *Peptides* 10:189–200.

Calogero AE, Bagdy G, Szemeredi K, Tartaglia ME, Gold PW, Chrousos GP. 1990. Mechanisms of serotonin receptor agonist-induced activation of the hypothalamic-pituitary-adrenal axis in the rat. *Endocrinology* 126:1888–1894.

Carroll LS, Penn DJ, Potts WK. 2002. Discrimination of MHC-derived odors by untrained mice is consistent with divergence in peptide-binding region residues. *Proc Natl Acad Sci USA* 99:2187–2192.

Carter R, Cheuvront SN, Kolka MA, Sawka MN. 2003. *Hydration Status Monitoring*. Presented at the Institute of Medicine, Committee on Metabolic Monitoring Technologies for Military Field Applications Workshop on Metabolic Monitoring Technologies for Military Field Applications, San Antonio, Texas, January 8–9.

Casa DJ, Armstrong LE. 2001. Letters to the editor. Hyponatremia or hype? *Phys Sportsmed* 29:21–22.

Casa DJ, Armstrong LE, Hillman SK, Montain SJ, Reiff RV, Rich BSE, Roberts WO, Stone JA. 2000. National Athletic Trainers' Association position statement: Fluid replacement for athletes. *J Athlet Train* 35:212–224.

Chailurkit LO, Ongphiphadhanakul B, Piaseu N, Saetung S, Rajatanavin R. 2001. Biochemical markers of bone turnover and response of BMD to intervention in early postmenopausal women: An experience in a clinical laboratory. *Clin Chem* 47:1083–1088.

Chan JT, Cheeks L, Slagle T, Green K. 1990. Relationship between plasma and tear fluoride levels in rabbit and man. *Ophthalmic Res* 22:39–44.

Chen D, Haviland-Jones J. 1999. Rapid mood change and human odors. *Physiol Behav* 68:241–250.

Chen D, Haviland-Jones J. 2000. Human olfactory communication of emotion. *Percept Mot Skills* 91:771–781.

Chilibeck PD. 2000. Hormonal regulations of the effects of exercise on bone. Positive and negative effects. In: Warren MP, Constantini NW. *Sports Endocrinology*. Totowa, NJ: Humana Press. Pp. 239–252.

Chrousos GP. 1998. Stressors, stress, and neuroendocrine integration of the adaptive response. The 1997 Hans Selye Memorial lecture. *Ann NY Acad Sci* 851:311–335.

Chrousos GP, Gold PW. 1992. The concepts of stress and stress system disorders. Overview of physical and behavioral homeostasis. *J Am Med Assoc* 267:1244–1252.

Church J, Williams H. 2001. Another sniffer dog for the clinic? *Lancet* 358:930.

Cizza G, Ravn P, Chrousos GP, Gold PW. 2001. Depression: A major, unrecognized risk factor for osteoporosis? *Trends Endocrinol Metab* 12:198–203.

Cizza G, Eskandari F, Phillips T, Sternberg EM. 2003. *Sweat Patch as a Novel Approach to Monitor the Level of Activity of the Stress System: Potential Application for Studies Conducted in the Field.* Presented at the Institute of Medicine, Committee on Metabolic Monitoring Technologies for Military Field Applications Workshop on Metabolic Monitoring Technologies for Military Field Applications, San Antonio, Texas, January 8–9.

Clarkson PM, Nosaka K, Braun B. 1992. Muscle function after exercise-induced muscle damage and rapid adaptation. *Med Sci Sports Exerc* 24:512–520.

Cocke R, Moynihan JA, Cohen N, Grota LJ, Ader R. 1993. Exposure to conspecific alarm chemosignals alters immune responses in BALB/c mice. *Brain Behav Immun* 7:36–46.

Cohen H, Matar MA, Kaplan Z, Kotler M. 1999. Power spectral analysis of heart rate variability in psychiatry. *Psychother Psychosom* 68:59–66.

Cohen N, Kinney KS. 2001. Exploring the phylogenetic history of neural-immune system interactions. In: Ader R, Felten DL, Cohen N, eds. *Psychoneuroimmunology.* Vol 1, 3rd ed. San Diego: Academic Press. Pp. 21–54.

Cohen O, Fine I, Monashkin E, Karasik A. 2003. Glucose correlation with light scattering patterns—A novel method for non-invasive glucose measurements. *Diabetes Technol Ther* 5:11–17.

Concepción Cerrato Oliveros M, Luis Pérez Pavón J, García Pinto C, Esther Fernández Laespada M, Moreno Cordero B, Fornia M. 2002. Electronic nose based on metal oxide semiconductor sensors as a fast alternative for the detection of adulteration of virgin olive oils. *Anal Chim Acta* 459:219–228.

Conover CA. 1996. The role of insulin-like growth factors and binding proteins in bone cell biology. In: Bilezikian JP, Raisz LG, Rodan GA, eds. *Principles of Bone Biology*. San Diego: Academic Press. Pp. 607–618.

Costill DL, Cote R, Fink W. 1976. Muscle water and electrolytes following varied levels of dehydration in man. *J Appl Physiol* 40:6–11.

Cummings SR, Black DM, Nevitt MC, Browner W, Cauley J, Ensrud K, Genant HK, Palermo L, Scott J, Vogt TM. 1993. Bone density at various sites for prediction of hip fractures. The Study of Osteoporotic Fractures Research Group. *Lancet* 341:72–75.

Darmaun D, Matthews DE, Bier DM. 1988. Physiological hypercortisolemia increases proteolysis, glutamine, and alanine production. *Am J Physiol* 255:E366–E373.

Das BN, Sengupta S, Das BK, Goswami NR. 1995. Tear glucose estimation—An alternative to blood glucose estimation. *J Indian Med Assoc* 93:127–128.

Das UN. 2000. Beneficial effects of *n*-3 fatty acids in cardiovascular diseases: But, why and how? *Prostaglandins Leukot Essent Fatty Acids* 63:351–362.

Davies CTM, White MJ. 1981. Muscle weakness following eccentric work in man. *Pflungers Arch* 392:168–171.

Davis JM. 1995. Central and peripheral factors in fatigue. *J Sports Sci* 13:S49–S53.

de Kerviler E, Leroy-Willig A, Jehenson P, Duboc D, Eymard B, Syrota A. 1991. Exercise-induced muscle modifications: Study of healthy subjects and patients with metabolic myopathies with MR imaging and P-31 spectroscopy. *Radiology* 181:259–264.

Dhabhar FS. 1998. Stress-induced enhancement of cell-mediated immunity. *Ann NY Acad Sci* 840:359–372.

Dhabhar FS. 2002. Stress-induced augmentation of immune function—The role of stress hormones, leukocyte trafficking, and cytokines. *Brain Behav Immun* 16:785–798.

Dhabhar FS, McEwen BS. 1997. Acute stress enhances while chronic stress suppresses cell-mediated immunity in vivo: A potential role for leukocyte trafficking. *Brain Behav Immun* 11:286–306.

Dhabhar FS, McEwen BS. 1999. Enhancing versus suppressive effects of stress hormones on skin immune function. *Proc Natl Acad Sci USA* 96:1059–1064.

Dhabhar FS, McEwen BS. 2001. Bidirectional effects of stress and glucorticoid hormones on immune function: Possible explanations for paradoxical observations. In: Ader R, Felten DL, Cohen N, eds. *Psychoneurimmunology*. Vol 1, 3rd ed. San Diego: Academic Press. Pp. 301–338.

Doty RL, Orndorff MM, Leyden J, Kligman A. 1978. Communication of gender from human axillary odors: Relationship to perceived intensity and hedonicity. *Behav Biol* 23:373–380.

Edwards RHT. 1981. Human muscle function and fatigue. In: Porter R, Wheland J, eds. *Human Muscle Fatigue: Physiological Mechanisms*. Ciba Foundation Symposium. London: Pitman Medical. Pp. 1–18.

Elenkov IJ, Wilder RL, Chrousos GP, Vizi ES. 2000. The sympathetic nerve—An integrative interface between two supersystems: The brain and the immune system. *Pharmacol Rev* 52:595–638.

Eliakim A, Brasel JA, Cooper DM. 2000. Exercise and the growth hormone–insulin-like growth factor-1 axis. In: Warren MP, Constantini NW, eds. *Sports Endocrinology*. Totowa, NJ: Humana Press. Pp. 77–95.

Epstein Y, Armstrong LE. 1999. Fluid-electrolyte balance during labor and exercise: Concepts and misconceptions. *Int J Sport Nutr* 9:1–12.

Ershler WB, Keller ET. 2000. Age-associated increased interleukin-6 gene expression, late-life diseases, and frailty. *Ann Rev Med* 51:245–270.

Eskandari F, Sternberg EM. 2002. Neural-immune interactions in health and disease. *Ann NY Acad Sci* 966:20–27.

Esterling BA, Kiecolt-Glaser JK, Glaser R. 1996. Psychosocial modulation of cytokine-induced natural killer cell activity in older adults. *Psychosom Med* 58:264–272.

Etkind P, Du J, Khan A, Pillitteri J, Wiernik PH. 2000. House mammary tumor virus-like *ENV* gene sequences in human breast tumors and in a lymphoma of a breast cancer patient. *Clin Cancer Res* 6:1273–1278.

Evans WJ. 2001. Protein nutrition and resistance exercise. *Can J Appl Physiol* 26:S141–S152.

Evans WJ, Cannon JG. 1991. The metabolic effects of exercise-induced muscle damage. *Exerc Sport Sci Rev* 19:99–125.

Fan W, Cai W, Parimoo S, Lennon GG, Weissman SM. 1996. Identification of seven new human MHC class I region genes around the HLA-F locus. *Immunogenetics* 44:97–103.

Fernstrom JD. 1990. Aromatic amino acids and monoamine synthesis in the central nervous system: Influence of the diet. *J Nutr Biochem* 1:508–517.

Ferrando AA, Williams BD, Stuart CA, Lane HW, Wolfe RR. 1995. Oral branched-chain amino acids decrease whole-body proteolysis. *J Parenteral Enteral Nutr* 19:47–54.

Ferrando AA, Lane HW, Stuart CA, Davis-Street J, Wolfe RR. 1996. Prolonged bed rest decreases skeletal muscle and whole body protein synthesis. *Am J Physiol* 270:E627–E633.

Fielding RA, Manfredi TJ, Ding W, Fiatarone MA, Evans WJ, Cannon JG. 1993. Acute phase response in exercise. III. Neutrophil and IL-1 beta accumulation in skeletal muscle. *Am J Physiol* 265:R166–R172.

Fitts RH. 1994. Cellular mechanisms of muscle fatigue. *Physiol Rev* 74:49–94.

Flinn SD, Sherer RJ. 2000. Seizure after exercise in the heat. *Physician Sportsmed* 28:61–65.

Forner MA, Barriga C, Rodriguez AB, Ortega E. 1995. A study of the role of corticosterone as a mediator in exercise-induced stimulation of murine macrophage phagocytosis. *J Physiol* 488:789–794.

Friedl KE, Moore RJ, Hoyt RW, Marchitelli LJ, Martinez-Lopez LE, Askew EW. 2000. Endocrine markers of semistarvation in healthy lean men in a multistressor environment. *J Appl Physiol* 88:1820–1830.

Friedman BH, Thayer JF. 1998a. Anxiety and autonomic flexibility: A cardiovascular approach. *Biol Psychol* 49:303–323.

Friedman BH, Thayer JF. 1998b. Autonomic balance revisited: Panic anxiety and heart rate variability. *J Psychosom Res* 44:133–151.

Fry AC, Kraemer WJ. 1997. Resistance exercise overtraining and overreaching. Neuroendocrine responses. *Sports Med* 23:106–129.

Fry RW, Morton AR, Keast D. 1991. Overtraining in athletes. An update. *Sports Med* 12:32–65.

Fukuoka H, Kiriyama M, Nishimura Y, Higurashi M, Suzuki Y, Gunji A. 1994. Metabolic turnover of bone and peripheral monocyte release of cytokines during short-term bed rest. *Acta Physiol Scand* 150:37–41.

Gardner JW, Bartlett PN. 1999. *Electronic Noses: Principles and Applications.* New York: Oxford University Press.

Gelfand RA, Matthews DE, Bier DM, Sherwin RS. 1984. Role of counterregulatory hormones in the catabolic response to stress. *J Clin Invest* 74:2238–2248.

Giger JM , Haddad F, Qin AX , Baldwin KM. 2002. Functional overload increases beta-MHC promoter activity in rodent fast muscle via the proximal MCAT (βe3) site. *Am J Physiol Cell Physiol* 282:C518–C527.

Glaser R, Kiecolt-Glaser JK, Bonneau RH, Malarkey W, Kennedy S, Hughes J. 1992. Stress-induced modulation of the immune response to recombinant hepatitis B vaccine. *Psychosom Med* 54:22–29.

Gluer CC, Cummings SR, Bauer DC, Stone K, Pressman A, Mathur A, Genant HK. 1996. Osteoporosis: Association of recent fractures with quantitative US findings. *Radiology* 199:725–732.

Gold PW, Chrousos GP. 2002. Organization of the stress system and its dysregulation in melancholic and atypical depression: High vs low CRH/NE states. *Mol Psychiatry* 7:254–275.

Gold PW, Goodwin FK, Chrousos GP. 1988. Clinical and biochemical manifestations of depression. Relation to the neurobiology of stress (2). *N Engl J Med* 319:413–420.

Goldstein DS. 1995. Clinical assessment of sympathetic responses to stress. *Ann NY Acad Sci* 771:570–593.

Gollnick PD, Piehl K, Saubert CW 4th, Armstrong RB, Saltin B. 1972. Diet, exercise, and glycogen changes in human muscle fibers. *J Appl Physiol* 33:421–425.

Gomez SA, Fernandez GC, Vanzulli S, Dran G, Rubel C, Berki T, Isturiz MA, Palermo MS. 2003. Endogenous glucocorticoids attenuate shiga toxin-2-induced toxicity in a mouse model of haemolytic uraemic syndrome. *Clin Exp Immunol* 131:217–224.

Gonzalez-Alonso J, Calbet JA, Nielsen B. 1999. Metabolic and thermodynamic responses to dehydration-induced reductions in muscle blood flow in exercising humans. *J Physiol* 520:577–589.

Graeff FG. 1997. Serotonergic systems. *Psychiat Clin N Am* 20:723–739.

Greenleaf JE. 1992. Problem: Thirst, drinking behavior, and involuntary dehydration. *Med Sci Sports Exerc* 24:645–656.

Guyton AC, Hall JE. 1997. The autonomic nervous system; cerebral blood flow; and cerebrospinal fluid. In: *Human Physiology and Mechanisms of Disease*. 6th ed. Philadelphia: W.B. Saunders Co. Pp. 495–507.

Habib GB. 1999. Reappraisal of heart rate as a risk factor in the general population. *Eur Heart J Suppl* 1:H2–H10.

Hackney AC, Viru A. 1999. Twenty-four-hour cortisol response to multiple daily exercise sessions of moderate and high intensity. *Clin Physiol* 19:178–182.

Harper WJ. 2001. The strengths and weaknesses of the electronic nose. *Adv Exp Med Biol* 488:59–71.

Hay P, Tummon A, Ogunfile M, Adebiyi A, Adefowora A. 2003. Evaluation of a novel diagnostic test for bacterial vaginosis: 'The electronic nose.' *Int J STD AIDS* 14:114–118.

Hedrick PW, Black FL. 1997. Random mating and selection in families against homozygotes for HLA in South Amerindians. *Hereditas* 127:51–58.

Heymsfield SB, Arteaga C, McManus C, Smith J, Moffitt S. 1983. Measurement of muscle mass in humans: Validity of the 24-hour urinary creatinine method. *Am J Clin Nutr* 37:478–494.

Hoffer LJ. 1999. Metabolic consequences of starvation. In: Shils ME, Olson JA, Shike M, Ross AC, eds. *Modern Nutrition in Health and Disease*. 9th ed. Baltimore: Williams & Wilkins. Pp. 645–665.

Holsboer F, Von Bardeleben U, Gerken A, Stalla GK, Muller OA. 1984. Blunted corticotropin and normal cortisol response to human corticotropin-releasing factor in depression. *N Engl J Med* 311:1127.

Houtkooper LB, Lohman TG, Going SB, Howell WH. 1996. Why bioelectrical impedance analysis should be used for estimating adiposity. *Am J Clin Nutr* 64:436S–448S.

Ingle BM, Hay SM, Bottjer HM, Eastell R. 1999. Changes in bone mass and bone turnover following distal forearm fracture. *Osteoporos Int* 10:399–407.

IOM (Institute of Medicine). 1993. *Nutritional Needs in Hot Environments: Applications for Military Personnel in Field Operations*. Marriott BM, ed. Washington, DC: National Academy Press.

IOM. 1994. *Fluid Replacement and Heat Stress: Proceedings of a Workshop*. Marriott BM, ed. Washington, DC: National Academy Press.

IOM. 1998. *Reducing Stress Fracture in Physically Active Military Women*. Washington, DC: National Academy Press.

IOM. 1999. *Military Strategies for Sustainment of Nutrition and Immune Function in the Field*. Washington, DC: National Academy Press.

Irwin M, Daniels M, Risch SC, Bloom E, Weiner H. 1988. Plasma cortisol and natural killer cell activity during bereavement. *Biol Psychiatry* 24:173–178.

Jacob S, McClintock MK. 2000. Psychological state and mood effects of steroidal chemosignals in women and men. *Horm Behav* 37:57–78.

Jacob S, McClintock MK, Zelano B, Ober C. 2002. Paternally inherited HLA alleles are associated with women's choice of male odor. *Nat Genet* 30:175–179.

Jakeman PM, Hawthorne JE, Maxwell SR, Kendall MJ, Holder G. 1994. Evidence for downregulation of hypothalamic 5-hydroxytryptamine receptor function in endurance-trained athletes. *Exp Physiol* 79:461–464.

Jaspers SR, Tischler ME. 1986. Role of glucorticoids in the response of rat leg muscles to reduced activity. *Muscle Nerve* 9:554–561.

Jose AD, Collison D. 1970. The normal range and determinants of the intrinsic heart rate in man. *Cardiovasc Res* 4:160–167.

Kang DH, Coe CL, McCarthy DO, Ershler WB. 1997. Immune responses to final exams in healthy and asthmatic adolescents. *Nur Res* 46:12–19.

Kasl SV, Evans AS, Niederman JC. 1979. Psychosocial risk factors in the developmental of infectious mononucleosis. *Psychosom Med* 41:445–466.

Kavaliers M, Colwell DD. 1992. Exposure to the scent of male mice infected with the protozoan parasite, *Eimeria vermiformis,* induces opoid-and nonopoid-mediated analgesia in female mice. *Physiol Behav* 52:373–377.

Kavaliers M, Colwell DD. 1995. Discrimination by female mice between the odours of parasitized and non-parasitized males. *Proc R Soc Lond B Biol Sci* 261:31–35.

Kell RT, Bhambhani Y. 2003. Cardiorespiratory and hemodynamic responses during repetitive incremental lifting and lowering in healthy males and females. *Eur J Appl Physiol* 90:1–9.

Kelly PJ, Eisman JA. 1992. Osteoporosis: Genetic effects on bone turnover and bone density. Editorial. *Ann Med* 25:100–101.

Kelsey JL, Browner WS, Seeley DG, Nevitt MC, Cummings SR. 1992. Risk factors for fractures of the distal forearm and proximal humerus. The Study of Osteoporotic Fractures Research Group. *Am J Epidemiol* 135:477–489.

Kiecolt-Glaser JK, Kennedy S, Malkoff S, Fisher L, Speicher CE, Glaser R. 1988. Marital discord and immunity in males. *Psychosom Med* 50:213–229.

Kiecolt-Glaser JK, Malarkey WB, Chee M, Newton T, Cacioppo JT, Mao HY, Glaser R. 1993. Negative behavior during marital conflict is associated with immunological down-regulation. *Psychosom Med* 55:395–409.

Kiecolt-Glaser JK, Marucha PT, Malarkey WB, Mercado AM, Glaser R. 1995. Slowing of wound healing by psychological stress. *Lancet* 346:1194–1196.

Kiecolt-Glaser JK, McGuire L, Robles TF, Glaser R. 2002. Emotions, morbidity, and mortality: New perspectives from psychoneuroimmunology. *Annu Rev Psychol* 53:83–107.

Kleerekoper M. 2003. *Biomarkers for Monitoring Bone Turnover and Predicting Bone Stress*. Presented at the Institute of Medicine, Committee on Metabolic Monitoring Technologies for Military Field Applications Workshop on Metabolic Monitoring Technologies for Military Field Applications, San Antonio, Texas, January 8–9.

Kleinman LI, Lorenz JM. 1996. Physiology and pathophysiology of body water and electrolytes. In: Kaplan LA, Pesce AJ, Kazmierczak SC, eds. *Clinical Chemistry. Theory, Analysis, and Correlation.* 3rd ed. St. Louis: Mosby. Pp. 439–463.

Kohrt WM, Jankowski CM. 2003. *Biomarkers to Predict the Occurrence of Bone Stress and Matrix Abnormalities Due to Sustained and Intensive Physical Activity*. Presented at the Institute of Medicine, Committee on Metabolic Monitoring Technologies for Military Field Applications Workshop on Metabolic Monitoring Technologies for Military Field Applications, San Antonio, Texas, January 8–9.

Kopple JD. 1999. Renal disorders and nutrition. In: Shils ME, Olson JA, Shike M, Ross AC, eds. *Modern Nutrition in Health and Disease.* 9th ed. Baltimore: Williams & Wilkins. Pp. 1439–1472.

Kovacs EM, Senden JM, Brouns F. 1999. Urine color, osmolality and specific electrical conductance are not accurate measures of hydration status during postexercise rehydration. *J Sports Med Phys Fitness* 39:47–53.

Krantz DS, McCeney MK. 2002. Effects of psychological and social factors on organic disease: A critical assessment of research on coronary heart disease. *Ann Rev Psychol* 53:341–369.

Kronfol Z, Remick DG. 2000. Cytokines and the brain: Implications for clinical psychiatry. *Am J Psychiat* 157:683–694.

Kusnecov AW, Sved A, Rabin BS. 2001. Immunologic effects of acute versus chronic stress in animals. In: Ader R, Felten DL, Cohen N, eds. *Psychoneuroimmunology.* Vol 2, 3rd ed. San Diego: Academic Press. Pp. 265–278.

Ladlow JF, Hoffmann WE, Breur GJ, Richardson DC, Allen MJ. 2002. Biological variability in serum and urinary indices of bone formation and resorption in dogs. *Calcif Tissue Int* 70:186–193.

Lai SY, Deffenderfer OF, Hanson W, Phillips MP, Thaler ER. 2002. Identification of upper respiratory bacterial pathogens with the electronic nose. *Laryngoscope* 112:975–979.

Lakier Smith L. 2003. Overtraining, excessive exercise, and altered immunity. Is this a T helper-1 versus T helper-2 lymphocyte response? *Sports Med* 33:347–364.

Latner AL. 1975. *Cantarow and Trumper Clinical Biochemistry*. 7th ed. Philadelphia: WB Saunders.

LeBlanc AD, Evans HJ, Marsh C, Schneider V, Johnson PC, Jhingran SG. 1986. Precision of dual photon absorptiometry measurements. *J Nucl Med* 27:1362–1365.

LeBlanc AD, Schneider VS, Evans HJ, Pientok C, Rowe R, Spector E. 1992. Regional changes in muscle mass following 17 weeks of bed rest. *J Appl Physiol* 73:2172–2178.

LeBlanc A, Schneider V, Spector E, Evans H, Rowe R, Lane H, Demers L, Lipton A. 1995. Calcium absorption, endogenous excretion, and endocrine changes during and after long-term bed rest. *Bone* 16:301S–304S.

LeBlanc AD, Driscol TB, Shackelford LC, Evans HJ, Rianon NJ, Smith SM, Feeback DL, Lai D. 2002. Alendronate as an effective countermeasure to disuse induced bone loss. *Musculoskel Neuron Ineract* 2:335–343.

Levo Y, Harbeck RJ, Kirkpatrick CH. 1985. Regulatory effect of hydrocortisone on the in vitro synthesis of IgE by human lymphocytes. *Int Arch Allergy Appl Immunol* 77:413–415.

Lieberman HR, Falco CM, Slade SS. 2002. Carbohydrate administration during a day of sustained aerobic activity improves vigilance, as assessed by a novel ambulatory monitoring device, and mood. *Am J Clin Nutr* 76:120–127.

Ligier S, Sternberg EM. 2001. The neuroendocrine system and rheumatoid arthritis: Focus on the hypothalamo-pituitary-adrenal axis. In: Ader R, Felten DL, Cohen N, eds. *Psychoneuroimmunology*. Vol 2, 3rd ed. San Diego: Academic Press. Pp. 449–469.

Lipsitz LA, Goldberger AL. 1992. Loss of 'complexity' and aging. Potential applications of fractals and chaos theory to senescence. *J Am Med Assoc* 267:1806–1809.

Lohman TG. 1992. *Advances in Body Composition Assessment. Current Issues in Exercise Science*. Monograph Number 3. Champaign, IL: Human Kinetics. Pp. 1–5, 7–23, 65–77, 79–89.

Lueken SA, Arnaud SB, Taylor AK, Baylink DJ. 1993. Changes in markers of bone formation and resorption in a bed rest model of weightlessness. *J Bone Miner Res* 8:1433–1438.

Macías N, Calderón de la Barca AM, Bolaños AV, Alemán H, Esparza J, Valencia ME. 2002. Body composition in Mexican adults by air displacement plethysmography (ADP) with the BOD-POD and deuterium oxide dilution using infrared spectroscopy (IRS-DOD). *Food Nutr Bull* 23:99–102.

MacKinnon LT. 2000. Chronic exercise training effects on immune function. *Med Sci Sports Exerc* 32:S369–S376.

Maier SF, Watkins LR, Fleshner M. 1994. Psychoneuroimmunology. The interface between behavior, brain, and immunity. *Am Psychol* 49:1004–1017.

Malliani A, Pagani M, Lombardi F. 1994. Physiology and clinical implications of variability of cardiovascular parameters with focus on heart rate and blood pressure. *Am J Cardiol* 73:3C–9C.

Manfredi TG, Fielding RA, O'Reilly KP, Meredith CN, Lee HY, Evans WJ. 1991. Plasma creatine kinase activity and exercise-induced muscle damage in older men. *Med Sci Sports Exerc* 23:1028–1034.

Manore M, Thompson J. 2000. *Sport Nutrition for Health and Performance.* Champaign, IL: Human Kinetics. Pp. 136–137, 148–149, 219–220, 224, 225, 228.

Margolis RN, Canalis E, Partridge NC. 1996. Invited review of a workshop: Anabolic hormones in bone: Basic research and therapeutic potential. *J Clin Endocrinol Metab* 81:872–877.

Marshall D, Johnell O, Wedel H. 1996. Meta-analysis of how well measures of bone mineral density predict occurrence of osteoporotic fractures. *Br Med J* 312:1254–1259.

Marucha PT, Sheridan JF, Padgett D. 2001. Stress and wound healing. In: Ader R, Felten DL, Cohen N, eds. *Psychoneuroimmunology.* Vol. 2, 3rd ed. San Diego: Academic Press. Pp. 613–626.

Mason D, MacPhee I, Antoni F. 1990. The role of the neuroendocrine system in determining genetic susceptibility to experimental allergic encephalomyelitis in the rat. *Immunology* 70:1–5.

Massip C, Riollet P, Quemener E, Bayle C, Salvayre R, Couderc F, Causse E. 2002. Choice of different dyes to label tyrosine and nitrotyrosine. *J Chromatogr A* 979:209–215.

Matkovic V, Heaney RP. 1992. Calcium balance during human growth: Evidence for threshold behavior. *Am J Clin Nutr* 55:992–996.

Maughan RJ. 1992. Fluid balance and exercise. *Int J Sports Med* 13:S132–S135.

Maughan RJ, Shirreffs SM. 1997. Recovery from prolonged exercise: Restoration of water and electrolyte balance. *J Sports Sci* 15:297–303.

Maul F, Sargent SA, Sims CA, Baldwin EA, Balaban MO, Huber DJ. 2000. Tomato flavor and aroma quality as affected by storage temperature. *J Food Sci* 65:1228–1237.

Maw GJ, Mackenzie IL, Taylor NA. 1998. Human body-fluid distribution during exercise in hot, temperate and cool environments. *Acta Physiol Scand* 163:297–304.

McClelland EE, Penn DJ, Potts WK. 2003. Major histocompatibility complex heterozygote superiority during coinfection. *Infect Immun* 71:2079–2086.

McClintock MK. 2000. Human pheromones: Primers, releasers, signalers, or modulators? In: Wallen K, Schneider JE, eds. *Reproduction in Context. Social and Environmental Influences on Reproductive Physiology and Behavior*. Cambridgs, MA: MIT Press. Pp. 355–420.

Melton LJ 3rd, Atkinson EJ, O'Fallon WM, Wahner HW, Riggs BL. 1993. Long-term fracture prediction by bone mineral assessed at different skeletal sites. *J Bone Miner Res* 8:1227–1233.

Meyer RA, Foley JM. 1996. Cellular processes integrating the metabolic response to exercise. In: Rowell LB, Shepherd JT, eds. *Handbook of Physiology: A Critical, Comprehensive Presentation of Physiological Knowledge and Concepts*. New York: Oxford University Press. Pp. 841–869.

Mills PJ, Ziegler MG, Dimsdale JE, Parry BL. 1995. Enumerative immune changes following acute stress: Effect of the menstrual cycle. *Brain Behav Immun* 9:190–195.

Mohamed EI, Linder R, Perriello G, Di Daniele N, Poppl SJ, De Lorenzo A. 2002. Predicting type 2 diabetes using an electronic nose-based artificial neural network analysis. *Diabetes Nutr Metab* 15:215–221.

Monaco F, Mutani R, Mastropaolo C, Tondi M. 1979. Tears as the best practical indicator of the unbound fraction of an anticonvulsant drug. *Epilepsia* 20:705–710.

Monaco F, Piredda S, Mastropaolo C, Tondi M, Mutani R. 1981. Diphenylhydantoin and primidone in tears. *Epilepsia* 22:185–188.

Monaco F, Piredda S, Mutani R, Mastropaolo C, Tondi M. 1982. The free fraction of valproic acid in tears, saliva, and cerebrospinal fluid. *Epilepsia* 23:23–26.

Monaco F, Mele G, Meloni T, Franca V, Sotgia A, Mutani R. 1984. A longitudinal study of valproate free fraction in the specific age group at greatest risk for febrile convulsions (children below 3 years). *Epilepsia* 25:240–243.

Montag S, Frank M, Ulmer H, Wernet D, Göpel W, Rammensee HG. 2001. "Electronic nose" detects major histocompatibility complex-dependent prerenal and postrenal odor components. *Proc Natl Acad Sci USA* 98:9249–9254.

Montain SJ, Coyle EF. 1992. Influence of graded dehydration on hyerthermia and cardiovascular drift during exercise. *J Appl Physiol* 73:1340–1350.

Morgan WP, Costill DL, Flynn MG, Raglin JS, O'Connor PJ. 1988. Mood disturbance following increased training in swimmers. *Med Sci Sports Exerc* 20:408–414.

Moynihan JA. 2003. Mechanisms of stress-induced modulation of immunity. *Brain Behav Immun* 17:S11–S16.

Müns G. 1994. Effect of long-distance running on polymorphonuclear neutrophil phagocytic function of the upper airways. *Int J Sports Med* 15:96–99.

Murphy PM. 1995. Blood, sweat, and chemotactic cytokines. *J Leukoc Biol* 57:438–439.

Murray R. 1995. Fluid needs in hot and cold environments. *Int J Sport Nutr* 5:S62–S73.

Musselman DL, Evans DL, Nemeroff CB. 1998. The relationship of depression to cardiovascular disease. *Arch Gen Psychiatry* 55:580–592.

Nabors-Oberg RE, Niaura RS, Sollers JJ, Thayer JF. 2002. The effect of controlled smoking on heart period variability. *IEEE Eng Med Biol* 21:65–70.

Nakajima M, Yamato S, Shimada K, Sato S, Kitagawa S, Honda A, Miyamoto J, Shoda J, Ohya M, Miyazaki H. 2000. Assessment of drug concentrations in tears in therapeutic drug monitoring: I. Determination of valproic acid in tears by gas chromatography/mass spectrometry with EC/NCI mode. *Ther Drug Monit* 22:716–722.

Neary JP, McKenzie DC, Bhambhani YN. 2002. Effects of short-term endurance training on muscle deoxygenation trends using NIRS. *Med Sci Sports Exerc* 34:1725–1732.

Newsholme EA. 1994. Biochemical mechanisms to explain immunosuppression in well-trained and overtrained athletes. *Int J Sports Med* 15:S142–S147.

Newsholme EA, Actworth IN, Blomstrand E. 1987. Amino acids, brain neruotransmitters and a functional link between muscle and brain that is important in sustained exercise. *Adv Myochem* 1:127–133.

Nguyen TV, Sambrook PN, Eisman JA. 1997. Source of variability in bone mineral density measurement: Implications for study design and analysis of bone loss. *J Bone Miner Res* 44:424–442.

Nieman DC. 2000. Is infection risk linked to exercise workload? *Med Sci Sports Exerc* 32:S406–S411.

Niess JH, Monnikes H, Dignass AU, Klapp BF, Arck PC. 2002. Review on the influence of stress on immune mediators, neuropeptides and hormones with relevance for inflammatory bowel disease. *Digestion* 65:131–140.

Nishimura Y, Fukuoka H, Kiriyama M, Suzuki Y, Oyama K, Ikawa S, Higurashi M, Gunji A. 1994. Bone turnover and calcium metabolism during 20 days bed rest in young healthy males and females. *Acta Physiol Scand* 150:27–35.

Noakes TD, Norman RJ, Buck RH, Godlonton J, Stevenson K, Pittaway D. 1990. The incidence of hyponatremia during prolonged ultraendurance exercise. *Med Sci Sports Exerc* 22:165–170.

Nose H, Morimoto T, Ogura K. 1983. Distribution of water losses among fluid compartments of tissues under thermal dehydration in the rat. *Jpn J Physiol* 33:1019–1029.

Nose H, Mack GW, Shi X, Nadel ER. 1994. Role of osmolality and plasma volume during rehydration in humans. In: Marriott BM, ed. *Fluid Replacement and Heat Stress*. Washington, DC: National Academy Press. Pp. 143–160.

NWS (National Weather Service). 2003. *Heat Index*. Online. National Oceanic and Atmospheric Administration. Available at http://www.crh.noaa.gov/pub/ heat.htm. Accessed September 24, 2003.

Ober C, Weitkamp LR, Cox N, Dytch H, Kostyu D, Elias S. 1997. HLA and mate choice in humans. *Am J Hum Genet* 61:497–504.

Obminski Z, Wojtkowiak M, Stupnicki R, Golec L, Hackney AC. 1997. Effect of acceleration stress on salivary cortisol and plasma cortisol and testosterone levels in cadet pilots. *J Physiol Pharmacol* 48:193–200.

O'Connor PJ, Morgan WP, Raglin JS. 1991. Psychobiologic effects of 3 d of increased training in female and male swimmers. *Med Sci Sports Exerc* 23:1055–1061.

Oh MS, Uribarri J. 1999. Electrolytes, water, and acid-base balance. In: Shils ME, Olson JA, Shike M, Ross AC, eds. *Modern Nutrition in Health and Disease.* 9th ed. Baltimore: Williams & Wilkins. Pp. 105–139.

Ohira Y, Jiang B, Roy RR, Oganov V, Ilyina-Kakueva E, Marini JF, Edgerton VR. 1992. Rat soleus muscle fiber responses to 14 days of spaceflight and hindlimb suspension. *J Appl Physiol* 73:51S–57S.

Olff M. 1999. Stress, depression and immunity: The role of defense and coping styles. *Psychiat Res* 85:7–15.

Pavlou AK, Magan N, McNulty C, Jones JM, Sharp D, Brown J, Turner APF. 2002. Use of an electronic nose system for diagnoses of urinary tract infections. *Biosens Bioelectron* 17:893–899.

Pearse-Pratt R, Schellinck H, Brown R, Singh PB, Roser B. 1999. Soluble MHC antigens and olfactory recognition of genetic individuality: The mechanism. *Genetica* 104:223–230.

Pedersen BK, Bruunsgaard H, Jensen M, Toft AD, Hansen H, Ostrowski K. 1999. Exercise and the immune system—Influence of nutrition and ageing. *J Sci Med Sport* 2:234–252.

Peng CK, Buldyrev SV, Hausdorff JM, Havlin S, Mietus JE, Simons M, Stanley HE, Goldberger AL. 1994. Non-equilibrium dynamics as an indispensable characteristic of a healthy biological system. *Integr Physiol Behav Sci* 29:283–293.

Penn D, Potts WK. 1998a. Chemical signals and parasite-mediated sexual selection. *Trends Ecol Evol* 13:391–396.

Penn D, Potts W. 1998b. How do major histocompatibility complex genes influence odor and mating preferences? *Adv Immunol* 69:411–436.

Penn D, Schneider G, White K, Slev P, Potts W. 1998. Influenza infection neutralizes the attractiveness of male odor to female mice (*Mus musculus*). *Ethology* 104:685–694.

Persaud KC, Travers PJ. 1996. Arrays of broad specificity films for sensing volatile chemicals. In: Kress-Rogers E, ed. *Handbook of Biosensors and Electronic Noses: Medicine, Food, and the Environment.* Boca Raton, FL: CRC Press. Pp. 563–592.

Pette D, Staron RS. 1990. Cellular and molecular diversities of mammalian skeletal muscle fibers. *Rev Physiol Biochem Pharmacol* 116:1–76.

Pillonel L, Ampuero S, Tabacchi R, Bosset JO. 2003. Analytical methods for the determination of the geographic origin of Emmental cheese: Volatile compounds by GC/MS-FID and electronic nose. *Eur Food Res Technol* 216:179–183.

Puente-Maestu L, Tena T, Trascasa C, Pérez-Parra J, Godoy R, Garcia MJ, Stringer WW. 2003. Training improves muscle oxidative capacity and oxygenation recovery kinetics in patients with chronic obstructive pulmonary disease. *Eur J Appl Physiol* 88:580–587.

Quaresima V, Lepanto R, Ferrari M. 2003. The use of near infrared spectroscopy in sports medicine. *Sports Med Phys Fitness* 43:1–13.

Ravn P, Bidstrup M, Wasnich RD, Davis JW, McClung MR, Balske A, Coupland C, Sahota O, Kaur A, Daley M, Cizza G. 1999. Alendronate and estrogen-progestin in the long-term prevention of bone loss: Four-year results from the early postmenopausal intervention cohort study. A randomized, controlled trial. *Ann Intern Med* 131:935–942.

Recker RR, Davies KM, Hinders SM, Heaney RP, Stegman MR, Kimmel DB. 1992. Bone gain in young adult women. *J Am Med Assoc* 268:2403–2408.

Reed SF, Porges SW, Newlin DB. 1999. Effect of alcohol on vagal regulation of cardiovascular function: Contributions of the polyvagal theory to the psychophysiology of alcohol. *Exp Clin Psychopharmacol* 7:484–492.

Rendell M, Anderson E, Schlueter W, Mailliard J, Honigs D, Rosenthal R. 2003. Determination of hemoglobin levels in the finger using near infrared spectroscopy. *Clin Lab Haematol* 25:93–97.

Richards L. 1996. April 27. Disturbing trend: Hikers ill from too much water. *Arizona Republic* A1.

Robbins JA, Hirsch C, Whitmer R, Cauley J, Harris T. 2001. The association of bone mineral density and depression in an older population. *J Am Geriatr Soc* 49:732–736.

Rocha EM, Cunha DA, Carneiro EM, Boschero AC, Saad MJA, Velloso LA. 2002. Identification of insulin in the tear film and insulin receptor and IGF-1 receptor on the human ocular surface. *Invest Ophthalmol Vis Sci* 43:963–967.

Rosen CJ, Beamer WG, Donahue LR. 2003. *Biomarkers of Bone and Muscle Turnover: Effects of Exercise*. Presented at the Institute of Medicine, Committee on Metabolic Monitoring Technologies for Military Field Applications Workshop on Metabolic Monitoring Technologies for Military Field Applications, San Antonio, Texas, January 8–9.

Rosen NA, Charash WE, Hirsch EF. 2002. Near-infrared spectrometric determination of blood pH. *J Surg Res* 106:282–286.

Rossy LA, Thayer JF. 1998. Fitness and gender-related differences in heart period variability. *Psychosom Med* 60:773–781.

Roth SM, Ivey FM, Martel GF, Lemmer JT, Hurlbut DE, Siegel EL, Metter EJ, Fleg JL, Fozard JL, Kostek MC, Wernick DM, Hurley BF. 2001. Muscle size responses to strength training in young and older men and women. *J Am Geriatr Soc* 49:1428–1433.

Rothermundt M, Arolt V, Fenker J, Gutbrodt H, Peters M, Kirchner H. 2001. Different immune patterns in melancholic and non-melancholic major depression. *Eur Arch Psychiat Clin Neurosci* 251:90–97.

Rottman SJ, Snowdon CT. 1972. Demonstration and analysis of an alarm pheromone in mice. *J Comp Physiol Psychol* 81:483–490.

Rozanski A, Blumenthal JA, Kaplan J. 1999. Impact of psychological factors on the pathogenesis of cardiovascular disease and implications for therapy. *Circulation* 99:2192–2217.

Rülicke T, Chapuisat M, Homberger FR, Macas E, Wedekind C. 1998. MHC-genotype of progeny influenced by parental infection. *Proc R Soc Lond B Biol Sci* 265:711–716.

Ruzek MC, Pearce BD, Miller AH, Biron CA. 1999. Endogenous glucocorticoids protect against cytokine-mediated lethality during viral infection. *Immunology* 162:3527–3533.

Saltin B, Gollnick PD. 1983. Skeletal muscle adaptability: Significance for metabolism and performance. In: Peachey LD, Adrian RH, Geiger SR, eds. *Handbook of Physiology. A Critical, Comprehensive Presentation of Physiological Knowledge and Concepts. Section 10: Skeletal Muscle*. Bethesda, MD: American Physiological Society. Pp. 555–631.

Saul JP. 1990. Beat-to-beat variations of heart rate reflect modulation of cardiac autonomic outflow. *News Physiol Sci* 5:32–37.

Sawchenko PE, Arias C. 1995. Evidence for short-loop feedback effects of ACTH on CRF and vasopressin expression in parvocellular neurosecretory neurons. *J Neuroendocrinol* 7:721–731.

Sawchenko PE, Li HY, Ericsson A. 2000. Circuits and mechanisms governing hypothalamic responses to stress: A tale of two paradigms. *Prog Brain Res* 122:61–78.

Sawka MN, Montain SJ. 2000. Fluid and electrolyte supplementation for exercise heat stress. *Am J Clin Nutr* 72:564S–572S.

Sawka MN, Pandolf KB. 1990. Effects of body water loss on physiological function and exercise performance. In: Lamb DR, Gisolfi CV, eds. *Perspectives in Exercise Science and Sports Medicine. Fluid Homeostasis During Exercise*. Vol. 3. Carmel, IN: Benchmark Press. Pp. 1–38.

Schaefer ML, Young DA, Restrepo D. 2001. Olfactory fingerprints for major histocompatibility complex-determined body odors. *J Neurosci* 21:2481–2487.

Schoeller DA. 1996. Hydrometry. In: Roche AF, Heymsfield SB, Lohman TG, eds. *Human Body Composition*. Champaign, IL: Human Kinetics. Pp. 25–43.

Scott LV, Dinan TG. 1998. Vasopressin and the regulation of hypothalamic-pituitary-adrenal axis function: Implications for the pathophysiology of depression. *Life Sci* 62:1985–1998.

Sevick-Muraca EM, Houston JP, Gurfinkel M. 2002. Fluorescence-enhanced, near infrared diagnostic imaging with contrast agents. *Curr Opin Chem Biol* 6:642–650.

Sevier TL. 1994. Infectious disease in athletes. *Med Clin North Am* 78:389–412.

Shapiro Y, Seidman DS. 1990. Field and clinical observations of exertional heat stroke patients. *Med Sci Sports Exerc* 22:6–14.

Shephard RJ, Shek PN. 2001. Physical activity and upper respiratory infection. In: Ader R, Felten DL, Cohen N, eds. *Psychoneuroimmunology*. Vol 2, 3rd ed. San Diego: Academic Press. Pp. 511–523.

Shirreffs SM, Maughan RJ. 2000. Rehydration and recovery of fluid balance after exercise. *Exerc Sport Sci Rev* 28:27–32.

Shishehbor MH, Aviles RJ, Brennan ML, Fu X, Goormastic M, Pearce GL, Gokce N, Keaney JF Jr, Penn MS, Sprecher DL, Vita JA, Hazen SL. 2003. Association of nitrotyrosine levels with cardiovascular disease and modulation by statin therapy. *J Am Med Assoc* 289:1675–1680.

Simon AM, Manigrasso MB, O'Connor JP. 2002. Cyclo-oxygenase 2 function is essential for bone fracture healing. *J Bone Miner Res* 17:963–976.

Singer AG, Beauchamp GK, Yamazaki K. 1997. Volatile signals of the major histocompatibility complex in male mouse urine. *Proc Natl Acad Sci USA* 94:2210–2214.

Smith LL. 1991. Acute inflammation: The underlying mechanism in delayed onset muscle soreness? *Med Sci Sports Exerc* 23:542–551.

Smith LL. 2000. Cytokine hypothesis of overtraining: A physiological adaptation to excessive stress? *Med Sci Sports Exerc* 32:317–331.

Smith SM, Krauhs JM, Leach CS. 1997. Regulation of body fluid volume and electrolyte concentrations in spaceflight. *Adv Space Biol Med* 6:123–165.

Smith SM, Nillen JL, Leblanc A, Lipton A, Demers LM, Lane HW, Leach CS. 1998. Collagen cross-link excretion during space flight and bed rest. *J Clin Endocrinol Metab* 83:3584–3591.

Smith SM, Wastney ME, Morukov BV, Larina IM, Nyquist LE, Abrams SA, Taran EN, Shih CY, Nillen JL, Davis-Street JE, Rice BL, Lane HW. 1999. Calcium metabolism before, during, and after a 3-mo spaceflight: Kinetic and biochemical changes. *Am J Physiol* 277:R1–R10.

Soller BR, Cabrera M, Smith SM, Sutton JP. 2002. Smart medical systems with application to nutrition and fitness in space. *Nutrition* 18:930–936.

Song C, Kenis G, van Gastel A, Bosmans E, Lin A, de Jong R, Neels H, Scharpe S, Janca A, Yasukawa K, Maes M. 1999. Influence of psychological stress on immune-inflammatory variables in normal humans. Part II. Altered serum concentrations of natural anti-inflammatory agents and soluble membrane antigens of monocytes and T lymphocytes. *Psychiat Res* 85:293–303.

Speedy DB, Noakes TD, Schneider C. 2001. Exercise-associated hyponatremia: A review. *Emerg Med* 13:17–27.

Stanulis ED, Matulka RA, Jordan SD, Rosecrans JA, Holsapple MP. 1997. Role of corticosterone in the enhancement of the antibody response after acute cocaine administration. *J Pharmacol Exp Therapeut* 280:284–291.

Steensberg A, Toft AD, Bruunsgaard H, Sandmand M, Halkjaer-Kristensen J, Pedersen BK. 2001. Strenuous exercise decreases the percentage of type 1 T cells in the circulation. *J Appl Physiol* 91:1708–1712.

Stein PK, Kleiger RE. 1999. Insights from the study of heart rate variability. *Ann Rev Med* 50:249–261.

Stein TP. 2003. *Amino Acids as Biomarkers for Fatigue*. Presented at the Institute of Medicine, Committee on Metabolic Monitoring Technologies for Military Field Applications Workshop on Metabolic Monitoring Technologies for Military Field Applications, San Antonio, Texas, January 8–9.

Sternberg EM. 1997. Emotions and disease: From balance of humors to balance of molecules. *Nat Med* 3:264–267.

Sternberg EM. 1998. Overview of the conference and the field. *Ann NY Acad Sci* 840:1–8.

Sternberg EM. 2001. Neuroendocrine regulation of autoimmune/inflammatory disease. *J Endocrinol* 169:429–435.

Sternberg EM, Chrousos GP, Wilder RL, Gold PW. 1992. The stress response and the regulation of inflammatory disease. *Ann Intern Med* 117:854–866.

Stofan JR, Zacwieja JJ, Horswill CA, Murray R. 2002. Sweat and sodium losses during practice in professional football players: Field studies. *Med Sci Sports Exerc* 34:S113.

Stofan JR, Zachwieja JJ, Horswill CA, Lacambra M, Murray R, Eichner ER, Anderson S. 2003. Sweat and sodium losses in NCAA Division I football players with a history of whole-body muscle cramping. *Med Sci Sports Exerc* 35:S48.

Strachan AT, Maughan RJ. 1999. The hormonal response to a D-fenfluramine challenge in trained and sedentary men. *Med Sci Sports Exerc* 31:547–553.

Strickland P, Morriss R, Wearden A, Deakin B. 1998. A comparison of salivary cortisol in chronic fatigue syndrome, community depression and healthy controls. *J Affect Disord* 47:191–194.

Strüder HK, Weicker H. 2001. Physiology and pathophysiology of the serotonergic system and its implications on mental and physical performance. Part II. *Int J Sports Med* 22:482–497.

Strüder HK, Hollmann W, Platen P, Donike M, Gotzmann A, Weber K. 1998. Influence of paroxetine, branched-chain amino acids and tyrosine on neuroendocrine system responses and fatigue in humans. *Horm Metab Res* 30:188–194.

Sutton JR. 1990. Clinical implications of fluid imbalance. In: Lamb DR, Gisolfi CV, eds. *Perspectives in Exercise Science and Sports Medicine. Fluid Homeostasis During Exercise.* Vol 3. Carmel, IN: Benchmark Press. Pp. 425–455.

Suzuki Y, Murakami T, Haruna Y, Kawakubo K, Goto S, Makita Y, Ikawa S, Gunji A. 1994. Effects of 10 and 20 days bed rest on leg muscle mass and strength in young subjects. *Acta Physiol Scand* 150:5–18.

Suzuki K, Yamada M, Kurakake S, Okamura N, Yamaya K, Liu Q, Kudoh S, Kowatari K, Nakaji S, Sugawara K. 2000. Circulating cytokines and hormones with immunosuppressive but neutrophil-priming potentials rise after endurance exercise in humans. *Eur J Appl Physiol* 81:281–287.

Takahashi N, Yuasa S, Fukunaga M, Hara T, Moriwaki K, Shokoji T, Hitomi H, Fujioka H, Kiyomoto H, Aki Y, Hirohata M, Mizushige K, Kohno M. 2003.

Long-term evaluation of nutritional status using dual-energy X-ray absorptimetry in chronic hemodialysis patients. *Clin Nephrol* 59:373–378.

Task Force of the European Society of Cardiology the North American Society of Pacing Electrophysiology. 1996. Heart rate variability: Standards of measurement, physiological interpretation, and clinical use. *Circulation* 93:1043–1065.

Thayer JF, Friedman BH. 1997. The heart of anxiety: A dynamical systems approach. In: Vingerhoets AJJM, Bussel F, Boelhouwer J, eds. *The (Non)Expression of Emotions in Health and Disease*. Amsterdam: Tilburg University Press. Pp. 39–49.

Thayer JF, Lane RD. 2000. A model of neurovisceral integration in emotion regulation and dysregulation. *J Affect Disord* 61:201–216.

Thayer JF, Friedman BH, Borkovec TD. 1996. Autonomic characteristics of generalized anxiety disorder and worry. *Biol Psychiatry* 39:255–266.

Thayer JF, Smith M, Rossy LA, Sollers JJ, Friedman BH. 1998. Heart period variability and depressive symptoms: Gender differences. *Biol Psychiatry* 44:304–306.

Thygesen JEM, Bach B, Molhave L, Pedersen OF, Prause JU, Skov P. 1987. Tear fluid electrolytes and album in persons under environmental stress. *Environ Res* 43:60–65.

Totman R, Kiff J, Reed SE, Craig JW. 1980. Predicting experimental colds in volunteers from different measures of recent life stress. *J Psychosom Res* 24:155–163.

Valenta JG, Rigby MK. 1968. Discrimination of the odor of stressed rats. *Science* 161:599–601.

Valentic JP, Leopold IH, Dea FJ. 1980. Excretion of salicylic acid into tears following oral administration of asprin. *Ophthalmology* 87:815–820.

van Agtmaal EJ, Bloem MW, Speek AJ, Saowakontha S, Wchreurs WHP, van Haeringen NJ. 1988. The effect of vitamin A supplementation on tear fluid retinol levels of marginally nourished preschool children. *Curr Eye Res* 7:43–48.

van Beekvelt MCP, van Engelen BGM, Wevers RA, Colier WNJM. 2002. In vivo quantitative near-infrared spectroscopy in skeletal muscle during incremental isometric handgrip exercise. *Clin Physiol Func Imag* 22:210–217.

van der Pompe G, Antoni MH, Visser A, Heijnen CJ. 1998. Effect of mild acute stress on immune cell distribution and natural killer cell activity in breast cancer patients. *Biol Psychol* 48:21–35.

van Haeringen NJ. 1985. Secretion of drugs in tears. *Curr Eye Res* 4:485–488.

Vedhara K, Cox NK, Wilcock GK, Perks P, Hunt M, Anderson S, Lightman SL, Shanks NM. 1999. Chronic stress in elderly carers of dementia patients and antibody response to influenza vaccination. *Lancet* 353:627–631.

Verrier RL, Mittleman MA. 2000. The impact of emotions on the heart. *Prog Brain Res* 122:369–380.

Walser M. 1999. Effects of protein intake on renal function and on the development of renal disease. In: *The Role of Protein and Amino Acids in Sustaining and Enhancing Performance*. Washington, DC: National Academy Press. Pp. 137–154.

Wariar R, Gaffke JN, Haller RG, Bertocci LA. 2000. A modular NIRS system for clinical measurement of impaired skeletal muscle oxygenation. *J Appl Physiol* 88:315–325.

Watts NB. 1999. Clinical utility of biochemical markers of bone remodeling. *Clin Chem* 45:1359–1368.

Weaver CM, LeBlanc A, Smith SM. 2000. Calcium and related nutrients in bone metabolism. In: Lane HW, Schoeller DA, eds. *Nutrition in Spaceflight and Weightlessness Models*. Boca Raton, FL: CRC Press. Pp. 179–201.

Webster JI, Tonelli L, Sternberg EM. 2002. Neuroendocrine regulation of immunity. *Ann Rev Immunol* 20:125–163.

Wedekind C, Seebeck T, Bettens F, Paepke AJ. 1995. MHC-dependent mate preferences in humans. *Proc R Soc Lond B Biol Sci* 260:245–249.

Wei R, Listwak SJ, Sternberg EM. 2003. Lewis hypothalamic cells constitutively and upon stimulation express higher levels of mRNA for proinflammatory cytokines and related molecules: Comparison with inflammatory resistant Fischer rat hypothalamic cells. *J Neuroimmunol* 135:10–28.

Weise F, Krell D, Brinkhoff N. 1986. Acute alcohol ingestion reduces heart rate variability. *Drug Alcohol Depend* 17:89–91.

Weiss DW, Hirt R, Tarcic N, Berzon Y, Ben-Zur H, Breznitz S, Glaser B, Grover NB, Baras M, O'Dorisio TM. 1996. Studies in psychoneuroimmunology: Psychological, immunological, and neuroendocrinological parameters in Israeli civilians during and after a period of Scud missle attacks. *Behav Med* 22:5–14.

Westerblad H, Lee JA, Lannergren J, Allen DG. 1991. Cellular mechanisms of fatigue in skeletal muscle. *Am J Physiol* 261:C195–C209.

Wick G, Kromer G, Neu N, Fassler R, Ziemiecki A, Muller RG, Ginzel M, Beladi I, Kuhr T, Hala K. 1987. The multi-factorial pathogenesis of autoimmune disease. *Immunol Lett* 16:249–257.

Wiegers GJ, Reul JM, Holsboer F, de Kloet ER. 1994. Enhancement of rat splenic lymphocyte mitogenesis after short term preexposure to corticosteroids in vitro. *Endocrinology* 135:2351–2357.

Wilmore JH, Costill DL. 1994. *Physiology of Sport and Exercise*. Champaign, IL: Human Kinetics.

Wilson WM, Maughan RJ. 1992. Evidence for a possible role of 5-hydroxytryptamine in the genesis of fatigue in man: Administration of paroxetine, a 5-HT re-uptake inhibitor, reduces the capacity to perform prolonged exercise. *Exp Physiol* 77:921–924.

Wittert G. 2000. The effect of exercise on the hypothalamo-pituitary-adrenal axis. In: Warren MP, Constantini NW, eds. *Sports Endocrinology*. Totowa, NJ: Humana Press. Pp. 43–55.

Wolfe R, Børsheim E. 2003. *Biomarkers for Change in Protein Turnover of Muscle*. Presented at the Institute of Medicine, Committee on Metabolic Monitoring Technologies for Military Field Applications Workshop on Metabolic Monitoring Technologies for Military Field Applications, San Antonio, Texas, January 8–9.

Wong ML, Kling MA, Munson PJ, Listwak S, Licinio J, Prolo P, Karp B, McCutcheon IE, Geraicioti TD, DeBellis MD, Rice KC, Goldstein DS, Veldhuis JD, Chrousos GP, Oldfield EH, McCann SM, Gold PW. 2000. Pronounced and sustained central hypernoradrenergic function in major depression with melancholic features: Relation to hypercortisolism and corticotropin-releasing hormone. *Proc Natl Acad Sci USA* 97:325–330.

Wysocki CJ, Preti G. 2000. Human body odors and their perception. *Jpn J Taste Smell Res* 7:19–42.

Xu GD, Liu F, Gong H, Ge XF, Luo QM. 2003. Blood oxygen and lactate concentrations in skeletal muscles during exercise. *Space Med Med Engl (Beijing)* 16:41–43.

Yamaguchi M, Yamazaki K, Beauchamp GK, Bard J, Thomas L, Boyse EA. 1981. Distinctive urinary odors governed by the major histocompatibility locus of the mouse. *Proc Natl Acad Sci USA* 78:5817–5820.

Yamazaki K, Yamaguchi M, Baranoski L, Bard J, Boyse EA, Thomas L. 1979. Recognition among mice. Evidence for the use of a Y-maze differentially scented by congenic mice of different major histocompatibility types. *J Exp Med* 150:755–760.

Yamazaki K, Singer A, Curran M, Beauchamp GK. 1999. Origin, functions, and chemistry of H-2 regulated odorants. In: Johnston RE, Müller-Schwarze D, Sorensen PW, eds. *Advances in Chemical Signals in Vertebrates*. New York: Kluwer Academic/Plenum Publishers. Pp. 173–180.

Yamazaki K, Boyse EA, Bard J, Curran M, Kim D, Ross SR, Beauchamp GK. 2002. Presence of mouse mammary tumor virus specifically alters the body odor of mice. *Proc Natl Acad Sci USA* 99:5612–5615.

Yehuda R, Teicher MH, Trestman RL, Levengood RA, Siever LJ. 1996. Cortisol regulation in posttraumatic stress disorder and major depression: A chronobiological analysis. *Biol Psychiat* 40:79–88.

Yehuda R, Bierer LM, Schmeidler J, Aferiat DH, Breslau I, Dolan S. 2000. Low cortisol and risk for PTSD in adult offspring of holocaust survivors. *Am J Psychiat* 157:1252–1259.

Young VR, Haverberg LN, Bilmazes C, Munro HN. 1973. Potential use of 3-methylhistidine excretion as an index of progressive reduction in muscle protein catabolism during starvation. *Metabolism* 22:1429–1436.

Zhang M, Xuan S, Bouxsein ML, von Stechow D, Akeno N, Faugere MC, Malluche H, Zhao G, Rosen CJ, Efstratiadis A, Clemens TL. 2002. Osteoblast-specific knockout of the insulin-like growth factor (IGF) receptor gene reveals an essential role of IGF signaling in bone matrix mineralization. *J Biol Chem* 277:44005–44012.

Zhang X, Firestein S. 2002. The olfactory receptor gene superfamily of the mouse. *Nat Neurosci* 5:124–133.

Zhao G, Monier-Faugere MC, Langub MC, Geng Z, Nakayama T, Pike JW, Chernausek SD, Rosen CJ, Donahue LR, Malluche HH, Fagin JA, Clemens TL. 2000. Targeted overexpression of insulin-like growth factor I to osteoblasts of transgenic mice: Increased trabecular bone volume without increased osteoblast proliferation. *Endocrinology* 141:2674–2682.

Zhou GX, Ge Z, Dorwart J, Izzo B, Kukura J, Bicker G, Wyvratt J. 2003. Determination and differentiation of surface and bound water in drug substances by near infrared spectroscopy. *J Pharm Sci* 92:1058–1065.

Ziegler D, Laude D, Akila F, Elghozi JL. 2001. Time- and frequency-domain estimation of early diabetic cardiovascular autonomic neuropathy. *Clin Auton Res* 11:369–376.

Ziegler R, Kasperk C. 1998. Glucocorticoid-induced osteoporosis: Prevention and treatment. *Steroids* 63:344–348.

Zukowska Z, Pons J, Lee EW, Li L. 2003. Neuropeptide Y: A new mediator linking sympathetic nerves, blood vessels and immune system? *Can J Physiol Pharmacol* 81:89–94.

5

Strategies for Monitoring Cognitive Performance

Up to this point the central focus of this report has been on the assessment or monitoring of the combat service member's capacity to perform physical tasks. In this regard, the importance of factors that influence bone and muscle health, as well as other processes that underlie and optimize physical endurance and resistance to physical injury, have been highlighted, and for good reason. Clearly it is necessary to ensure that operational personnel are as physically fit as possible because success on the battlefield is to a great extent dependent on the ability of combat service members to carry and operate weapons, overcome physical obstacles, traverse distances in harsh environments, and endure a host of physical stresses and strains that could easily overwhelm unfit individuals. However, optimal performance in today's military also is increasingly dependent on a high level of cognitive fitness. The widespread use of computerized weapon systems; complicated communications and targeting devices; high-performance aircraft, tanks, and maritime vessels; and the technologically advanced diagnostic systems used in the maintenance of military equipment demands the highest levels of cognitive readiness.

In the following sections, operator cognitive fatigue, one of the principal threats to military readiness, is discussed. Also included is an overview of the primary operational causes of fatigue, followed by a brief synopsis of strategies that should be considered for monitoring the cognitive status of servicemembers.

The fact that the focus here is on the fatigue that results from sleep deprivation should in no way imply that this is the only stressor of concern in the operational environment. As noted earlier in this report, combat service members are routinely exposed to a wide variety of physical and environmental stresses that, if ignored, will ultimately degrade operational performance. Heat stress and dehydration pose major threats to the cognitive readiness of ground combat service members, and these factors can be expected to exacerbate the fatigue from sleep loss and strenuous work. In the aviation arena, uncomfortable levels of noise, heat, vibration, and mental workload must be dealt with by pilots on a day-to-day basis, and these stresses likewise can be expected to compromise cognitive capacity. However, since a detailed discussion of each of these areas is beyond the scope of this report, it is hoped that the reader can generalize many of the concepts from the forthcoming discussion of the most common cause of operator fatigue (sleep deprivation) to the fatigue stemming from other operational stressors.

THE PROBLEM OF SLEEPINESS AND COGNITIVE DEGRADATION IN MILITARY SETTINGS

Current military doctrine requires that units operate around the clock during times of conflict because the success of battlefield operations depends, at least in part, on maintaining the momentum of continuous day-night operations (U.S. Army, 1997). Technological advances, such as night vision devices, have enhanced the night-fighting capabilities of both ground and air combat military personnel, making around-the-clock missions a highly feasible component of the modern military strategy. Combining efficient day and night fighting capabilities across successive 24-hour periods places a significant strain on enemy resources and presents a clear tactical advantage for U.S. forces. In fact, the Air Force Chief of Staff recently noted that persistent and sustained operations "24 hours a day, seven days a week" are essential to attaining U.S. victory in today's battle space (Elliott, 2001).

However, there are difficulties inherent in maintaining effective around-the-clock operations. For example, aircraft can function for extended periods without adverse effects, but human operators need periodic sleep for the restoration of both body and cognitive function (Horne, 1978). Depriving humans of proper restorative sleep produces attention lapses and slower reaction times, which are associated with poor performance (Krueger, 1991). It has been determined that sleep-deprived personnel lose approximately 25 percent of their ability to perform useful mental work with each 24-hour period of sleep loss (Belenky et al., 1994). Thus by the end of 3 days without sleep, combat service members may be considered totally ineffective in the operational setting, especially if they are performing complex tasks, such as operating computerized command-and-control centers or flying an aircraft. This is a significant problem given that an Army manual makes it clear that "Soldiers in continuous operations can expect to be deprived of extended regular sleep, *possibly any sleep*, for as long as three to five days" (U.S. Army, 1991, P. 3-10).

Over the past several years the problem of sleep loss and fatigue has escalated because of increased requirements on military forces due to reductions in manpower and other resources. Over the past 10 to 15 years Army funding has been cut 38 percent and the number of personnel has been cut 35 percent, while missions have increased 300 percent (U.S. Army, 1996). A similar problem exists in the Air Force, where there has been a 37.7 percent reduction in military personnel and about a 50 percent reduction in the number of active Air Force tactical wings (Daggett and Belasco, 2002), while the operational tempo has increased by as much as 400 percent (Correll, 1998). U.S. military capabilities are increasingly strained as understaffed units strive to accomplish more work with fewer resources. The ultimate result has been diminished military combat readiness (Spencer, 2000), in part because of increased levels of physical and cognitive fatigue.

Although reductions in available resources do not guarantee that sleep deprivation will be a problem in the operational environment, they create a situation in which the available personnel are more likely to work prolonged shifts without the benefit of sufficient rest. Krueger (1991) reported that the efficiency of combatants in sustained operations can be significantly compromised by inadequate sleep. Vigilance and attention suffer, reaction time is impaired, mood declines, and some personnel begin to experience perceptual disturbances. Naitoh and Kelly (1992) warned that poor sleep management in extended operations quickly leads to motivational decrements, impaired attention, short-term memory loss, carelessness, reduced physical endurance, degraded verbal communication skills, and impaired judgment. Angus and Heslegrave (1985) noted that cognitive abilities suffer 30 percent reductions after only 1 night without sleep, and 60 percent reductions after a second night.

Although all types of performance are not affected to the same degree by sleep loss, the fatigue from prolonged duty periods clearly is a threat to unit readiness in the operational context. This is especially the case for tasks that are lengthy, devoid of performance feedback, and boring. Caldwell and Ramspott (1998), Wilkinson (1969), and Wilkinson and colleagues (1966) found that when task durations extend beyond 15 to 20 minutes, performance deteriorations from fatigue become far more pronounced than when the task durations are shorter. Wilkinson (1961) found that knowledge of results alone can significantly attenuate the effects of sleep deprivation on some types of vigilance tasks. In addition, Wilkinson (1964) reported that while reaction-time tasks and vigilance tasks are most degraded by sleep loss, more interesting learning tasks and performance tasks often are less affected, presumably because the subject's level of interest provides greater motivation and ability to resist attention lapses or outright sleep episodes (although, as warned by Dinges and Kribbs [1991], this works only up to a point).

In addition to the impact of task characteristics, it should be noted that there are individual differences in resiliency to sleep loss. Although this is an area that has not been sufficiently researched at this point, Van Dongen and colleagues (2003) found that there are basic interindividual differences in vulnerability to sleep debt that cannot be explained on the basis of differences in sleep need (i.e., short vs. long sleepers). This source of variability no doubt contributes to findings that there are wide differences in the accuracy with which several currently available methods can predict performance decrements. As the reader later reviews the strategies proposed to monitor alertness in the field, a recent U.S. Highway Traffic Safety report should be kept in mind (Dinges et al., 1998). In that report, even the eye-closure measure PERCLOS, which was found to be one of the most predictive indicators of fatigue-related performance lapses under laboratory conditions ($r = 0.7$), sometimes correlated with performance only at about $r = 0.3$ in some individuals. Two electroencephalographic (EEG) algorithms showed a *median* predictive capability of only 0.3 to 0.4, and one type of eye-blink monitoring device correlated with minute-to-minute lapse frequency at a median level of 0.17. Thus despite the known dangers of fatigue and the established need to accurately measure it in some contexts, it is clear that much work remains to be done on monitoring technologies that can accurately predict moment-to-moment performance fluctuations. Clearly sleep loss from prolonged duty periods is a major threat to unit readiness in the operational environment. In addition, factors related to the requirement for shift work or night operations also pose difficulties.

During military operations a number of personnel are rotated from the day shift to the night shift so that operations can be continuous. Night-shift work in and of itself presents problems associated with insufficient sleep, increased fatigue, and sleepiness on the job because people are working at times when their bodies are programmed for sleep (Åkerstedt, 1988; Åkerstedt and Gillberg, 1982; Härmä, 1995; Penn and Bootzin, 1990). These same people are trying to sleep at times when their bodies are accustomed to being awake. Studies have shown that even small amounts of shift-work-related sleep disruption can decrease sleep length by 2 or more hours per night, and even this small amount of sleep loss can lead to significant performance and alertness decrements (Gillberg, 1995; Rosenthal et al., 1993; Taub and Berger, 1973). The initial period of adjustment from days to nights is particularly problematic since work must still be accomplished despite the fact that the human body is incapable of changing its internal sleep/wake rhythms quickly. Thus, personnel are faced with the problem of performing during their circadian low points until their internal rhythms adapt to the new schedule. In addition, impaired alertness and performance can result from the requirement for personnel to awaken at inopportune times. For example, early-morning report times require personnel to rise while their core body temperatures are still low, leading to difficulties in awakening and feelings of being inadequately rested (Åkerstedt et al., 1991).

Clearly, one of the greatest threats to military readiness is the insufficient sleep that results from prolonged duty periods, shift work, and a related phenomenon, jet lag. Dinges (1995) summarized the impact of sleepiness/fatigue by pointing out that people who work when overly tired must expend increased energy simply to remain awake while suffering from poor, inefficient, and variable performance; impaired attention, information processing, and reaction time; reduced short-term memory capacity; and increased involuntary lapses into varying durations of actual sleep episodes. Momentary episodes of sleep and the periods of drowsiness preceding these "sleep attacks" are thought to underlie many serious accidents and incidents that are typically attributed to "insufficient operator attention."

USEFUL APPROACHES FOR PREDICTING OPERATOR ALERTNESS

Sleep

As indicated previously, sleep quality and quantity are important determinants of operator cognitive status. Frequent sleep disturbances can adversely affect next-day mood and performance as much as severely truncated sleep periods can.

Sleep Quality

Examination of the structure and sequence of an individual's sleep cycles offers crucial information about the restorative value of the sleep period. Although adequate sleep duration exerts a substantial impact on subsequent cognitive function, it is also important that the sleep be of high quality. The precise impact of changes in sleep content (i.e., distribution and amount of the sleep stages described below) remains a matter of some debate, since some investigators have shown that the loss of slow-wave sleep adversely impacts alertness (Walsh et al., 1994), whereas others have reported that neither slow-wave sleep restriction nor rapid-eye-movement (REM) sleep restriction lead to performance decrements (Agnew et al., 1967). Nonetheless, it is clear that sleep fragmentation (one aspect of sleep quality) exerts an important influence on next-day alertness (Roehrs et al., 2000). Many clinical sleep disorders are characterized by frequent sleep disruptions (Roehrs et al., 2000), and experimentally induced sleep fragmentation has been shown to degrade the recuperative value of sleep (Gillberg, 1995).

The usual sleep cycle is characterized by a series of stages that can be distinguished using polygraphic techniques. Attenuation of alpha activity (8–12 Hz) is the first sign of a transition from wakefulness to sleep. This is followed by increased theta (3–7 Hz) and vertex sharp waves accompanied by slow eye movements and loss of facial muscle tone. Next, during stage 2 sleep, there are bursts of K-complexes (a special type of delta wave) and 12 to 14 Hz activity (sleep spindles) in the virtual absence of typical delta waves (0.5–2 Hz). After stage 2 sleep, there is a progression into slow-wave sleep (stages 3 and 4) that is characterized by increasing amounts of delta activity (0.5–2 Hz). Stages 1 through 4 sleep are all generally considered to be non-REM sleep. These stages are interspersed with REM periods, which consist of a desynchronized, low-amplitude EEG with no K-complexes or spindles, sporadic rapid eye movements, and the virtual absence of muscle activity. As the night progresses, the REM periods typically become more numerous, whereas the amount of very deep (slow-wave) sleep decreases. Adults typically cycle through non-REM and REM sleep approximately every 90 minutes during an 8-hour sleep period.

Disruptions to normal sleep architecture have been correlated with daytime sleepiness. Frequent transitions into a very light stage of sleep during the night clearly impact the restorative value of the sleep period. Several studies in which subjects have been aroused (but not necessarily awakened) by auditory stimuli have shown that next-day performance deteriorates and both subjective and objective measures of sleepiness increase (Roehrs et al., 1994; Thiessen, 1988). It is important to note that these are sleep disturbances that may not produce behavioral arousals, so the affected individuals are often unaware that their sleep is being disrupted. In a military field environment there are obviously many factors that can produce such disruptions. Although a discussion of each of these is beyond the scope of this report, the presence of high levels of ambient light, excessive environmental noise, temperature extremes, and uncomfortable sleep surfaces rank high on the list. Often these problems create outright sleep fragmentation (which produces shortened sleep periods) but, in many cases, they produce their deleterious effects by simply degrading sleep quality. Unfortunately it is unlikely that in the near future it will be possible to precisely monitor sleep-quality decrements in the field. Thus more attention has been aimed at monitoring sleep quantity, another major contributor to on-the-job alertness.

Sleep Quantity

As noted earlier, sleep restriction and sleep deprivation impair mood and performance. Balkin and colleagues (2000) found that chronic sleep reductions of even 2 hours per night result in performance decrements on vigilance tasks, and that even after 7 consecutive days of shortened sleep, there is no evidence of an adaptive response. Furthermore, these authors reported that severe sleep restriction not only hampered a wide variety of functions during the deprivation period itself (including the ability to accurately drive through a simulated course), but it continued to adversely affect performance capabilities for several days after full 8-hour sleep periods were once again permitted. Bonnet (1994) found that total sleep deprivation exerted especially noticeable effects on tasks that were lengthy, tasks that did not offer immediate performance feedback, and tasks that were externally paced. Sleep loss had a greater effect on newly learned skills as opposed to well-established skills, and it degraded complex tasks more than simple ones and those that had short-term memory requirements. Subjective feelings of sleepiness and fatigue often begin to appear before actual performance decrements, as do EEG indications of increased slow-wave activity, and thus may have value as predictors of performance decrements.

Circadian Effects

Regardless of the exact nature of the effects of insufficient sleep on different types of activities or physiological processes, it is clear that insufficient sleep quality or quantity degrades performance. In addition, working at times that are incompatible with circadian rhythms can produce problems that are separate from those associated with simply being awake or being on the job for a long period of time. Performance on the night shift is often less optimal than performance on the day shift regardless of the nature of the work. The probability of accidents on the highways, in industry, and in aviation is higher at night in part because of increased sleepiness (Åkerstedt, 1995). Monk and Folkard (1985) have shown that nighttime work impairs even the simplest tasks. Night workers are slower to handle a telephone switchboard, more error prone when reading meters, more sluggish at the task of spinning thread, less able to remain alert while driving, and less vigilant at operating freight trains. Dinges (1995) has shown that nontraditional work hours, in combination with increased automation, have substantially increased the risk of fatigue-related problems throughout the industrialized world. Furthermore, there is evidence that a number of high-profile catastrophes (i.e., the grounding of the Exxon Valdez, the Space Shuttle Challenger accident, the crash of Korean Air flight 801, and the near meltdown at Three Mile Island) were at least partially attributable to the fatigue associated with night work (Mitler et al., 1988; NTSB, 1990, 2000).

Of particular concern to the military aviation community is the considerable evidence that night flights are especially vulnerable to cognitive lapses, or "micro sleeps" (i.e., brief periods during which sleep uncontrollably intrudes into wakefulness). Moore-Ede (1993) found that while micro sleeps occurred in the cockpits of flight simulators regardless of the time of day, there was a tenfold increase between the hours of 0400 and 0600; pilots made the greatest number of errors during this time. Wright and McGown (2001) found that long-haul pilots were especially compromised by sleepiness on flights that departed late in the night compared with those that departed earlier. Furthermore, many of the micro sleeps experienced by these pilots were so short (less than 20 seconds) that the crewmembers may not have been aware that they had fallen asleep. Rosekind and colleagues (1994) also found a substantial increase in microevents (slow-wave EEG activity and slow eye movements) on long-haul flights, with night flights being particularly affected compared with day flights. Vigilance performance and subjective alertness ratings were degraded more at night as well. Caldwell and colleagues (2002) found that the combination of sleep loss and night flying significantly accentuated the type of slow-wave EEG activity that has been associated with insufficient alertness, while concurrently causing the types of mood and cognitive deteriorations that impair crew coordination and responses to system deviations or failures.

Because of findings like these it has become clear that both sleep and circadian effects must be considered in any attempt to estimate the impact of work and sleep schedules on performance. Circadian cycles can be fairly well tracked by continuously measuring core body temperature, and sleep quantity and quality can be assessed by EEG techniques (see below). However, besides utilizing direct measures of physiological indices to help predict performance, predictive computerized models have been developed to estimate fatigue and cognitive performance capacity based on what is generally known about sleep and circadian influences.

Computerized Cognitive Performance Prediction Models

Several organizations and individual scientists in the United States and abroad have developed computerized models (and scheduling tools based on these models) that predict cognitive performance decrements using known information about sleep and circadian rhythms. Such tools do not actually monitor any aspect of individual physiology, but they make predictions via keyboard or actigraphic inputs about work and sleep schedules.

Two related prediction models are the Sleep Performance Model and the Sleep, Activity, Fatigue and Task Effectiveness (SAFTE) model, both of which were developed by Dr. Hursh of Science Applications International Corporation under Army and Air Force sponsorship (Eddy and Hursh, 2001). An additional model is the System for Aircrew Fatigue Evaluation (SAFE), which was developed at QinetiQ Centre for Human Sciences in the United Kingdom (Belyavin and Spencer, 2004). The Sleep Performance Model is an early version of the SAFTE model that was designed to be used in conjunction with wrist actigraphy. Both the SAFTE and SAFE versions are models that are applied to proposed work/sleep schedules (based on operator input provided via a computer keyboard) in order to identify the changes in cognitive readiness that would be expected to occur in personnel at various times during select work cycles. (SAFTE can also take "after-the-fact" scheduling input from actigraphic recordings.)

Although other models and implementations are available, a complete review is beyond the scope of this report. However, this subject is treated in detail in a special edition of *Aviation, Space, and Environmental Medicine* (2004, Vol 75, Sup 3). The present state of the art permits only general predictions about the impact of specific work/rest schedules on the cognitive alertness of personnel, and additional work will be needed before such models can accurately predict the performance of any specific individual. This is because the models do not account for individual differences and because they do not monitor any physiological parameter to make their predictions. Since, for instance, the models do not actually monitor body temperature, they must rely on averaged data to predict circadian phase. In addition, since they do not examin physiological sleep quality, they can only make assumptions about the restorative value and amount of sleep that is being obtained. Thus, even if all of the prediction equations are perfect, guesswork remains due to the absence of direct physiological inputs, especially with regard to sleep quality and quantity.

SAFTE

A schematic of the SAFTE model appears in Figure 5-1. Note that SAFTE is based on the concept of a sleep reservoir that quantifies the impact of sleep-related processes on cognitive readiness, or "cognitive effectiveness." Sufficient sleep time fills the sleep reservoir, and hours of wakefulness deplete the reser-

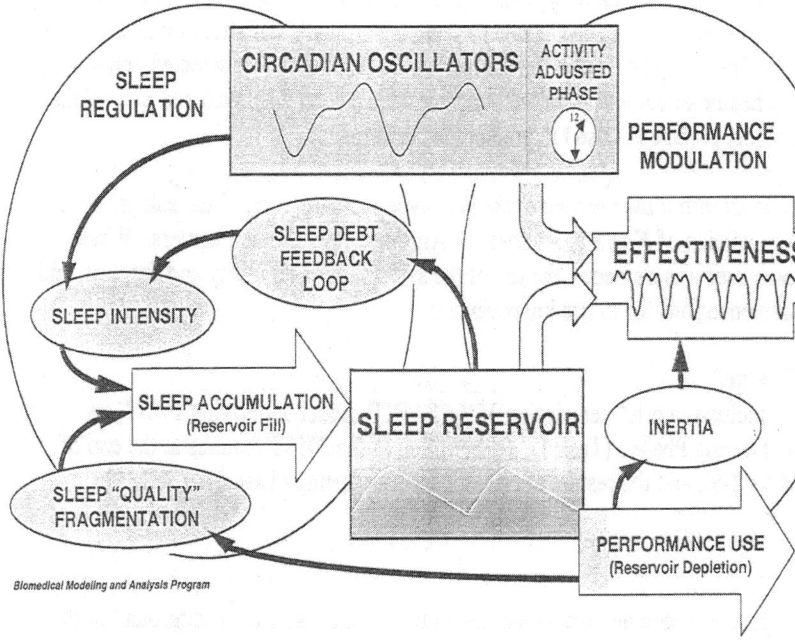

FIGURE 5-1 A schematic of the Sleep, Activity, Fatigue, and Task Effectiveness (SAFTE) model.
SOURCE: Eddy and Hursh (2001). Figure reprinted with permission of Biodynamics and Protection Division, Human Effectiveness Directorate.

voir. The sleep accumulation process is affected by sleep intensity (which is modulated by existing sleep debt and circadian factors) and quality of sleep (which is affected by sleep continuity). Cognitive readiness or effectiveness is predicted based on the level of the sleep reservoir and the time of day (circadian phase), as well as on the potential influence of short-term, postsleep grogginess (referred to as "sleep inertia").

This model has been implemented through the Fatigue Avoidance Scheduling Tool. This tool is useful for identifying times at which performance might be compromised within a given work/sleep schedule, and it is useful for optimizing schedule development because it allows an operator/planner to ask a series of "what if" questions. For example, as shown in Figure 5-2, a planner can view the predicted effects of 2 days without sleep, and then ask "What if we placed a 4-hour nap during this 40-hour period of otherwise continuous wakefulness?" As the figure indicates, such a napping strategy could offer a 20 percent

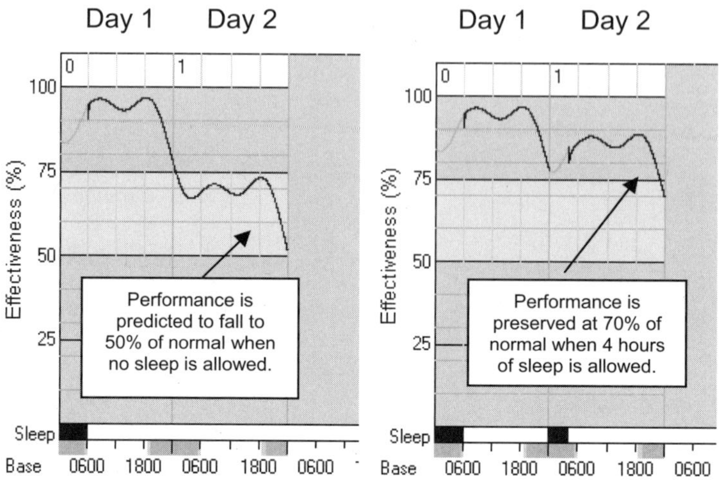

FIGURE 5-2 An example of output from a Fatigue Avoidance Scheduling Tool (FAST) to help predict cognitive effectiveness (%). Example: 2 days with no sleep compared with 2 days with 4 hours of sleep.

improvement in cognitive effectiveness over what would be expected with no sleep at all.

The predictive capability of the SAFTE model has been established by comparing the model's output with laboratory data collected during various sleep-deprivation studies. For example, model predictions accounted for 89 percent of the variance (degradations) in throughput on serial addition-subtraction across 72 hours of sleep loss in one study, and 98 percent of the variance in throughput on a variety of cognitive tests across 54 hours of sleep deprivation in another (Hursh et al., 2004). Throughput is a combined speed/accuracy measure that on many basic cognitive tests is presumed to reflect the individual's capacity to perform mental discriminations, react to incoming stimuli, think logically, process information, and comprehend language. Although the tasks on which SAFTE was validated are not typical military tasks, it is assumed that anything that degrades such basic mental facilities would also degrade operationally relevant performance. Future studies will validate the relationship between SAFTE model predictions and decrements in a variety of "real-world" performances.

SAFE

The SAFE model (Belyavin and Spencer, 2004) is similar to SAFTE in that it takes keyboard input about specific work/rest schedules and estimates performance risk based on what is known about the impact of the body's clock and time since sleep on alertness. In addition, the model accounts for the effects of sleep inertia. SAFE predictions were initially validated via comparisons with laboratory data collected during several studies of sleep deprivation and shift work. Select variables were used from tests of visual vigilance, continuous memory recall, psychomotor tracking, and the Multi-Attribute Task Battery. The results indicated that the basic model effectively predicted group performance on most aspects of these basic tasks.

Later, SAFE predictions were compared with the subjective alertness ratings of a sample of commercial airline pilots across 72 flights (comprised of long-haul international trips). On some schedules, the model predicted mean alertness levels moderately well, with the exception of a sudden increased arousal that occurred at the end of some of the return flights. On other schedules, although the model tracked fatigue-related changes fairly well from the beginning to the end of each flight segment, the model underestimated alertness on outbound flights and overestimated alertness on return flights. Because of these discrepancies, the designers of SAFE performed additional studies and ultimately included prediction modifiers that considered not only the three basic alertness processes (time since sleep, circadian rhythms, and sleep inertia), but added the effects of: (a) multiple flight legs, (b) duration of time on duty, (c) the effects of consecutive and/or long tours of duty, (d) the impact of early report times, (e) the impact of daytime vs. nighttime sleep, and (f) the effects of sleep degradations during on-board rest periods. The addition of these factors substantially increased the predictive accuracy of the model.

Sleep Monitoring

There are two basic approaches for monitoring human sleep. The first, and most accurate, consists of electrophysiological recordings (polysomnograms). The second, and most practical for nonlaboratory settings, consists of activity-based recording (actigraphy).

Polysomnography

Polysomnographic recordings involving the collection of EEG, electromyographic (EMG), and electrooculographic (EOG) data from skin-mounted electrodes represent the most accurate way to monitor sleep parameters. For clinical and research purposes, sleep recordings are usually made in a sleep laboratory because of the available level of environmental control and the instrumentation required. EEG data are acquired with silver-silver chloride or gold electrodes attached to the scalp with collodion before the person retires for the night. A minimum of one or two EEG electrodes are attached, along with a mastoid (or ear-lobe) reference, two EOG electrodes, and two EMG electrodes placed underneath the subject's chin. Amplification of the signals is accomplished via highly sensitive polygraph amplifiers. The signals are recorded on paper, usually at a speed of 10 mm/sec, or by a computerized system configured for sleep polygraphy. Using standard guidelines, the stages of sleep (stages 1 through 4, REM, awake, and movement) are determined by scoring each epoch (20–30 second period) throughout the record. Most data are scored visually following standardized criteria set forth by Rechtschaffen and Kales (1968). New computer systems have been developed to score the data using mathematical functions but, at present, there is no widely accepted automatic scoring procedure that can take the place of a human sleep scorer.

Polysomnographic sleep evaluation is the "gold standard" in sleep science. These standard recordings have been used for years to document and understand "normal sleep," as well as to investigate a wide array of clinical complaints, including excessive daytime sleepiness, insomnia, and a number of sleep disorders (Carskadon and Dement, 1994; Dement, 1976; Hauri and Orr, 1982; Roffwarg, 1979). The polysomnographic approach avoids the pitfall of making potentially erroneous assumptions that behaviorally quiescent people are asleep when, in fact, they may simply be lying still. This approach also offers a wealth of information about the depth (or quality) of sleep than cannot easily be determined by other means. However, these advantages are offset by recording and instrumentation requirements that make in-the-field sleep recordings at best, impractical, and at worst, impossible. Although various types of ambulatory physiological recorders are available for nonstandard recording applications, it is unlikely that these will be used on a widespread basis (for large groups of personnel) any time in the near future. First of all, there is significant overhead involved in the attachment and maintenance of suites of recording electrodes and, second, the necessity of downloading and processing the data recorded from large numbers of people on a daily basis is impractical. These are the reasons that actigraphic approaches to estimations of sleep quantity have received increased attention.

Actigraphy

Actigraphs are battery-powered, wristwatch-like units that are programmed via a microcomputer interface. The wristwatch contains a three-axis accelerometer sensor with a preamplifier and filter that are interfaced to a microprocessor by a multiplexed analog-digital converter. The microprocessor uses storage memory to record the collected data. The actigraph is programmed by a microcomputer to start and end data collection at specific time points; the same microcomputer interface is used for periodic data retrieval. Once downloaded, the activity data are processed by analysis software that permits sleep-state scoring, basic statistics, and several forms of visual presentation. Raw graphic depictions of data show different levels of activity using a series of discrete vertical lines of different amplitudes. Typically these graphs are scored by both computer algorithms and a human observer (who checks the computer scoring).

Recent investigations have shown that actigraphy is a fruitful approach to the study of sleep in nonlaboratory settings. Pollak and colleagues (2001) compared actigraphically measured sleep/wakefulness with standard polysomnographic measures and found that actigraphs could correctly identify periods of sleep versus wakefulness. Furthermore, the actigraphs offered a general indication of sleep quality in that lower actigraphic counts corresponded to deeper sleep stages. Monk and colleagues (1999) found that actigraphic recordings were useful for determining the sleep onset and offset of four astronauts engaged in 17-day Space Shuttle missions. There was a high correlation between high activity counts and polygraphically identified light stages of sleep. Wrist actigraphy is a promising monitoring strategy for military field applications—it may be used in numerous operational contexts since the required equipment is small, and it is a measure that can be obtained without disturbing the ongoing mission.

Actigraphy in Combination with Performance Prediction Models

In addition to using actigraphy to record sleep/wake cycles and to estimate sleep quality and quantity, efforts are underway to integrate these data with computerized performance prediction algorithms. One of the best developed of these applications is the Walter Reed Army Institute of Research Sleep Watch Actigraph (Balkin et al., 2000). The Sleep Watch is a wrist-worn device that predicts the wearer's cognitive performance status based on the level of sleep debt and the phase of the circadian cycle (as calculated via actigraph activity counts). The actigraphically determined sleep/circadian information is fed into an on-board computer model that includes a "charging function" for recuperative sleep, a "discharging function" for the amount of time awake, and a "circadian function" for the specific phase of the wearer's estimated circadian rhythm. (This is the Sleep Performance Model that was mentioned earlier.) The face of the Sleep Watch contains a "fuel gauge" that displays a performance prediction ranging from 0 to 100 percent of well-rested levels and a simple red-yellow-green analog scale that can alert the wearer of the need to acquire additional sleep. The Sleep Watch is still under development to include individual differences in sleep needs and performance capabilities and the effects of time-zone transitions and variations in light exposure levels (which influence circadian adaptation). The Sleep Watch predictions have been validated to some extent on numerous tasks collected during sleep-deprivation and sleep-restriction studies in the laboratory, and further work along these lines is currently underway. There are plans to employ the Sleep Watch in upcoming field exercises so that Watch-based alertness measures can be correlated with aspects of real-world performance. Once this tool is optimized, it will offer a field-useable method for monitoring operator fatigue levels and for warning wearers of impending cognitive performance failures associated with insufficient sleep.

Spontaneous Electroencephalography

Operational personnel are required to perform even if they are fatigued. In these situations it is desirable to have the capability to continuously monitor the cognitive status of combat service members without interfering with the accomplishment of their primary mission. Although there are cognitive tests that are exquisitely sensitive to the presence of fatigue stemming from sleep loss, circadian disruptions, and a host of other factors, it is difficult to continuously administer such tests on an hourly or daily basis without disrupting job performance. Thus a more unobtrusive monitoring strategy is required. One possibility is to take advantage of the spontaneous EEG because the data can be obtained and to some extent, examined, in real time, and the results are considered to be objective, valid, and related to operational readiness (Caldwell et al., 1994, 1997, 2002). As mentioned earlier, one of the key advantages of the EEG is that it is a psychophysiological measure that can be collected without interfering with the primary task.

EEG Measures

EEG signals are detectable from a variety of scalp locations using small electrodes (8 mm) that are attached with tape, collodion, or paste and are filled with an electrolyte solution. Electrical activity is then recorded with two or more electrodes (depending on how much of the brain's surface activity is of interest) by amplifiers capable of amplifying 5- to 100-μV signals that oscillate at 0.5 to 100 Hz. Amplified data are usually stored on an ambulatory or laboratory recording device and/or displayed on an ink-writing polygraph or a computer cathode-ray tube. Recorded data may be scored via visual inspection or by computerized procedures, such as power spectral analysis. In either case, the recording is usually reduced to a table of values that represents the relative amount of EEG falling within each of four distinct bands: delta (1–3.9 Hz), theta (4–7.9 Hz), alpha (8–13 Hz), and beta (>13–20 or 30 Hz). Also, the dominant or peak frequency observed during specified time frames can be determined. The normal adult waking EEG contains each of these different rhythms, but the most easily recognizable one is the alpha rhythm that is blocked by opening the eyes, cognitive activation, sudden arousal, and sleep. Beta waves also contribute substantially to the normal awake EEG, but slower activity (below 8 Hz) is usually predominant only during sleep (Cooper et al., 1980) or under conditions of severe drowsiness.

Numerous studies have established the sensitivity of EEG activity to work-related stressors (e.g., sleep deprivation). For instance, Caldwell and colleagues (1996), Comperatore and colleagues (1992), Lorenzo and colleagues (1995), and Pigeau and colleagues (1987) have all shown that slow-wave EEG activity (i.e., delta and theta) is significantly elevated by even moderate sleep loss (i.e., sleep loss resulting from 18–20 hours of continuous wakefulness), and research has repeatedly established that the fatigue from insufficient sleep affects both EEG activity and nonconcurrently measured flight performance (Caldwell et al., 2000a, 2000b, 2003; LeDuc et al., 2000). Based on these findings, it is reasonable to suspect that EEG data should show a predictive relationship to operationally relevant cognitive performance. However, while several investigators have offered evidence that EEG is useful for describing an operator's general status during tasks such as flights (Blanc et al., 1966; Caldwell et al., 2002; Howitt et al., 1978; Maulsby, 1966) and driving simulations (Balkin et al., 2000), correlations with actual task performance are often weaker than desired except in cases of extreme drowsiness.

It should also be noted that while a strong link between EEG and drowsiness has been demonstrated, there have been a host of problems related to real-time EEG monitoring in operational environments. These include the necessity of highly trained technicians, cumbersome and fragile instrumentation, and a rather time-consuming preparation period for EEG recordings. Additionally, the acquired data is susceptible to contamination by physiological and instrumental artifacts, such as movements, muscle activity, eye blinks, or heartbeats. Also, while much progress has been made in overcoming these obstacles, there is no general consensus on what aspects of EEG are sufficiently sensitive and reliable to serve as general indicators of fatigue (Gevins et al., 1995).

Nonetheless, the utility of EEG continues to be explored because of a logical association between brain electrical activation and brain function. New analysis routines, better equipment, automated artifact-correction algorithms, and new types of high-impedance electrodes will ultimately make widespread real-time monitoring of cognitive readiness (via measures of brain activity) feasible in field settings. As Gevins and colleagues (1995) have pointed out, "the EEG has one or more advantages over other [central-nervous system monitoring] approaches, including millisecond temporal resolution, complete harmlessness and noninvasiveness…and [the fact that] EEG is the only brain imaging modality suitable for use in operational environments or from ambulatory subjects."

A SMART HELMET, designed to provide inputs for 32 channels of low-level electrophysiological signals, including EEG, EOG, EMG, and heart activity (electrocardiogram [ECG]) (Gevins et al., 1995) was once available. Additional channels offered the capability to record measures such as respiration, blood volume, skin conductance, and head and body movements. In conjunction with preamplifier circuits and electrically driven shielding built directly into a flight helmet, a stretchable fabric hat was used for rapidly positioning EEG, EOG, and EMG electrodes on the head and face for recording data. The SMART HELMET successfully collected data from subjects in a centrifuge, airplane, and car with the use of ruggedized laptop personal computers (Gevins et al., 1995). However, the requirement for low-impedance sensors (e.g., skin preparation, electrolyte solution) limited the usefulness of such a technique, and at present, the SMART HELMET is no longer available (although it may pave the way for similar, more modern technology). In all probability, newer devices will strive to actually embed EEG (and possibly EOG) sensors into an integrated helmet configuration (as opposed to using a stretchable hat worn under the helmet liner). In this way, physiological data reflecting pilot alertness may soon be available every time a pilot dons his or her flight gear. A small Ohio-based company (SRICO) is currently working to overcome one of the major obstacles to using such an embedded-sensor approach by developing a high-impedance, dry-contact EEG sensor (the Photrode) (Kingsley et al., 2003) that can be mounted inside of a flight helmet or a duty uniform. Photrode is still under refinement, but it should be widely available within 2 to 3 years. Once this technology can be coupled with high-capacity recording devices equipped with software routines that can remove contaminating artifacts from movements, muscle tension, eye blinks, and heart beats, the feasibility of continuous real-time EEG monitoring in the field will improve. Ultimately these data could be used to feed performance prediction models, such as the one currently used for Sleep Watch. This should be an available option in 5 to 7 years.

EEG Measures Combined with Performance Measures

Sleep-watch measures, EEG assessments, or other physiological parameters may be the ultimate strategy to monitor the cognitive states of ground combat service members, but combined physiological and performance measures may be a better alternative for vehicle operators. Caldwell and Roberts (2000) have shown that objective, integrated flight-performance assessments are sensitive to the impact of fatigue and specific types of antifatigue medications, and others have noted the sensitivity of EEG measures to the effects of fatigue in a variety of situations (Balkin et al., 2000; Hossain et al., 2003; Miller, 1997). However, little work has been done to develop status predictors that rely on the integrated combination of continuous performance assessments and concurrent evaluations of physiological status. Petit and colleagues (1990) have shown that steering wheel functions and EEG alpha power correlate, and de Waard and Brookhuis (1991) found that the standard deviation of steering wheel movements increased and the number of steering wheel reversals per minute decreased in conjunction with a gradual decrease in relative EEG energy. Brookhuis and de Waard (1993) identified the co-occurrence of changes in physiology and in behavior and demonstrated the feasibility of monitoring a vehicle operator's status by monitoring driving performance. In part, this led Brookhuis (1995) to contend, "Measuring physiological parameters could be considered from the point of view of validating non-obtrusive in-vehicle measures that might be used to monitor driver state continuously through vehicle parameters." However, it may be unwise to rely on either type of measure (physiological vs. performance) alone in situations where both could be integrated to predict impending cognitive decrements. Integrated monitoring of both categories of measures appears to be a more fruitful approach for future monitoring efforts.

Electrooculographic and Other Eye-Movement Measures

The sensitivity of the oculomotor control system to fatigue, boredom, and lapses in attention has also been noted. The process of monitoring eye movements, EOG, is concerned with measuring fluctuations in electrical potentials during movement of the eyes. EOG measurements have been used in a wide range of applications, such as the recording of REM during sleep research (Andreassi, 1989). It has also been found that long-duration eye closures during blinking are related to reduced alertness (Stern, 1980).

General Ocular Measures

Stern and Ranney (1999) identified a series of oculomotor measures that may be potentially useful for detecting lapses in attention. The first of these is saccadic eye movements. These are the types of eye movements that quickly transition the eyes from one point of focus to another, such as when reading text. Surrounding the occurrence of the saccade is a brief period during which information intake is inhibited. The latency between stimulus presentation and the saccade, the saccade duration, and the distance of the saccade have been suggested as indicators of fatigue. Although saccades are initiated under voluntary control, once they are underway their speed is not within the individual's control. Fatigued conditions can cause a longer latency period, reduce the velocity of the saccade, or result in saccades that either undershoot or overshoot the target. Russo and colleagues (2003) found that saccadic velocity is particularly sensitive to an increase in sleepiness in response to prolonged periods of partial sleep deprivation.

Another type of oculomotor measure is blinks. Eye blinks can be measured in terms of blink frequency, timing in respect to stimulus presentation, and duration of the closing and reopening movement of the eyelid. It has been found that fatigue can cause smaller-amplitude eye blinks. Similarly, the frequency of eyelid closures has been shown to increase under fatiguing conditions.

A third type of oculomotor measure is pupil diameter. Stern and Ranney (1999) point out that a decrease in pupil diameter or a slow fluctuation in pupil diameter coincides with feelings of fatigue. Similarly, Russo and colleagues (1999) found that decreases in saccadic velocity and increases in pupil constriction latency correlated with an increase in the rate of crashes seen in simulated driving conditions during periods of sleep deprivation.

PERCLOS

Research in the area of slow eye closures has given rise to PERCLOS, a measure defined as the "percentage of time that the eyes are 80% to 100% closed over a defined time interval" (Wierwille, 1999). This type of measurement has the advantage of being physiologically based, and it has a great deal of face validity since drooping or slow eyelid closures are not usually seen in alert individuals. Furthermore, performance decrements on a variety of tasks are virtually certain to occur when slow eye closures impair an individual's ability to gather visual information. Early research developed algorithms that combined estimations of ocular measures (PERCLOS) with a direct measurement of performance (Wierwille, 1999). Dinges and colleagues (1998) have determined that there is a high degree of coherence between PERCLOS and performance lapses on the psychomotor vigilance test (an accepted test of fatigue). At present, PERCLOS is a labor-intensive monitoring technology that involves the human scoring of eye closures from video footage of volunteers' faces. However, a direct on-line PERCLOS system that uses infrared illumination to compare retinal reflections against a dark background and automatically calculates a real-time PERCLOS value is being developed. This has led to a dash-mounted Copilot, a "low-cost drowsiness monitor intended for use in commercial operations involving nighttime driving" and "designed for robust operation in a heavy truck environment" (Grace and Steward, 2001). This is a technique that may one day be useful for monitoring vehicle operators in field environments, but the equipment involved makes it unlikely that PERCLOS can be employed to assess the operational readiness of ground combat service members.

Other Ocular Measures

There are a number of commercial products available that measure fatigue. One such device is the FIT Fatigue Analyzer (PMI, Inc., Rockville, Maryland). This particular device can assess the degree of fatigue by analyzing involuntary pupillary responses to brief flashes of light and by analyzing eye movements in response to moving light targets. Measures of pupil size, constriction latency, constriction amplitude, and saccadic velocity are combined into a weighted score that purportedly assesses fatigue levels. There are efforts underway to miniaturize this device for operational use.

Similarly, MTI Research Inc. has developed a device designed to detect and track fatigue using eye-blink analysis. Using optical electronics, the Alertness Monitor determines the level of alertness or drowsiness by measuring the ratio of eyelid closures to eyelid openness. Mounted unobtrusively on safety glasses, the research models emit an infrared beam along the axis of the eye blink where the beam cannot be broken by the eyelashes during an eye blink and will not shine directly into the operator's eye (Dinges et al., 1998). Meanwhile, IM Systems, Inc. has developed the Blinkometer, an ambulatory device that records eye blinks using an algorithm reported to be sensitive to drowsiness. The Blinkometer can record in one of two modes: either blinks per minute or the intervals between blinks. The device detects blinks using a sensor attached to the outer canthus of one eye with a double-sided adhesive disk and a small recording device clipped to the operator's person. IM Systems reports that by using a fairly straightforward algorithm (the fewer the number of blinks, the greater the level of drowsiness), the Blinkometer detects a decreased alertness within 20 to 30 seconds (Dinges et al., 1998). Both the Alertness Monitor and the Blinkometer were tested for validation, alongside PERCLOS, by comparison with lapses in a psychomotor vigilance task. While the "result for PERCLOS was uniformly high coherence" to these attention lapses as seen in the psychomotor vigilance task, the result for the Alertness Monitor was "at the other end of the spectrum, averaging the lowest bout-to-bout coherence for lapse frequency" (Dinges et al., 1998). The Blinkometer had a moderate bout-to-bout coherence for lapse frequency, but was problematic due to difficulties with the unit's data storage and retrievability functions (Dinges et al., 1998). While most of these technologies have potential, Dinges and colleagues (1998) pointed out that "more validation studies of this type are needed to sort out from the wide variety of biobehavioral fatigue monitors those that have the highest validity and reliability for predicting actual hypo-vigilance performance."

Another device, originally developed as a home sleep-monitoring system, also shows promise in this area. The Nightcap, developed by Healthdyne Technologies, detects eyelid movements through a small, piezoelectric film sensor, which is attached to the upper eyelid. This method allows the detection of both active movements of the eyelid and passive movements caused by movement of the eyeball. The Nightcap detects decreases in vigilance as lowered levels of eyelid movements (Stickgold et al., 1995). Using the Nightcap, Stickgold found decreased eyelid movements during periods of decreased vigilance resulting from inadequate sleep on the previous night. Stickgold and colleagues (1995) concluded that "the Nightcap would appear to be potentially useful for the real-time monitoring of vigilance in a variety of work environments."

A similar method for measuring eyelid movements originally developed by Evinger and colleagues (1991), in which a very small piece of insulated wire coil is taped to the upper eyelid while the operator sits in a 3-D magnetic field, has been used by Leder and colleagues (1996) to study the relationship between eyelid activity and alertness/vigilance. They report that the magnetic sensor followed the wire coil well and responded to every blink. Additionally, this method was able to distinguish spontaneous blinks from vertical lid saccades and horizontal eye saccades. As a result, Leder and colleagues (1996) "...expect to be able to unobtrusively collect spontaneous eyelid activity in ambulatory subjects engaged in their routine activities," including "changes in blink rate associated with fatigue and loss of alertness or vigilance."

OTHER CENTRAL NERVOUS SYSTEM MONITORING TECHNOLOGIES

In addition to the technologies described above, there are other methods of studying central nervous system changes that may offer information about cognitive status. However, none of these are suitable for field applications in which continuous, real-time assessment is the goal.

Positron Emission Tomography

Wu and colleagues (1991), with the use of positron emission tomography (PET), found that about 32 hours of total sleep deprivation decreased metabolism in the thalamus, basal ganglia, white matter, and cerebellum. Sleep deprivation further reorganized regional cerebral metabolic activity by decreasing temporal lobe activation and increasing activity in the visual cortex. As a result, visual vigilance on a continuous performance test was degraded. Thomas and colleagues (2000) reported that 24 hours of sleep deprivation produced significant decreases in relative regional glucose metabolism in the thalamus and prefrontal and posterior-parietal cortices of the brains of 17 volunteers. Once again, both alertness and cognitive performance declined in conjunction with changes in brain activity. Although not within the context of sleep deprivation, Pietrini and colleagues (2000) have asserted that PET is also useful for tracking the changes in neural activity that accompany the cognitive declines associated with Alzheimer's disease. Scans of patients revealed a progressive decline in the magnitude of brain response to audiovisual stimulation with progressive worsening of cognitive dementia. Thus PET offers important information about the levels of brain activation that underlie cognitive performance; however, the instrumentation and testing requirements for this method cannot be met in an operational context.

Functional Magnetic Resonance Imaging

Downing and coworkers (2001) have used neuroimaging techniques, such as functional magnetic resonance imaging (fMRI) and magneto-EEG, to identify the neural substrates of visual attention. The results indicated that these techniques are able to identify markers of face processing and place processing. Likewise, Rees (2001) has addressed the relationship among selective attention, neural activity, and visual awareness through fMRI research. Portas and coworkers (1998) have used fMRI to help delineate the role of specific brain areas in attention and arousal (both of which are important for cognitive performance). The authors identified differences associated with the performance of an attention task as a function of arousal decrements. Sleep deprivation produced an increase in attention-related thalamic activity compared with what was observed after administration of caffeine to improve arousal. Drummond and colleagues (2000) observed that while sleep deprivation increased subjective sleepiness, prefrontal cortex activation was actually more responsive after 1 night of sleep deprivation than after normal sleep. Sleep deprivation also impaired performance on a free-recall task, but it was observed that free-recall was improved in subjects with greater parietal lobe activation. The prefrontal cortex results from this study appear to partially agree with a later finding that sleep deprivation was associated with greater activation in the bilateral prefrontal cortex and parietal lobes during the performance of verbal learning and divided attention tasks (Drummond and Brown, 2001). However, the fact that sleep deprivation led to decreased activity in these same areas during the performance of an arithmetic task suggested that the brain's response patterns are dependent on the type of cognitive processing required. Clearly, fMRI can offer useful information about the brain areas involved in specific types of task processing, as well as about the effects of fatigue on basic central nervous system functioning. However, as is the case with PET, fMRI is not suitable for field applications.

Transcranial Doppler Sonography

Transcranial doppler (TCD) sonography is a method for noninvasively monitoring cerebral blood flow levels that can serve as an indicator of metabolic activation in the brain. TCD has been used in the study of vigilance, as well as to understand the cerebral processes underlying various cognitive tasks (Hollander et al., 2002). For instance, Hitchcock and colleagues (2003) found that there were performance-related changes in right hemisphere blood flow as a result of manipulations that increased or decreased the demands of a 40-minute, simulated air traffic control task. Other investigations have demonstrated the potential utility of TCD in understanding the cerebral organization of cognition. However, Stroobant and Vingerhoets (2000) indicated that additional standardization of procedural methodologies will be required before the full utility of TCD can be realized. In any event, it remains unlikely that such a technique will ever be feasible for monitoring foot-soldier status in the field.

HEART-RATE MEASURES

Although heart-rate measures typically have not been used to assess aspects of cognitive readiness associated with fatigue or sleepiness, heart rate has often been employed to assess other aspects of operator state. The heart is innervated by both the sympathetic and the parasympathetic nervous systems and, as such, it is influenced by higher cortical centers. The sympathetic nervous system increases the firing rate of the heart's pacemaker and also modulates the constriction and dilation of the blood vessels. The parasympathetic nervous system inhibits the firing rate of the pacemaker cells via the vagal nerve, and this reduces heart rate. Of course heart rate has long been used as an indicator of physical effort, but it has also been proven useful for studying mental effort and other aspects of psychological and cognitive status. Thus the monitoring of heart rate as an indicator of cognitive stress may be useful for optimizing task demands with the aim of avoiding levels of cognitive fatigue that could lead to a breakdown in alertness or performance capacity.

As described by Caldwell and coworkers (1994), numerous studies have found systematic relations between cognitive demands and heart rate in both laboratory and real-world environments (for reviews, see Kramer, 1991; Roscoe, 1992; and Wilson and Eggemeier, 1991). In addition, the operational relevance of heart-rate measures has been well established in demanding performance contexts, such as flying combat missions (Lewis et al., 1967), flying surface-attack training missions (Comens et al., 1987; Wilson, 1993), flying aircraft test missions (Roscoe, 1980), and landing at different airports (Nicholson et al., 1970; Ruffell-Smith, 1967). Heart-rate changes have been shown to discriminate between pilot vs. copilot flying (Hart and Hauser, 1987; Kakimoto et al., 1988; Roscoe, 1978) and flying in the lead versus the wing position (Wilson et al., 1987). Simulated flight studies have also reported increases in heart rate associated with increases in task difficulty (Lindholm et al., 1984; Opmeer and Krol, 1973; Wierwille and Connor, 1983).

Heart-rate variability (HRV) is also a sensitive indicator of task demands. Several studies have reported decreases in HRV with increasing cognitive workload. Specifically, it has been found that after performing a spectral analysis on the ECG signal, an examination of the midfrequency band (the 0.10 Hz component) offers information about the amount of mental effort that has to be invested to meet the task demands (Mulder, 1992; Mulder and Mulder, 1980). The tasks evaluated have included simulated and actual flight (Lindholm et al., 1984; Lindqvist et al., 1983; Opmeer and Krol, 1973; Sekiguchi et al., 1979; Wilson, 1993). Opmeer and Krol (1973) reported that HRV and respiration were sensitive to simulated flight task demands. Itoh and coworkers (1989) found HRV in the 0.10 band to decrease during take off and landing (high workload) when compared with cruise segments (low workload).

Recently, researchers have also found that HRV in the high-frequency band (0.15–0.40 Hz) can be used to predict cognitive performance. Tasks that have been examined include the Stoop color-word conflict task, continuous performance tasks, and working memory tasks. Johnsen and coworkers (2003) found that dental phobics with higher HRV had faster reaction times to incongruent color and threat-related words than did dental phobics with lower HRV. Importantly, Hansen and colleagues (2003) recently reported the results of a study in a military sample. Naval cadets in the Royal Norwegian Navy were divided in to high- and low-HRV groups based on their resting HRV. These researchers reported that those individuals with high HRV performed better on tasks that used executive functions, such as working memory, compared with those with low HRV.

Since monitoring ECG is in many ways easier than monitoring EEG (due to greater signal strength and subsequent improvement in signal-to-noise ratio), the collection and analysis of heart rate and HRV is actually quite feasible at this point. With the introduction of high-impedance sensors that can be mounted in standard clothing, it is likely that these cardiac variables will soon be routinely monitored, at least in some specialized training environments. After all, commercially available systems consisting of chest straps and wrist-worn receivers (such as the Polar systems) are already widely used by athletes.

OTHER MEASURES

It should be noted that there are several other types of psychophysiological measures besides EEG, EOG, and ECG that hold promise for assessing aspects of operator cognitive status. For instance, changes in body temperature not only reflect different levels of physical energy expenditure and changing environmental conditions, but also fluctuations in psychological arousal. Differences in muscle activation measured by EMG recordings can indicate increased or decreased physical activity or elevations or reductions in psychological tension. Fluctuations in respiration rate can suggest either changes in physical energy expenditure or changes in mental stress. These and other psychophysiological measures are not widely used for the assessment of cognitive readiness per se, but they can provide insight into psychological or work-related factors that ultimately can influence operator status. Since all of them can be assessed via nonintrusive, skin-mounted sensors, their potential utility for future applications should not be dismissed; however, each measure poses different challenges in terms of both recording and analysis. A complete discussion of all of the available psychophysiological measures is beyond the scope of this report, but interested readers may wish to consult one of more of the authoritative texts that have already compiled and synthesized detailed information on this topic, such as Andreassi (1989), Cacioppo and Tassinary (1990), and Coles and colleagues (1986).

Head-Position Monitoring

Head-position monitoring, although not considered psychophysiological, is another method that has been thought to hold promise as a measure of fatigue. One of the self-assessment indicators of fatigue that many operators watch for is increased head bobs or other involuntary movements that occur due to loss of neck muscle tone. Stern and Ranney (1999) suggest that an increase in the amount of reactive head movements (as opposed to eye movements) when attempting to react to some event may be a sign of fatigue. This is thought to indicate an increase in passive responding. Some research suggests that there may in fact be a relationship between micromotion of the head and fatigue and, because of this, Advanced Safety Concepts, Inc. has developed the Proximity Array Sensing System (PASS). This apparatus records the x, y, and z coordinates of the head, using an array of three capacitive sensors that are mounted overhead in a vehicle or other fixed location. The position of the head is triangulated by determining the proximity of the head to each capacitive sensor through partial blocking of the sensing fields. It is hypothesized that changes in head-movement patterns may indicate fatigue onset. It has been reported that in laboratory tests, "the PASS system has detected changes in head position as little as 0.01," while providing absolute x-y-z resolution of head position to about 0.1" (Dinges et al., 1998). "Beta" systems that can be used in simulator research and in real-world trials are under development (Kithil et al., 2001).

Voice Analysis as a Monitoring Approach

For some time the law enforcement community has utilized methods of speech examination as a source of information on intoxication from alcohol and drugs. In the highly publicized Exxon Valdez accident, speech analysis was used to help determine that the responsible individual's judgment was impaired by alcohol (Brenner and Cash, 1991). Brenner and Cash (1991) note that alcohol ingestion produces slowed speech, speech errors, misarticulation of difficult sounds, and changes in vocal quality. It is possible that speech analysis might also be useful during fatigued conditions, as presumably many aspects of fatigued speech would be similar to speech under the influence of alcohol (a depressant of the central nervous system).

Brenner and colleagues (1994) have suggested that analyzing an operator's physiological state with speech-based analyses would be useful in the aerospace environment since speech analysis, unlike many other measures, is unobtrusive and does not require the pilot to be attached to any equipment. Speech measurements can be obtained through preexisting, on-board communications equipment (Brenner et al., 1994). These authors have identified six aspects of speech that may be applicable for determining psychological state (at least stress and possibly fatigue): (a) speaking fundamental frequency (pitch), which increases under stress; (b) speaking rate, which increases under stress; (c) vocal intensity (loudness), which increases in decibels as a function of the increased thoracic air pressure that occurs under stress; (d) vocal jitter, a subtle measure of the minute changes in the period of successive fundamental frequency cycles, which decreases in response to stress; (e) vocal shimmer, which is analogous to jitter and reflects the cycle-by-cycle differences in vocal intensity; and (f) derived speech measure, which combines properties of several speech measures and may provide a more sensitive indicator of stress. It was found by Brenner and coworkers (1994) that speaking fundamental frequency, vocal intensity, and speaking rate all increased in response to changing workload demands.

Johannes and coworkers (2000) point out that vocal pitch is affected by changes in autonomic nervous system arousal and that, in general, an increase in fundamental pitch is associated with emotional excitation. However, these authors go on to point out that useful voice-based state predictions are hampered by considerable individual differences in fundamental pitch, as well as by differing reactions to stressful events. In addition, some type of initial state calibration is required to differentiate the effects of stress versus fatigue. Whitmore and Fisher (1996) found that speech signals (word duration and fundamental frequency) recorded from aircrews in B-1B long-range bomber simulators tended to fluctuate parallel to the circadian cycle, like subjective and cognitive performance, during sleep deprivation. Word duration lengthened and fundamental frequency decreased as a function of fatigue. Griffin and Williams (1987) determined that an increase in peak amplitude and a decrease in word duration during conditions of increased workload were indicative of task complexity.

Additional research on the manner in which speech degrades under fatigued conditions may enable the development of new strategies to monitor both cognitive load and fatigue. However, it remains to be seen whether this technology will ever be applicable to military or other operational settings. In fact, a 1990 review of 50 years of research on voice analysis techniques indicated that while this is a promising area of research, the results have not shown voice analyses to be reliable techniques for determining the type or degree of reaction to stress or workload in operational settings (Ruiz et al., 1990). Studies on the utility of voice analysis for the prediction of changes in cognitive readiness are virtually nonexistent.

Self-Assessment

Standardized assessments of basic cognitive skills and periodic self-ratings of alertness and performance capabilities can provide valuable insight into the functional status of personnel as long as basic standardization (and a few other criteria) are met. With regard to cognitive assessments, Santucci and colleagues (1989) point out that cognitive tests are useful for monitoring the impact of environmental stressors and for evaluating the information-processing capabilities of individuals. However, these authors also caution that it is difficult to interpret the results of mental performance tests in uncontrolled, rapidly changing environments, across individuals who may show wide (and unknown) individual differences, and in circumstances in which the effects of practice cannot be controlled. Also, deciding which tests are best for each military job specialty may be difficult. Psychomotor tasks may seem optimal for monitoring the performance status of vehicle operators, whereas visual-attention tasks may appear to be a better choice for predicting decrements in radar, sonar, and radio operators. However, validation procedures must substantiate such assumptions, and there are no doubt extensive interactions among test requirements and test characteristics that will complicate the selection of the most appropriate choice for each occupational specialty. Subjective self-ratings appear more straightforward as long as their implementation is feasible and there is little chance that the personnel being assessed will be motivated to over-report or under-report the subjective symptoms of interest. For instance, Dorrian and coworkers (2000) have reported that research subjects were globally able to self-assess neurobehavioral performance decrements attributable to increases in fatigue with a high degree of accuracy. Gillberg and colleagues (1994) likewise found that three different subjective sleepiness scales were highly correlated with performance on a visual vigilance and a reaction-time task over the course of a night shift. More relevant to the military operational context, Caldwell and coworkers (2003) reported that preflight self-ratings of fatigue (from the Profile of Mood States) correlated highly (–0.72) with pilots' abilities to accurately complete simulator flight maneuvers during a 37-hour period of continuous wakefulness. In addition, as described in Chapter 3, self-assessments have proven useful for predicting the levels of optimal physical performance and the extent of performance deteriorations that would be of concern to combat service members engaged in demanding physical tasks. Thus self-ratings of operational status deserve serious consideration for their potential usefulness in status monitoring.

SUMMARY

No doubt there are strategies under development (and under refinement) that may contribute significantly to a further understanding of the basis of cognitive processing, as well as to the effects of fatigue, workload, and other factors that influence human performance. In all probability most will be useful only in laboratory environments or in fixed-based operational facilities (such as posts in which radar and sonar equipment are monitored or stations from which remote-controlled vehicles are piloted) where complex equipment can be housed, lengthy recording procedures can be conducted, and rigid controls can be maintained. Only a small subset of the strategies will likely be suitable for operational settings.

Based on a general review of the literature, it appears that the most promising techniques for accomplishing real-time, continuous assessments of foot-soldier cognitive readiness in military field settings are: (1) actigraphy based, or (2) EEG based, although neither technique is currently ready for widespread application. As noted, the Walter Reed Army Institute of Research has made substantial progress in the development and validation of an actigraph-based, sleep/fatigue monitor that could be worn like a wristwatch in almost any environment. This device may be available by 2005. Concurrent work with high-impedance EEG and ECG electrodes will soon make it possible to continuously record brain activity, heart-rate data, and other electrophysiological parameters and, as noted above, both the EEG and ECG offer useful information about operator status. However, once these new sensors are sufficiently refined, work will remain in terms of mounting them in combat helmets or integrating them into combat clothing. Speech-pattern analysis at one time seemed to hold promise for the future since there is a fair amount of verbal radio communication in the modern operational environment, but the work on this particular measure has not been particularly encouraging.

The most promising techniques for accomplishing real-time, continuous evaluations of the operators of military vehicles; the personnel responsible for manning radar, sonar, or other monitoring equipment; and those whose jobs consist of interfacing with computers and communications devices are: (1) EEG based, or (2) eye-movement based. The recording and evaluation of EEG activity becomes much more straightforward in settings in which operators are physically stationary and quiet because muscle and movement artifacts are attenuated. Furthermore, military aviators are required to wear flight helmets in which newly developed, high-impedance sensors could be mounted. Eye movement parameters (i.e., PERCLOS) have already proven feasible for the detection of changes in truck driver alertness, and efforts are underway to establish an automated PERCLOS that could be used in aviation settings. Since many eye monitoring systems require the use of cameras that are aimed at the faces of the operators, this is a technology that is clearly more applicable for stationary operators who are already staring straight ahead (at least most of the time) in order to complete some type of monitoring or computer-based task.

Questions about where these new monitoring approaches will be implemented are best considered first by assessing the feasibility of using them in specific environments (as noted above), and second by performing an analysis of the cost of the technology versus the cost of the mishap that the technology would be expected to prevent. Obviously, it is likely to be quite expensive to put some of the newest and most complicated monitoring devices in the hands of every foot soldier or to mount them in every military vehicle, and this in and of itself will pose a substantial barrier to widespread implementation. Thus a jeep driver or a member of a rifle platoon probably will not see the common use of operational alertness monitors for several years after such monitors first become available because of the initial expenses. Furthermore, a performance failure on the part of such individuals is unlikely to be a multimillion dollar catastrophe, so it would ultimately take the military years to reap sufficient savings from the technology to justify implementation in these segments of the overall force structure.

The pilot of a B-2 bomber, however, or those operating other highly complex modern aircraft may be among the first to benefit from newly developed status-monitoring approaches because there are relatively few of these aircraft, and the cost of losing even one would be significant by any standard. Each B-2 aircraft costs more than $1 billion, and the expenses likely to result from a single B-2 air mishap would no doubt be far greater depending on what type of munitions were on board and what the aircraft crashed into during the mishap. On top of these considerations is the fact that B-2s are long-range, two-crew bombers in which aircrew fatigue is known to be an operational hazard (some missions extend well beyond 33 hours of continuous flight time). In light of these facts, automated, onboard alertness monitors would be an obvious choice for fulfilling a much-needed fatigue countermeasure role. Therefore, the costs associated with instrumentation of such a platform are easily justifiable based on the aircraft's mission and the savings that would result from the prevention of even a single mishap. Such considerations and calculations will no doubt be applied to every potential site for future monitoring applications, at least until a relatively inexpensive and easy solution to the general status monitoring problem is found.

While the search is underway, individuals and their commanders will be forced to rely upon the same types of general alertness predictions (based on group data) and the same subjective impressions about "go" and "no-go" status that have been used for years. A great deal of progress has been made toward helping the armed forces address fatigue-related cognitive decrements once they have been identified. However, highly reliable, efficient, and cost-effective technological means of initially detecting and predicting those decrements remain to be developed.

REFERENCES

Agnew HW Jr, Webb WB, Williams RL. 1967. Comparison of stage four and 1-REM sleep deprivation. *Percept Mot Skills* 24:851–858.

Åkerstedt T. 1988. Sleepiness as a consequence of shift work. *Sleep* 11:17–34.

Åkerstedt T. 1995. Work hours, sleepiness and the underlying mechanisms. *J Sleep Res* 4:15–22.

Åkerstedt T, Gillberg M. 1982. Displacement of the sleep period and sleep deprivation. *Hum Neurobiol* 1:163–171.

Åkerstedt T, Kecklund G, Knutsson A. 1991. Spectral analysis of sleep electroencephalography in rotating three-shift work. *Scand J Work Environ Health* 17:330–336.

Andreassi JL. 1989. *Psychophysiology: Human Behavior and Physiological Response*. 2nd ed. Hillsdale, NJ: Lawrence Erlbaum Associates.

Angus RG, Heslegrave RJ. 1985. Effects of sleep loss on sustained cognitive performance during a command and control simulation. *Behav Res Methods Instrum Comput* 17:55–67.

Balkin J, Thorne D, Sing H, Thomas M, Redmond D, Wesensten N, Williams J, Hall S, Belenky G. 2000. *Effects of Sleep Schedules on Commercial Motor Vehicle Driver Performance*. Federal Motor Carrier Safety Administration. DOT-MC-00-133. Washington, DC: U.S. Department of Transportation.

Belenky G, Penetar DM, Thorne D, Popp K, Leu J, Thomas M, Sing H, Balkin T, Wesensten N, Redmond D. 1994. The effects of sleep deprivation on performance during continuous combat operations. In: Marriott BM, ed. *Food Components to Enhance Performance*. Washington, DC: National Academy Press. Pp. 127–135.

Belyavin AJ, Spencer MB. 2004. Modelling performance and alertness: The QinetiQ approach. *Aviation Space Environ Med* 75:A93–A103.

Blanc C, LaFontaine E, Medvedeff M. 1966. Radiotelemetric recordings of the electroencephalograms of civil aviation pilots during flight. *Aerospace Med* 37:1060–1065.

Bonnet MH. 1994. Sleep deprivation. In: Kryger MH, Roth T, Dement WC, eds. *Principles and Practice of Sleep Medicine*. 2nd ed. Philadelphia: W.B. Saunders. Pp. 50–67.

Brenner M, Cash JR. 1991. Speech analysis as an index of alcohol intoxication—The Exxon Valdez accident. *Aviat Space Environ Med* 62:893–898.

Brenner M, Doherty ET, Shipp T. 1994. Speech measures indicating workload demand. *Aviat Space Environ Med* 65:21–26.

Brookhuis K. 1995. Driver impairment monitoring by physiological measures. In: Hartley L, ed. *Fatigue and Driving: Driver Impairment, Driver Fatigue and Driver Simulation*. Bristol, PA: Taylor & Francis. Pp. 181–188.

Brookhuis KA, de Waard D. 1993. The use of psychophysiology to assess driver status. *Ergonomics* 36:1099–1110.

Cacioppo JT, Tassinary LG, eds. 1990. *Principles of Psychophysiology: Physical, Social, and Inferential Elements*. New York: Cambridge University Press.

Caldwell JA, Ramspott S. 1998. Effects of task duration on sensitivity to sleep deprivation using the multi-attribute task battery. *Behav Res Methods Instrum Comput* 30:651–660.

Caldwell JA, Roberts KA. 2000. Differential sensitivity of using simulators versus actual aircraft to evaluate the effects of a stimulant medication on aviator performance. *Mil Psychol* 12:277–291.

Caldwell JA, Wilson GF, Cetingue M, Gaillard AWK, Gunder A, Lagarde D, Makeig S, Myhre G, Wright NA. 1994. *Psychophysiological Assessment Methods*. AGARD-AR-324. Neuilly-Sur-Seine, France: North Atlantic Treaty Organization.

Caldwell JA, Caldwell JL, Crowley JS. 1996. Sustaining helicopter pilot alertness with Dexedrine during sustained operations. In: *Advisory Group for Aerospace Research and Development Conference Proceedings CP-579, Aerospace Medical Symposium on Neurological Limitations of Aircraft Operations: Human Performance Implications*. Neuilly-Sur-Seine, France: North Atlantic Treaty Organization. Pp. 38-1–38-11.

Caldwell JA, Kelly CF, Roberts KA, Jones HD, Lewis JA, Woodrum L, Dillard RM, Johnson PP. 1997. *A Comparison of EEG and Evoked Response Data Collected in a UH-1 Helicopter to Data Collected in a Standard Laboratory Environment*. USAARL 97-30. Fort Rucker, AL: U.S. Army Aeromedical Research Laboratory.

Caldwell JA, Caldwell JL, Smythe NK, Hall KK. 2000a. A double-blind, placebo-controlled investigation of the efficacy of modafinil for sustaining the alertness and performance of aviators: A helicopter simulator study. *Psychopharmacology* 150:272–282.

Caldwell JA, Smythe NK, LeDuc PA, Caldwell JL. 2000b. Efficacy of Dexedrine® for maintaining aviator performance during 64 hours of sustained wakefulness: A simulator study. *Aviat Space Environ Med* 71:7–18.

Caldwell JA, Hall KK, Erickson BS. 2002. EEG data collected from helicopter pilots in flight are sufficiently sensitive to detect increased fatigue from sleep deprivation. *Int J Aviat Psychol* 12:19–32.

Caldwell J, Caldwell JL, Brown D, Smythe N, Smith J, Mylar J, Mandichak M, Schroeder C. 2003. *The Effects of 37 Hours of Continuous Wakefulness on the Physiological Arousal, Cognitive Performance, Self-Reported Mood, and Simulator Flight Performance of F-117A Pilots*. AFRL-HE-BR-TR-2003-0086. Brooks City Base, TX: U.S. Air Force Research Laboratory.

Carskadon MA, Dement WC. 1994. Normal human sleep: An overview. In: Kryger MH, Roth T, Dement WC, eds. *Principles and Practice of Sleep Medicine*. 2nd ed. Philadelphia: WB Saunders. Pp. 16–25.

Coles MGH, Donchin E, Porges SW, eds. 1986. *Psychophysiology: Systems, Processes, and Applications*. New York: Guilford Press.

Comens P, Reed D, Mette M. 1987. Physiologic responses of pilots flying high-performance aircraft. *Aviat Space Environ Med* 58:205–210.

Comperatore CA, Caldwell JA, Stephans RL, Chiaramonte JA, Pearson JY, Trast ST, Mattingly AD. 1992. *The Use of Electrophysiological and Cognitive Variables in the Assessment of Degradation During Periods of Sustained Wakefulness*. USAARL 93-5. Fort Rucker, AL: U.S. Army Aeromedical Research Laboratory.

Cooper R, Osselton JW, Shaw JC. 1980. *EEG Technology*. 3rd ed. London: Butterworths.

Correll JT. 1998. Strung out. We have too few forces and too little money chasing too many open-ended deployments. Online. *Air Force Magazine*. Available at http://www.afa.org/magazine/sept1998/09edit98_print.html. Accessed November 3, 2003.

Daggett S, Belasco A. 2002. *Defense Budget for FY2003: Data Summary*. CRS Report for Congress, RL31349. Washington, DC: Congressional Research Service.

de Waard D, Brookhuis KA. 1991. Assessing driver status: A demonstration experiment on the road. *Accid Anal Prev* 23:297–307.

Dement WC. 1976. *Some Must Watch While Some Must Sleep*. New York: WW Norton & Co.

Dinges DF. 1995. An overview of sleepiness and accidents. *J Sleep Res* 4:4–14.

Dinges DF, Kribbs NB. 1991. Performing while sleepy: Effects of experimentally-induced sleepiness. In: Monk TH, ed. *Sleep, Sleepiness, and Performance*. New York: John Wiley & Sons. Pp. 97–128.

Dinges DF, Mallis MM, Maislin G, Powell JW. 1998. *Evaluation of Techniques for Ocular Measurement as an Index of Fatigue and as the Basis for Alertness Management*. DOT-HS-808-762. Washington, DC: National Highway Traffic Safety Administration. Pp. 42–47, 79–80.

Dorrian J, Lamond N, Dawson D. 2000. The ability to self-monitor performance when fatigued. *J Sleep Res* 9:137–144.

Downing P, Liu J, Kanwisher N. 2001. Testing cognitive models of visual attention with fMRI and MEG. *Neuropsychologia* 39:1329–1342.

Drummond SPA, Brown GG. 2001. The effects of total sleep deprivation on cerebral responses to cognitive performance. *Neuropsychopharmacology* 25:S68–S73.

Drummond SPA, Brown GG, Gillin JC, Stricker JL, Wong EC, Buxton RB. 2000. Altered brain response to veral learning following sleep deprivation. *Nature* 403:655–657.

Eddy DR, Hursh SR. 2001. *Fatigue Avoidance Scheduling Tool (FAST)*. AFRL-HE-BR-TR-2001-0140. Brooks City Base, TX: U.S. Air Force Research Laboratory.

Elliott S. 2001. *Chief of Staff Shares Views on Global Strike Task Force*. Online. U.S. Air Force. Available at http://www.af.mil/news/Oct2001/n20011029_1543.shtml. Accessed November 4, 2003.

Evinger C, Manning KA, Sibony PA. 1991. Eyelid movements. *Invest Ophthalmo Vis Sci* 32:387–400.

Gevins A, Leong H, Du R, Smith ME, Le J, Du Rousseau D, Zhang J, Libove J. 1995. Towards measurement of brain function in operational environments. *Biol Psychol* 40:169–186.

Gillberg M. 1995. Sleepiness and its relation to the length, content, and continuity of sleep. *J Sleep Res* 2:37–40.

Gillberg M, Kecklund G, Åkerstedt T. 1994. Relations between performance and subjective ratings of sleepiness during a night awake. *Sleep* 17:236–241.

Grace R, Steward S. 2001. *Drowsy Driver Monitor and Warning System*. Online. Public Policy Center, University of Iowa. Available at http://ppc.uiowa.edu/driving-assessment/2001/Summaries/Driving%20Assessment%20Papers/ 11_Grace_Richard.htm. Accessed October 10, 2003.

Griffin GR, Williams CE. 1987. The effects of different levels of task complexity on three vocal measures. *Aviat Space Environ Med* 58:1165–1170.

Hansen AL, Johnsen BH, Thayer JF. 2003. Vagal influence on working memory and attention. *Int J Psychophysiol* 48:263–274.

Härmä M. 1995. Sleepiness and shiftwork: Individual differences. *J Sleep Res* 4:57–61.

Hart SG, Hauser JR. 1987. Inflight application of three pilot workload measurement techniques. *Aviat Space Environ Med* 58:402–410.

Hauri P, Orr WC. 1982. *The Sleep Disorders*. 2nd ed. Kalamazoo, MI: Upjohn.

Hitchcock EM, Warm JS, Matthews G, Dember WN, Shear PK, Tripp LD, Mayleben DW, Parasuraman R. 2003. Automation cueing modulates cerebral blood flow and vigilance in a simulated air traffic control task. *Theor Issues Ergon Sci* 4:89–112.

Hollander TD, Warm JS, Matthews GR, Dember WN, Parasuraman R, Hitchcock EM, Beam CA, Tripp LD. 2002. Effects of signal regularity and salience on vigilance performance and cerebral hemovelocity. In: *Proceedings of the Human Factors and Ergonomics Society 46th Annual Meeting*. Santa Monica: Human Factors and Ergonomics Society. Pp. 1654–1658.

Horne JA. 1978. A review of the biological effects of total sleep deprivation in man. *Biol Psychol* 7:55–102.

Hossain JL, Reinish LW, Kayumov L, Bhuiya P, Shapiro CM. 2003. Underlying sleep pathology may cause chronic high fatigue in shift-workers. *J Sleep Res* 12:223–230.

Howitt JS, Hay AE, Shergold GR, Ferres HM. 1978. Workload and fatigue—Inflight EEG changes. *Aviat Space Environ Med* 49:1197–1202.

Hursh SR, Redmond DP, Johnson ML, Thorne DR, Belenky G, Balkin TJ, Storm WF, Miller JC, Eddy DR. 2004. Fatigue models for applied research in warfighting. *Aviat Space Environ Med* 75:A44–A53.

Itoh Y, Hayashi Y, Tsukui I, Saito S. 1989. Heart rate variability subjective mental workload in flight task validity of mental workload measurement using the H.R.V. method. In: Smith MJ, Salvendy G, eds. *Work With Computers: Organizational, Management, Stress and Health Aspects*. Amsterdam: Elsevier. Pp. 209–216.

Johannes B, Salnitski VP, Gunga HC, Kirsch K. 2000. Voice stress monitoring in space—Possibilities and limits. *Aviat Space Environ Med* 71:A58–A65.

Johnsen BH, Thayer JF, Laberg JC, Wormnes B, Raadal M, Skaret E, Kvale G, Berg E. 2003. Attentional and physiological characteristics of patients with dental anxiety. *J Anxiety Disord* 17:75–87.

Kakimoto Y, Nakamura A, Tarui H, Nagasawa Y, Yagura S. 1988. Crew workload in JASDF C-1 transport flights: I. Change in heart rate and salivary cortisol. *Aviat Space Environ Med* 59:511–516.

Kingsley SA, Sriram S, Pollick A, Marsh J. 2003. Photrode™ optical sensor for electrophysiological monitoring. *Aviat Space Environ Med* 74:1215–1216.

Kithil PW, Jones RD, MacCuish J. 2001. *Development of Driver Alertness Detection System Using Overhead Capacity Sensor Array*. Online. Available at http://www.lascruces.com/~rfrye/complexica/d/ASCI%20drowsy%20driver%20paper%2011-20-01.doc. Accessed November 4, 2003.

Kramer AF. 1991. Physiological metrics of mental workload: A review of recent progress. In: Damos DL, ed. *Multiple-Task Performance*. Washington, DC: Taylor & Francis. Pp. 279–328.

Krueger GP. 1991. Sustained military performance in continuous operations: Combatant fatigue, rest and sleep needs. In: Gal R, Mangelsdorff AD, eds. *Handbook of Military Psychology*. New York: John Wiley & Sons. Pp. 255–277.

Leder RS, Gale H, Stamp C, Yamasaki DS, Webster JG. 1996. Eyelid activity measurement: A new retroreflective sensor. *Sleep Res* 25:509.

LeDuc PA, Caldwell JA, Ruyak PS. 2000. The effects of exercise as a countermeasure for fatigue in sleep-deprived aviators. *Mil Psychol* 12:249–266.

Lewis CE, Jones WL, Austin F, Roman J. 1967. Flight research programs: IX. Medical monitoring of carrier pilots in combat—II. *Aerosp Med* 38:581–592.

Lindholm E, Cheatham C, Koriath J, Longridge TM. 1984. *Physiological Assessment of Aircraft Pilot Workload in Simulated Landing and Simulated Hostile Threat Environments*. AFHRL-TR-83-49. Williams Air Force Base, AZ: U.S. Air Force Human Resources Laboratory.

Lindqvist A, Keskinen E, Antila K, Halkola L, Peltonen T, Valimaki I. 1983. Heart rate variability, cardiac mechanics, and subjectively evaluated stress during simulator flight. *Aviat Space Environ Med* 54:685–690.

Lorenzo I, Ramos J, Arce C, Guevara MA, Corsi-Cabrera M. 1995. Effect of total sleep deprivation on reaction time and waking EEG activity in man. *Sleep* 18:346–354.

Maulsby RL. 1966. Electroencephalogram during orbital flight. *Aerosp Med* 37:1022–1026.

Miller JC. 1997. Quantitative analysis of truck driver EEG during highway operations. *Biomed Sci Instrum* 34: 93–98.

Mitler MM, Carskadon MA, Czeisler CA, Dement WC, Dinges DF, Graeber RC. 1988. Catastrophes, sleep, and public policy: Consensus report. *Sleep* 11:100–109.

Monk TH, Folkard S. 1985. Shiftwork and performance. In: Folkard S, Monk TH, eds. *Hours of Work. Temporal Factors in Work-Scheduling*. New York: John Wiley & Sons. Pp. 239–252.

Monk TH, Buysse DJ, Rose LR. 1999. Wrist actigraphic measures of sleep in space. *Sleep* 22:948–954.

Moore-Ede M. 1993. Aviation safety and pilot error. In: *Twenty-Four Hour Society*. Reading, MA: Addison-Wesley Publishing. Pp. 81–95.

Mulder G, Mulder LJM. 1980. Coping with mental work load. In: Levine S, Ursin H, eds. *Coping and Health*. New York: Plenum Press. Pp. 233–258.

Mulder LJM. 1992. Measurement and analysis methods of heart rate and respiration for use in applied environments. *Biol Psychol* 34:205–236.

Naitoh P, Kelly TL. 1992. *Sleep Management User's Guide for Special Operations Personnel*. Naval Health Research Center Report No. 92-28. Bethesda, MD: Naval Medical Research and Development Command.

Nicholson AN, Hill LE, Borland RG, Ferres HM. 1970. Activity of the nervous system during the let-down, approach and landing: A study of short duration high workload. *Aerosp Med* 41:436–446.

NTSB (National Transportation Safety Board). 1990. *Marine Accident Report-Grounding of the U.S. Tankship Exxon Valdez on Bligh Reef, Prince William Sound, Near Valdez, Alaska, 24 Mar 1989*. Report No. NTSB/Mar-90/04. Washington DC: NTSB.

NTSB. 2000. *Aircraft Accident Report: Controlled Flight into Terrain, Korean Air Flight 801, Boeing 747-300, HL7468, Nimitz Hill, Guam, August 6, 1997*. Report No. NTSB/AAR-00-01. Washington, DC: NTSB.

Opmeer CHJM, Krol JP. 1973. Towards an objective assessment of cockpit workload: I. Physiological variables during different flight phases. *Aerosp Med* 44:527–532.

Penn PE, Bootzin RR. 1990. Behavioural techniques for enhancing alertness and performance in shift work. *Work Stress* 4:213–226.

Petit C, Chaput D, Tarriere C, LeCoz JY, Planque S. 1990. Research to prevent the driver from falling asleep behind the wheel. In: *34th Annual Proceedings, Association of the Advancement of Automotive Medicine Conference, October 1–3, 1990*. Barrington, IL: Association of the Advancement of Automotive Medicine. Pp. 505–522.

Pietrini P, Alexander GE, Furey ML, Hampel H, Guazzelli M. 2000. The neurometabolic landscape of cognitive decline: In vivo studies with positron emission tomography in Alzheimer's disease. *Int J Psychophysiol* 37:87–98.

Pigeau RA, Heslegrave RJ, Angus RG. 1987. Psychophysiological measures of drowsiness as estimators of mental fatigue and performance degradation during sleep deprivation. In: *Electrical and Magnetic Activity of the Central Nervous System: Research and Clinical Applications in Aerospace Medicine*. Paris, France: NATO Advisory Group for Aerospace Research and Development. Pp. 21-1–21-16.

Pollak CP, Tryon WW, Nagaraja H, Dzwonczyk R. 2001. How accurately does wrist actigraphy identify the states of sleep and wakefulness? *Sleep* 24:957–965.

Portas CM, Rees G, Howseman AM, Josephs O, Turner R, Frith CD. 1998. A specific role for the thalamus in mediating the interaction of attention and arousal in humans. *J Neurosci* 18:8979–8989.

Rechtschaffen A, Kales A, eds. 1968. *A Manual of Standardized Terminology, Techniques and Scoring System for Sleep Stages of Human Subjects*. Washington, DC: U.S. Government Printing Office.

Rees G. 2001. Neuroimaging of visual awareness in patients and normal subjects. *Curr Opin Neurobiol* 11:150–156.

Roehrs T, Merlotti L, Petrucelli N, Stepanski E, Roth T. 1994. Experimental sleep fragmentation. *Sleep* 17:438–443.

Roehrs T, Carskadon MA, Dement WC, Roth T. 2000. Daytime sleepiness and alertness. In: Kryger MH, Roth T, Dement WC, eds. *Principles and Practice of Sleep Medicine*. Philadelphia: WB Saunders. Pp. 43–52.

Roffwarg HP. 1979. Diagnostic classification of sleep and arousal disorders. *Sleep* 2:5–15.

Roscoe AH. 1978. Stress and workload in pilots. *Aviat Space Environ Med* 49:630–636.

Roscoe AH. 1980. Heart-rate changes in test pilots. In: Kitney RI, Rompelman O, eds. *The Study of Heart-Rate Variability*. Oxford, England: Clarendon Press. Pp. 178–190.

Roscoe AH. 1992. Assessing pilot workload. Why measure heart rate, HRV and respiration? *Biol Psychol* 34:259–287.

Rosekind MR, Gander PH, Miller DL, Gregory KB, Smith RM, Weldon KJ, Co EL, McNally KL, Lebacqz JV. 1994. Fatigue in operational settings: Examples from the aviation environment. *Hum Factors* 36:327–338.

Rosenthal L, Roehrs TA, Rosen A, Roth T. 1993. Level of sleepiness and total sleep time following various time in bed conditions. *Sleep* 16:226–232.

Ruffell-Smith HP. 1967. Heart rate of pilots plying aircraft on scheduled airline routes. *Aerosp Med* 38:1117–1119.

Ruiz R, Legros C, Guell A. 1990. Voice analysis to predict the psychological or physical state of a speaker. *Aviat Space Environ Med* 61:266–271.

Russo M, Thomas M, Sing H, Thorne D, Balkin T, Wesensten N, Redmond D, Welsh A, Rowland L, Johnson D, Cephus R, Hall S, Belenky G, Krichmar J. 1999. Sleep deprivation related changes correlate with simulated motor vehicle crashes. In: Carroll RJ, ed. *Ocular Measures of Driver Alertness: Technical Conference Proceedings*. FHWA-MC-99-136. Washington, DC: Office of Motor Carrier and Highway Safety/Federal Highway Administration. Pp. 119–124.

Russo M, Thomas M, Thorne D, Sing H, Redmond D, Rowland L, Johnson D, Hall S, Krichmar J, Balkin T. 2003. Oculomotor impairment during chronic partial sleep deprivation. *Clin Neurophysiol* 114:723–736.

Santucci G, Boer L, Farmer E, Goeters KM, Grissett JD, Schwartz E, Wetherall A, Wilson G. 1989. *Human Performance Assessment Methods*. AGARDograph No. 308. Neuilly-Sur-Seine, France: NATO Advisory Group for Aerospace Research and Development.

Sekiguchi C, Handa Y, Gotoh M, Kurihara Y, Nagasawa Y, Kuroda I. 1979. Frequency analysis of heart rate variability under flight conditions. *Aviat Space Environ Med* 50:625–634.

Spencer J. 2000. *The Facts about Military Readiness*. Online. The Heritage Foundation Backgrounder: No. 1394. Available at http://www.heritage.org/Research/MissileDefense/loader.cfm?url=/commonspot/security/getfile.cfm&PageID=10734. Accessed November 7, 2003.

Stern A, Ranney T. 1999. Ocular based measures of driver alertness. In: Carroll RJ, ed. *Ocular Measures of Driver Alertness: Technical Conference Proceedings*. FHWA-MC-99-136. Washington, DC: Office of Motor Carrier and Highway Safety/Federal Highway Administration. Pp. 4–23.

Stern JA. 1980. *Aspects of Visual Search Activity Related to Attentional Processes and Skill Development*. AFOSR-TR-81-0119. Washington, DC: U.S. Air Force Office of Scientific Research.

Stickgold R, Neri DF, Pace-Schott E, Juguilon A, Czeisler CA, Hobson JA. 1995. Nightcap detection of decreased vigilance. *Sleep Res* 24:500.

Stroobant N, Vingerhoets G. 2000. Transcranial Doppler ultrasonography monitoring of cerebral hemodynamics during performance of cognitive tasks: A review. *Neuropsychol Rev* 10:213–231.

Taub JM, Berger RJ. 1973. Performance and mood following variations in the length and timing of sleep. *Psychophysiology* 10:559–570.

Thiessen GJ. 1988. Effect of traffic noise on the cyclical nature of sleep. *J Acoust Soc Am* 84:1741–1743.

Thomas M, Sing H, Belenky G, Holcomb H, Mayberg H, Dannals R, Wagner H, Thorne D, Popp K, Rowland L, Welsh A, Balwinski S, Redmond D. 2000. Neural basis of alertness and cognitive performance impairments during sleepiness. I. Effects of 24 h of sleep deprivation on waking human regional brain activity. *J Sleep Res* 9:335–352.

U.S. Army. 1991. *Soldier Performance in Continuous Operations*. FM 22-9. Washington, DC: U.S. Department of the Army.

U.S. Army. 1996. *Force of Decision: Capabilities for the 21st Century*. White paper. Washington, DC: U.S. Department of the Army.

U.S. Army. 1997. *Army Aviation Operations*. FM 1-100. Washington, DC: U.S. Department of the Army.

Van Dongen HPA, Rogers NL, Dinges DF. 2003. Sleep debt: Theoretical and empirical issues. *Sleep Biol Rhythms* 1:5–13.

Walsh JK, Hartman PG, Schweitzer PK. 1994. Slow-wave sleep deprivation and waking function. *J Sleep Res* 3:16–25.

Whitmore J, Fisher S. 1996. Speech during sustained operations. *Speech Commun* 20:55–70.

Wierwille WW. 1999. Historical perspective on slow eyelid closure: Whence PERCLOS? In: Carroll RJ, ed. *Ocular Measures of Driver Alertness: Technical Conference Proceedings*. FHWA-MC-99-136. Washington, DC: Office of Motor Carrier and Highway Safety/Federal Highway Administration. Pp. 31–53.

Wierwille WW, Connor SA. 1983. Evaluation of 20 workload measures using a psychomotor task in a moving-base aircraft simulator. *Hum Factors* 25:1–16.

Wilkinson RT. 1961. Interaction of lack of sleep with knowledge of results, repeated testing, and individual differences. *J Exp Psychol* 62:263–271.

Wilkinson RT. 1964. Effects of up to 60 hours' sleep deprivation on different types of work. *Ergonomics* 17:175–186.

Wilkinson R. 1969. Some factors influencing the effect of environmental stressors upon performance. *Psychol Bull* 72:260–272.

Wilkinson RT, Edwards RS, Haines E. 1966. Performance following a night of reduced sleep. *Psychonomic Sci* 5:471–472.

Wilson GF. 1993. Air-to-ground training missions: A psychophysiological workload analysis. *Ergonomics* 36:1071–1087.

Wilson GF, Eggemeier FT. 1991. Psychophysiological assessment of workload in multi-task environments. In: Damos DL, ed. *Multiple-Task Performance*. Washington, DC: Taylor & Francis. Pp. 329–360.

Wilson GF, Purvis B, Skelly J, Fullenkamp P, Davis I. 1987. Physiological data used to measure pilot workload in actual flight and simulator conditions. *Proceedings of the Human Factors Society*, 31st Annual Meeting. Pp. 779–783.

Wright N, McGown A. 2001. Vigilance on the civil flight deck: incidence of sleepiness and sleep during long-haul flights and associated changes in physiological parameters. *Ergonomics* 44:82–106.

Wu JC, Gillin JC, Buchsbaum MS, Hershey T, Hazlett E, Sicotte N, Bunney WE. 1991. The effect of sleep deprivation on cerebral glucose metabolic rate in normal humans assessed with positron emission tomography. *Sleep* 14:155–162.

6

Conclusions and Recommendations

Trends in the conduct of military operations will continue toward the use of smaller operational units deployed more frequently and equipped with advanced technology, weaponry, and communications. Monitoring metabolic status is a way of optimizing the functioning of the individual service member and minimizing risk of fatigue and illness through the observation, interpretation, and transmission of physiological data both to the individual and to the command unit. The use of an array of sensors to monitor both the biomarkers of the individual's physiological and cognitive status and the ambient environment can allow metabolic irregularities to be anticipated in a manner that will permit timely feedback and initiation of corrective actions. These same systems can continue to monitor the individual for compliance with recommendations and provide information on the efficacy of the corrective action taken.

It is important to look forward a decade or two to imagine what might be possible with the evolution of new technologies in regard to metabolic monitoring. It is quite certain that sensors will get smaller, faster, more mobile, more versatile, and perhaps more affordable. However, this forecasting is hampered when only the technological tools available today are considered. One needs to stretch the imagination to make predictions in two major areas: (1) What will be the new biomarkers that will enhance monitoring of individual health and performance? and (2) What will be the new sensor technologies that will facilitate rapid assessment of individual status? Clearly, improvement in monitoring metabolic status requires significant research investments in the identification and validation of new biomarkers, the field validation of existing sensor technologies, the development of new sensor devices, and the enhancement of bioinformatics to evaluate the data.

For example, in the last two decades biotechnology has provided great benefits to medicine, agriculture, criminology, and environmental sciences and holds great promise for future advancements in these fields. Biotechnology can be defined as using living material or molecular components of living material, to interact with small amounts of environmental substances, resulting in a physical or chemical change that can be measured by a detection system. A recent report (NRC, 2001) extensively reviewed the state of the art of biochips that might use proteins, nucleic acids, deoxyribonucleic acid, or even living cells to detect a wide array of chemical toxins in the environment, biochemical substances excreted by the body in response to stress, or exposure to toxins or pathogenic organisms. Although this technology is in its infancy and now is only reliable in the laboratory, some embedded sensors, such as glucose monitors, are already available and the committee envisions that externally worn sensors can be developed in the near future.

Finally, the integration of self- (or peer-) reported and objective measures through a single wrist-worn device should be a priority in the military. Software and hardware are available to create such a device that would integrate information from ratings of perceived exertion, muscle soreness, fatigue scores, weight changes, urine specific gravity, as well as physical activity data from an accelerometer or pedometer.

The implementation of any new approaches, however, should first be evaluated for feasibility of using them in specific environments and for the cost of the technology versus the cost of the mishap that the technology would be expected to prevent.

Also, the effectiveness of monitoring, including physiological and self- (and peer-) assessments, depends largely on the standardized use of methodology and on taking appropriate decisions; therefore, it is important that military personnel be educated in basic physiology and psychology and monitoring methods.

This chapter provides suggestions on which research efforts for monitoring metabolic status should take priority, along with the committee's answers to the five questions posed by the military.

QUESTION 1

What are the most promising biomarkers for the prediction of: (a) excessive rates of bone loss and muscle turnover, (b) reduced glucose and energy metabolism (e.g., bioelectrical indicators of muscle and mental fatigue), (c) dehydration, and (d) decrements in cognitive function?

Irrespective of the biological or cognitive markers selected, there is a need for baseline measurements of individual combat service members so that it can be determined, on an individual basis, if a marker is significantly altered under stress. The committee recommends that, initially, simple protocol data of normal/abnormal ranges may be used. However, these ranges may be sufficiently imprecise to make individual-based predictions dubious. By evaluating a marker's deviation from the individual's baseline, rather than by comparing it with a population-based norm, an individual's condition can be much more accurately described.

Biomarkers for Bone and Muscle Metabolism

Bone

There are no groups of intermediate markers of bone health that can provide a one-time identification of risk of fractures, including stress fracture. Bone remodeling is a relatively slow biological process and thus not amenable to monitoring in field situations. Prediction of bone changes that increase fracture risk may be of greater importance in initial entry training, when individuals are transitioning to a greater state of fitness, than in combat.

Markers should be used both pre- and post-training and should include bone density (as measured by dual-energy X-ray absorptiometry), sensation of bone pain, menstrual status, and mental state as related to cortisol responsiveness. Bone turnover can be assessed by increases in 24-hour urinary n-telopeptide excretion over baseline. The role of cortisol in bone health during military exercises, however, may be transient and may not have long-term effects on bone health.

Bone mineral density (BMD) is the most predictive measure of risk of fractures; this measure should be used in determining medical suitability for training and combat-related activities. Strategies should be developed to determine the BMD levels that are required to meet medical standards, and approaches should be identified to prevent significant loss of bone mass. In this sense, adequate countermeasures for preventing bone loss and fractures should be implemented prior, during, and after intensive physical training.

Muscle

Muscle fatigue is related to decreases in oxygen availability to muscle cells. This decrease in oxygen availability may result from, for example, decreases in cardiovascular function, decreased hemoglobin concentrations, or inadequate intravascular volume due to excessive water loss (dehydration). There are a number of biomarkers that may be indicative of muscle fatigue or increased catabolism (see Appendix A). Some of these include protein turnover and 24-hour urinary 3-methylhistidine. Protein turnover measures use stable or radioisotopes when amino acids, such as N15 glycine or C13 leucine, are infused and appearance and disappearance rates are measured. Twenty-four-hour urinary 3-methylhistidine, which is not metabolized, indicates rates of muscle protein catabolism. This speaks to the importance of renal function (see discussion below). However, there is insufficient evidence that can specifically correlate these biomarkers with actual decrements in muscle performance during activities such as weight lifting, timed running trials, and endurance running. In general, markers of muscle catabolism will overemphasize negative changes in muscle and must be coupled with markers of muscle protein synthesis. However, even with an imbalance of protein breakdown to synthesis, a loss of as much as 15 percent of muscle mass may occur without significant effects on muscle performance.

There is substantial evidence in the sports medicine literature that self- (or peer-) reported measures, such as perceived exertion, muscle soreness, muscle pain, ratings of sleep quality, and mood states, possess efficacy in predicting both physical performance and deterioration in performance and, in fact, have often been found to be superior to any physiological measures. Validation of these measurements in the field is necessary.

Renal Function

Potential markers of renal function deserve attention due to the essential role of the kidneys in maintaining protein status, hydration status, and electrolyte balance. Also, the loss of large amounts of nitrogen end products through the kidneys would be indicative of a negative protein balance. There are a number of markers and technologies now available that could be adapted for self- (or peer) monitoring during training or field operations. In order to assess renal function, it is suggested that the field measures presented in Figure 4-4 be taken at mid-day and in the evening after the day's exertion.

The military should consider providing and training personnel in the use of simple urine dipstick-type test strips that would provide information on levels of urine protein (a marker for potential kidney damage), ketones and glucose (potential markers for energy metabolism), and leukocyte esterase and nitrates (indicators of urinary tract infections) as indicators of muscle damage and hydration status.

Biomarkers for Reduced Glucose Metabolism

The development of specific biomedical markers under other situations, such as chemical exposures or psychological threats, would require an understanding of the metabolic processes resulting from such circumstances. The potential biomarkers for anaerobic glucose metabolism are: Borg's 6–20 scale of perceived exertion (local, central, and overall); muscle soreness; tissue levels of lactate measured by near-infrared spectroscopy (NIRS); muscle biopsy for glycogen, cytokines, and enzymes; actigraphy; electroencephalography (EEG); heart-rate variability; profile of mood state; and visual analog scale. The use of these biomarkers for this purpose needs to be validated in the field.

Biomarkers of Dehydration

Heightened physical activity under adverse environmental conditions causes dehydration, which impacts exercise performance and other physiological functions. Even 1 percent dehydration can cause obvious signs of heat exhaustion if strenuous exercise occurs in hot (41°C or 105°F) environments. Dehydration increases hemoconcentration, blood viscosity and osmolality, core body temperature, and heart rate, while causing a decrease in stroke volume. Dehydration also increases the onset of fatigue and makes any given exercise intensity appear harder than it would be if the individual was well hydrated. However, the most serious effect of progressive dehydration is that due to a lower cardiac output, the body decreases its ability to sweat via decreased blood flow to the skin. This in turn decreases the body's ability to cool itself, which leads to an increased core body temperature and the risk of heat illness and collapse and, in rare situations, life-threatening heat stroke.

In the military setting, changes in water and osmotic balance are usually synergistic with increases in water loss (dehydration reflected by reductions in body volume and increases in osmolality). One of the most sensitive indicators of hydration status is short-term changes in body weight since most day-to-day variation in body weight is due to hydration status. The assessment of weight loss or loss of body mass, plasma sodium or plasma osmolality, urinary specific gravity, fluid balance, and the recovery of weight 24 hours after dehydration can be used for the identification of extent and type of dehydration. In the military setting, where dehydration is the most common condition, weight changes over a short period of time reflect fluid changes and loss of body water coupled with measures of serum sodium or serum osmolality can define the degree of concomitant salt loss. Renal function is also a good indicator of hydration status.

Biomarkers of Cognitive Function

The most promising techniques for accomplishing continuous assessments of ground combat service member cognitive readiness in field settings are actigraphy, EEG, and heart-rate variability. Actigraphy is useful because it offers a field-practical way of monitoring the sleep of combat service members, and insufficient sleep is the primary cause of cognitive degradations in operational environments. EEG is useful because it offers a relatively noninvasive assessment of the brain activity that underlies all types of performance, including vigilance and judgment. Heart-rate variability is a peripheral nervous system measure that also reflects the brain activity that underlies performance attention and mood. In vehicle operators or in radar or other fixed-based system operators, eye-movement monitoring is also promising. Saccadic velocity and percentage-of-eye-closure measures have been shown to reflect the status of the central nervous system. In all probability, most of these measures will be useful only in laboratory environments or in fixed-based operational facilities (such as posts in which radar or sonar equipment is monitored or stations from which remote-controlled vehicles are piloted) where complex equipment can be housed, lengthy recording procedures can be conducted, and rigid controls can be maintained. Only a small subset of these methods will likely be suitable for operational settings.

Besides these objective measures, subjective ratings of alertness and fatigue should be considered for use in the field since these have been shown to correlate with performance changes in some situations. However, it should be recognized that self-report data can be influenced by peer pressure (or supervisor pressure); also, there is evidence that self-reports may lose a degree of sensitivity when the stress or fatigue becomes so chronic that the individual has difficulty referencing his or her present feelings to more normal past experiences.

QUESTION 2

What monitoring technologies would be required (that may not currently exist) to predict these intermediate targets in critical metabolic pathways?

New biomarkers are likely to be identified in the future; still, the greater need lies in: (1) the development of easier systems to measure and transmit data, and (2) the development of new mathematical models to provide enhanced data integration and analysis by using nonlinear discriminant algorithms. Future monitoring technologies should consist of an integrated system that incorporates noninvasive or minimally invasive sensor technology, communication interface and integration, data analysis tools, and local area networks. This infrastructure should be both redundant and noncentralized. A "black box" or "medical hub" is needed to gather data from multiple sensors or devices, standardize the outputs, and submit these data to a data reduction system or decision-making tool for the creation of both prioritized alarm signals and recommended interventions.

In summary, the major obstacles likely to be encountered in the implementation of future monitoring technologies will be the selection of variables and the building of models that truly predict health performance status.

QUESTION 3

What tools currently exist for monitoring metabolic status that could be useful in the field?

Metabolic status can be defined in part by energy metabolism, intermediary fuels (glucose, fatty acids, and amino acids), acid/base and hydration status, and psychophysiological data. One methodology that can examine many different biomarkers of metabolism and shows great promised in the field is NIRS. NIRS can concurrently monitor muscle oxygenation and deoxygenation, intramuscular pH, lactate, and skin hydration status. With NIRS, muscle function and hydration status can be measured under field conditions with telemetry units.

Muscle Fatigue

Individuals experience fatigue when muscle energy sources are inadequate or when faced with inadequate energy substrates when oxygen delivery falls below the point for lactate accumulation. One measure that could be useful in the field, after validation in military settings, is self-perception, as described in Chapter 3. Predictors of fatigue at an earlier state have also been proposed. The challenge remains to differentiate diagnosis between acute damage from muscle injury, fatigue due to overuse or overconditioning, exercise until exhaustion, hydration, and nutritional status given the interactions of these factors in the subjective feeling of fatigue.

Renal Function and Hydration

Simple methods that measure renal function and hydration already exist. As mentioned previously, the military should train personnel in the use of simple urine dipstick-type test strips that would provide information on levels of urine protein, ketones and glucose, and leukocyte esterase and nitrates as indicators of muscle damage and hydration status. Also, a practical method of monitoring weight changes in the field would be of value for monitoring hydration.

Energy Expenditure

An individual is said to be in energy balance if energy input (calories consumed) matches energy expenditure and weight is maintained. Research has focused on measuring the energy expenditure side of the energy balance equation as a measurement of total energy needs since these methods may not rely on individual data recording. If energy balance is not maintained, weight is lost and available energy is decreased. This situation can dramatically impair physical performance and cognitive ability in high-stress situations.

Several field methods have been tested for predicting total daily energy expenditure, including heart-rate monitors, pedometers, and accelerometers. Accelerometer- and pedometer-based monitors provide valid indicators of overall physical activity, but they are less accurate at predicting energy expenditure. In addition, single-axis accelerometers or pedometers and most multidimensional accelerometers are not useful in detecting the increased energy costs of high-intensity exercise, upper-body exercise, carrying a load, or changes in surface or terrain.

The combination of doubly labeled water, as a measure of total energy expenditure, and hand-held indirect calorimetry to assess resting energy expenditure could be used to monitor metabolic status and assess energy metabolism over periods of up to 2 weeks. Self-selected pace, foot-strike devices, and activity monitors that integrate pulse, temperature, and movement can estimate activity and total energy expenditure and may be useful in the field.

If predicting total energy expenditure is the goal of monitoring the activity of the combat service member, then more sophisticated devices must be developed (multidimensional devices that include multiple types of metabolic measurements). Accurate measurement of total daily energy expenditure in military personnel will require the development of motion sensors that are inexpensive, but more convenient and reliable than current pedometers or accelerometers.

Stress and Immune Function

The precise combination of measures chosen to monitor stress and immune function depends on the flexibility of the collection of the measures in the field setting. There is a substantial body of research that conclusively links both physical and psychological stress to derangements in immune function. In both military and civilian populations, immunosuppression has been reported after exhaustive aerobic exercise. It is hypothesized that trauma in muscle and connective tissue stimulates the production of cytokines that suppress cellular immune responses consistent with reported higher levels of stress hormones. Higher levels of stress hormones also occur in response to psychological stress. A full evaluation of the effects of activation of stress response systems on immune function requires measures of multiple functional and molecular biomarkers at multiple time points prior to, during, and after the stress exposure. Monitoring biomarkers of the stress response should include molecular and functional measures of the hypothalamic-pituitary-adrenal (HPA) axis, the adrenergic response systems, and the immune system at multiple levels. The HPA axis can be monitored by measuring levels of the corticotropin-releasing hormone adrenocorticotropin and cortisol in plasma, cerebrospinal fluid, urine, saliva, and sweat.

Measuring heart-rate variability should be considered as an accurate, sensitive, and noninvasive way to measure the relative activity of the sympathetic and parasympathetic nervous systems.

Immunological evaluation could include measuring the numbers, maturity, activation, and function of immune cells, including such measures as macrophage phagocytosis, lymphocyte proliferation in stimulation test, natural killer-cell activity, cytokine production patterns, expression of genes and receptors, antibody production, skin delayed-type hypersensitivity, antibody response to vaccine, wound healing, and infection rate.

Indicators of stress and immune responses that are currently in use and in development include cortisol levels (measured from saliva, sweat, or urine), and heart-rate variability as measured with high-impedance electrocardiogram (ECG) electrodes that are currently available and are being further developed.

Sleep

Several companies currently offer wrist-worn actigraphs that are capable of estimating the quantity and quality of sleep in a variety of environments. These devices can collect data for periods ranging from a few hours to several weeks. Associated software can present sleep/wake histories in a number of user-friendly formats.

Electrophysiological measures (EEG and ECG) are more difficult to collect in field settings because of the requirement to attach sensors to the body and to maintain low sensor impedance. However, significant progress has already been made in developing and validating high-impedance sensors that could soon be mounted in helmets or clothing. The technology for field-portable, individual-worn systems for amplifying, recording, and to some extent analyzing these data already exist.

Assessment of eye movements and eye closures will only be possible in limited situations in which monitoring equipment can be mounted and aimed at the combat service member. A substantial amount of literature has already shown that a subset of oculomotor measures is sensitive to cognitive fatigue, but further work is necessary to validate the utility of these measures for predicting performance.

Self-assessments, on the other hand, are quite easy to collect. Questionnaires can be administered via paper and pencil or hand-held computer. As noted above, there are a variety of self-assessments available, and many have been shown to be sensitive to operational stressors, such as mental and physical fatigue. However, readers are cautioned that self-assessments can be significantly confounded by motivational factors or peer pressure or in chronic-demand conditions (e.g., people who are very tired for several days at a time may lose their subjective ability to determine how tired they actually are).

As with other measurements, when deciding where new objective, physiologically based cognitive monitoring approaches (e.g., EEG-based or eye-movement based strategies) will be implemented, an assessment of the feasibility of using these approaches in specific environments and an analysis of the cost of the technology versus the cost of the prevented mishap should be performed.

QUESTION 4

What algorithms are available that might provide useful predictions from combined sensor signals? What additional measurements would improve specificity of the predictions?

Simple algorithms that are already in use include wet bulb globe temperature and cold strain-wind chill index. Other models, such as the Acute Physiologic and Chronic Health Evaluation Scores and the simpler Simplified Applied Physiological Score, also use physiological variables to predict health outcomes. Although these tools have worked quite well in the intensive care unit setting where pathological changes in physiological parameters are the rule, there is little compelling evidence that similar algorithms would be equally effective in the military setting where such parameters vary over a narrower range. NASA (National Aeronautics and Space Administration) also has undertaken a major research effort in this area (see Appendix B), the design of which may be quite compatible with the military environment. Although it would be reasonable to explore whether new variables made possible by new field technologies, such as serum osmolality, sodium concentration, or tissue pH, would be predictive using simpler algorithms, a parallel initiative to explore presently available physiological measurements with more complex models seems appropriate.

The future development of algorithms must include the development of nonlinear models that allow discrimination of more complex decision surfaces (e.g., a graphical representation of a problem space). Given the enormous number of variables present, nonlinear models may permit improved optimization of the solution. Generally, univariate analysis is overly simplistic and thus impractical for such situations because it fails to capture significant interactions among the numerous variables. For example, more complex models involving artificial neural networks are needed.

Although it is often thought that additional measures enhance the validity to discriminate between metabolic status, depending on the desired purpose of the algorithms, different or additional measurements may not be needed. However, additional work is clearly required to create models that comprise variables in nonlinear ways, utilizing modeling such as neural networks. For example, more complex algorithms can be developed that result in more accurate predictions to prescribe actions (e.g., rest, hydration, or active cooling) and prevent the unwelcome result. In this case, additional research will be needed to better understand the nature and mechanism of the outcome so that interventions can be targeted.

In addition, as described in the responses to questions 2 and 5, the technology must evolve to permit the integration of data in multiple forms from different devices. Like in all analysis programs, the value of complex, multivariate, nonlinear analysis relies upon the data provided. Until all available information from multiple sensors can be utilized by the algorithms, the system will remain constrained.

Last, it is crucial to develop baseline data for each individual (combat service member) in order to implement effective field strategies for monitoring metabolic status. Repeated measures of individuals to determine and validate individual normal response patterns are essential.

QUESTION 5

What is the committee's "blue sky" forecast for useful metabolic monitoring approaches (i.e., 10- to 20-year projection)? What are the current research investments that may lead to revolutionary advances?

Evolution of New Cognitive Measurement Approaches

Stress and fatigue can be induced by high physical and cognitive workloads, such as exercise, extreme environmental temperature, dehydration, heat exhaustion, constant battlefield threats to personal safety, sleep deprivation, circadian-rhythm disruptions, and other common operational demands. The prediction of cognitive responses to stress and fatigue needs to be improved. In addition to performing more research on the utility of traditional approaches that use self-reported data, a significant focus should be placed on further developing and implementing new psychophysiological methods for monitoring brain activity, heart-rate variability, eye movements, and metabolites and validating these techniques as predictors of cognitive responses to stress and fatigue. New performance-assessment methodologies may soon be available for computerized tasks in which cognitive probes can be unobtrusively introduced during the completion of primary operational demands. In addition, the use of hand-held computers to record ecological momentary assessments of cognitive function should be further developed.

In addition to developing new psychophysiological methods, more work needs to be undertaken on the mathematical integration of these data and the computer models that will synthesize numerous inputs into a field-useable status assessment.

Optimization of Markers to Monitor Stress and Immune Function

A limited battery of selected stress-response and immune markers should be validated to monitor physiological adaptations to changes in the environment and to evaluate the readiness of individuals for impending deployment.

Odors as Biomarkers

Since odors evolved to communicate distinct information about individuals, it would seem to be an ideal system for monitoring organic states of individual combat service members in the field. Further studies on the role of human odors as a future source of biomarkers should be performed. These studies should assess the role of the major histocompatability complex and other gene expressions on odor profiles. Studies should also identify the specific information that human odor profiles convey, and should determine their predictive value in assessing individual identity, stress, cognitive performance, and health status. Further development of sensor technologies, such as the e-nose or other methodologies, for monitoring in the field should also be pursued.

Studies linking human perception of odors with emotion and cognitive states are currently in their infancy and need to be encouraged in order to ascertain the full range of information that human odors might convey. The military should promote innovative research in chemical signaling that will accelerate these advances. Also, research in the development of sensor technology is likely to yield smaller, more automated devices that reduce analysis time and increase reliability—two factors that are critical for field applications. These advances will go hand-in-hand with the development of sweat patches that can be uniquely designed to capture the substances of interest. It seems highly plausible that new insights from these diverse areas will converge in 5 to 10 years, making odor biomarkers a viable technology for military field applications.

Human Tears as Sources of Biomarkers

Bodily excretions and secretions that are noninvasively accessible and that reflect actual internal concentrations of substances within physiologically relevant systems represent possible targets of metabolic monitoring technology. An often overlooked external secretion is lachrymal fluid, or tears. Although there appears to be little currently accepted clinical analytic use of tears as indicators of nonophthalmic internal status, a number of disparate studies suggest that there may be merit in examining tears as a possible medium for monitoring relevant aspects of metabolic status. For example, it has been reported that tear glucose concentrations are related to blood glucose levels. This is an area where little research has been done, but one that may have significant potential as a noninvasive monitoring technology for a variety of physiological biomarkers.

New Algorithms to Integrate Complex Biological Information

The use of technology and "smart systems" are required to bridge the cognitive gap created by the lack of skilled clinicians in the field to provide individualized recommendations to support end users. Predictive medical algorithms can be utilized to generate specific recommendations and interventions from complex biological information gathered by metabolic monitoring systems. Further research is needed to develop and validate these models, with a particular emphasis on identifying prognostic factors in asymptomatic subjects.

The Impact of Biological and Chemical Hazards on Traditional Biomarkers of Health

It is largely unknown how hazards and toxins encountered during deployment will affect the biomarkers used by the military for monitoring. For example, low chronic exposure to a bacterial toxin or a heavy metal may alter serum electrolytes, glucose, or enzymes and confound usual interpretation of these values. In contrast, other biomarkers might serve as critical indicators for biological or chemical toxin exposure; for example, pulse rate alterations may be used as an indication of (sublethal) nerve toxin exposure.

Metabolomics/Nutrigenomics

The human genome has essentially been sequenced and is estimated to contain about 35,000 genes. It is the differential expression of genes that creates individual differences or phenotypes. Gene arrays show differences in the expression of genes under various conditions. The long-term goal is to understand how the expression of groups of genes and the production of proteins affect performance. It is known that the single nucleotide polymorphisms can affect the way individuals respond to drugs, can affect individuals' vulnerability to microbiological infections, and can have the potential to cause long-term degenerative diseases in individuals. Such knowledge is envisioned to enhance a combat service member's performance and lower the risk of life-threatening injury. Further, it is possible that such determinations would allow for prophylactic vaccinations, prescription of preventative pharmaceuticals, and the possible use of special monitoring sensors. Although it may be a number of years before it becomes possible, it would be ideal to be able to predict how a single combat service member will perform under a variety of different dietary and other environmental conditions based upon his or her phenotype. In this manner, the identification of differences among individuals by the use of genomic and metabolomic information collected on each combat service member is the ultimate "blue sky."

RESEARCH RECOMMENDATIONS

- To develop new algorithms that employ currently measurable biomarkers and nonlinear modeling techniques. In circumstances where average group data may not appropriately correlate with the performance of an individual, prediction models will need to be based on data from repeated measures from individuals.
- To develop patterns of rates of changes and resiliency. For example, research is needed to elucidate individual patterns of rates of change of stress hormones and to determine the resiliency of these stress responses in returning to baseline after the stressors have been removed.
- To conduct research to evaluate and validate available technology in the field. For example, technology related to self-assessment of perceived exertion, preferred exertion, and mood states that have been tested extensively in sports settings but needs to be evaluated and validated in military settings. Optimal combinations for use with physiological markers need to be determined.
- To further perform research activities in areas with the greatest long-range benefits, such as genomics/metabolomics, odors as biomarkers, tears as a new media for potential biomarkers, new cognitive measurements approaches, optimization of monitoring stress and immune function markers, the development of new algorithms to integrate complex biological information, and the impact of biological and chemical hazards on traditional biomarkers of health.
- To continue military activities in bone research. These should include studies of markers of bone loss, especially related to fracture risk and the prevention of lost duty time during initial entry training, advanced training, and combat operations.
- To continue to study cortisol levels during training and operations to ensure that its elevation is not a contributor to bone loss.

- To develop non- and minimally invasive technologies, particularly for the determination of muscle metabolism, hydration status, and cognitive function.
- To develop motion sensors that are inexpensive but more convenient and reliable than current pedometers and accelerometers.
- To conduct research to validate the use of self- (and peer-) assessment tools (e.g., the Borg 6–20 rating scale of perceived exertion) in the field as indicators of fatigue and cognitive ability.
- To continue research on the use of NIRS to monitor muscle oxygenation and deoxygenation, intramuscular pH, and skin hydration status concurrently. This particular technology also has the potential for detecting the occurrence of inflammation.
- To develop simple field-friendly tests for urine specific gravity as an indicator of hydration status.
- To develop a practical method of monitoring body-weight change in the field.
- To conduct research to be able to mount or integrate high impedance EEG and ECG electrodes in helmets or into combat clothing. Although this technology will soon make it possible to continuously record brain activity, heart-rate data, and other electrophysiological parameters, some remaining challenges limit its use in the field.

REFERENCE

NRC (National Research Council). 2001. *Opportunities in Biotechnology for Future Army Applications*. Washington, DC: National Academy Press.

A

Examples of Physiological and Cognitive Markers of Performance

TABLE A-1 Examples of Metabolic Markers

Tissue, Organ, Function	Intermediate Marker	Source
Body temperature	Cold strain index Esophageal telemetry device Galvanic skin response Heart rate Heat flux Oral temperature Reaction time Skin temperature Physiological strain index	
Hydration	Aldosterone Arginine Blood pressure Heart rate Hydration status from bioelectrical impedance Sodium Total body water Vasopressin	Blood Saliva Urine
Physical activity/energy expenditure	Accelerometers Activity logs Activity monitors (integrated, i.e., body movement, heart rate, and core temperature) Dietary questionnaires Doubly labeled water Foot-ground contact/body weight Glucose Heart rate monitors Insulin Insulin-like growth factor-1 Lactate	Blood

NOTE: Metabolic monitoring biomarkers can be categorized according to outcome function or intermediate measure that can be quantified to reflect the outcome function. This table summarizes outcome functions of various organs/systems/physiological/psychological states and some intermediate biomarkers that might be used to predict or quantify these outcome functions and optimal performance. In general, it was felt that

Performance, Outcome	Measure
Heat stress Hypo- and hyperthermia	Core temperature
Cognitive performance De- and overhydration Fatigue Heat exhaustion Heat tolerance Muscular endurance	Body-weight change Eye pressure Plasma volume, osmolarity Saliva flow Skin turgor Urine color Urine specific gravity, osmolarity Urine volume
Cognition Hypo- and hyperglycemia Heat cramps Heat exhaustion Sunstroke	Body weight Calorimetry (direct and indirect) Lean body mass

no single intermediate biomarker accurately predicts outcome function. Accurate measures of outcome function are often invasive and not applicable to field situations. More emphasis should be placed on developing noninvasive measures that accurately predict peak performance or catastrophic failure of a given organ/system or physiological/psychological state.

TABLE A-2 Examples of Brain Function Markers

Tissue, Organ, Function	Intermediate Marker	Source
Cognitive	Blood flow	
	Electrocardiogram	
	Functional magnetic resonance imaging	
	Imaging	
	Magneto-electroencephalography	
	Metabolism	
	Positron emission tomography	
	Spectroscopy	
Mood	Odor profiles	
Sleep	Ambulatory sleep monitor	
	Electrocardiogram pattern	
Stress response	Autonomic nervous system	Blood
	Cortisol	Saliva[a]
	Dehydroepiandrosterone	Urine[b]
	Growth hormones	
	Heart rate variability	
	Impedance	
	Insulin-like growth factor-1	
	Neuropeptide Y	
	Neurotransmitters	
	Norepinephrine	
	Other hormones	
	Prolactin	
	Stress hormones	
	Testosterone	

NOTE: Metabolic monitoring biomarkers can be categorized according to outcome function or intermediate measure that can be quantified to reflect the outcome function. This table summarizes outcome functions of various organs/systems/ physiological/psychological states and some intermediate biomarkers that might be used to predict or quantify these outcome functions and optimal performance. In general, it was felt that no single intermediate biomarker accurately predicts outcome function. Accurate measures of outcome function are often invasive and not applicable to field situations. More emphasis should be placed on developing noninvasive

Performance, Outcome	Measure
Focused attention Memory Problem solving	Ratings of perceived exertion Self-assessment scales
Appropriate relative to situation Fear	Modified STROOP Profile mood Self-assessment scales Visual analog
Reaction time Sleepiness/alertness Task performance	Self-assessment scales
Appropriate activation relative to situation	Self-assessment scales

measures that accurately predict peak performance or catastrophic failure of a given organ/system or physiological/psychological state.

[a] Salivary cortisol is an accurate measure of single plasma-free cortisol at the time point collected.

[b] Urinary cortisol measured in 24-hour urine reflects average cortisol secretion over 24 hours.

TABLE A-3 Examples of Bone Markers

Tissue, Organ, Function	Intermediate Marker	Source
Bone	Collagen breakdown products	Plasma
	Carboxy-terminal telepeptide	Urine
	Deoxypridinoline	
	Hydroproline	
	N-telepeptide	
	Pyridinoline	
	Cytokines	
	Interleukin-1 and -6	
	Tumor necrosis factor	
	Transforming growth factor	
	Endocrine markers	
	Calcitonin	
	Growth hormone	
	Insulin-like growth factor-1	
	Osteocalcin	
	Parathyroid hormone	
	Thyroid hormones	
	Enzymes	
	Alkaline phosphatase	
	Bone-specific alkaline	
	Phosphatase	
	Resorption markers	
	24-hour urinary calcium	
	Calcium balance	
	Phosphatase	
	Tartrate-resistant acid	

NOTE: Metabolic monitoring biomarkers can be categorized according to outcome function or intermediate measure that can be quantified to reflect the outcome function. This table summarizes outcome functions of various organs/systems/physiological/psychological states and some intermediate biomarkers that might be used to predict or quantify these outcome functions and optimal performance. In general, it was felt that

Performance, Outcome	Measure
Bone fracture, including stress fracture	Bone mineral density:
Edema	Dual-energy X-ray absorptiometry
Inflammation/damage	Ultrasound
Pain	Quantitative computed topography
Weakness	Histology
	Mono accumulation

no single intermediate biomarker accurately predicts outcome function. Accurate measures of outcome function are often invasive and not applicable to field situations. More emphasis should be placed on developing noninvasive measures that accurately predict peak performance or catastrophic failure of a given organ/system or physiological/psychological state.

TABLE A-4 Examples of Cardiac, Muscle, and Pulmonary Markers

Tissue, Organ, Function	Intermediate Marker	Source
Cardiac	Heart rate Heart rate variability Impedance	
Muscle	Amino acids (glutamine, histidine, 3-methyl-histidine)	
	Enzymes/molecules Carbonic anhydrase Isoenzymes of creatine kinase Myoglobin Myosin heavy chains Phosphocreatine levels Ubiquitin	Muscle
	Immune Circulatory polymorphonuclear leukocytes Insulin-like growth factor-1 Interleukin-1, -6 Tumor necrosis factor	Blood Saliva[a] Urine[b]
	Metabolism/catabolism/anabolism Lactate Glycogen Blood ammonia	Blood Urine
	Protein turnover	Blood Urine
	Structure/metabolism 3-methyl-/histidine excretion Glycogen Trace metals	Muscle
Pulmonary	Expired air	Oxygen and carbon dioxide saturation

NOTE: Metabolic monitoring biomarkers can be categorized according to outcome function or intermediate measure that can be quantified to reflect the outcome function. This table summarizes outcome functions of various organs/systems/physiological/psychological states and some intermediate biomarkers that might be used to predict or quantify these outcome functions and optimal performance. In general, it was felt that no single intermediate biomarker accurately predicts outcome function. Accurate measures of outcome function are often invasive and not applicable

Performance, Outcome	Measure
Cardiac output	
Relative sympathetic and parasympathetic control	
	Dynamometers
	Ergometers
	Strain gauges
	Ratings of perceived exertion
Decreased endurance	Delayed onset muscle soreness
Decreased performance	Increased muscle atrophy
Decreased strength	
Fatigue	
Pulse oximeter	
Capnograph	

to field situations. More emphasis should be placed on developing noninvasive developing noninvasive measures that accurately predict peak performance or catastrophic failure of a given organ/system or physiological/psychological state.

[a] Salivary cytokine concentrations vary according to salivary gland source from which saliva is collected and presence and degree of periodontal disease.

[b] 24-hour urine for Interleukin-6 and soluble receptors for tumor necrosis factor normalized to creatine are currently used and are sensitive measures of cytokine production.

B

Metabolic Monitoring at NASA: A Concept for the Military

Kira Bacal, M.D., Ph.D., M.P.H., Wyle Laboratories and Life Sciences, and Johnson Space Flight Center, NASA, Houston, Texas

NASA's (National Aeronautics and Space Administration) Johnson Space Center (JSC) Office of Space Medicine, in collaboration with NASA's Ames Research Center and the Stanford University Medical Center, has been interested in the field of metabolic monitoring for some time. In the aerospace environment crew time is a very precious commodity due to limited resources and limited personnel; metabolic monitoring can be used to optimize crew function and minimize the risk of fatigue and illness through the observation and interpretation of physiological data. By using a variety of sensors to monitor both the individual's biomarkers and the ambient environment, data can be captured and then correlated and analyzed using software models. These tools anticipate metabolic irregularities, provide feedback to the operator, and advise appropriate interventions to prevent unwanted consequences. The same systems also monitor the user for compliance with the recommendations and evaluate the efficacy of the recommendations.

Given its operational milieu, NASA is particularly interested in remote metabolic monitoring. The majority of aerospace operations take place at sites far distant from clinical care providers and decision makers, thus any system that enhances the situational awareness of the control team is helpful. The astronaut and warfighter share many similar traits: both are highly trained individuals who are engaged in prolonged and exhausting efforts in a hostile environment. Whether the individual is searching for enemy patrols in the desert or repairing a satellite during a spacewalk, there is a similar level of both effort expended and physiological demands. In addition, both individuals are engaged in time-critical tasks and are far from medical support. For these reasons prevention of illness or injury, rather than its care, is desirable.

In the space environment, as in the military, operations can be divided into two categories: nominal and contingency. The latter category contains unscheduled events, such as illness or injury, and the medical resources brought to bear should be those that best conform to an adapted terrestrial standard of care. In contingency conditions, therefore, only approved medical devices and accepted treatment guidelines are employed, while unproven equipment or monitoring of novel parameters is eschewed as the information thus provided lacks an appropriate clinical context. Given the numerous confounding factors and unknowns about pathology and pathophysiology in the microgravity environment, it is imperative that, to the greatest extent possible, medical care on orbit proceeds from accepted practices.

Conversely, nominal operations, which can include activities such as spacewalks, exercise, or research studies to define "space-normal" physiology, can and often do use new tools and monitor novel parameters. Often associated with research activities, nominal operations utilize both proven and innovative technologies to gather data, develop predictive models, and validate these predictions.

Under nominal operations the goal of metabolic monitoring is to intervene before a medical event occurs. Some of the on-orbit conditions that could be prevented in this way include dehydration, fatigue, heat stress, hyperventilation, and hypothermia. In addition, monitoring can also assist in the evaluation of specific performance metrics, such as cognition, workload, situational awareness, memory, and concentration, to ensure that critical or complex tasks are performed by competent operators. Fatigue is a constant concern in space operations because circadian cues are disrupted and sleep shifting is common, and it is thus considered ideally suited to monitoring. Fatigue was implicated as a factor in the collision of a Progress resupply rocket with the Mir space station, and crewmembers aboard the International Space Station (ISS) have also cited occasions where they performed complex and dangerous tasks (e.g., moving a Soyuz from one docking port to another) when extremely fatigued. The applicability of these concerns to military operations is readily apparent.

Also similar to military operations, space missions have very limited personnel. Space shuttle missions generally have seven-person crews, while the ISS crew complement is only three. (In the wake of the Columbia tragedy, there are currently only two crewmembers aboard the ISS. When the Shuttle fleet returns to flight status, it is anticipated that the program will return to a three-person crew.) Because of these tight personnel constraints, any tasks that can be transferred from human to artificial intelligence will free crewmembers for other mission-critical tasks. In addition, by transferring skill sets from personnel to equipment, medical decision-making, targeted assessment, and clinical judgment can be standardized and moved farther forward (onto the battlefield or on orbit) than otherwise possible. During nominal operations this "smart" technology can utilize predictive algorithms in order to analyze captured data and avoid preventable medical events.

As shown in Figure B-1, the concept of operations for this technology calls for the acquisition of data from a variety of sensors. This information is then integrated and delivered to an analytic program that can provide immediate

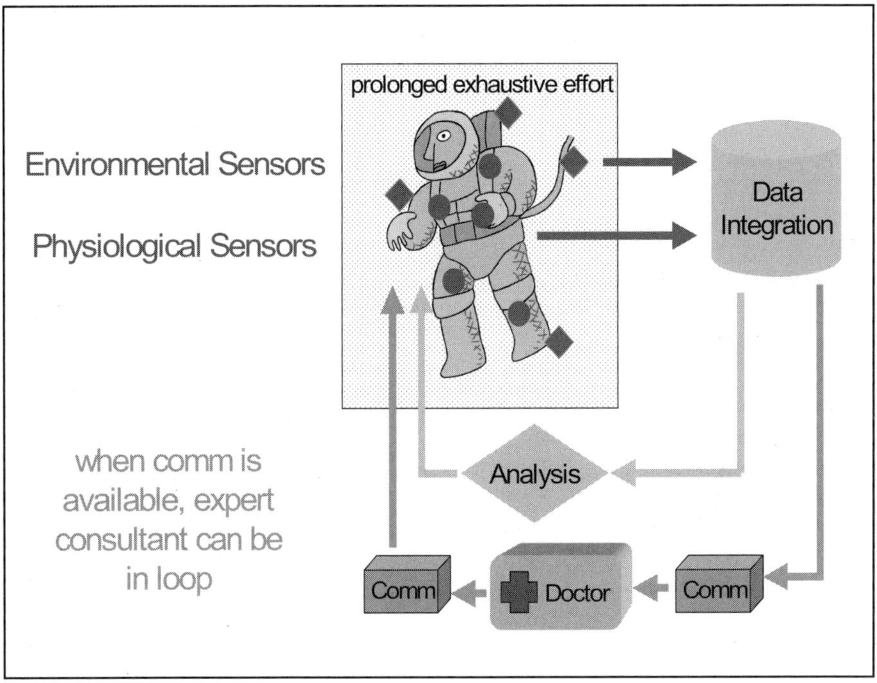

FIGURE B-1 Concept of operations.

feedback to the operator. In addition, when skilled personnel are available at a remote site, the data can be packaged and sent down a communications relay for human-based interpretation, and guidance based on the information can be provided.

There are numerous parameters that can be monitored. The selection will vary depending on the mission, the personnel, and the areas of interest. In addition, the level and type of parameter must be specified, such as individual data, group information, environmental details, and/or interactive information. For example, monitoring of an individual could report basic vital signs (e.g., body temperature, pulse oximetry, heart rate, respiratory rate, blood pressure, heart rate variability, electrocardiogram tracing) or less conventional measures (e.g., lactate levels, tissue pH, muscle creatine kinase). Individual monitoring might also focus on trends, describing specific changes within a single person over a period of time, such as a spacewalk, exercise period, or forced march. Data could also be grouped to provide critical information about the status of the crew or squad as a whole; this knowledge might be of more utility if gaining mission objectives is a higher priority than preserving individual health. Similarly, the selection of environmental parameters will likewise vary depending on the mission, but the parameters might include items such as ambient temperature, barometric pressure, or individual activity level. Self-reported criteria (e.g., perceived exertion or interpretation of mission or task success) can also be handled in a similar fashion, with the information thus obtained being integrated with data from other sensors to provide a more global picture of the condition of the individual or team.

In order to maximize efficacy, a "smart system" is needed to obtain and present information in the most efficient way to both the end user (astronaut or warfighter) and the remote consultants (e.g., a ground-based flight surgeon or a commanding officer). In addition, analysis techniques for rapid diagnosis and intervention are required—data without a relevant context will be unusable to most operators. The components of such a system include:

- *Sensors*. Many of these, particularly those for standard physiological parameters, are readily available, commercial off-the-shelf items.
- *Data integration*. Information derived from multiple sensors will usually be packaged in different ways; currently there are few standards for medical data management. As a result, the monitoring system must have a way to standardize the data, integrate it, and then extract relevant parameters. In addition, trends for individual subjects need to be identified and the standardized data needs to be exported to both the algorithm library and a data store.
- *Data storage*. At each stage the data must be stored for future (or real-time) downloads and review.
- *Algorithm library*. In the absence of a clinician to process the information, this software provides the initial guidance to interpret the data and act upon it. In this component, the data is sent to a store of executable algorithms and decision trees, including both diagnostic and therapeutic protocols, which "crunch" the data and pass it to the next step.
- *Feedback/recommendation generation*. Analysis by the algorithms or decision trees will in turn generate recommendations to prevent, mitigate, diagnose, or treat a medical event since the simple relay of data from the sensors to the average crewmember will not be of value. Prioritized alarms must also be provided, as the operator will not have the medical training to know which of several abnormal readings are most pressing. In a military example, if a casualty sustains a penetrating injury to the chest, the caregiver's top priority may initially be to address hemorrhage and a falling blood pressure. However, if respiratory arrest then occurs, a new alarm must intervene and guide the caregiver to direct attention to that problem, otherwise his or her lack of medical training may lead to prioritizing tasks inappropriately.
- *Displays*. In order to provide feedback to the operator, a local display of some kind is necessary. In addition, display of the information at a remote location enables clinicians at this site to supervise and intercede as appropriate.

Perhaps the most innovative hardware required by such a system is the data integration piece. This device must accept input from diverse data streams and packets (e.g., RS-232, RS-485, USB, 1394, Ethernet) that originate from a wide variety of sensors and medical equipment, repackage these inputs into a homogeneous format, and send the concatenated information on for integration into the algorithm library. For the ISS environment, a concept of operations has been developed that makes use of a common interface established through network appliances rather than via computers (which require human intervention). In this way, the crew needs to attach the patient, power, and communication interfaces, but does not need to establish, maintain, or troubleshoot the connections. Instead, the connections are automatically established and maintained by dedicated embedded microprocessors that are programmed to work with the specific hardware. The main goal of the device is to ensure that medical data is quickly, reliably, and accurately transmitted with a minimum amount of effort by the crew.

Toward this end, the Medical Informatics Branch of Space Medicine at NASA-JSC, in conjunction with the NASA-Ames Research Center and Stanford University, has commenced development of a Medical Communications Interface Adapter (MCIA), which is envisioned as a "smart hub," or universal adapter for processing and downloading data from all medical devices, for accepting inputs from multiple sensors, and for providing output as multiplexed telemetry data. Three primary subsystems have been identified: an external data interface that receives information from the various devices, a data-handling subsystem that processes the information into a homogeneous format, and a ground communications subsystem that transmits the information to an algorithm library, to a data storage device, to a local display, and to remote sites (e.g., the Flight Surgeon console in the Mission Control Center). Among the medical devices currently on board or proposed for the ISS with which the MCIA would interface are a physiological monitor/defibrillator, a blood analyzer, an intravenous pump, and a ventilator. Medical teams in the military (e.g., the USAF Critical Care Air Transport Team) often use similar equipment, so this configuration may be of interest to the military as well.

Once the sensors have gathered the data and the MCIA (or equivalent) has processed it into a standard, integrated form, the data needs to be put into a clinical context. Raw data, or even consolidated information, is of little utility to a nonexpert. Telling nonclinicians that "serum lactate values have increased 20 percent within 5 minutes" does not provide them with information they can use. However, that same data, in conjunction with an algorithm library and a recommendation store, can generate useful instructions, such as "Rest in the shade for 3 minutes" or "A 5-minute break in upper arm activities is advised." Information in this form can be utilized by any nonclinician as it requires no specialized knowledge to interpret or implement.

The value of analysis is thus twofold. On a local level, analysis can provide specific advice to an individual. This tactical advice (e.g., eat, rest, hydrate) allows the warfighter or astronaut to maximize his or her work capacity. When an analysis is performed remotely on groups, it can permit strategic planning by providing flight control teams, squad leaders, or other decision makers the means by which to assess group strength and condition. In developing the best way to analyze the data, numerous factors must be considered. Generally speaking, terrestrial, validated medical algorithms and guidelines should be used whenever possible for diagnostic and therapeutic purposes. There are numerous medical algorithms (broadly defined as "any computation, formula, survey, or look-up table useful in health care") and treatment guidelines available in the medical literature. In addition, there are commercially available, validated, off-the-shelf diagnostic tools and medical information couplers. To the greatest extent possible, these existing tools should be used rather than attempting to develop new tools as the validation process can be prohibitive in terms of both cost and time. Naturally, all of these tools are intended for terrestrial, often hospital-based, use, and they will require adaptation to an austere environment, be it military or aerospace.

Desirable features of a real-time analysis tool include smart agent-based software, multiple parameters (including environmental and physiological data), prescribed trend analysis, model-based predictions, voice-based interaction (a dialogue system), operator-initiated inquiries, and unsolicited audible suggestions or advice.

Under contingency operations the main focus of data analysis should be directed toward diagnostic and therapeutic algorithms. For example, in the context of an episode of abdominal pain, the system can send sensor data to diagnostic tools in order to obtain first a presumptive diagnosis of, for example, appendicitis, and then use this diagnosis to select appropriate treatment guidelines and algorithms that will in turn generate recommendations regarding stabilizing care and the need for immediate surgery. The system can then monitor the casualty's response to these measures and update or modify the diagnosis and treatment recommendations accordingly.

Algorithms and guidelines for contingency operations are in varying stages of development. For treatment guidelines, there is a great deal of published material—perhaps almost too much—that can be adapted. However, because these guidelines and algorithms are derived from and developed by different medical specialties, different approaches, and even different nations, additional work is required to integrate them into a single consensus position on the best treatment modality. Diagnostic algorithms are less widely available and tend to be least helpful for illnesses with vague or general symptoms and signs. For example, as any clinician would attest, determining the cause of "abdominal pain" or "dizziness" can be very difficult. By contrast, diagnostic tools can be more easily applied to conditions with a clear mechanism or pathognomonic findings, such as "mechanical airway obstruction" or "tension pneumothorax."

There is likely to be only minor use of predictive algorithms in contingency operations for space compared with the use of diagnostic and treatment guidelines. Once an event has occurred, more attention will be focused on addressing it than on predicting its course. One exception might be in the case of a serious traumatic injury. In the absence of care from a surgical intensive care unit, a trauma scoring system might be employed to predict the patient's condition so that this information could assist in a decision about the timing of a crew evacuation.

For nominal operations, however, predictive and preventive algorithms will be more widely used. For example, these algorithms could determine whether a continuing trend in body temperature presages imminent heat exhaustion, which interventions in the short term could prevent this from occurring, and which intervention would be most appropriate. Unfortunately, these algorithms are generally in the very early stages of development, and it will be necessary to develop and test research models before these tools become operational.

To perform research into the early tracking of signs and symptoms and their predictive value in describing the condition's ultimate outcome or natural history, data gathering must occur at the outpatient- or family practice-based level, rather than at the inpatient- or subspecialty-based level. Research that is primarily located in the hospital will focus on the later stages of pathology and thus be less useful to our needs. Our interest lies in the earliest (perhaps asymptomatic) stages of a potentially disabling condition, and thus data must be gathered from primary caregivers or even from the lay public (as in, "What makes you go to the doctor for some headaches but not for others?").

Like predictive algorithms, preventive algorithms and guidelines are also in very rudimentary form. They are often anecdotal or qualitative (e.g., "Stay out of the sun!") rather than quantitative (e.g., "Rest in shade for 5 minutes."), and a relatively small number have been rigorously validated. Given that the system sensors gather information about physiological parameters in a highly quantified manner, it may be that the data they obtain can be fed back into predictive algorithm models so that the algorithms will also (eventually) be able to anticipate the onset of symptoms quite precisely.

Algorithm development by the Office of Space Medicine is at an early stage. Rules must be established for both format and content. For authoring activities, a standard, user-friendly format is needed for all algorithm developers. In addition, the format must be able to integrate into the current informatics system so as to avoid lengthy data-entry steps. In terms of the content contained in the algorithms, it is necessary to ensure a standardized approach across authors with clear logic flow, shared assumptions, appropriate evidence, and explicit decision points. A process must be established for thorough review by all stakeholders, and an evidence-based rationale for each point must be included. Ideally, the format should lend itself to easy incorporation of content references. Lastly, the algorithm must be displayed in such a way as to permit easy use by the operators.

The work being conducted by the Medical Informatics and Health Care Systems branch (led by Dr. James Logan) is called the Global Onboard Detailed

Diagnostic and Evaluation Systemic Survey (GODDESS). It is divided into two subtasks: one to provide an initial evaluation and stabilization of the patient, the other to initiate more detailed diagnostic and therapeutic activities.

In the ISS Systemic Initial Survey (ISIS), the goal is to identify and address any immediate, life-threatening conditions and then to direct the caregiver to the appropriate diagnostic and treatment pathway. The content (see Figure B-2) and format for ISIS have been developed and are currently in the validation process. The Astronaut Total Health Network Algorithms section (ATHeNA) will contain both diagnostic and treatment pathways. A format for ATHeNA is in development, and several treatment guidelines are currently in draft form. Once the guidelines have been written and validated, the section will be integrated with ISIS and the entire system validated in an end-to-end fashion.

As shown in Figure B-3, the ISIS interface is to be immediately activated upon recognition of a medical event. The standardized questions begin with "Are they conscious?" (A). For example, in a case of anaphylaxis, the caregiver would answer "Yes." ISIS would then ask the caregiver, "Can they speak?" (B). Subsequent questions are designed to rule out an obstructed airway (C) and to initiate care (D). Within a few moments, additional questions discriminate among various conditions (E) until anaphylaxis is identified as the presumptive diagnosis (F). At this point, ISIS has completed its role and ATHeNA takes over, although this transition is transparent to the user.

Using the same interface, ATHeNA guides the caregiver through the proper treatment guidelines, providing inventory locations, supplemental information, and additional guidance as required. If the chief complaint had been of lower acuity than anaphylaxis (e.g., abdominal pain, headache, or nausea), ISIS would simply have ruled out the life-threatening conditions and ATHeNA would have initiated a secondary survey in which the caregiver (or patient himself, depending on his condition) would have answered a series of diagnostic questions designed to lead to a presumptive diagnosis. The patient's individual medical history would have been automatically fed into the software so that if, for example, a person with abdominal pain had an appendectomy in the past, appendicitis would have automatically been removed from the differential, but pain due to adhesions would have been added.

Once a presumptive diagnosis is reached through ISIS or ATHeNA, appropriate treatment begins and the patient's response is monitored. In addition to the data obtained through the medical devices (such as blood pressure, heart rate, or temperature), the system also prompts the caregiver to reassess the patient at regular intervals and information regarding response to analgesics, appetite, nausea, and other subjective parameters is entered, so constant review and revision of the diagnosis and treatment occurs. For a ventilated patient, ATHeNA makes use of closed-loop algorithms to adjust the ventilator settings so as to ensure maximum efficacy. Eventually, perhaps tasks such as medication administration (e.g., sedatives, antibiotics, analgesics) will be automatically

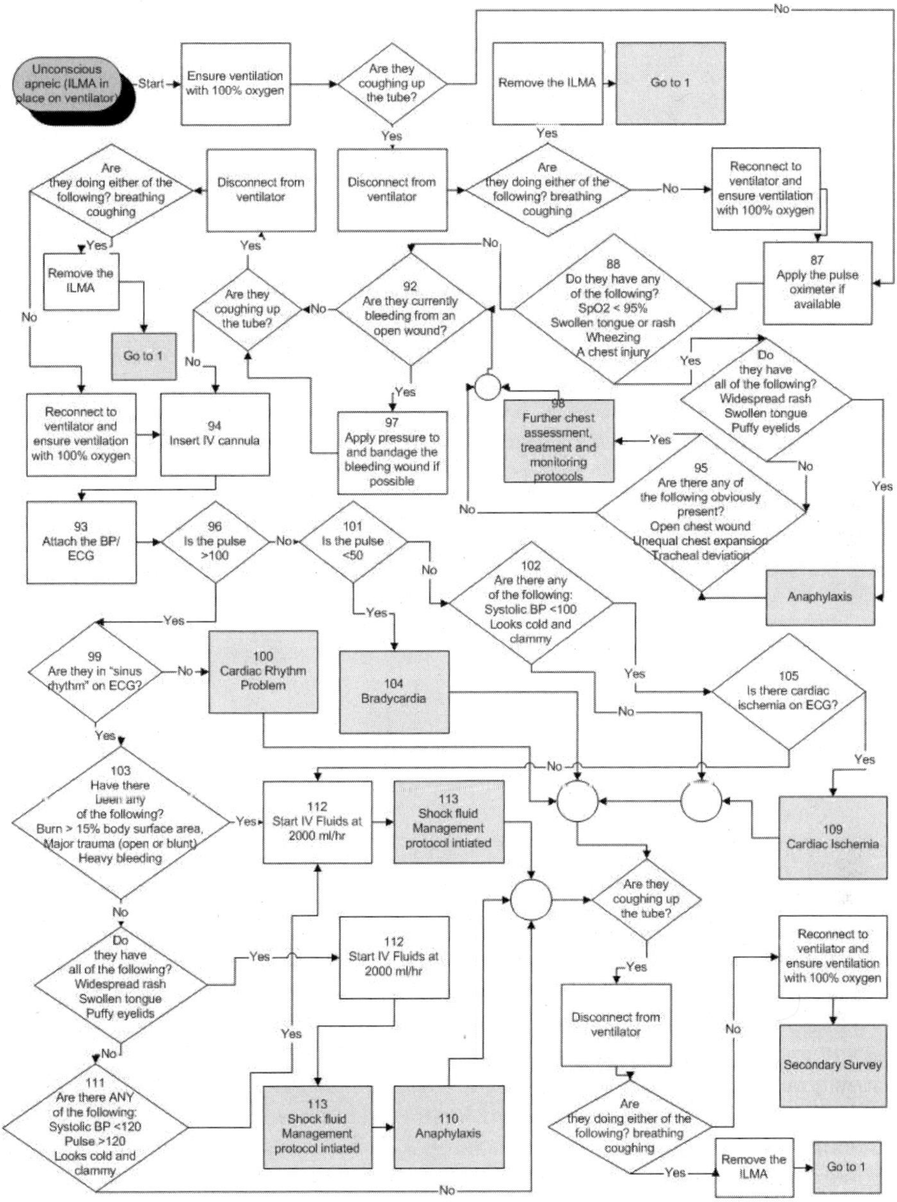

FIGURE B-2 Example of International Space Station Systemic Initial Survey content.

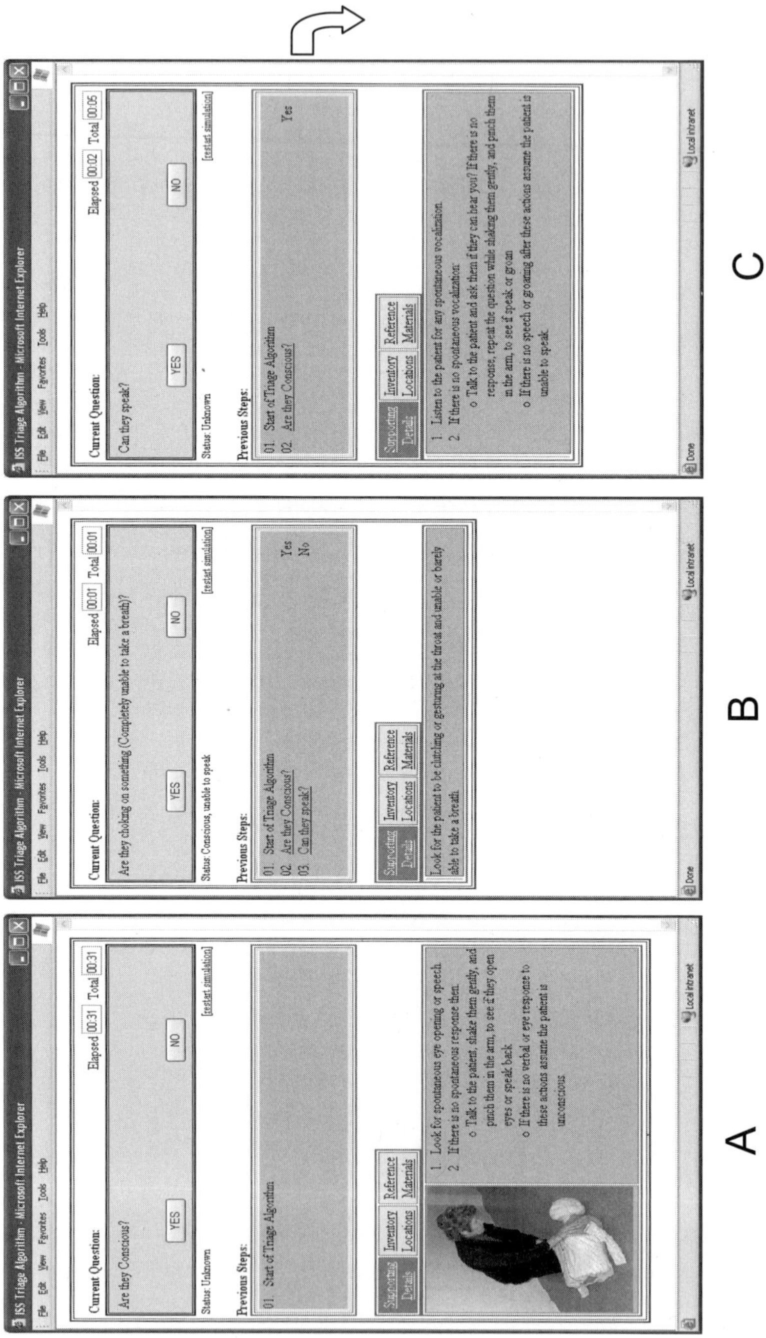
ISS Triage Algorithm - Microsoft Internet Explorer
Current Question:
Are they Conscious?
YES
NO
Elapsed 00:31 Total 00:31
Status: Unknown
[restart simulation]
Previous Steps:
01. Start of Triage Algorithm
Supporting Details
Inventory Locations
Reference Materials
1. Look for spontaneous eye opening or speech.
2. If there is no spontaneous response then:
o Talk to the patient, shake them gently, and pinch them in the arm, to see if they open eyes or speak back
o If there is no verbal or eye response to these actions assume the patient is unconscious.
A
ISS Triage Algorithm - Microsoft Internet Explorer
Current Question:
Are they choking on something (Completely unable to take a breath)?
YES
NO
Elapsed 00:01 Total 00:01
Status: Conscious, unable to speak
[restart simulation]
Previous Steps:
01. Start of Triage Algorithm
02. Are they Conscious? Yes
03. Can they speak? No
Supporting Details
Inventory Locations
Reference Materials
Look for the patient to be clutching or gesturing at the throat and unable or barely able to take a breath.
B
ISS Triage Algorithm - Microsoft Internet Explorer
Current Question:
Can they speak?
YES
NO
Elapsed 00:02 Total 00:05
Status: Unknown
[restart simulation]
Previous Steps:
01. Start of Triage Algorithm
02. Are they Conscious? Yes
Supporting Details
Inventory Locations
Reference Materials
1. Listen to the patient for any spontaneous vocalization.
2. If there is no spontaneous vocalization:
o Talk to the patient and ask them if they can hear you? If there is no response, repeat the question while shaking them gently, and pinch them in the arm, to see if speak or groan
o If there is no speech or groaning after these actions assume the patient is unable to speak
C

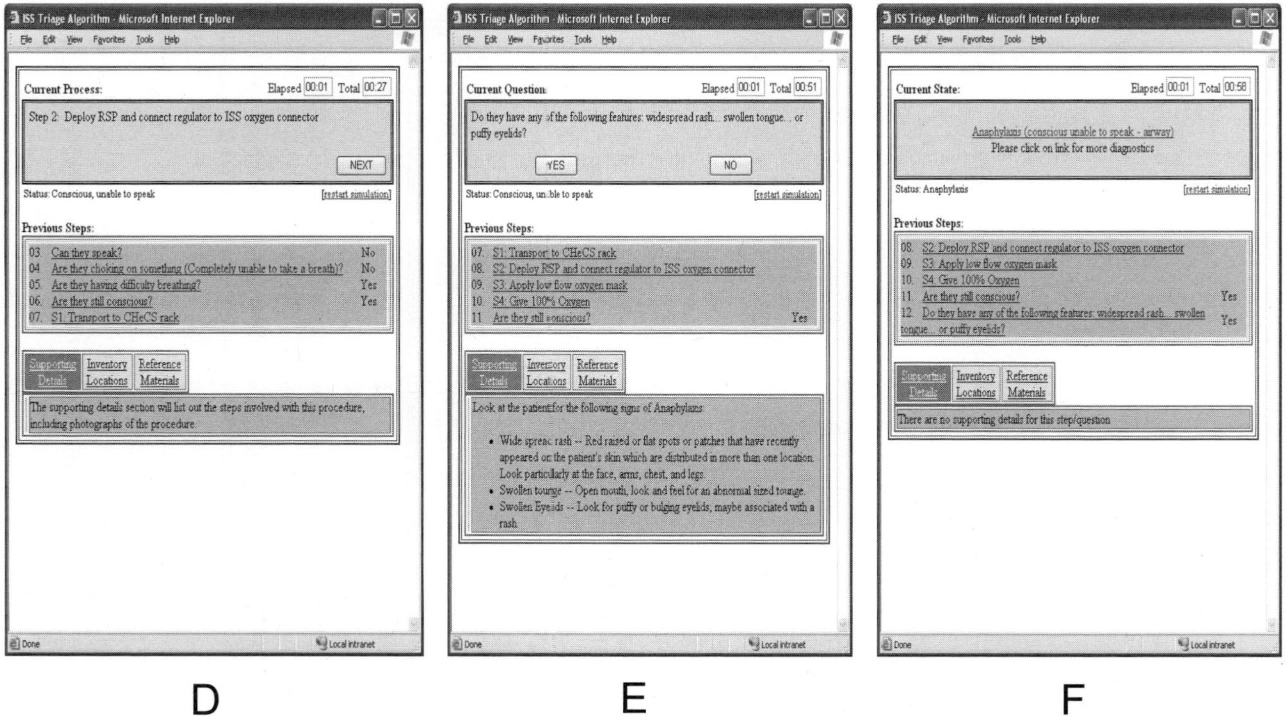

FIGURE B-3 Sample screen shots from the International Space Station Systemic Initial Survey.

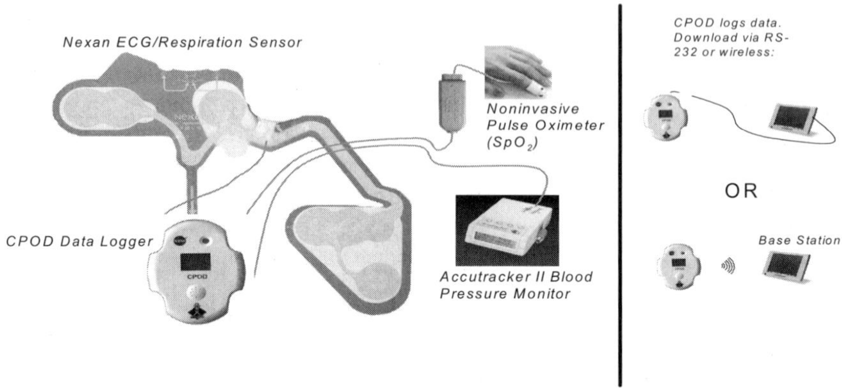

FIGURE B-4 A schematic of the LifeGuard Monitoring System.

performed by ATHeNA, though in the short term it is likely that this will continue to require human intervention, presumably with guidance from ATHeNA.

The GODDESS project is obviously intended for use in contingency operations. An example of a project intended for use under nominal conditions is Stanford and NASA-Ames' LifeGuard Monitoring System, which is in its final stages of testing. LifeGuard is an example of a novel system designed to obtain, aggregate, and analyze physiological data, display it locally, transmit it, and recommend interventions. The current model can interface with a variety of commercially available sensors (e.g., the Nexan ECG/respiration sensor, the Accutracker II blood pressure monitor, and a noninvasive pulse oximeter) that all connect to a CPOD Data Logger. The CPOD then logs the data and-downloads it via an RS-232 or a wireless (see Figure B-4). Table B-1 contains an example of the functional and performance requirements levied against the device.

In summary, remote metabolic monitoring systems are of utility in multiple operational environments, including aerospace and military activities. To create such tools, it is first necessary to identify the parameters of interest (e.g., physiological, environmental), then to capture, process, and transmit the data. Following analysis, in which potential or actual medical conditions are diagnosed and appropriate interventions are developed, these data (with recommended actions) can be displayed both locally and remotely. The system then continues to monitor the intervention and its outcome and provides updated advice. In this way,

TABLE B-1 Sample Requirements for the LifeGuard Monitoring System

Measured Parameters	Device Functionality	Derived Parameters	Base Station Functions	Data Transfer Requirements
Electrocardiogram (2 channels)	Acquisition/signal conditioning of all sensor data	Respiration rate (from respiration waveform)	Download data from wearable device	Wired (RS-232) and short-range (10 m) wireless
Respiration (raw waveform)	Analog to digital conversion	Heart rate (from electrocardiogram)	Store downloaded data on storage media	Data is downloaded to base station one user at a time
Body temperature	Data logging (internal memory in wearable device)		Display downloaded data	Single base station
Activity (2-axis acceleration)	Data transmission to base station on demand		Derive parameters (respiration and heart rates)	Minimum operational lifetime of wearable device: 8 hr
Pulse oximetry	Status display			Wearable device, pager-size
Blood pressure (noninvasive)				

technology can move specialized knowledge farther forward operationally, providing artificial substitutes for the skilled professionals who are so often in short supply. Work of this nature must be interdisciplinary in approach, utilizing engineers, information specialists, and clinicians in order to build a functional, validated, and user-friendly system.

Acknowledgments: NASA-Johnson Space Center/National Space Biomedical Research Institute: Jim Logan, Rick Pettys, Subhajit Sarkar, M.G. Sriram, Christopher Stokes; NASA-Ames Research Center/Stanford University: Sekou Crawford, John Hines, Kevin Montgomery.

C

Workshop Agenda

Metabolic Monitoring Technologies for
Military Field Applications

Committee on Military Nutrition Research
Food and Nutrition Board
Institute of Medicine
The National Academies

January 8–9, 2003
School of Aerospace Medicine
Brooks Air Force Base, San Antonio, Texas

Wednesday January 8, 2003

8:45 Welcome on Behalf of Brooks Air Force Base
Commander, Brooks Air Force Base

8:50 Welcome on Behalf of the Committee on Military Nutrition Research
Dr. John Vanderveen, Chair, Committee on Military Nutrition Research

9:00 Overview of Military Interest in Technologies for Metabolic Monitoring
COL *Karl E. Friedl, U.S. Army Research Institute of Environmental Medicine*

9:30 Overview of Field Applications of Physiological Monitoring
Dr. Reed W. Hoyt, U.S. Army Research Institute of Environmental Medicine (USARIEM)

Part I: Biomarkers and Monitoring Technologies for Heat Production and Hydration Status and Carbohydrate Metabolism (Moderator: Johanna Dwyer)

10:00 Biomarkers of Physiological Strain During Exposure to Hot and Cold Environments
Dr. Andrew J. Young, USARIEM

10:30 Hydration Status Monitoring
Dr. Michael N. Sawka, USARIEM

11:00 Break

11:10 Technologies for Monitoring Glucose and Lactate
Dr. David C. Klonoff, Mills-Peninsula Health Services

11:40 Utility of Insulin-like Growth Factor-I for Assessing Metabolic Status
Dr. Bradley C. Nindl, USARIEM

12:10 Discussion

12:30 Lunch

Part II: Biomarkers and Technologies for Monitoring Physiological Status and Work Capacity (Moderator: William Morgan)

1:30 The Use of Portable Accelerometers in Predicting Activity Energy Expenditure
Dr. Kong Y. Chen, Vanderbilt University Medical Center

2:00 Humans, Hills, and the Metabolic Cost of Locomotion: Simple Explanations from Putting Foot-Ground Contact Times to Work
Dr. Peter G. Weyand, Rice University

Part III: Biomarkers and Technologies for Monitoring Muscle Protein Turnover and Metabolism (Moderator: Bruce Bistrian)

2:30 Biomarkers for Changes in Protein Turnover of Muscle and Other Tissues
Dr. Robert R. Wolfe, University of Texas Medical Branch

3:00 Break

3:10 Potential Real-Time Markers: Muscle Fatigue or Environmental Stress
Dr. T. Peter Stein, University of Medicine and Dentistry of New Jersey

3:40 Muscle Protein Biomarkers to Predict the Occurrence of Physical Stress and Muscle Fatigue or Muscle Inflammatory Responses to Extreme Levels of Physical Activity
Dr. William J. Evans, University of Arkansas for Medical Sciences

Part IV: Biomarkers and Technologies for Predicting Bone Turnover (Moderator: Helen Lane)

4:10 Biomarkers of Bone and Muscle Turnover: Effects of Exercise
Dr. Clifford J. Rosen, Maine Center for Osteoporosis Research and Education, St. Joseph Hospital

4:40 Discussion

5:00 Adjourn

Thursday January 9, 2003

9:00 Biomarkers for Monitoring Bone Turnover and Predicting Bone Stress
Dr. Michael Kleerekoper, School of Medicine, Wayne State University

9:30 Biomarkers to Predict the Occurrence of Bone Stress and Matrix Abnormalities Due to Sustained and Intensive Physical Activity
Dr. Wendy M. Kohrt, University of Colorado Health Sciences Center

10:00 Discussion

10:15 Break

Part V: Biomarkers and Technologies for Monitoring Cognitive and Physiological Status in Relation to Stress (Moderator: Esther Sternberg)

10:30 Technologies for Monitoring Cognitive Status to Predict the Occurrence of Mental and Physical Stress
Dr. Julian F. Thayer, National Institute on Aging

11:00 Use of Sweat Patch Technology to Monitor Neuroendocrine Status
Dr. Giovanni Cizza, National Institute of Mental Health

11:30 Discussion

11:45 Lunch

Part VI: Biomarkers and Technologies for Monitoring Mental Status, Cognitive Function, and Alertness (Moderator: Patrick O'Neil)

1:00 Biomarkers for Brain Hypometabolism Due to Sleep Deprivation
Dr. Nancy J. Wesensten, Walter Reed Army Institute of Research

1:30 Electroencephalographic Indicators of Impaired Aviator Status During Sleep Deprivation
Dr. John A. Caldwell, Air Force Research Laboratory, Brooks Air Force Base

2:00 Circulating Plasma Markers of Cognitive Status
Dr. Harris R. Lieberman, USARIEM

2:30 Discussion

3:00 Break

Part VII: Future Possibilities for Monitoring Physiological and Cognitive Function (Moderator: Beverly Tepper)

3:15 Odors as Biomarkers to Predict the Occurrence of Mental and Physical Stress
Dr. Gary K. Beauchamp, Monell Chemical Senses Center

4:15 Molecular Markers of Mechanical Activity- and Inactivity-Induced Anabolic and Catabolic States in Striated Muscle
Dr. Kenneth M. Baldwin, University of California, Irvine

4:45 Discussion

5:00 Summary of the Workshop
Dr. John Vanderveen, Chair, Committee on Military Nutrition Research

5:30 Adjourn

D

Workshop Manuscripts

PREDICTING AND PROTECTING PERFORMANCE USING METABOLIC MONITORING STRATEGIES: IT'S ALL WET STUFF ANYWAY, ISN'T IT?

COL Karl E. Friedl, U.S. Army Research Institute of Environmental Medicine

The ultimate reductionistic view of the Military Operational Medicine Research Program (MOMRP) centers on metabolism as the answer to all questions. For every problem we are trying to solve in the MOMRP, we will someday complete the connection to a metabolic basis. This includes soldier performance problems that range from extended physical stamina to sustaining optimal mood and behavior. While this first-principles approach is not likely to provide many near-term solutions to MOMRP problems, we can exploit the emerging physiology to develop monitoring technologies. Insight into this metabolic activity should help predict individual status and physiological reserve. This is based on the premise that these metabolic processes are the basis of the responses that allow organisms to survive in the face of environmental challenges and are the earliest indicators of a change in physiological status. This calls for a thoughtful review of currently known regulatory mechanisms that suggest promising predictive markers of status and impending failure of adaptive response capabilities. We should also consider applications of the most promising monitoring technologies that are currently available. The focus of this workshop is to address: what are the best metabolic targets for monitoring and what are the most promising monitoring technologies?

This information is needed for predictions about the readiness status of individuals in training and in operational settings where human performance is important. We have formidable monitoring capabilities on military systems, but lack real-time information on the status of our own troops. This serves U.S. defense priorities to "assure readiness of the Armed Forces" and to "transform the Department of Defense" (including experimenting with new approaches to warfare).

RESEARCH REQUIREMENTS FOR PHYSIOLOGICAL MONITORING

Monitoring soldier status has become increasingly important because of new lethal and complex technologies that require high reliability of the human operator and new tactics that reduce line-of-sight contact with team members and increase geographical distance and isolation. No longer is soldier monitoring just a nice-to-have technological replacement for common sense or for good leadership that includes understanding the signs of soldier limits. Soldiers may not know they are reaching dangerous levels of overheating and dehydration and, if they are fully encapsulated in protective suits and operating in a remote site, their team leaders also may not know they are heading for trouble. An alert to the individual on their future helmet visor display and/or an automatic "911" message to their squad leader can provoke a prompt intervention and save a mission.

The Navy is designing ships with substantially reduced crew sizes, which calls for greater reliance on each individual. Monitoring the status of these sailors becomes especially important if they are incapacitated in an isolated crew compartment during high-risk damage control operations, such as fighting fires or flooding. The concept of the Reduced Ships-Crew by Virtual Presence is for smart ships to continuously receive data on the status of the ship, as well as on the crew within the ship (Street et al., 2002).

Today's high performance aircraft can easily exceed the limits of human physiological tolerances, and one concept for physiological monitoring includes detection of an approaching loss of consciousness to trigger an automatic take over of the controls (Forster et al., 1994). This calls for a rapidly responsive system that, with high reliability, identifies a major lapse in pilot capabilities.

Monitoring in training is at least as important as in operational environments. It may be most useful for leaders to use physiological monitoring to learn the limits of their own soldiers during training operations. Then, during an actual operational mission, they might use monitoring only for specific warnings about real-time status. Other aspects of metabolic monitoring may not require a wearable system, but simply periodic testing to determine, for example, if individuals have reached a high state of bone and muscle remodeling during their training and can reduce a high probability of injury by resting the next day. This kind of feedback will be broadly useful to learning limits of individuals and units.

Physiological monitoring is being explored for a wide variety of other military applications, including the forensic "black box" flight recorder-type of analysis of a pilot's mental state after a class A accident, in order to prevent future accidents (Forster, 2002). There is also a need for overall "whole body" health markers for easy assessment of global indices of service members' health at regular intervals throughout their career. This could eventually represent some combination of psychological and physiological health, using markers such as brain metabolites monitored via magnetic resonance spectroscopy (MRS) scans, whole-body oxidative stress load assessments, and mitochondrial redox potential of critical brain cells.

RECENT EVOLUTION OF MONITORING RESEARCH

Physiological monitoring concepts are not new, but the measurement technologies have advanced more rapidly than our understanding of what the measurements mean to health and performance. Fifty years ago, the Office of Naval Research and the Army Surgeon General cooperatively studied infantrymen in combat to identify metabolic predictors of mental status (Davis et al., 1952). Using neuropsychological testing (including visual flicker fusion and auditory flutter fusion tests) and blood and urine testing, they assessed hydration status, adrenal stress markers, and corresponding changes in cognitive functioning. Studies by the Air Force explored the use of an electroencephalogram (EEG) to monitor pilot performance as early as the 1950s (Sem-Jacobsen, 1959). Current studies are examining many of the same factors and relationships that were tested in the studies 50 years ago. Although these newer empirical studies have some technological advantages, most notably electronic computing power, the studies have largely relied on available technologies instead of exploring the most suitable measurement targets and developing specifically needed monitoring technology. Many of the available technologies are simply telemetered applications of clinical monitoring systems, limiting advances to spin offs from standards of medical care. We have spent too much time trying to find uses for new measurement technologies instead of pushing the development of technology to systematically test what we understand about physiology and to predict outcomes of greatest importance.

The greatest barrier to advances in performance monitoring has been the lack of suitably defined performance outcome measures. Until recently, aviator performance has been the most extensively studied model for physiological monitoring. Military aviators have been a logical focus because of the need (i.e., the high costs associated with catastrophic performance failures) and because of the experimental advantages. Performance outcome measures are better defined for aviator tasks, especially the ultimate outcome of successful landing versus disaster. The cockpit also provides a friendly setting for clunky prototype monitoring systems that are power hungry and tethered to heavy equipment. Aviator studies can provide early proof of concept for systems that are later reduced in size, weight, power, and invasiveness for untethered applications in soldiers, marines, and sailors. Nevertheless, the aviator monitoring studies are not generalizable without the further development of performance assessment methods and metrics.

Without suitable performance measures, results from lab-based studies cannot be translated into militarily relevant outcomes. These measures are also needed for field studies that are otherwise forced to rely on simple dichotomies of "no bad outcome" or catastrophic failure (e.g., heat stroke, serious injury, or mission failure). The MOMRP has invested heavily in the development and standardization of practical neuropsychological tests (e.g., the Automated Neuropsychological Assessment Metric) (Kane and Kay, 1992), and current field studies are attempting to link these test results with military performance. For example, simple reaction time remained impaired following sports concussions in military cadets even after they were cleared for return to duty by clinical criteria; the significance of this finding to other performance measures is being further investigated. Cold water immersion reliably affected the matching-to-sample test; what this means to Navy diver performance capabilities is also being further investigated (Thomas et al., 1989). One eventual monitoring application would be to embed informative tests into common military tasks that could be monitored in order to obtain unobtrusive periodic assessments of an individual's performance status. We are currently sponsoring a Department of Defense (DOD) review of methods and metrics for performance assessment that synthesizes the current state of the knowledge on militarily relevant performance assessments and models (Ness et al., In preparation). We have also launched a new research initiative on the development of military performance assessment methods based on measures of neurological function, such as voice stress analysis and eye saccades (Science Technology Evaluation Package 3.C).

Physiological monitoring moved from a research sidelight to a central objective in the Army research program under the guidance of Dr. Fred Hegge in 1996. The goal of the Warfighter Physiological Status Monitoring (WPSM) initiative is to make real-time performance predictions that leaders can use to assess the readiness status of their forces. The concept is to develop a soldier-acceptable, minimally invasive sensor set with on-the-soldier analysis. The output (which can be queried for further information) will be a simple "green" (within normal limits), "amber" (physiological challenges are present), or "red" (systems have failed and the soldier is a casualty). This relies on the vast trove of environmental physiology and psychological data collected and modeled in DOD research programs for many years. A key feature of the approach is that these systems must also learn the usual range of responses for its soldier, accounting for individual variability. Currently, WPSM is a research "tool kit" to learn more about normal and abnormal physiological signals encountered in real soldier environments; these include a range of responses that routinely exceed those that can be obtained in an ethically developed experimental laboratory setting. WPSM will ultimately be reduced to the minimal sensor set needed for highly reliable and important predictions. Reed Hoyt currently leads this program with the development of experimental signal acquisition and data handling systems and data collection studies with marines and soldiers in challenging training environments (Hoyt et al., 1997a, 2001). The immediate requirements for WPSM are to provide status for thermal strain, live-dead detection, sleep history, and energy expenditure for the Land Warrior system. In later iterations of this system (e.g., the Objective Force Warrior), more sophisticated monitoring capabilities and performance predictions are planned that will also include early casualty triage capabilities.

EXAMPLES OF CURRENT RESEARCH EFFORTS, AND LEVERAGING FROM RELATED PROGRAMS

We have chosen several critical areas for review: hydration and heat production, substrate utilization and energy metabolism, muscle and bone remodeling, and brain function. These traditionally separate research areas are interrelated through metabolic processes. For example, exertional rhabdomyolysis has elements of hydration and heat exposure, energy flux, and muscle remodeling, with early effects on mental status (Gardner and Kark, 1994). The topics are also closely interrelated through common measures that might signal changes in one or more of these physiological categories. For example, shivering may indicate a variety of threats that, when combined with one or two other measurements, can unambiguously distinguish impending hypothermia risk, exposure to a neurotoxic chemical, or intense psychological fear. Brain function reflected in cognitive, mood, or psychomotor measures (e.g., speed of mental processing, irritability, and marksmanship) may be a common and sensitive marker of deficits of all the other stressors and functional deficits of interest. These may include each of the topics in this workshop, including carbohydrate metabolism in physical exhaustion (Frier, 2001), dehydration or significant fluid shifts such as those observed in the brain with acute mountain sickness (Singh et al., 1990), and perhaps even cytokine-mediated changes in brain function following intense muscular exertion (Febbraio and Pedersen, 2002). Brain function is both an early indicator of many stressors of concern and a direct reflection of specific performance capabilities.

Early changes to defend critical functions are likely to be more promising prognostic indicators than awaiting change in the critical function itself (e.g., blood glucose, serum osmolality, core body temperature). The critical function may be so well defended, such as serum osmolality and sodium concentration, that when a significant change is detected, homeostatic mechanisms have failed and the individual is already a casualty. Earlier changes in interstitial fluid or osmoregulatory hormones may signal a heroic defense against a threat to intravascular volume, even while other measures appear to indicate that all is still well. There are also conditions under which the critical function measurement, such as body temperature, may have a wider range of "normal" at performance extremes in healthy individuals than previously recognized. This reflects highly appropriate compensation to sustain peak performance, defying definitive classification of an impending performance failure until regulatory mechanisms fail. For example, core body temperature may be as low as 35°C at the circadian

TABLE D-1 Technology Forecast for Practical Metabolic Assessment Measures (Measured Endpoints and Conceivable Technologies)

Past	Present[a]
Energy balance and fuel availability	
• Blood and urine biochemistry • Ratings of perceived exertion • Home test glucose monitors, lab tests	• "Gluco-watch" • Activity-based predictions • Reverse iontophoresis, actigraphy
Brain metabolic function	
• Paper and pencil tests	• Computerized neuropsychological testing • EEG spectral analysis • Palm-top test, dry electrodes in a hat band
Hydration and water balance	
• Urine specific gravity	• Balance based on intake and predicted losses • Whole body water estimates • Instrumented canteen/camelbak, bioelectrical resistance
Bone and muscle turnover	
• Loss of strength and delayed onset muscle soreness • "Hot spots" • Thermography	• Specific blood and urinary markers (e.g., telopeptides, myoglobin, CPK, IGF-1) • Lab tests

[a] EEG = electroencephalogram, CPK = creatine phosphokinase, IGF-1 = insulin-like growth factor-1.

nadir in Ranger students who have lost most of their insulative fat and have metabolically adjusted to a reduced energy intake (Hoyt et al., 1997b), and it may be sustained at 40°C for several hours in marathoners during their race (Maron et al., 1977). Monitoring the signs of compensation (e.g., changes in heat flux, activation of sweating or shivering mechanisms, cardiac responses, and mental functioning) may predict a trajectory to danger (amber) well in advance of the unambiguous changes in core body temperature (red).

Bone and muscle turnover studies are important to the military to solve near-term problems of high rates of injury during physical training, most importantly during the rapid train-up phase of the 8- to 12-week initial entry training course conducted in every service (half of all female soldiers incur musculoskeletal injury during basic training). A peak incidence of stress fractures by about the third week of training was hypothesized to be associated with high rates of bone remodeling stimulated by the training. This led to a major Army

Near Future[b]	Far Future[c]
• Subdermal continuous glucose, lactate, pH, free fatty acids • Semi-invasive implantable sensors and "tattoos"	• Functional outcome (e.g., EMG, nerve conduction, changes in thermal flux) • Noninvasive physiological sensors built into clothing
• Saccades and pupil responses • Voice analysis • Task embedded psychological tests • Doppler etc. in soldier helmet/spectacles	• Sweat/exhaled cytokines • Volatile compounds/pheromones • Brain blood flow • Chemical nose, respiratory sampling, personal intrahelmet brain imaging systems
• Intercellular fluid assessment • Whole body water changes	• Changes in skin properties • Endocrine changes in defense of water volume
• Subdermal wicks, boot-sensor body weight tracking with electrolyte and BIA sensors	• Skin mechanical/electrical changes, semi-invasive sensing of osmoregulatory hormones
• Sweat markers of calcium and protein metabolism • Altered biomechanics • Practical field test systems	• Changes in redox status • Regional metabolism/blood flow changes • Deep muscle biochemical sensors

[b] BIA = bioelectrical impedance analysis.
[c] EMG = electromyogram.

study that examined the benefits of a physical training rest period in the third week of training (Popovich et al., 2000). Unfortunately, this did not modify the injury profile, suggesting a more complicated pathogenesis, including individual variability. The development of specific markers of susceptibility and impending injury in individuals is still urgently needed.

Table D-1 suggests some of the outcomes that might be logical targets for monitoring within the next decade and some of the technologies that exist or could be developed for such monitoring. The boundary between current and near-term approaches is slightly blurred by the overlap of current technologies that require far more validation and projected near-term technologies that are just beginning to demonstrate promise. For example, fitness for duty based on various peripheral indicators of brain function is an important but elusive goal. In the past, there was a hope that performance could be predicted from recent sleep history measured by wrist-worn actigraphy (Redmond and Hegge, 1985); the current status of fatigue-performance models is too immature and individual responses to this single measure are too variable to make this useful by itself (Friedl et al., In press). Potentially noninvasive measurement methods that could be mounted in a helmet, such as pupillometry and saccadic eye movements, are being explored but have so far not held up well compared with lab measures such as the psychomotor vigilance task (Russo et al., 2003). A method developed by the National Aeronautics and Space Administration (NASA) that follows slow eye closure ("droopy" eyelids) shows great promise, but will have to be proven in a helmet-type platform that keeps the monitor in line with the subject's eyes (Dinges et al., 1998). Voice analysis is specifically affected by emotional load in soldiers, returning to normal with psychological adaptation even while general activation (e.g., accelerated heart rate) continues (Wittels et al., 2002); however, this measure has not yet been demonstrated to correspond to specific performance decrements. EEG analyses in fatigued subjects or during sustained vigilance tasks have been studied in at least three military laboratories and show promise, but they remain to be demonstrated as strong predictors of impending deficits (Caldwell et al., 2002).

Far-future technologies are concepts that might be achievable but have not been seriously explored and remain "marks on the wall." Mitochondrial redox state in specific brain tissues has been suggested as the key marker of brain function status, based on the importance of neural cell bioenergetics. Perhaps the far-future final common pathway to monitor would be something like this and everyone will submit to a minor transsphenoidal surgical procedure for a rice grain-sized monitor of brain status! Intracerebral monitoring of energy-related metabolites is being done with neurosurgical patients now to follow acute conditions involving hypoxia and ischemia. As we learn more about what we need to measure, the technologists may be able to develop the noninvasive monitoring devices to our emerging specifications. For example, with the higher powered magnets, researchers are now detecting glutamate peaks in MRS brain pixels. An elevated frontal lobe glutamate might signify a range of acute metabolic insults that would be very important to detect and countermand. We now have transcranial magnetic stimulation systems that operate with very low power; why not a technology for brain spectroscopy built into a helmet in the future? Nearer term approaches to monitoring brain metabolic activity includes applications of existing near infrared and Doppler probes to estimate fron lobe activity and monitor middle cerebral artery blood flow (Hitchcock et al., 2003).

The current military research programs are leveraged with special Congressional appropriations that accelerate basic metabolic research in specific topic areas. The Bone Health and Military Medical Readiness research program (supported by the National Osteoporosis and Related Bone Disorders Coalition) is focused on the improved understanding of bone remodeling processes and includes projects that are exploring markers of impending stress fracture injury. The Technologies for Metabolic Monitoring research program (supported by the Juvenile Diabetes Research Foundation) is testing novel approaches to measure functional outcomes related to biochemical status and energy metabolism, notably glucose regulation, but including also the development of lactate sensors and the exploration of physiological indicators of metabolic status. Projects supported by the Force Health Protection research program examine methods to monitor global health status in soldiers, including the use of breath condensates to measure cytokines and other markers of lung function following blast or toxic inhalation exposures. Two large projects are assessing the association of brain magnetic resonance spectroscopy measures (Schuff et al., 1999) and symptom reporting in chronic multisymptom illnesses to determine objective markers of well-being. Another program is dedicated to the investigation of eye saccades and pupil responses as indices of fatigue and fitness for duty, as described in a recent review by Major General (ret.) Gary Rapmund (2002). The Neurotoxin Exposure Treatment Research Program (sponsored by the Parkinson's Action Network) includes exploration of voice analysis and neuropsychological testing methods for early detection of neurological changes.

Disclaimer: The opinions and assertions expressed in this paper are those of the author and do not necessarily express the official views of the Department of the Army or other Services.

REFERENCES

Caldwell JA, Hall KC, Erickson BS. 2002. EEG data collected from helicopter pilots in flight are sufficiently sensitive to detect increased fatigue from sleep deprivation. *Int J Aviation Psychol* 12:19–32.

Davis SW, Elmadjian F, Hanson LF, Liddell HS, Zilinsky AA, Johnston ME, Killbuck JH, Pace N, Schaffer FL, Walker EL, Minard D, Kolovos ER, Longley GH. 1952. *A Study of Combat Stress, Korea 1952.* Technical Memorandum ORO-T-41(FEC). Chevy Chase, MD: Operations Research Office, The Johns Hopkins University.

Dinges DF, Mallis MM, Maislin G, Powell JW. 1998. *Evaluation of Techniques for Ocular Measurement as an Index of Fatigue and the Basis for Alertness Management.* Technical Report DOT-HS-808-762. Washington, DC: National Highway Traffic Safety Administration.

Febbraio MA, Pedersen BK. 2002. Muscle-derived interleukin-6: Mechanisms for activation and possible biological roles. *FASEB J* 16:1335–1347.

Forster EM. 2002. *Safety of Flight: The Physiologic Aspect of the Weapon System.* Patuxent River, MD: Naval Air Warfare Center Aircraft Division.

Forster EM, Morrison JG, Hitchcock EM, Scerbo MW. 1994. *Physiologic Instrumentation in the Naval Air Warfare Center Human-use Centrifuge to Determine the Effects of Cumulative +Gz on Cognitive Performance.* Technical Report NAWCADWAR-956006-4.6. Warminster, PA: Naval Air Warfare Center Aircraft Division.

Friedl KE, Mallis MM, Ahlers ST, Popkin SM, Larkin W. In press. Research requirements for operational decision making using fatigue and performance. *Aviat Space Environ Med.*

Frier BM. 2001. Hypoglycaemia and cognitive function in diabetes. *UCP Suppl* 123:30–37.

Gardner JW, Kark JA. 1994. Fatal rhabdomyolysis presenting as mild heat illness in military training. *Mil Med* 159:160–163.

Hitchcock EM, Warm JS, Matthews G, Dember WN, Shear PK, Tripp LD, Mayleben DW, Parasuraman R. 2003. Automation cueing modulates cerebral blood flow and vigilance in a simulated air traffic control task. *Theor Issues Ergon Sci* 4:89–112.

Hoyt RW, Buller M, Redin MS, Poor RD, Oliver SR. 1997a. *Soldier Physiological Monitoring—Results of Dismounted Battlespace Battle Lab Concept Experimentation Program Field Study*. Natick, MA: U.S. Army Research Institute of Environmental Medicine.

Hoyt RW, Young AJ, Matthew WT, Kain JE, Buller M. 1997b. *Warfighter Physiological Status Monitoring (WPSM): Body Core Temperatures During 96 h of Swamp Phase Ranger Training*. Natick, MA: U.S. Army Research Institute of Environmental Medicine.

Hoyt RW, Buller MJ, DeLany JP, Stultz D, Warren K. 2001. *Warfighter Physiological Status Monitoring (WPSM): Energy Balance and Thermal Status During a 10-day Cold Weather U.S. Marine Corps Infantry Officer Course Field Exercise*. Technical Note. Natick, MA: U.S. Army Research Institute of Environmental Medicine.

Kane RL, Kay GG. 1992. Computerized assessment in neuropsychology: A review of tests and test batteries. *Neuropsychol Rev* 3:1–117.

Maron MB, Wagner JA, Horvath SM. 1977. Thermoregulatory responses during competitive marathon running. *J Appl Physiol* 42:909–914.

Popovich RM, Gardner JW, Potter R, Knapik JJ, Jones BH. 2000. Effect of rest from running on overuse injuries in army basic training. *Am J Prev Med* 18:147–155.

Rapmund G. 2002. The limits of human performance: A point of view. *Aviat Space Environ Med* 73:508–514.

Redmond DP, Hegge FW. 1985. Observations on the design and specification of a wrist-worn human activity monitoring system. *Behav Res Methods Instrum Comput* 17:659–669.

Russo M, Thomas M, Thorne D, Sing H, Redmond D, Rowland L, Johnson D, Hall S, Krichmar J, Balkin T. 2003. Oculomotor impairment during chronic partial sleep deprivation. *Clin Neurophysiol* 114:723–736.

Schuff N, Amend DL, Knowlton R, Norman D, Fein G, Weiner MW. 1999. Age-related metabolite changes and volume loss in the hippocampus by magnetic resonance spectroscopy and imaging. *Neurobiol Aging* 20:279–285.

Sem-Jacobsen CW. 1959. Electroencephalographic study of pilot stresses in flight. *J Aviat Med* 30:787–801.

Singh MV, Rawal SB, Tyagi AK. 1990. Body fluid status on induction, reinduction and prolonged stay at high altitude of human volunteers. *Int J Biometeorol* 34:93–97.

Street TT, Nguyen X, Williams FW. 2002. *Wireless Communication Technologies on Ex-USS Shadwell.* Technical Report NRL/MR/6180-02-8631. Washington, DC: Naval Research Laboratory.

Thomas JR, Ahlers ST, House JF, Schrot J. 1989. Repeated exposure to moderate cold impairs matching-to-sample performance. *Aviat Space Environ Med* 60:1063–1067.

Wittels P, Johannes B, Enne R, Kirsch K, Gunga HC. 2002. Voice monitoring to measure emotional load during short-term stress. *Eur J Appl Physiol* 87:278–282.

CURRENT STATUS OF FIELD APPLICATIONS OF PHYSIOLOGICAL MONITORING FOR THE DISMOUNTED SOLDIER

Reed W. Hoyt, COL Karl E. Friedl, U.S. Army Research Institute of Environmental Medicine

The dismounted warfighter's workplace is fairly unique within the variety of occupational challenges encountered by the American population. Modern foot soldiers commonly engage in intense, mentally and physically demanding 3- to 10-day missions, often in rugged terrain or complex urban settings. These warriors carry heavy loads (35–65 kg) and are often food and sleep restricted. Environmental conditions—ambient temperature, humidity, wind speed, solar load, and barometric pressure—can vary widely. Consider as recent examples of the operational environment the desert heat conditions of the Persian Gulf, the cold, wet weather in Bosnia, and the cold and high altitude challenges in the mountains of Afghanistan.

WARFIGHTER PHYSIOLOGICAL STATUS MONITORING CONCEPT

Why is physiological monitoring in the field needed? Wearable metabolic and physiological status monitoring can play important roles in: (a) sustaining physical and mental performance, (b) reducing the likelihood of nonbattle injuries, such as heat stroke, frostbite, and acute mountain sickness, and (c) improving casualty management in remote situations.

Ambulatory warfighter physiological status monitoring (WPSM) technologies are being developed to provide useful performance and health status indicators for warfighters, medics, commanders, and logisticians. The goal is to maximize the operational effectiveness of soldiers, to reduce the occurrence of non-battle casualties, and to improve remote casualty management. Currently, the WPSM program is using a novel research "tool kit" to collect ambulatory physiological data from soldiers operating in stressful field environments. Analysis of these data sets is providing a better understanding of the physiological strains associated with operations in a multi-stressor environment. The data are also guiding the development a soldier-acceptable WSPM system for advanced combat systems for dismounted warfighters, including land warriors and objective force warriors.

The WPSM effort risks being driven by technology rather than the biological needs of the warfighter, resulting in inappropriate technologies lack scalability, adaptability, reliability, and ease of use. Indeed, sensor hardware often first comes to mind when thinking about ambulatory metabolic and physiological monitoring. In practice, however, sensor development is one of a series of steps needed to reliably generate a useful flow of health-state information in a harsh and highly constrained wearable environment. These steps include: reliable sensor data collection, data cleaning, data reduction and interpretation, and the communication, synthesis, interpretation, and presentation of the data. Key technologies that support this process, including posthoc time-series data management and the medical Personal Area Network, are reviewed elsewhere (Hoyt et al., 2002).

Power, weight, and volume constraints, and the need for truly "wear-and-forget" comfort, limit the functionality of wearable sensors. What can be sensed may be unconventional. For example, estimating sleep by monitoring activity is practical, but it is not currently practical to do so by electroencephalogram. Furthermore, wearable sensors are usually less reliable than their laboratory counterparts due to factors such as motion artifact and environmental effects (water, temperature, pressure). An intelligent sensor network that reliably generates useful information from a number of disparate sources is needed to provide a holistic, rather than a "keyhole," view of the physiological status of the individual.

CURRENT COMPONENTS OF PHYSIOLOGICAL STATUS

A prototype WPSM user interface (display) for the medic or field commander (Figure D-1) illustrates relevant types of contextual and physiological information. This heuristic display shows: (1) thermal/work strain as the physiological strain index (PSI) (Moran et al., 1998), (2) hydration state or water balance (water intake relative to water requirements), (3) metabolic rate, (4) environmental conditions, (5) cognitive/sleep status (hours of sleep, etc.), and (6) clinical status and location information. This knowledge display requires data from multiple sources, including a baseline characterization of the individual,

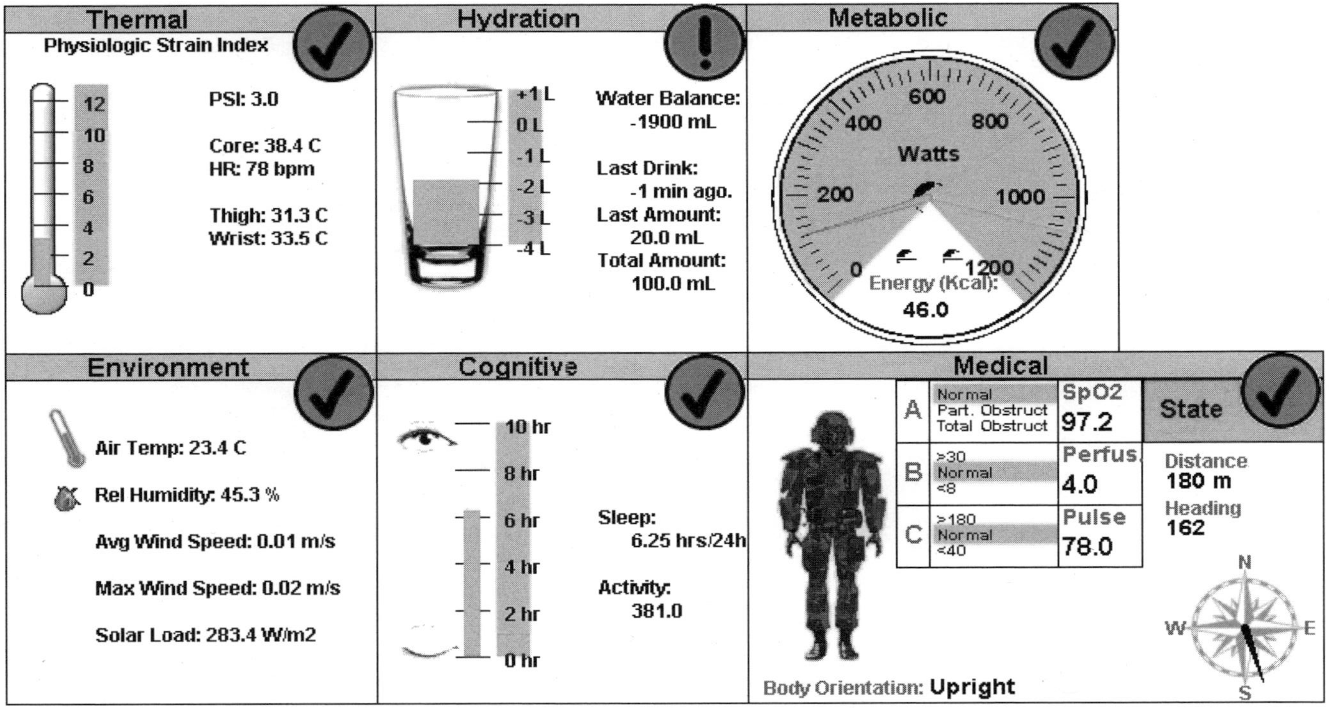

FIGURE D-1 Prototype warfighter physiological status monitoring user interface (display) for the medic or field commander illustrating contextual and physiological information. This heuristic display shows: (1) thermal/work strain as physiological strain index (PSI), (2) hydration state or water balance, (3) metabolic rate, (4) environmental conditions, (5) cognitive/sleep status (hours of sleep, etc.), and (6) clinical status and location information. HR = heart rate.

real-time soldier and environmental sensor input, and historical and group mean data.

Warfighter Characteristics

Warfighter characteristics, along with clothing, diet, load, geolocation, and meteorological conditions (air temperature, solar load, wind speed, humidity), are important determinants of the individual's physiological and pathophysiological responses to environmental stresses and trauma. Relevant warfighter characteristics include: job type (military occupational specialty), gender, ethnicity, age, height, body weight, percent body fat, thermal and altitude acclimation history, and aerobic fitness. These factors change slowly, if at all, and can be recorded well before any training or combat mission. Body fat percent can be estimated simply from waist circumference (Wright and Wilmore, 1974). Simple field techniques for characterizing thermal and altitude acclimation states are currently not well defined. Aerobic fitness can be estimated from the Army Physical Fitness Test 2-mile run for time score (Mello et al., 1988), or from foot-ground contact time and heart rate using the method of Weyand and colleagues (2001).

Heat Strain

Understanding why hot weather injuries occur and developing ways to prevent these injuries are important concerns given the approximately 120 heat stroke/sun stroke injuries that occur per year and the associated $10 million cost per year (Sawka et al., 1996; http://amsa.army.mil). The graphical display in Figure D-2 shows core temperature, measured by an ingested thermometer pill (O'Brien et al., 1998) and heart rate, typically derived from an electrocardiogram. The PSI, a lumped core temperature/heart rate index that reflects thermal/work strain on a scale of 0 to 10 (Moran et al., 1998), is currently used to generate green/amber/red alerts as thresholds are passed. PSI values may prove useful in assessing acclimation status, guiding heat acclimation routines, and in setting the timing and duration of work/rest cycles. A first-principles thermal strain model, called Scenario, estimates core temperature from work rate, clothing characteristics, and ambient meteorological conditions (Kraning and Gonzalez, 1997). This and other surrogate measures of core temperature may be appropriate when risk of hypo- or hyperthermia is moderate and more precise core temperature measurements, such as those provided by an ingested radio thermometer pill, are not needed. The core temperature requirement is likely to be replaced by improvements in heat flux modeling from measures of cutaneous responses and temperatures; combined with other sensor measurements, this may provide strong inferences not only about thermal status, but also about shock and hemorrhage.

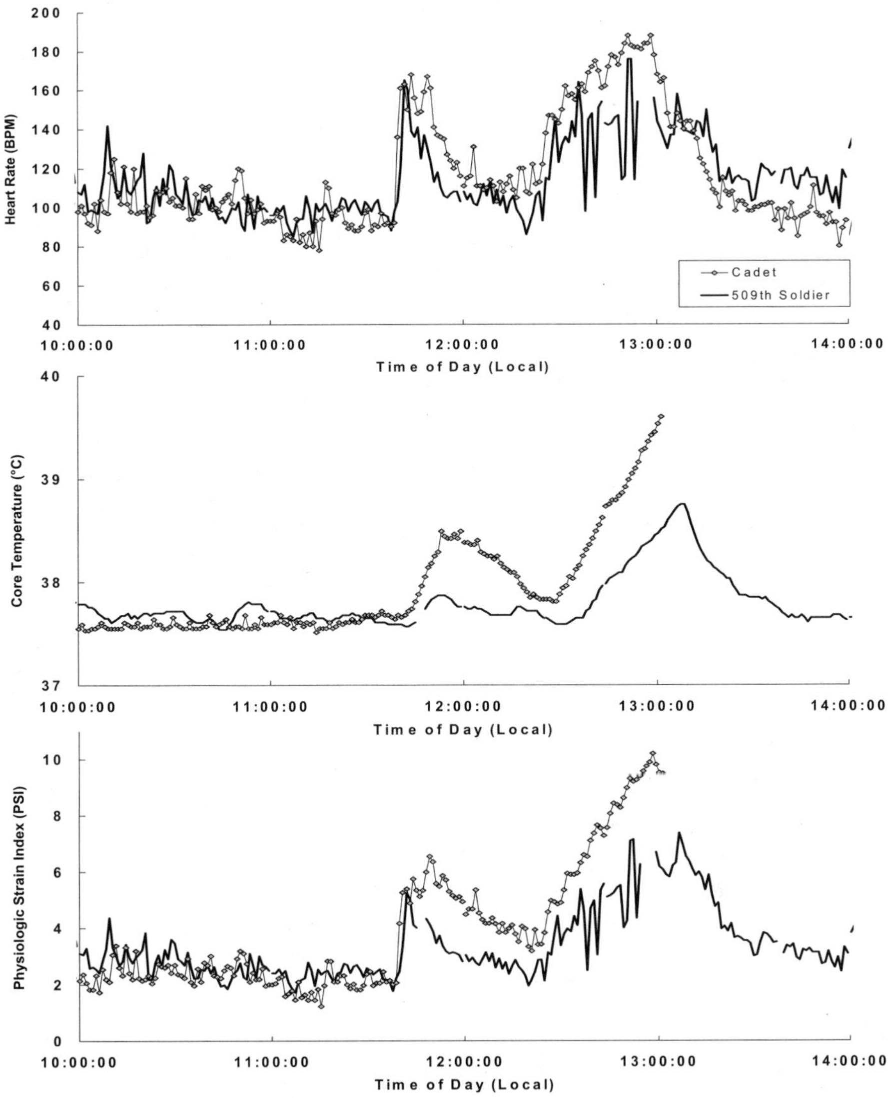

FIGURE D-2 Heart rate, core temperature, and physiological strain index (Moran et al., 1998) in two soldiers engaged in similar training activities during a hot-weather field exercise at the Joint Readiness Training Center, Fort Polk, Louisiana. The thermal/work strain levels associated with two bouts of marching (1145–1200 h and 1230–1300 h) were more pronounced in the heat exhaustion casualty (cadet) than in the less-affected 509th soldier. The heat casualty had a higher body fat percent, carried a heavier load, was less physically fit, and was not heat acclimated, as compared with his 509th cohort.

Cold Strain

Cold injuries, that is, hypothermia and peripheral cold injuries, are also a major concern for soldiers (King and Lum, 2002). Temperature pills can be used to monitor for hypothermia (O'Brien et al., 1998). Peripheral temperature and heat flux sensors can be used to assess the risk of peripheral cold injury and to guide improvements in clothing, boots, and gloves. The Cold Strain Index (Moran et al., 1999) uses core and peripheral temperatures to track cold strain. However, this algorithm needs to be modified to account for altered thermoregulation during underfeeding and sleep. (See Toner and McArdle [1988] for a discussion of the physiological adjustment of humans to the cold.)

Hydration

Under- or overhydration can lead to decrements in physical and cognitive performance, increased risk of heat injury, hyponatremia, or death (Montain et al., 2001; Pandolf et al., 1988). Mission water requirements, which are largely driven by basal water needs and sweat losses, can be predicted based on the anticipated weather, clothing, load weight, and metabolic rate during the mission (Kraning and Gonzalez, 1997). Technologies to monitor water intake from bladder-type canteens, the "drink-o-meter" concept, can help ensure adequate water intake (water discipline). However, practical field methods to assess overall hydration (total body water content), or to monitor chronic hydration state through adequacy of hourly urine output, have yet to be developed. Tests of the use of body resistance measurements have consistently failed to demonstrate accurate tracking of water changes, perhaps in part because of the inability to control for variability in electrolyte concentrations during various types of dehydration (Berneis and Keller, 2000; Koulmann et al., 2000). It may be possible in the future to improve electrical resistance-derived estimates of hydration with minimally invasive subdermal electrolyte sensors. Alternatively, future automatic monitoring of urinary excretion rates and solute concentrations may provide valuable insight into hydration status and other aspects of acute soldier health.

Metabolic Status/Energy Reserve—Modeling the Metabolic Fuel Requirements of Soldiers

Field rations may not always meet the nutritional needs of soldiers (Friedl and Hoyt, 1997). Negative fat balance, commonly associated with undereating in the field, can usually be managed with little consequence by drawing on substantial body-fat reserves. Body-fat energy reserves can be calculated from percent body fat, as estimated from waist circumference less the 5 percent absolute minimum body-fat levels attainable in underfed healthy male soldiers (Friedl et al., 1994). However, negative carbohydrate balance, which is common in the field and associated with decreased endurance capacity and loss of lean mass, is more difficult to manage due to the body's limited carbohydrate reserves. Can monitoring technologies help ensure that field rations meet the fuel requirements of physically active soldiers?

Carbohydrate requirements of soldiers can be estimated from aerobic fitness, daily activity patterns, and the metabolic cost of locomotion (Hoyt et al., 1997). Maximum aerobic capacity can be derived from the Army's Annual Physical Fitness Test 2-mile run for time results (Mello et al., 1988). Daily activity patterns can be derived from heart rate or actigraphy (Redmond and Hegge, 1985). The metabolic cost of locomotion can be derived from total weight and foot-ground contact times (pedometry) (Hoyt and Weyand, 1996; Kram and Taylor, 1990) or from the Pandolf equation and body weight, load weight, and geolocation (including velocity of movement, grade, and footing) (Pandolf et al., 1977). Knowing the metabolic rate and the maximum aerobic capacity for each individual, an exercise intensity profile can be generated (i.e., percent of maximum aerobic capacity over time). Oxygen consumption can be partitioned into carbohydrate and fat combustion by assuming a given relationship between resting or exercise intensity and the nonprotein respiratory exchange ratio (RER = carbon dioxide production/oxygen consumption) and using standard conversion factors. The exercise intensity-RER relationship chosen might be more fat-predominant than that of fully fed individuals (Åstrand and Rodahl, 1986) due to practical limits on the amount of food soldiers can carry.

Remote Trauma Triage

Warfighters are expected to be widely dispersed on the battlefield and minimal medical care will be available to combat casualties. To help improve remote casualty management, a remote trauma triage system is being developed. This remote triage system, part of the WPSM system, will contain sensors and algorithms that allow medics to remotely detect ballistic wounding events and to determine casualty life signs and the need for a major surgical life-saving intervention (Holcomb et al., In press). Parameters important in life-sign detection after wounding include responsiveness to radio contact, motion, body position, cardiac activity, and systolic blood pressure. Distilled health-state information will help the medic use medical resources (time, equipment, supplies) effectively.

Altitude Acclimatization

Soldiers deploying to elevations above 2,800 m (~ 8,000 ft) may experience Acute Mountain Sickness (AMS) (Pandolf et al., 1988). AMS is characterized by headache, nausea, fatigue, decreased appetite, and poor sleep, often with signs of poor balance and mild swelling of the face, hands, and feet. Without special preparation, a large proportion of a military unit rapidly inserted at high altitude is likely to develop acutely debilitating symptoms. Normally, AMS is

TABLE D-2 Age, Physical Characteristics, Total Load Carried, and Maximal Aerobic Capacity of Two Soldiers—A Heat Exhaustion Casualty (Cadet), and an Unaffected 509th Soldier from the 1/509th Infantry Brigade (Airborne)

Soldier	Age (y)	Height (cm)	Weight (kg)	Body Fat (%)	Load (kg)	VO_{2max} (ml O_2/kg^1 min^{-1})
Cadet	21	175	79.3	18	45.3	47
509th soldier	22	170	68	13.3	35.3	53

NOTE: These soldiers were engaged in similar hot-weather training activities at the Joint Readiness Training Center, Fort Polk, Louisiana. During a road march, the nonheat-acclimated, less lean, more burdened, less physically fit cadet became a heat casualty, while the heat-acclimated, leaner, less-burdened, more-fit soldier from the 1/509th Infantry Brigade (Airborne) tolerated the thermal/work stress.

either absent or resolves within 3 to 4 days following ascent. However, maladaptation can lead to life-threatening, high-altitude pulmonary or cerebral edema. Individual acclimatization state can be assessed by comparing blood-oxygen saturation for a given ascent profile (i.e., SaO_2 for the reported or measured exposure to hypobaric hypoxia), with that expected with normal acclimatization. An ability to monitor and model acclimatization status will make it easier to plan high-altitude missions and minimize altitude illnesses.

AN EXAMPLE APPLICATION—CHARACTERISTICS OF A HEAT CASUALTY

Heat strain provides a demonstration of nascent capabilities for physiological monitoring. Reliable predictions of soldier mental status and performance capabilities are not yet available, while the assessment of frank casualties has been possible for some time through the use of clinical monitoring technologies. Progressive heat strain moves on a continuum from impaired cognitive function to frank casualty and presents one of the first opportunities to provide commanders with useful predictions of failing performance before a soldier becomes an environmental stress casualty. Collection of field data that includes clear medical outcomes makes it possible to backtrack to earlier indicators of the impending health risk and develop more precise predictive thresholds of individual risk.

A pair of soldiers was engaged in similar training activities during a hot-weather field exercise at the Joint Readiness Training Center, Fort Polk, Louisiana. Although the two soldiers performed similar activities from about 1130 to 1400 h (ambient temperature = 32°–34°C; relative humidity = 46–55 percent; solar load = 800–875 W/m^2; wind speed = 1–2 ms^{-1}), and both were fed and hydrated, only one became a heat casualty. Soldier characteristics, including maximal aerobic capacity determined using the method of Weyand and colleagues (2001), are shown in Table D-2. Geolocation data (not shown) was collected using a Global Positioning System and Dead Reckoning Module (Model

DRM III, Point Research Corp., Fountain Valley, California). Ambulatory heart-rate data, from an electrocardiography, and core temperature data, via an ingested temperature radio telemetry pill (Human Technologies Inc., St. Petersburg, Florida), were also collected. PSI was calculated (Moran et al., 1998). Posthoc data analysis showed that the difference in response to heat stress was due to a number of factors. The heat casualty had a higher body-fat percent, carried a heavier load, was less physically fit, and was not heat acclimated (by interview) as compared with his unaffected cohort. In this instance, integrating multiple data streams was essential to the process of understanding a multistressor physiological events. In contrast, experiences in the intensive care unit (ICU), where equally or more complex biological challenges present themselves, suggests multiple data streams may not always be necessary. For example, decades ago Dr. Hans Weil introduced the great toe temperature as an effective integrator of many complex physiologic variables (Joly and Weil, 1969; Vincent et al., 1988). This has resulted in more explicit ICU protocols that have favorably changed both clinician compliance and patient outcome. The minimum number and type of data streams needed for useful physiological status monitoring in the field, where noise, sensor failure, and changeable biophysical conditions are common, deserves further investigation.

In conclusion, physiological and metabolic monitoring offers a number of potential benefits for dismounted warfighters. However, achieving these benefits is scientifically and technically challenging.

Acknowledgments: The authors express their gratitude to Drs. S.R. Muza and W.R. Santee for useful discussions and to Mr. Mark Buller for preparing the innovative data displays. The authors are also indebted to Mr. Tom Thcaux, Captain William P. Gaffney, and the soldier test volunteers from the 1/509th Infantry Battalion (Airborne), Fort Polk, Louisiana, for making the hot weather study possible.

Disclaimer: The opinions and assertions expressed in this paper are those of the authors and do not necessarily express the official views of the Department of the Army. The study data presented is from volunteers who gave their free and informed consent. Investigators adhered to AR 70-25 and USAMRMC Regulation 70-25 on Use of Volunteers in Research.

REFERENCES

Åstrand PO, Rodahl K. 1986. *Textbook of Work Physiology, Physiological Bases of Exercise*. 3rd ed. New York: McGraw-Hill.

Berneis K, Keller U. 2000. Bioelectrical impedance analysis during acute changes of extracellular osmolality in man. *Clin Nutr* 19:361–366.

Friedl KE, Hoyt RW. 1997. Development and biomedical testing of military operational rations. *Ann Rev Nutr* 17:51–75.

Friedl KE, Moore RJ, Martinez-Lopez LE, Vogel JA, Askew EW, Marchitelli LJ, Hoyt RW, Gordon CC. 1994. Lower limit of body fat in healthy active men. *J Appl Physiol* 77:933–940.

Holcomb JB, Niles SE, Hinds D, Aoki N, Salinas J, Flannigan TJ, Macaitis JM, Duke JH, Moore FA. In press. Prehospital physiologic data and life saving interventions in trauma patients. *J Trauma.*

Hoyt RW, Weyand PG. 1996. Advances in ambulatory monitoring: Using foot contact time to estimate the metabolic cost of locomotion. In: Marriott BM, Carlson SJ, eds. *Emerging Technologies for Nutrition Research: Potential for Assessing Military Performance Capability*. Washington, DC: National Academy Press. Pp. 1–29.

Hoyt RW, Young AJ, Matthew WT, Kain JE, Buller M. 1997. *Warfighter Physiological Status Monitoring (WPSM): Body Core Temperatures During 96 H of Swamp Phase Ranger Training*. Natick, MA: U.S. Army Research Institute of Environmental Medicine.

Hoyt RW, Reifman J, Coster TS, Buller MJ. 2002. Combat medical informatics: Present and future. In: Kohane IS, ed. *Biomedical Informatics: One Discipline. Proceedings of the 2002 AMIA Annual Symposium.* Bethesda, MD: American Medical Informatics Association.

Joly HR, Weil MH. 1969. Temperature of the great toe as an indication of the severity of shock. *Circulation* 39:131–138.

King CN, Lum G. 2002. Cold weather injuries among active duty Soldiers, US Army, January 1997–July 2002. *Med Surveill Mon Rep* 7:2–5.

Koulmann N, Jimenez C, Regal D, Bolliet P, Launay JC, Savourey G, Melin B. 2000. Use of bioelectrical impedance analysis to estimate body fluid compartments after acute variations of the body hydration level. *Med Sci Sports Exerc* 32:857–864.

Kram R, Taylor CR. 1990. Energetics of running: A new perspective. *Nature* 346:265–267.

Kraning KK, Gonzalez RR. 1997. A mechanistic computer simulation of human work in heat that accounts for physical and physiological effects of clothing, aerobic fitness, and progressive dehydration. *J Therm Biol* 22:331–342.

Mello RP, Murphy MM, Vogel JA. 1988. Relationship between a two mile run for time and maximal oxygen uptake. *J Appl Sports Sci Res* 2:9–12.

Montain SJ, Sawka MN, Wenger CB. 2001. Hyponatremia associated with exercise: Risk and pathogenesis. *Exerc Sports Sci Rev* 29:113–117.

Moran DS, Shitzer A, Pandolf KB. 1998. A physiological strain index to evaluate heat stress. *Am J Physiol* 275:R129–R134.

Moran DS, Castellani JW, O'Brien C, Young AJ, Pandolf KB. 1999. Evaluating physiological strain during cold exposure using a new cold strain index. *Am J Physiol* 277:R556–R564.

O'Brien C, Hoyt RW, Buller MJ, Castellani JW, Young AJ. 1998. Telemetry pill measurement of core temperature in humans during active heating and cooling. *Med Sci Sports Exer* 30:468–472.

Pandolf KB, Givoni B, Goldman RF. 1977. Predicting energy expenditure with loads while standing and walking very slowly. *J Appl Physiol* 43:577–581.

Pandolf KB, Sawka MN, Gonzalez RR, eds. 1988. *Human Performance Physiology and Environmental Medicine at Environmental Extremes*. Traverse City, MI: Cooper Publishing Group.

Redmond DP, Hegge FW. 1985. Observations on the design and specification of a wrist-worn human activity monitoring system. *Behav Res Methods Instrum Comput* 17:659–669.

Sawka MN, Wenger CB, Pandolf KB. 1996. Thermoregulatory responses to acute exercise-heat stress acclimation. In: Fregley MJ, Blatteis CM, eds. *Handbook of Physiology, Section 4: Environmental Physiology*. New York: Oxford University Press. Pp. 157–185.

Toner MM, McArdle WD. 1988. Physiological adjustments of man to the cold. In: Pandolf KB, Sawka MN, Gonzalez RR, eds. *Human Performance Physiology and Environmental Medicine at Environmental Extremes*. Traverse City, MI: Cooper Publishing Group.

Vincent JL, Moraine JJ, van der Linden P. 1988. Toe temperature versus transcutaneous oxygen tension monitoring during acute circulatory failure. Intensive Care Med. 14:64–68.

Weyand PG, Kelly M, Blackadar T, Darley JC, Oliver SR, Ohlenbusch NE, Joffe SW, Hoyt RW. 2001. Ambulatory estimates of maximal aerobic power from foot-ground contact times and heart rates in running humans. *J Appl Physiol* 91:451–458.

Wright HF, Wilmore JH. 1974. Estimation of relative body fat and lean body weight in a United States Marine Corps population. *Aerospace Med* 45:301–306.

BIOMARKERS OF PHYSIOLOGICAL STRAIN DURING EXPOSURE TO HOT AND COLD ENVIRONMENTS

Andrew J. Young, Michael N. Sawka, Kent B. Pandolf
U.S. Army Research Institute of Environmental Medicine

Soldiers experience thermal (heat and cold) stress arising from the combined effects of environment, clothing insulation, and body heat production. Alterations in body temperatures (core, skin, and muscle) above and below normal levels can lead to thermal illness and injury and also degrade performance. Humans regulate core temperature within a narrow range (35°–41°C) through both behavioral and physiological responses to thermal stress. When conscious actions to minimize or avoid thermal stress by modifying activity levels, changing clothes, and seeking shelter do not completely negate thermal stress,

TABLE D-3 Core Temperature Measures

Site	Advantage	Disadvantage
Esophageal	Accurate, rapid response	Uncomfortable, affected by swallowing
Rectal	Accurate, measurement ease	Slow response, uncomfortable, cultural objections
Auditory canal - tympanic membrane	Measurement ease	Inaccurate (biased by skin and ambient temperature), uncomfortable
Oral	Measurement ease	Inaccurate (affected by mouth breathing)
"Pill"	Accurate, measurement ease	Pill movement influences measurement, signal "cross talk" between subjects in close proximity

physiological responses are activated that enhance dissipation or conservation of body heat stores, as appropriate, through alterations in metabolic rate, blood flow between the core and the skin, and sweating. Activation of these responses works to maintain temperature homeostasis, but it also results in physiological strain. In this brief review, human physiological responses elicited in response to exposure to extremes of hot and cold will be summarized with a view to identifying potential biomarkers of physiological strain. Further, an example of how such biomarkers can be used collectively to assess physiological strain and warn of impending health and performance degradation during exposure to heat and cold will be presented.

CORE TEMPERATURE

Thermal strain is most commonly assessed by the measurement of body core temperature. There is no one "true" core temperature because of temperature differences among different sites in the core. Core temperature is often measured at the esophagus, rectum, mouth, tympanum, and auditory meatus. Measurement methods employed for each of these sites and the relative advantages and disadvantages of each are discussed in detail by Sawka and colleagues (1996) and summarized in Table D-3. In brief, most thermal physiologists consider esophageal temperature to be the most accurate and reliable noninvasive index of core temperature for humans, followed in preference by rectal temperature and gastrointestinal tract temperature measured using ingestible temperature sensor pills, the latter of which is ideally suited for ambulatory monitoring outside of laboratories (O'Brien et al., 1998). Oral (sublingual), tympanic, and auditory meatus temperatures are widely used as reflections of core temperature, but all are influenced to some degree by head and face skin temperatures, as well as by ambient temperature, and are sensitive to inaccuracies related to proper placement of the sensor.

HEAT STRAIN

Heat Stress

Heat stress increases the requirements for sweating and circulatory responses to dissipate body heat. When the ambient temperature is warmer than skin, the body gains heat from the climate, which increases the heat the body must dissipate. In addition, exercise increases metabolic rate and thus increases the rate that heat must be dissipated to keep core temperature from increasing to dangerous levels. Climatic heat stress and exercise interact synergistically.

The Wet Bulb Globe Temperature (WBGT) is widely used as a quantitative index of climatic heat stress for use in regulating permitted physical activity level and strategies to minimize the risk of heat injury. WBGT is an empirical index of climatic heat stress but does not quantify physiological strain. It is calculated as outdoor WBGT = 0.7 natural wet bulb + 0.2 black globe + 0.1 dry bulb, or as indoor WBGT = 0.7 natural wet bulb + 0.3 black globe. High WBGT values can be achieved either through high humidity, as reflected in high wet bulb temperature, or through high air (dry bulb) temperature and solar load, as reflected in black globe temperature. While useful, WBGT underestimates the risk of heat injury for humid conditions, and the index was originally developed for predicting resting comfort conditions and does not consider clothing or exercise intensity (metabolic rate), so it cannot predict heat exchange between a person and the climate or the physiological strain of thermoregulation (Sawka and Young, 2000). The National Weather Service uses a similar index, referred to as the Heat Index, which, in theory, provides the temperature sensed by the body when the ambient temperature and humidity are combined (NWS, 2003). This index, like the WBGT, does not consider the level of physical activity or cloth ing in estimating strain.

Thermoregulatory Responses to Heat Stress

During exercise, core temperature initially increases rapidly and subsequently increases at a reduced rate until heat loss equals heat production and steady-state values are achieved. The core temperature increase represents the storage of metabolic heat that is produced as a by-product of skeletal muscle contraction. At the beginning of exercise, the metabolic rate increases immediately, while thermoregulatory effector responses that enable heat dissipation respond more slowly, but eventually heat loss increases sufficiently to balance metabolic heat production, allowing a new steady-state core temperature to be achieved. Within a range of conditions known as the "prescriptive zone," the magnitude of the increase in core temperature is independent of climatic conditions and proportional to the metabolic rate (Sawka et al., 1996).

Outside the prescriptive zone, the increase in core temperature is no longer independent of ambient conditions (Sawka and Young, 2000). During compensable heat stress, thermoregulatory responses may still dissipate heat at a rate allowing a steady-state core temperature to be maintained, albeit at a higher level than within the prescriptive zone. However, there are biophysical limits to heat exchange between the climate and the body, and the relative contributions of dry and evaporative heat exchange to total heat loss varies with climatic conditions. As ambient temperature increases, the gradient for dry heat exchange diminishes and evaporative heat exchange becomes more important. When the ambient temperature equals or exceeds skin temperature, evaporative heat exchange will account for virtually all heat loss. Evaporation is limited by the vapor pressure of water in air, thus, increasing humidity constrains evaporative heat loss. Uncompensable heat stress occurs when the maximal evaporative cooling capacity of the ambient environment exceeds the amount of evaporative cooling required to dissipate metabolic heat production, and a steady-state core temperature cannot be achieved.

Core temperature provides a reliable physiological index to predict the incidence of exhaustion from heat strain (Sawka and Young, 2000). Figure D-3 presents the relationships between core temperature and incidence of exhaustion from heat strain for heat-acclimated persons exercising in uncompensable or compensable heat stress. During uncompensable heat stress, exhaustion was rarely associated with a core temperature below 38°C, and exhaustion always occurred before a temperature of 40°C was achieved, whereas during compensable heat stress, there are many reports of individuals whose core temperatures exceed 40°C at exhaustion (Sawka and Young, 2000). For example, Joy and Goldman (1968) reported that 35 of 63 (56 percent) elite soldiers were still performing military tasks when core temperature reached 39.5°C, and Pugh and colleagues (1967) observed that the core temperature of 7 out of 47 marathon runners exhibited core temperatures > 40°C (highest value was 41°C) immediately upon completion of the race. Thus, increasing core temperatures may be useful for predicting onset of heat exhaustion within a group of individuals, but the relationship between core temperature and time to exhaustion is greatly influenced by the environment (compensable versus uncompensable heat stress) and individual variability due to fitness and other factors.

Other commonly measured physiological responses indicative of thermal strain during heat stress include skin temperature, sweating rate, and heat rate. Increases in both skin temperature and sweat rate do occur with increasing heat strain, but both skin temperature and sweat rate vary considerably depending on the site of the body where the measurements are made. Further, the ambient air/water temperature surrounding the body can influence temperature measured at the skin unless steps are taken to carefully insulate the sensor from the environment. Similarly, sweating rate at a given metabolic rate varies with environmental conditions, fitness, hydration, and acclimatization status of the individual. Therefore, while skin temperature and sweat rate are useful measurements for laboratory studies of thermoregulation, these variables are probably of limited value for use as generalized biomarkers for monitoring an individual's heat strain.

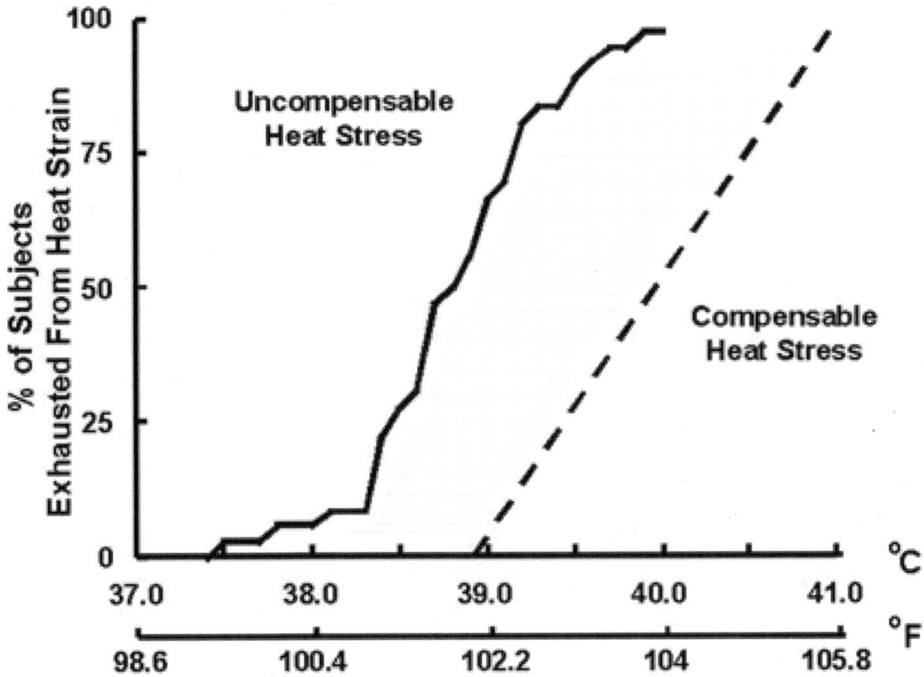

FIGURE D-3 Relationships between core temperature and incidence of exhaustion from heat strain.
SOURCE: Reprinted, with permission Sawka and Young (2000), *Exercise and Sport Science*, Lippincott Williams & Wilkins©.

Heart rate, on the other hand, is easy to measure and is a useful index of thermal strain. During exercise, metabolic rate and heat production may be ten times their levels at rest, and delivery of heat to the skin to achieve core-to-skin heat transfer sufficient for thermal balance must increase proportionately in order to reestablish thermal balance. Since skin temperature increases in warmer environments, the core-to-skin temperature gradient becomes relatively narrow in hot environments, and skin blood flow must be rather high to achieve sufficient heat transfer to maintain thermal balance during exercise. During exercise in the heat, the primary cardiovascular challenge is to provide simultaneously enough blood flow to exercising skeletal muscle to support its metabolism and enough blood flow to the skin to dissipate heat. High skin blood flow often is associated with reduced cardiac filling and with stroke volume, which require a higher heart rate to maintain cardiac output. Therefore, elevation of the heart rate response to exercise is an index of the increased cardiovascular strain required for thermoregulation during heat stress. The ease of measuring heart rate makes it a good candidate for monitoring thermal strain during exercise heat stress.

Metabolic Responses to Heat Stress

Exercise in the heat also reportedly increases plasma or muscle lactate levels, and accelerated muscle glycogenolysis during exercise is sometimes observed, suggesting that glycolytic metabolism has been increased (Young, 1990). Whether this metabolic effect reflects Q_{10} effects, reduced oxygenation due to reduced perfusion of metabolically active tissue, reduced hepatic removal of plasma lactate, or some combination of those effects remains contentious. However, changes in blood lactate levels are too nonspecific to be useful as indexes of thermal strain.

There is growing evidence in both humans and animals of a role for serotonin (5-HT) accumulation in the brain for the genesis of fatigue from exercise hyperthermia (Cheuvront and Sawka, 2001). Monitoring changes in brain 5-HT levels is not feasible, but peripheral measurements of prolactin (PRL) concentrations are an accepted marker for brain serotonergic activity. The most recent findings indicate that an increase in PRL in response to exercise heat strain is only observed above a core temperature threshold of 38°C. Thus, while PRL release may provide useful information regarding the development of serotonergic fatigue, the apparent existence of a 38°C temperature threshold for PRL suggests that PRL may be a useful metabolic marker to denote early thermal strain in the heat.

COLD STRAIN

Cold Stress

Humans usually rely on behavioral strategies like wearing clothing or remaining in shelters to protect themselves against the cold. However, the nature of most outdoor winter-time military activities limits the efficacy of behavioral strategies. When behavioral thermoregulation provides inadequate protection from the cold, physiological responses are elicited.

When ambient temperature is colder than body temperature, the resulting thermal gradient favors body heat loss. Besides ambient temperature, wind speed, solar radiation, and humidity also influence the heat loss potential. No single cold-stress index integrates all these effects with respect to the heat loss potential of the environment, but one, the Wind Chill Index (WCI), has achieved widespread acceptance and use. The WCI estimates the environmental cooling rate from the combined effects of the wind and air temperature. Lacking any better tool for quantifying cold stress, these tables are useful to help guide decisions concerning the conduct or cancellation of outdoor activities, but the computational formula for the WCI probably overestimates the risk of tissue freezing as wind speed increases, while underestimating the effect of decreasing air temperature. Further, the WCI estimates the risk of tissue freezing only for the exposed skin of sedentary persons, and wearing windproof clothing greatly reduces wind chill effects.

Water has a much higher thermal capacity than air, and the cooling power of the ambient environment is greatly enhanced under cold-wet conditions. During water immersion, conductive and convective heat transfer can be 70-fold greater than in air of the same temperature, depending on the water depth or body surface immersed in the water and the individual's metabolic rate. Thus, even when water temperatures are relatively mild, persons swimming, wading streams, swamps, or through surf can lose considerable amounts of body heat. Furthermore, when clothing becomes wet due to rain or accidental immersion, its insulative value is compromised, and wetting of the skin facilitates heat loss by conduction, convection, and evaporation.

Physiological Responses to Cold Stress

Since the exposed body surface loses heat faster than it is replaced, skin temperature declines upon exposure to cold. When skin temperature falls below about 35°C, a peripheral vasoconstriction is elicited, mediated by increased sympathetic nervous activity that decreases peripheral blood flow and reduces convective heat transfer between the body's core and shell (skin, subcutaneous fat, and skeletal muscle). This effectively increases insulation, retarding heat loss and defending core temperature, but at the expense of a decline in temperature of peripheral tissue that can contribute to the etiology of cold injuries. If tissue temperature falls below 0°C, freezing tissue injury will ensue, the severity of which will be related to the extent of freezing. Thus, monitoring skin temperature during cold exposure can provide information regarding the likelihood of developing freezing tissue injury.

The vasoconstrictor response to cold is pronounced in the hands and fingers, making them particularly susceptible to cold injury and a loss of manual dexterity. In these areas, another vasomotor response, cold-induced vasodilation (CIVD), develops (characterized by transient increases in blood flow to the cooled finger to periodically rewarm skin following the initial decline during cold exposure). The CIVD is thought to be beneficial in maintaining dexterity and preventing cold injury, suggesting that by monitoring the presence or absence of such a response during cold exposure might be useful for predicting cold effects, but no clear evidence exists to support this idea.

The other major physiological mechanism elicited during cold exposure is an increased metabolic heat production that helps offset heat losses. Muscle is the principal source of this thermogenic response in humans. Shivering, an involuntary series of rhythmically repeated muscle contractions, may start immediately or after several minutes of cold exposure, usually beginning in torso muscles and then spreading to the limbs. During muscular contraction, approximately 70 percent of total energy expended is liberated as heat. Certain animals can increase in metabolic heat production by noncontracting tissue in response to cold exposure (such as nonshivering thermogenesis), but no clear evidence indicates that humans share this mechanism.

As cold stress becomes more severe, shivering intensity increases and more muscles are recruited to shiver. Oxygen uptake increases as a result of the increasing metabolic requirement of shivering, and the increase in oxygen uptake is related to the intensity of shivering. As mentioned above, heat losses and body cooling are generally more pronounced during cold-water immersion than during exposure to cold air, and the stimulus for shivering is greater in the water. As a result, whole body oxygen uptake usually increases more during immersion in cold water, often reaching 25–45 percent maximal oxygen uptake or higher, than during exposure to cold air where oxygen uptakes of 15 percent of maximal are more common (Sawka and Young, 2000). This might suggest that measuring oxygen uptake could provide a means to assess shivering intensity, and this is the case for inactive, nonexercising persons. However, muscular contractions associated with exercise also increase heat production, and this heat production can mitigate the need for shivering (see Figure D-4).

At low exercise intensities in the cold, metabolic heat production is not high enough to prevent shivering. Thus, oxygen uptake is higher, with the increased oxygen uptake representing the added requirement for shivering activity. As metabolic heat production rises with increasing exercise intensity, core and skin temperatures are maintained and the afferent stimulus for shivering declines, causing the shivering-associated component of total oxygen uptake during exercise to also decline. At high intensities, exercise metabolism is high enough to completely prevent shivering, and oxygen uptake during exercise is the same in cold and temperate conditions. The exercise intensity at which metabolic heat production is sufficient to prevent shivering depends on the severity of cold stress, which, in any given environment, will vary among individuals (see below). As a result, the utility of using oxygen uptake/metabolic rate measurements as an quatitative index of shivering activity is limited. On the other hand, more direct measurements of muscular contractile activity via actigraphy, accelerometry, or even electromyography might provide useful quantitative indices of shivering activity.

Cold exposure also influences metabolism. For example, the increased sympathetic nervous activity that mediates the cold-induced vasoconstrictor response described above also results in a pronounced rise in circulating norepinephrine concentrations. Increased norepinephrine concentrations are thought to promote glycogenolysis and glycolytic metabolism (Young, 1990), and some evidence suggests that glycogenolysis and blood lactate accumulation during light-intensity exercise can be higher in the cold than in temperate conditions. The increased glycogen use during low-intensity exercise has been attributed to the additional metabolic cost of shivering, but it is also possible that high circulating norepinephrine levels favor a shift in energy substrate metabolism favoring carbohydrate utilization. Unfortunately, a myriad of exercise, environmental,

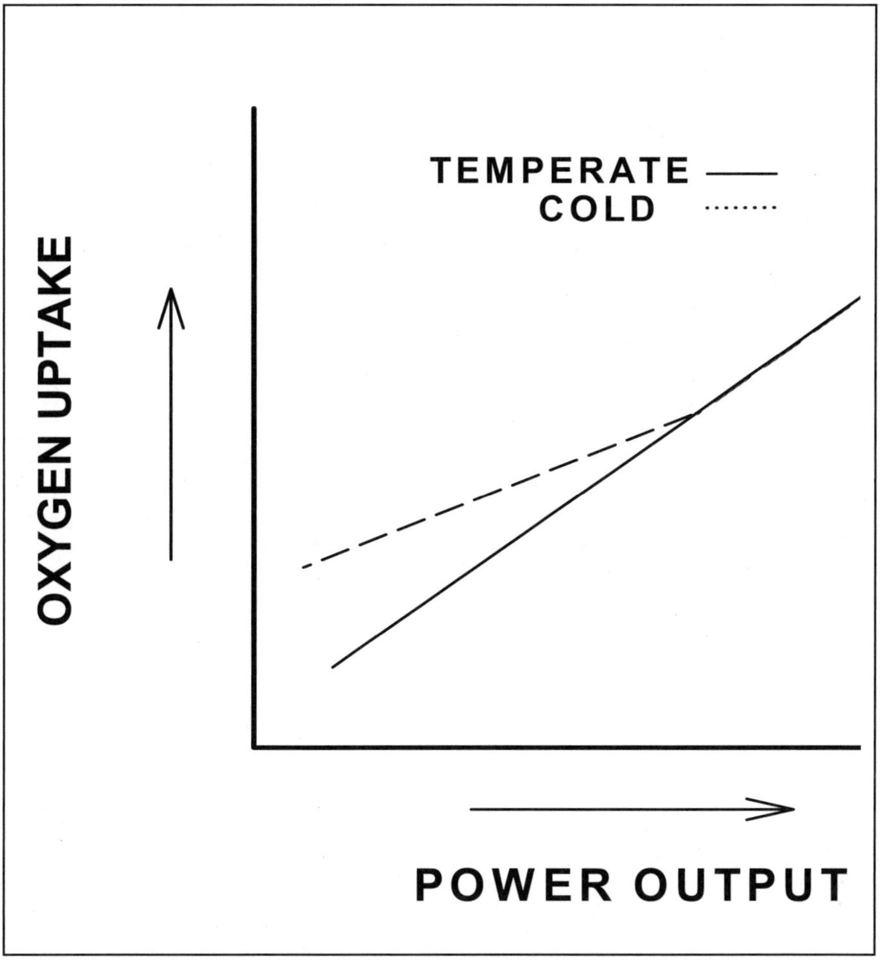

FIGURE D-4 Effect of cold-induced shivering on oxygen uptake during exercise at different intensities.
SOURCE: Adapted from Young et al. (1996)

and dietary factors can cause norepinephrine and lactate concentrations to increase and muscle glycogen breakdown to accelerate, so these responses are too nonspecific to provide any useful information about thermal strain during cold exposure.

Factors Modifying Thermoregulatory Responses to Cold

Although measuring skin temperature and shivering activity during cold exposure are feasible, and monitoring skin temperature might provide a means to predict the danger of freezing tissue injury, neither of these indices appear entirely reliable as indices of whole-body thermal strain. For example, while blunted shivering contributes to the impaired ability to maintain core temperature during cold exposure observed with exertional fatigue (Young et al., 1998) or prolonged cold exposures (Castellani et al., 1998), there are patterns of cold acclimatization in which shivering responses to cold also become blunted but, simultaneously, other adjustments develop to mitigate heat loss and enhance body heat conservation (Young, 1996). Also, fatter persons shiver less but experience smaller declines in body temperature than lean persons exposed to the same cold conditions because subcutaneous fat provides significant insulation against heat loss in the cold (Gagge and Gonzalez, 1996). Thus, differences in shivering response to cold may not always reflect important differences in thermal strain. Similarly, while the decline in skin temperature during cold exposure does reflect the cold-induced vasoconstrictor response, it is well known that the steady-state skin temperature maintained during exposure to a given cold condition can be influenced by the thickness of subcutaneous fat, fitness level, acclimatization state, and level of exercise or activity, not to mention clothing (Gagge and Gonzalez, 1996; Young, 1996). Thus, if only a single parameter is to be monitored to assess overall thermal strain in the cold, core temperature probably provides more meaningful information than measurements of either shivering or skin temperature.

Integrative Approach to Predicting Thermal Strain

Measuring or monitoring any single parameter to reflect thermal strain may be of limited value. To address this limitation, indices that integrate information from several parameters have been developed. For example, WBGT and Wind Chill both attempt to combine multiple climatic measurements into a single value reflective of the environmental stress level. Those indices predict the capacity of the environment to induce physiological strain, but not the strain actually experienced. However, Moran and colleagues (1998, 1999) have described an approach to integrate multiple physiological parameters into a single value reflective of the thermal strain experienced during exposure to heat or cold stress.

Two separate equations, one for use with heat stress and the other for cold stress, have been derived using a similar conceptual basis (Moran et al., 1998, 1999). The equations are constructed to compute the strain value, which can range from 0 (no/little strain) to 10 (very high strain) from the measured values of the physiological input parameters. Both equations assume that core temperature (both the absolute and the change from the normal resting level) is of fundamental importance in assessing the strain. Further, the Physiological Strain

Index (PSI) equation derived to predict strain in heat stress conditions incorporates a heart rate parameter because it was assumed that, with heat stress, cardiovascular strain associated with meeting thermoregulatory requirements would contribute to the overall physiological strain. PSI is calculated as

$$\mathrm{PSI} = 5(T_{Ct} - T_{C0})/(39.5 - T_{C0}) + 5(HR_t - HR_0)/(180 - HR_0)$$

in which T_{Ct} and HR_t are simultaneous measurements of core temperature and heart rate at a particular time during the heat stress exposure, and T_{C0} and HR_0 are initial (pre-stress) measurements. The weighting factors for core temperature and heart rate are the same, reflecting the assumption that each contributes equally to the strain.

The Cold Strain Index (CSI), derived to predict physiological strain during exposure to cold, replaces the heart rate parameter with a skin temperature parameter because heart rate is little affected by cold, per se, whereas skin temperature does change quickly in response to the environmental stress and is known to provide afferent stimulus for shivering and vasoconstriction. The parameter weighting used in CSI differ from those in PSI and were chosen to mimic the weightings used to calculate mean body temperature from core and skin temperature (Pandolf and Moran, 2002). Thus, CSI is calculated

$$\mathrm{CSI} = 6.67(T_{Ct} - T_{C0})/(35 - T_{C0}) + 3.33(T_{SKt} - T_{SK0})/(20 - T_{SK0})$$

in which, again, T_{Ct} and T_{SKt} are the simultaneously measured values for core and skin temperature at a particular time during cold exposure, and T_{C0} and T_{SK0} are the initial (pre-stress) values.

Moran evaluated PSI values calculated using databases from six independent experimental studies in which human volunteers experienced exercise/heat stress and reported that PSI very adequately reflects the heat strain experienced for different climatic conditions, clothing ensembles, hydration states, and exercise intensities, and between subjects of differing ages and genders (Pandolf and Moran, 2002). A similar approach to evaluate CSI calculated using databases from three independent experimental studies in which human volunteers were exposed to different cold air or cold water immersion conditions also indicated that CSI effectively depicted cold strain (Pandolf and Moran, 2002), but the authors acknowledged that the evaluation of CSI needed to consider a wider range of ambient conditions. Further development of CSI appears necessary to consider the effects of exercise on the calculated strain value (Castellani et al., 2001).

SUMMARY

Climatic heat stress and exercise interact synergistically and may strain physiological systems to their limits, impairing performance and increasing susceptibility to heat injury. Heat stress increases requirements for sweating and circulatory responses to dissipate body heat, and these physiological adjustments combined with rising body temperatures may have metabolic effects. Core body temperature and heart rate are considered reliable physiological parameters for monitoring heat strain, while monitoring skin temperature and sweat rates probably provide less important information due to the wide variability in these responses. The possibility that changes in peripheral metabolites, such as circulating prolactin levels, may provide information about central nervous system heat strain remain to be definitively examined.

In the cold, the ability to maintain body heat balance and normal body temperatures will depend primarily on the severity of climatic cold stress and clothing insulation and to a lesser extent on the influence of physiological responses. Exposure to cold elicits shivering thermogenesis, but the response to a given environment varies widely among individuals depending on their clothing, acclimatization, activity level, and body composition. Thus, monitoring the intensity of shivering may not provide useful information regarding cold strain being experienced by individuals exposed to cold. Cold-induced vasoconstriction decreases blood flow to peripheral tissues, favoring conservation of body heat at the expense of a decline in skin temperature and increased susceptibility to cold injury; thus, monitoring skin temperature, particularly in unprotected skin regions exposed to cold or areas receiving poor circulation, can provide prediction regarding development of freezing tissue injury. Changes in core temperature provide a reliable index of whole-body cooling and cold strain experienced by individuals, and reduced core temperature can degrade the ability to achieve maximal metabolic rate and submaximal endurance performance.

Possibly, no one parameter can provide a complete assessment of thermal strain under all conditions. Information from multiple physiological parameters is likely to be the best approach to quantitatively assessing thermal strain to predict injury or performance degradation. More research is needed to identify the most appropriate parameters to assess physiological strain during exposure to heat and cold strain, and to formulate the appropriate weighting and calculations to integrate the information from these multiple inputs.

REFERENCES

Castellani JW, Young AJ, Sawka MN, Pandolf KB. 1998. Human thermoregulatory responses during serial cold water immersions. *J Appl Physiol* 85:204–209.

Castellani JW, Young AJ, O'Brien C, Stulz DA, Sawka MN, Pandolf KB. 2001. Cold strain index applied to exercising men in old-wet conditions. *Am J Physiol* 281:R1764–R1768.

Cheuvront SN, Sawka MN. 2001. Physical exercise and exhaustion from heat strain. *J Korean Soc Living Environ System* 8:134–145.

Gagge AP, Gonzalez RR. 1996. Mechanisms of heat exchange: Biophysics and physiology. In: Fregly MJ, Blatteis CM, eds. *Handbook of Physiology. Section 4: Environmental Physiology*. New York: Oxford University Press. Pp. 45–84.

Joy RJT, Goldman RF. 1968. A method of relating physiology and military performance: A study of some effects of vapor barrier clothing in a hot climate. *Mil Med* 133:458–470.

Moran DS, Shitzer A, Pandolf KB. 1998. A physiological strain index (PSI) to evaluate heat stress. *Am J Physiol* 275:R129–R134.

Moran DS, Castellani JW, O'Brien C, Young AJ, Pandolf KB. 1999. Evaluating physiological strain during cold exposure using a new cold strain index. *Am J Physiol* 277:R556–R564.

NWS (National Weather Service). 2003. *Heat Index*. Online. National Oceanic and Atmospheric Administration. Available at http://www.crh.noaa.gov/pub/ heat. htm.

O'Brien C, Hoyt RW, Buller MJ, Castellani JW, Young AJ. 1998. Telemetry pill measurement of core temperature in humans during active heating and cooling. *Med Sci Sports Exerc* 30:468–472.

Pandolf KB, Moran DS. 2002. Relatively new heat and cold strain predictive indices. In: Tochihara XY, ed. *Environmental Ergonomics*. Fukuoka, Japan: Kyushu Inst. Design. Pp. 163–168.

Pugh LG, Corbett JL, Johnson RH. 1967. Rectal temperature, weight losses and sweat rates in marathon running. *J Appl Physiol* 23:347–352.

Sawka MN, Young AJ. 2000. Physical exercise in hot and cold climates. In: Garrett WE, Kirkendall DT, eds. *Exercise and Sports Science*. Baltimore, MD: Lippincott, Williams & Wilkins. Pp. 385–399.

Sawka MN, Wenger CB, Pandolf KB. 1996. Thermoregulatory responses to acute exercise-heat stress and heat acclimation. In: Fregly MJ, Blatteis CM, eds. *Handbook of Physiology. Section 4: Environmental Physiology*. New York: Oxford University Press. Pp. 157–186.

Young AJ. 1990. Energy substrate utilization during exercise in extreme environments. *Exerc Sport Sci Rev* 18:65–117.

Young AJ. 1996. Homeostatic responses to prolonged cold exposure: Human cold acclimatization. In: Fregly MJ, Blatteis CM, eds. *Handbook of Physi-*

ology. Section 4: Environmental Physiology. New York: Oxford University Press. Pp. 419–438.

Young AJ, Sawka MN, Pandolf KB. 1996. Physiology of Cold Exposure. In: Marriott BM, Carlson SJ, eds. *Nutritional Needs in Cold and in High-Altitude Environments*. Washington, DC: National Academy Press. Pp. 127–147.

Young AJ, Castellani JW, O'Brien C, Shippee RL, Tikuisis P, Meyer LG, Blanchard LA, Kain JE, Cadarette BS, Sawka MN. 1998. Exertional fatigue, sleep loss and negative energy balance increase susceptibility to hypothermia. *J Appl Physiol* 85:1210–1217.

HYDRATION STATUS MONITORING

Robert Carter III, Samuel N. Cheuvront, Margaret A. Kolka, Michael N. Sawka,
U.S. Army Research Institute of Environmental Medicine

DEFINITION AND DOCUMENTATION

This paper reviews widely used indices of hydration status in humans. For the purposes of this review, euhydration will refer to "normal" total body water (TBW), whereas hypohydration will refer to a body water deficit. The term dehydration will be used to refer to the dynamic process of body water loss (i.e., the transition from euhydration to hypohydration) (Greenleaf and Sargent, 1965; Sawka, 1992). The term hypovolemia will define when blood volume is less than "normal."

IMPACT ON HUMAN PERFORMANCE

Both physical and cognitive performance are impaired proportionally to the magnitude of body water loss incurred (Gopinathan et al., 1988; Sawka, 1988) However, even small losses of body water (1–2 percent body mass [BM]) have a detrimental impact on physical work and negatively impact human thermoregulation (Sawka, 1988; Sawka et al., 2001). Accordingly, dehydration may be the greatest nonadversary threat to military operations.

FLUID BALANCE, DISTRIBUTION, AND EXCHANGE

Adequate hydration is essential for maintaining effective military field operations. Several common operational stresses can result in relatively large alterations in TBW content and distribution. During most normal conditions, humans have little trouble maintaining optimal fluid balance. However, many factors, such as sickness, physical exercise, climatic exposure (heat, cold, altitude), and psychological strain, can lead to significant disturbances in water balance. Perhaps the best example of this is the combination of heat stress and physical activity. For sedentary persons in temperate conditions, water requirements usually range from 2 to 4 L/day, and water balance is regulated primarily by the kidneys. For physically active persons exposed to heat stress, water requirements can often more than double (Sawka et al., 2001), and it would not be unusual for physically active, heat-stressed individuals to incur water deficits of several liters.

Water is the largest single constituent of the body (50–70 percent of body weight) and is essential for supporting the cardiovascular and thermoregulatory systems and cellular homeostasis. TBW is distributed into intracellular fluid (ICF) and extracellular fluid (ECF) compartments. The ICF and ECF contain ~ 65 percent and ~ 35 percent of TBW, respectively (Guyton et al., 1975). The ECF is further divided into the interstitial and plasma spaces. The average 75 kg male has ~ 45 L of TBW; therefore, ICF contains ~ 30 L of water, whereas the ECF contains ~ 15 L of water with ~ 3.4 L in plasma and ~ 11.6 L in the interstitium. These volumes are not static, but represent the net effect of dynamic fluid exchange and turnover between compartments (Guyton et al., 1975). Exercise heat stress not only stimulates fluid loss, primarily by sweating, but also it induces electrolyte imbalances and changes in renal function. As a result, fluid deficits with and without proportionate solute changes can occur. In addition, exercise heat stress alters transcompartmental and transcapillary forces that redistribute fluids between various compartments, organs, and tissues (Sawka et al., 2001). For these reasons, the accuracy of most methods used to assess hydration status is limited by the circumstances in which they are measured and the purposes for which they are intended.

DEHYDRATION AND MUSCLE WATER

Incomplete fluid replacement decreases total body water and, as a consequence of fluid exchange, affects each fluid space. For example, Nose and colleagues (1983) determined the distribution of body water loss among the fluid spaces as well as among different body organs during dehydration. They thermally dehydrated rats by 10 percent of body weight, and the fluid deficit was apportioned between the intracellular (41 percent) and extracellular (59 percent) spaces. The distribution of organ fluid loss was muscle (40 percent), skin (30 percent), viscera (14 percent), and bone (14 percent). However, no significant changes occurred in liver and brain water content. Nose and colleagues (1983) concluded that dehydration results in water distribution largely from the intra and extracellular spaces of muscle and skin.

The measurement of TBW is the "gold standard" to assess hydration status (Aloia et al., 1998; Lesser and Markofsky, 1979). TBW can be directly measured with doubly labeled water (DLW) or other dilution techniques. The major drawbacks of the DLW and other dilution methodologies are the cost and the technical difficulties associated with isotope analyses. The requirement for an isotope ratio mass spectrometer and sample preparation systems often limits the use of this method in most military scenarios. In addition, to obtain accurate changes in TBW with these methodologies, serial measurements are required, which further limits their use for routine assessment of TBW changes for hydration assessment. Although the choice of specific biomarker for assessing hydration status should ideally be sensitive and accurate enough to detect relatively small fluctuations in body water, the practicality of its use (time, cost, and technical expertise) is also of significant importance.

Estimates of hydration status are commonly done using (1) bioelectrical impedance analysis, (2) plasma markers and fluid regulatory hormones, (3) urine indices, (4) changes in body weight, or (5) signs and symptoms. Given consideration to military field operational use, hydration assessment measurements are presented in order of increasing assessability and practicality.

METHODS FOR HYDRATION STATUS MONITORING

Bioelectrical Impedance

Recently, bioelectric impedance (BIA) has gained attention because it is simple to use and allows rapid, inexpensive, and noninvasive estimates of TBW (O'Brien et al., 2002). In practice, a small constant current, typically 800 μA at a fixed frequency, usually 50 kHz, is passed between electrodes spanning the body. The voltage drop between these electrodes provides a measure of bioimpedance. Prediction equations, previously generated by correlating impedance measures against an independent estimate of TBW, may be used subsequently to convert a measured impedance to a corresponding estimate of TBW (Kushner et al., 1992). Absolute BIA values are well correlated with dilution TBW techniques (Kushner et al., 1992; Van Loan, 1990).

BIA does not have sufficient accuracy to assess dehydration (~ 7 percent TBW) and loses resolution with isotonic fluid loss (O'Brien et al., 2002; Van Loan, 1990). In addition, since fluid and electrolyte concentrations can have independent effects on the BIA signal, it can often provide grossly misleading values regarding hydration status (O'Brien et al., 2002). Therefore, BIA has little application for the field assessment of hydration status.

Plasma Markers

Plasma volume changes can be estimated from hemoglobin and hematocrit changes; however, accurate measurement of these variables requires considerable control for posture, arm position, skin temperature, and other factors (Sawka, 1988). If adequate controls are employed, plasma volume decreases in proportion with the level of exercise-heat mediated dehydration. Likewise, plasma volume decreases with dehydration, and this response varies due to the type of dehydration (isoosmotic or hyperosmotic), physical activity, physical fitness, and heat acclimatization status (Sawka, 1988).

Plasma osmolality is controlled around a set-point of 280–290 mOsmol/kg in euhydrated volunteers (Senay, 1979). This narrow range increases ~ 5 mOsmol/kg for every 1 to 2 percent BM of dehydration incurred (Popowski et al., 2001). Figure D-5 presents the effects of body water loss on resting plasma osmolality and plasma volume in heat acclimated persons undergoing exercise-heat mediated dehydration (Sawka and Coyle, 1999). These same levels will be maintained during subsequent physical exercise. If an isoosmotic dehydration occurs, such as with altitude or cold exposure (O'Brien et al., 1998; Sawka, 1992), then plasma osmolality changes will not follow TBW changes and much larger plasma volume reductions will occur.

Plasma sodium concentration provides an alternative to measuring osmolality (as most of the osmolality changes are usually reflective of sodium changes). However, that linear relationship may not be as strong as expected (Senay, 1979).

Osmolarity is sensed in the hypothalamus by osmoreceptors, and those neurons, in turn, stimulate the production of antidiuretic hormone. When plasma osmolarity is below threshold, the osmoreceptors are not activated and antidiuretic hormone secretion is suppressed. When osmolarity increases above the threshold for alcohol dehydrogenase release, the osmoreceptors recognize this as the cue to stimulate the neurons that secrete antidiuretic hormone. Figure D-6 shows that antidiuretic hormone concentrations rise steeply and linearly with increasing plasma osmolarity (Robertson and Athar, 1976). If hydration status changes are the result of water loss, the plasma solute concentration (osmolality) will change proportionately. However, the relationship of plasma osmolarity and vasopression concentrations is confounded by exercise, hyperthermia, nausea, and fluid volume changes (Norsk, 1996).

Aldosterone, secreted by the adrenal cortex, is a potent hormone regulating electrolyte balance. Aldosterone acts directly on the kidney to decrease the rate of sodium-ion excretion with accompanying retention of water and to increase the rate of potassium-ion excretion. Dehydration-mediated elevations in aldosterone secretion are confounded by heat acclimation status and exercise (Francesconi et al., 1983). The measurement of plasma volume, osmolality, sodium, aldosterone, and adenovirus proteinase (AVP) requires phlebotomy (invasive), technical skill, and expensive instrumentation.

Urine

Urinalysis is a frequently used clinical measure to distinguish between normal and pathological conditions. Urinary markers of hydration status include urine specific gravity (USG), urine osmolality (U_{Osmol}), and urine color. Urine specific gravity and osmolality are quantifiable and threshold values can have some value, whereas color is subjective and can be influenced by many factors. It is important to recognize that the accuracy of these urinary indices in assessing chronic hydration status is improved when the first morning urine is used,

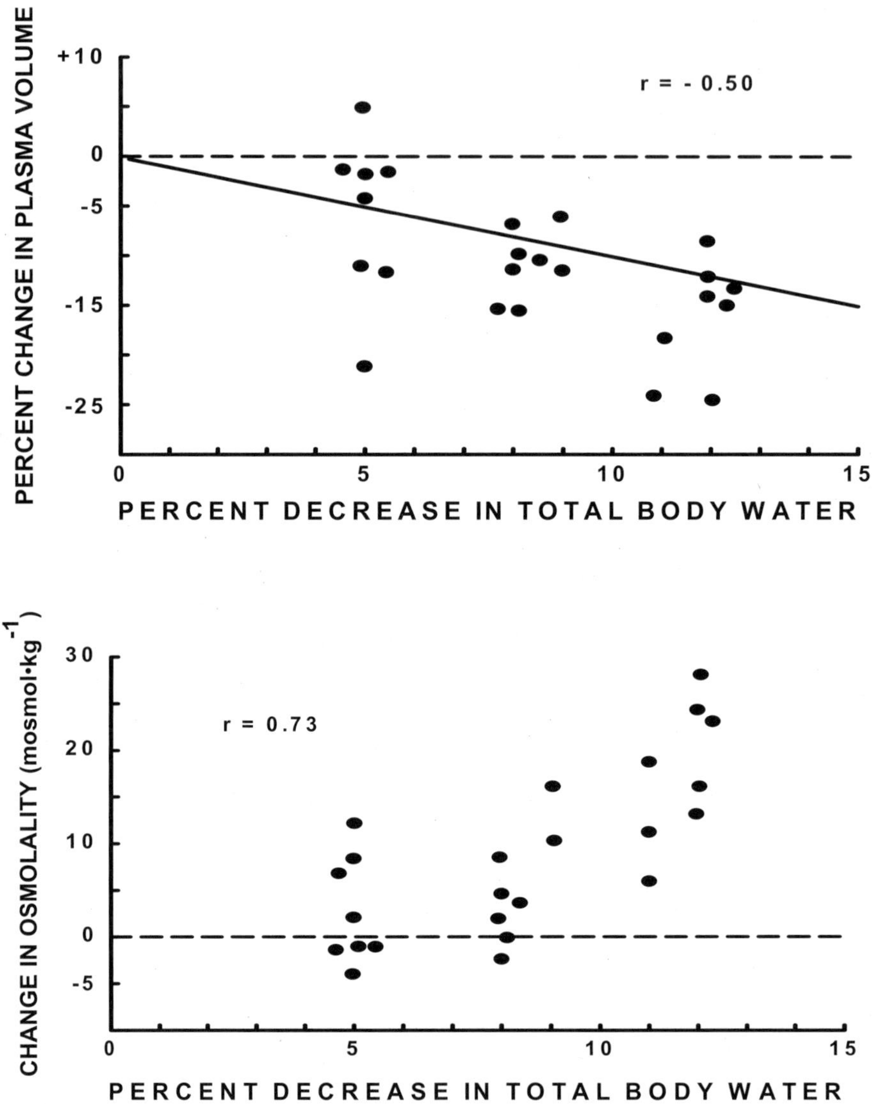

FIGURE D-5 The effects of body water loss on resting plasma osmolality and plasma volume in heat acclimated persons undergoing exercise-heat mediated dehydration. SOURCE: Reprinted, with permission Sawka and Coyle (1999). Influence of body water and blood volume on thermoregulation and exercise performance in the heat. *Exerc Sport Sci Rev* 27:167–218.

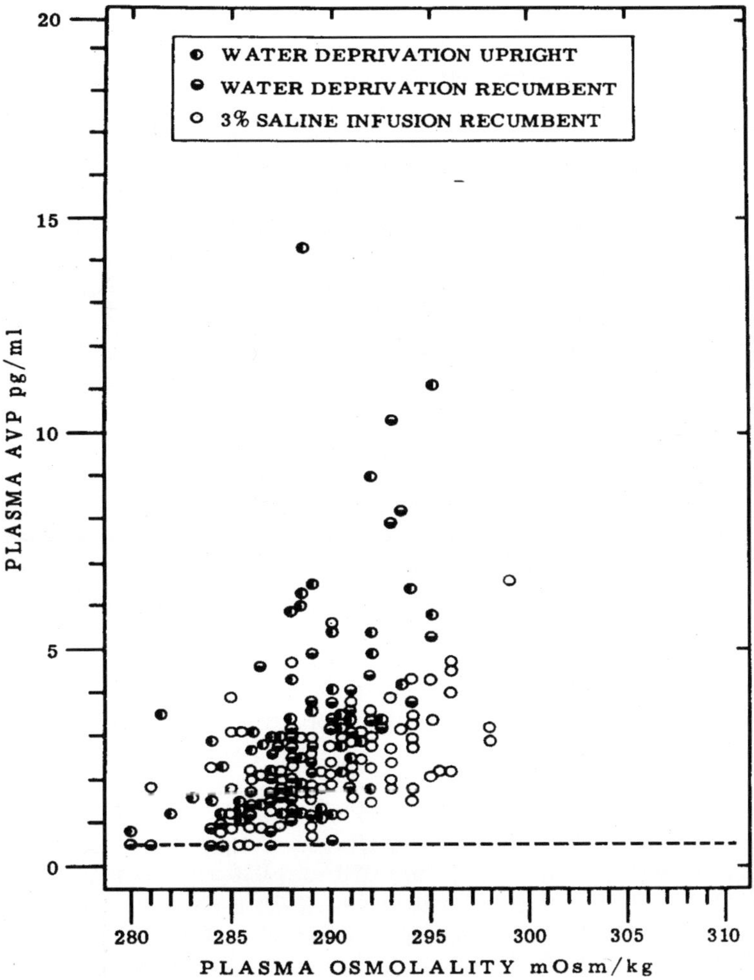

FIGURE D-6 Plasma vasopressin concentrations compared with plasma osmolarity. SOURCE: Reprinted, with permission, Robertson and Athar (1976). Copyright 1976, The Endocrine Society.

because this urine has a more uniform volume and concentration (Sanford and Wells, 1962; Shirreffs and Maughan, 1998). Likewise, many additional factors, such as diet, medications, exercise, and previous climatic exposure, can confound these indices.

The most widely used urine index is USG. Measured against water as a standard (1.000 g/ml), USG represents the concentration of particles dissolved in

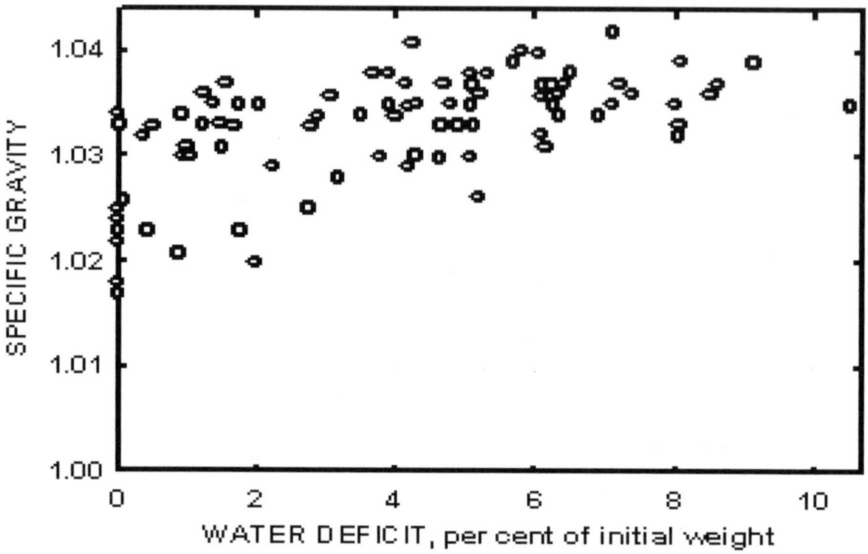

FIGURE D-7 Relation between specific gravity of urine and body water deficit.
SOURCE: Reprinted, with permission from Adolph et al. (1969).

urine and is a reflection of the kidney's ability to concentrate or dilute urine in relation to plasma. Because urine is a solution of water and various other substances, normal values range from 1.010 to 1.030 (Armstrong et al., 1994; Popowski et al., 2001; Sanford and Wells, 1962). It has been suggested that a USG of ≤ 1.020 represents a state of euhydration (Armstrong et al., 1994; Sanford and Wells, 1962). As a measure of chronic hydration status, USG appears to accurately reflect a hypohydrated state when in excess of 1.030 (Armstrong et al., 1994; Popowski et al., 2001; Sanford and Wells, 1962). However, considerable variability exists and no single value can be used to determine a specific hydration level (see Figure D-7). U_{Osmol} also can provide an approximation of hydration status (Shirreffs and Maughan, 1998) as it is highly correlated with, but more variable than, USG (Armstrong et al., 1994; Popowski et al., 2001).

Endocrine responses to dehydration stimulate water and electrolyte retention by the kidney. However, while the linear rise in plasma osmolality (with hypovolemia) that occurs with dehydration (Popowski et al., 2001) stimulates vasopressin and the tubular reabsorption of water at the kidney, the renal response lags behind changes in plasma osmolality during acute fluxes in body water (2–4 hr) brought on by dehydration-rehydration (Popowski et al., 2001). In fact, when large volumes of water are consumed, a pale-colored urine with low specific gravity is excreted long before euhydration is achieved (Shirreffs and Maughan, 1998) due to rapidly declining AVP levels triggered by the swallowing reflex. When water is consumed in excess of sweat losses during exercise, urine output increases and fluid balance is not restored unless sufficient electrolytes are also consumed (Maughan et al., 1996). Logically, U_{Osmol} is therefore also limited for assessing acute changes in body water (Kovacs et al., 1999; Popowski et al., 2001).

Body Mass

BM measurements represent the simplest technique for rapid assessment of changes in hydration status. In our laboratory, we observe very small (< 1 percent) fluctuations in first morning BM when measured over consecutive days in young men taking food and fluid ad libitum. The stability of this measurement, coupled with the known losses of fluid that occur with exercise-heat exposure (primarily eccrine sweat), allows rapid changes in BM (incurred over hours) to be correctly attributed to water loss. Acute changes in BM weight are therefore a popular and reasonable field estimate of dehydration (Cheuvront et al., 2002).

The level of dehydration is expressed as a percentage of starting body weight ($[\Delta BW/startBW] \times 100$) rather than as a percentage of TBW because TBW ranges from 50 to 70 percent of body weight. This technique assumes that (1) starting body weight represents a euhydrated state, and (2) 1 ml of sweat loss represents a 1 g change in weight (i.e., specific gravity of sweat is 1.000 g/ml). As an acute measure, first morning body weight is still limited by changes in bowel habits. Body weight is also limited as a tool for long-term assessment of hydration status since the changes in body composition (fat and lean mass) that may occur with chronic energy imbalance are also reflected grossly as changes in body weight. Clearly, the use of daily body weight should be used in combination with another hydration assessment technique to dissociate gross tissue losses from water losses if long-term hydration status is of interest.

Signs and Symptoms of Dehydration

In the early stages of dehydration, no signs or symptoms are apparent. However, as greater body water losses occur, increased thirst, increased pulse rate, and increased rectal temperature present. In addition, body-water loss of 1 to 5 percent can be associated with flushed skin, nausea, sleepiness, and reductions in economy of movement. Body-water losses of 6 to 10 percent are associated with dizziness, headache, tingling in limbs, decreased blood volume, and cyanosis. Severe dehydration, 11 to 20 percent body water, results in delirium, numb skin, deafness, and spasticity. Furthermore, death is likely as greater body-water loss occurs. Assessment of dehydration via signs and symptoms is easy and quick; however, these estimates are too imprecise to accurately

TABLE D-4 Biomarkers for Hydration Assessment

Marker	Advantages	Disadvantages
Signs and symptoms	Easy, quick	Imprecise
Total body water, dilution	Valid, reliable	Premeasurement, invasive, complex
Total body water, bioelectric impedance	Easy, rapid	Premeasurement, imprecise
Plasma volume	—	Premeasurement, invasive
Osmolality	Often valid, reliable	Imprecise
Sodium	Hyponatremia	Invasive, complex
Fluid reg. hormones	Often valid	Invasive, imprecise
Urine	Easy, rapid, screen	Invasive, sometimes confounded, complex
Saliva	Easy	Imprecise, easily confounded
Body weight	Easy, rapid	Invalid

determine hydration status. Nevertheless, if any of the signs and symptoms of dehydration present, rehydration should begin immediately.

CONCLUSIONS

Under most conditions, day-to-day BM changes (> 2 percent) and first morning urine specific gravity (> 1.030), when used together, provide an approximate indication that an individual is hypohydrated (see Table D-4). However, plasma osmolality changes can provide more reliable information regarding hydration when greater precision is required. Measurement of fluid regulatory hormones for routine hydration assessment are not necessary and are often confounding. Moreover, BIA has limited utility to assess hydration status in the field for reasons previously described. It is possible that other technological advances may allow evaluation of other measures (e.g., muscle water content) that hold promise as hydration indices.

Disclaimer: The views, opinions, and/or findings contained in this publication are those of the authors and should not be constructed as an official Department of the Army position, policy, or decision unless so designated by other documentation.

REFERENCES

Adolph EF. 1969. *Physiology of Man in the Desert*. New York: Hafner Publishing Co. P. 103.

Aloia JF, Vaswani A, Flaster E, Ma R. 1998. Relationship of body water compartments to age, race, and fat-free mass. *J Lab Clin Med* 132:483–490.

Armstrong LE, Maresh CM, Castellani JW, Bergeron MF, Kenefick RW, LaGasse KE, Riebe D. 1994. Urinary indices of hydration status. *Int J Sport Nutr* 4:265–279.

Cheuvront SN, Haymes EM, Sawka MN. 2002. Comparison of sweat loss estimates for women during prolonged high-intensity running. *Med Sci Sports Exerc* 34:1344–1350.

Francesconi RP, Sawka MN, Pandolf KB. 1983. Hypohydration and heat acclimation: Plasma renin and aldosterone during exercise. *J Appl Physiol* 55:1790–1794.

Gopinathan PM, Pichan G, Sharma VM. 1988. Role of dehydration in heat stress-induced variations in mental performance. *Arch Environ Health* 43:15–17.

Greenleaf JE, Sargent F 2nd. 1965. Voluntary dehydration in man. *J Appl Physiol* 20:719–724.

Guyton A, Taylor A, Granger H. 1975. *Circulatory Physiology II: Dynamics and Control of the Body Fluids*. Philadelphia: WB Saunders.

Kovacs EM, Senden JM, Brouns F. 1999. Urine color, osmolality and specific electrical conductance are not accurate measures of hydration status during postexercise rehydration. *J Sports Med Phys Fitness* 39:47–53.

Kushner RF, Schoeller DA, Fjeld CR, Danford L. 1992. Is the impedance index (ht2/R) significant in predicting total body water? *Am J Clin Nutr* 56:835–839.

Lesser GT, Markofsky J. 1979. Body water compartments with human aging using fat-free mass as the reference standard. *Am J Physiol* 236:R215–R220.

Maughan RJ, Leiper JB, Shirreffs SM. 1996. Restoration of fluid balance after exercise-induced dehydration: Effects of food and fluid intake. *Eur J Appl Physiol Occup Physiol* 73:317–325.

Norsk P. 1996. Role of arginine vasopressin in the regulation of extracellular fluid volume. *Med Sci Sports Exerc* 28:S36–S41.

Nose H, Morimoto T, Ogura K. 1983. Distribution of water losses among fluid compartments of tissues under thermal dehydration in the rat. *Jpn J Physiol* 33:1019–1029.

O'Brien C, Young AJ, Sawka MN. 1998. Hypohydration and thermoregulation in cold air. *J Appl Physiol* 84:185–189.

O'Brien C, Young AJ, Sawka MN. 2002. Bioelectrical impedance to estimate changes in hydration status. *Int J Sports Med* 23:361–366.

Popowski LA, Oppliger RA, Patrick Lambert G, Johnson RF, Kim Johnson A, Gisolf CV. 2001. Blood and urinary measures of hydration status during progressive acute dehydration. *Med Sci Sports Exerc* 33:747–753.

Robertson GL, Athar S. 1976. The interaction of blood osmolality and blood volume in regulating plasma vasopressin in man. *J Clin Endocrinol Metab* 42:613–620.

Sanford S, Wells B. 1962. *The Urine*. Philadephia: WB Saunders.

Sawka MN. 1988. *Body Fluid Responses and Hypohydration During Exercise-Heat Stress*. Indianapolis, IN: Cooper Publishing Group.

Sawka MN. 1992. Physiological consequences of hypohydration: Exercise performance and thermoregulation. *Med Sci Sports Exerc* 24:657–670.

Sawka MN, Coyle EF. 1999. Influence of body water and blood volume on thermoregulation and exercise performance in the heat. *Exerc Sport Sci Rev* 27:167–218.

Sawka MN, Montain SJ, Latzka WA. 2001. Hydration effects on thermoregulation and performance in the heat. *Comp Biochem Physiol A Mol Integr Physiol* 128:679–690.

Senay LC Jr. 1979. Effects of exercise in the heat on body fluid distribution. *Med Sci Sports* 11:42–48.

Shirreffs SM, Maughan RJ. 1998. Urine osmolality and conductivity as indices of hydration status in athletes in the heat. *Med Sci Sports Exerc* 30:1598–1602.

Van Loan MD. 1990. Bioelectrical impedance analysis to determine fat-free mass, total body water and body fat. *Sports Med* 10:205–217.

TECHNOLOGY FOR THE MEASUREMENT OF BLOOD LACTATE

David C. Klonoff, Mills-Peninsula Health Services

Glucose is metabolized by cells to produce energy. Glucose metabolism involves progressive oxidation plus breakage of carbon bonds. The oxidation process causes C-H and C-C bonds to be stripped of electrons (oxidized), which are then used to build adenosine triphosphate (ATP).

The initial steps in breakdown of glucose involve conversion of one 6-carbon molecule of glucose to two 3-carbon molecules of pyruvate. This process is known as glycolysis. Next, in the presence of oxygen, the carbon atoms in pyruvate are converted into three molecules of carbon dioxide in a process known as aerobic metabolism. When oxygen is available to serve as the final acceptor of electrons, then pyruvate is able to transfer electrons to the final acceptor, oxygen (or reduce), by way of a series of steps known as the Krebs cycle or the tricarboxylic acid cycle. When oxygen is totally reduced, it becomes water. Meanwhile, the carbon bonds of pyruvate all become oxidized to carbon dioxide.

Conversely, in the absence of oxygen, all the electron acceptors "downstream" from pyruvate are reduced and unable to offload electrons to mediators that will carry them toward oxygen. The carbon bonds are progressively oxidized in the Krebs cycle and the electrons' energy is drawn off in steps through a process known as oxidative phosphorylation. The process is analogous to water falling down a dam and turning turbines, and at the same time the turbines transfer energy to generators that produce electric power. The Krebs cycle is the dam, and the oxidative phosphorylation is the generator. Anaerobic metabolism is a state of water being backed up downstream so that there is no flow of water across the dam. Without oxygen, the backup of reduced substances reaches pyruvate, which cannot transfer its electrons into any chemicals within the Krebs cycle. Pyruvate itself then becomes reduced to lactate and broken down no further. The metabolic process that begins with glucose and ends with lactate is known as anaerobic metabolism. Lactate does not accumulate when oxygen is available.

Aerobic metabolism is preferable to anaerobic metabolism. More energy (defined as the number of ATP molecules generated per glucose molecule broken down) is derived from aerobic metabolism than from anaerobic metabolism. The combination of glucose ignition by way of glycolysis, the Krebs cycle, and oxidative phosphorylation in aerobic metabolism generates 36 ATP molecules per glucose molecule, whereas only two ATP molecules per glucose molecule are generated in anaerobic metabolism by glycolysis alone. When exercise is continued past the point of adequate oxygen delivery (such as during excessive training beyond the ability of cardiac output to supply adequate blood), then glucose breakdown switches from aerobic to anaerobic metabolism. Lactic acid builds up and the acid dissociates to lactate plus free hydrogen ions, which lower the pH of the blood. The acid load can damage muscles, including the heart, or even kill.

Currently, technology exists for portable monitoring of lactate to monitor people who are exercising heavily, such as athletes or soldiers in training. The technology is exclusively invasive and intermittent. Unlike the situation with portable monitoring of blood glucose, in which new monitors with advanced features are regularly introduced, there are only two portable lactate monitors on the market. No portable lactate monitors currently exist or are close to existing that are minimally invasive or noninvasive (only invasive), implanted (only external), continuous (only intermittent), or optical (only chemical).

The molecular weight of lactic acid is 90, while that of glucose is 180. Resting blood lactic acid concentrations normally range from 0.5 to 2.0 mmol/L, which are approximately one-fourth those of blood glucose. During anaerobic exercise, lactic acid levels may increase five- to tenfold up to 12 mmol/L.

Blood lactate levels can be used to determine the optimal workload for an athlete in training. Below the optimal workload, glucose metabolism is aerobic. At some point when the workload increases, the body's ability to supply increasing amounts of oxygen to working muscles becomes limited. This is the lactate threshold, or the workload whereby lactate levels no longer rise slowly with increasing exertion, but instead rise rapidly. At the lactate threshold, glucose metabolism begins to be anaerobic as well as aerobic. At the inflection point of the curve in which lactate concentration is plotted against workload, it is best for athletes to decrease their amount of exertion to get back to or just below the lactate threshold. For a given individual, over a short term, heart rate is proportionate to workload, and heart rate is much easier to measure than workload. To identify the optimal workload at which lactate is cleared approximately as fast as it is produced (without accumulation), an athlete's lactate level can be measured and plotted against varying heart rates.

With improved cardiovascular function (i.e., increased fitness), the heart can deliver sufficient oxygen to maintain aerobic metabolism for progressively greater workloads. Conversely, with deconditioning, at progressively lower workloads, the lactate threshold is met. Therefore, for an athlete in training, determination of the lactate threshold (expressed as a workload level or a heart rate) indicates (1) the state of fitness (proportionate to the lactate threshold workload), and (2) the optimal work load at which to exercise whereby the workload is challenging, but potentially dangerous lactic acidosis can be avoided. Knowledge of the optimal workload is useful for an athlete in training, such as a soldier, to optimize the exercise regimen.

The lactate threshold can be calculated by performing a series of workouts at varying workloads that can be estimated by the heart rates associated with these workloads. The strategy involves initially exercising well beyond the lactate threshold to build up the blood lactate level, then decreasing the exercise to allow the lactate level to fall, and finally increasing the workload slightly to a point where the lactate level starts to rise once again. That point where lactate generation exceeds lactate clearance is the lactate threshold. The specific steps of how to calculate the lactate threshold are as follows: First is the lactate buildup phase, consisting of three 6-minute workouts (easy, medium, and hard), followed by a blood lactate measurement. Second is the lactate clearance phase, consisting initially of a 5-minute workout at a heart rate of 40 beats per minute below that of the workout rate, followed by a blood lactate measurement. The 5-minute workout should be repeated at a greater workload defined as a heart rate of 10 beats per minute higher and the blood lactate should be rechecked. Then the workout and lactate measurement should be repeated each time with a heart rate of 5 beats per minute more. Initially, the blood lactate will fall from that of the heavy exercise peak value, but with increasing workloads, the blood lactate level will begin to rise. The point where lactate production comes to exceed clearance is the lactate threshold.

Lactate monitors can be classified by size and there are three types: First are portable handheld monitors that are good for monitoring athletes and workers in the field. These include the Accusport/Accutrend (two different names for the same monitor), manufactured by Roche Diagnostics of Germany, and the Lactate Pro, manufactured by Ankray of Japan. Second, there are small bench-top monitors that can run on batteries and are only slightly mobile. These include the Little Champion monitor, manufactured by Analox and the YSI 1500 Sport Lactate Analyzer. These devices are somewhat cumbersome to use in the field, but can be so used if the instrument is fairly stationary. There are several bench-top lactate monitors that are used for hospital and research purposes. These devices are not suitable for studying athletes outdoors, but can be used within an indoor training facility. They include the Analox Champion Lactate Analyzer, the YSI 2300 and 2700 Glucose plus Lactate Analyzers, the Kodak Ektachem DT60, and the Eppendorf Biosen 5130.

The portable lactate monitors resemble the blood glucose monitors of the late 1980s in their ease of use. The Accusport/Accutrend requires 20 μL of blood and 60 seconds of measuring time. The Lactate Pro requires 5 μL of blood and 50 seconds of measuring time. Neither monitor is approved for alternate site testing, and no portable lactate monitor has been developed for minimally invasive or noninvasive lactate testing and none has been developed for implantable, continuous, or optical lactate sensing.

If the need for faster and more convenient lactate measurement of soldiers, athletes, or other workers in the field is evident, then there is room for development of faster, more convenient lactate monitors using smaller volumes of blood. Because lactate has a structure similar to glucose, a goal for manufacturers of lactate monitors could be to produce lactate monitors as user-friendly as portable glucose monitors. There is an untapped potential for measuring lactate in more groups of exercising people and a need for better instruments to perform the monitoring.

UTILITY OF INSULIN-LIKE GROWTH FACTOR-I FOR ASSESSING METABOLIC STATUS DURING MILITARY OPERATIONAL STRESS

Bradley C. Nindl, Scott J. Montain, U.S. Army Research Institute of Environmental Medicine

MILITARY RELEVANCE OF MONITORING INSULIN-LIKE GROWTH FACTOR-I

Mission success in military tactical environments dictate that the warfighter be able to perform prolonged physical exertion in the face of food and sleep restriction (i.e., military operational stress). The physiological strain produced by these operational stressors can have deleterious effects on muscle mass, endocrine and metabolic function, as well as physical and mental performance (Friedl, 1999; Friedl et al., 2000; Nindl et al., 1997, 2002, 2003a, 2003b) (see Figure D-8). A goal of the U.S. Army Medical Research and Materiel Command's biomedical research program is to identity useful biomarkers that are indicative of nutritional and physiological status that can be assessed rapidly, with minimally or noninvasive collection methods. Once identified, these biomarkers could potentially be used to sustain warfighter readiness and aid in assessing the effectiveness of intervention and recovery strategies.

The growth hormone/insulin-like axis is a central endocrine axis and is thought to mediate many of the somatotropic changes that are observed when

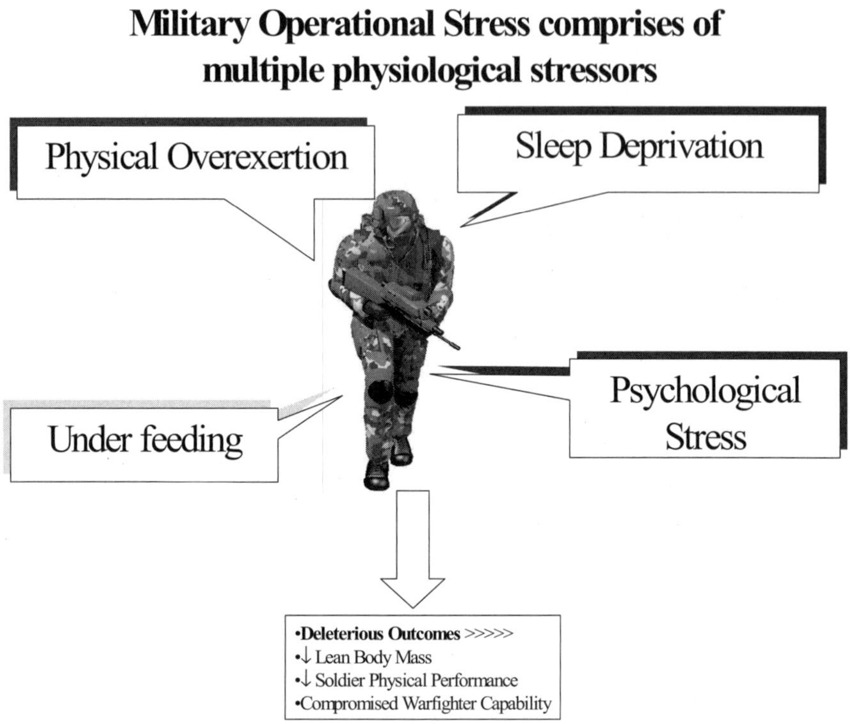

FIGURE D-8 Military operations place multiple stressors on the warfighter. These stressors typically occur simultaneously. The magnitude of the resulting strain is dependent on the severity of the stressors. The resulting physiological stain can result in deleterious outcomes on lean body mass ans soldier physical performance, and it can compromise warfighter readiness.

warfighters are exposed to harsh field environments (Florini et al., 1996; Friedl et al., 2000; Nindl et al., 2003a; Rosen, 1999; Rosendal et al., 2002). For this reason, periodic assessment of the growth hormone/insulin-like growth factor axis may have utility for sustaining warfighter health and performance. In direct support of the Objective Force Warrior's vision of revolutionizing soldier performance by aggressively employing science and technology efforts that enhance the warfighter's survivability, lethality, sustainment, and mobility on the modern battlefield, The Military Performance and Military Nutrition Division of the U.S. Army Research of Institute of Environmental Medicine have been evaluating insulin-like growth factor I (IGF-I) as a candidate biomarker for assessing nutritional stress. Our research has focused on (1) characterizing temporal response patterns of IGF-I and its family of binding proteins during military operational stress, (2) the influence of macronutrient and energy intake on the circulating IGF-I system responses to stress, and (3) assessment of minimally invasive and field expedient collections methods for determination of IGF-I.

The purpose of this short review paper is to summarize why IGF-I has been of interest as a potential biomarker and our experimental strategies for evaluating the merits of IGF-I as a biomarker of nutritional and operational stress. This paper initially describes the complex nature of IGF-I regulation and relevance for the military, then the initial work characterizing the IGF-I response to military operational stress. The experimental outcomes suggest that IGF-I has potential value as a biomarker of nutritional strain during operational stress.

INSULIN-LIKE GROWTH FACTOR-I PHYSIOLOGY AND REGULATORY COMPLEXITY

The primary source of circulating IGF-I is the liver, but local release from tissues that secrete IGF-I in an autocrine/paracrine manner also contribute. IGF-I itself is a 7.6-kDa polypeptide consisting of 70 amino acids with three intrachain disulfide bonds. Only a small amount (< 2 percent) of IGF-I, however, circulates in free form. Most circulates in either a binary (~ 20–25 percent) or ternary complex (~ 75 percent). When circulating in the binary form, IGF-I is complexed with one of six binding proteins (BPs 1–6), ranging in size from 22.8 to 31.4 kDa (see Figure D-9). The ternary complex consists of IGF-I, IGF BP-3, and an 80-86 kDa protein called the acid labile subunit (Baxter, 2000; Jones and Clemmons, 1995; Rajaram et al., 1997; Sara and Hall, 1990). An IGF-I specific protease is responsible for breaking the bonds holding the ternary complex together and making the IGF-I available for receptor binding. The IGF-I complexes are thought to regulate the availability of IGF-I to target tissues only the free and binary complexes can pass from the vascular compartment into the interstitial space. The different forms of BPs are also thought to play a role in transporting the IGF-I to the target tissue (Baxter, 2000; Sara and Hall, 1990).

IGF-I has several metabolic effects. It is known to promote amino acid uptake, enhance protein synthesis, and attenuate protein degradation (Florini et al., 1996; Rosen, 1999; Thissen et al., 1999). Additionally, IGF-I plays a role in stimulating cell growth and differentiation (Baxter, 2000; Florini et al., 1996).

The appeal of IGF-I as a biomarker is the dynamic nature in which circulating concentrations respond to nutritional stress. Underfeeding and protein-calorie malnutrition result in substantial reductions in IGF-I concentrations, and the response persists until the nutritional stress is removed (Friedl et al., 2000; Frystyk et al., 1999; Nindl et al., 2003a; Rand et al., 2003; Thissen et al., 1992, 1999). Additionally, IGF-I concentrations are relatively stable. Unlike hormones such as growth hormone, IGF-I displays little in the way of circadian variability, thus single time point samples are indicative of IGF-I status.

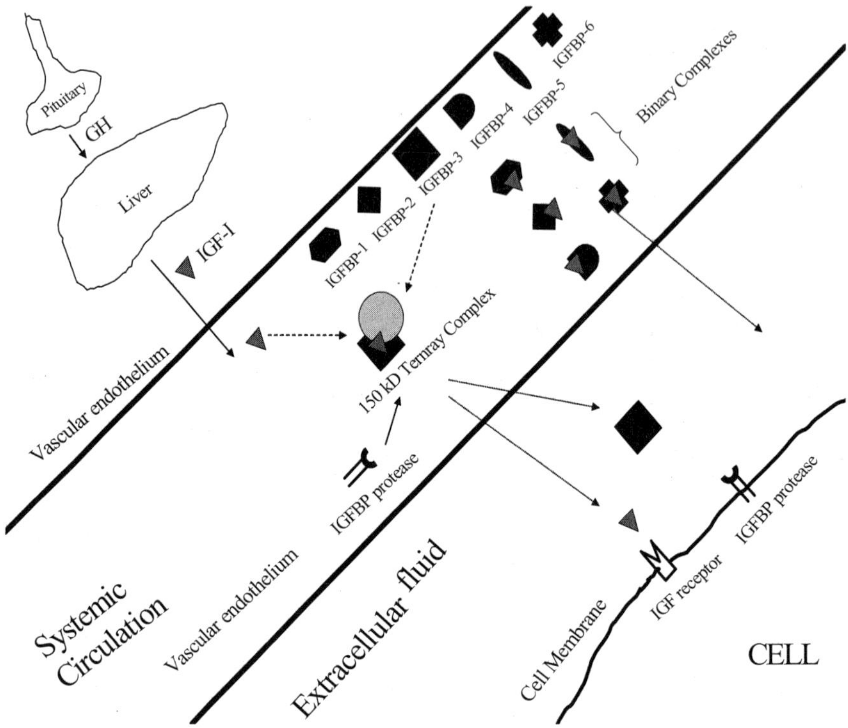

FIGURE D-9 Schematic of the IGF-I system showing the origin of release (i.e., liver), its family of binding proteins (BPs 1-6), ternary and binary complexes, and IGF-I trafficking from the circulation to the receptor.

EFFECTS OF MILITARY OPERATIONAL STRESS ON THE CIRCULATING IGF-I SYSTEM

U.S. Army Ranger Training

Friedl and colleagues performed experimental studies characterizing the physiological responses of soldiers participating in the U.S. Army Ranger Training Course (Friedl et al., 1994, 2000; Nindl et al., 1997). The data provide insight into the adaptive process that occurs as soldiers cope with sustained physical work, energy restriction, and sleep disruption. The U.S. Army Ranger training course is 62 days and is designed to teach and evaluate individual leadership and small-unit tactics under physically and mentally challenging conditions. The course includes multiday periods consisting of near-continuous physical activity, energy restriction and sleep deprivation. In the first investigation, energy intake was restricted to 1,300 kcal/day during the field-training portion

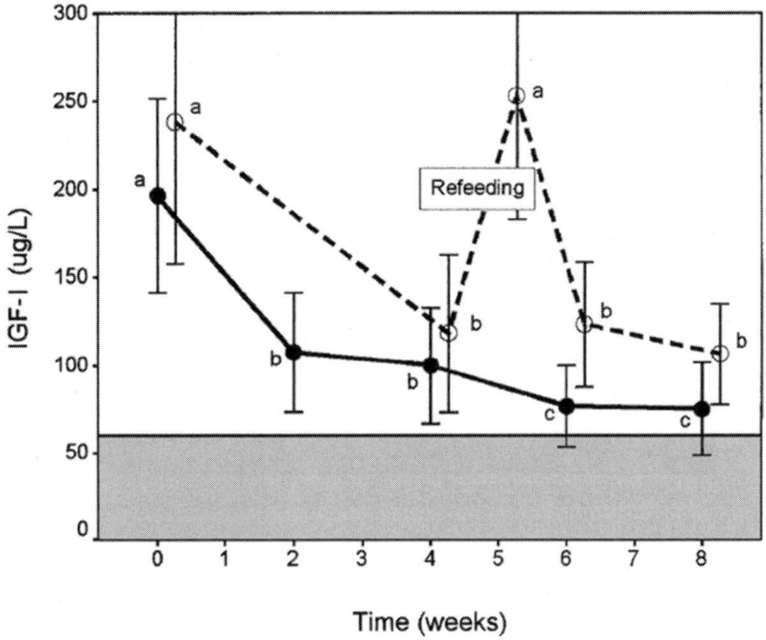

FIGURE D-10 Serum IGF-I concentrations over the 8-week U.S. Army Ranger Training Course. The solid lines represent the values from Study 1 and the dotted line represents the values from Study 2. Study 1 and Study 2 were conducted under identical conditions with the exception that during Study 2, the subjects received 400 more kcal/day than those in Study 1. Values are mean ± standard deviation. Different letters represent mean values that are statistically different; the shaded area represents values below normal for young men.
SOURCE: Reprinted, with permission Friedl et al. *JAP* (2000).

of the course, and the periods of underfeeding produced average energy deficits of ~ 1,000 kcal/day over the entire course (Friedl et al., 2000). Average energy expenditures were ~ 4,000 kcal/day. At the end of the course, the participants had lost 13 to 16 percent of their initial body mass, ~ 65 percent of their fat mass, and 7 percent of their initial lean body mass. IGF-I, measured every 2 weeks during the Training Course, progressively declined through the first 6 weeks, with no further reduction over the final 2 weeks of the course (Figure D-10). At the end of the course, IGF-I values had fallen 62 percent (pre: 198 ± 54 ng/mL^{-1} vs. post: 75 ± 25 ng/mL^{-1}). As Figure D-10 illustrates, most of the decrease in serum IGF-I occurred during the initial 2 weeks of the course. The potential of IGF-I as a discriminating variable for assessing nutritional and/or metabolic stress was the separate observation that the soldiers who had the greatest decline in IGF-I were those that lost the most weight ($r = -0.38$, $P < 0.01$).

A second study with the U.S. Army Ranger Training Course enabled investigators to study the effects of altering the energy content of the diet on the metabolic and hormonal responses to the course (Friedl et al., 2000). In the second study, the training conditions were nearly identical, but the participants received additional calories during the energy restriction periods embedded within the course (+ 400 kcal/day). Additionally, to gain information about short-term responses to refeeding (while other course stressors remained undiminished), a blood sample was obtained after a week of access to food that was preceded by multiple days of energy restriction (~ 1,700 kcal/day) coupled with high-energy expenditures (> 4,500 kcal/day). As illustrated in Figure D-10, the addition of 400 kcal/day significantly attenuated the decline in circulating IGF-I concentrations when compared with the group receiving fewer calories. Additionally, the investigators found that the brief period of refeeding was sufficient to temporarily restore IGF-I concentrations to baseline values. When food was again restricted after this brief refeeding period, IGF-I concentrations rapidly fell and remained low through the remainder of the course. These data demonstrate the sensitivity and responsiveness of IGF-I to energy and nutrient delivery. When energy is restricted, IGF-I values fall and remain low until energy restriction is removed. The provision of energy and the restoration of fuel stores are accompanied by an increase in IGF-I.

The traditional evaluation of nutritional status uses a global assessment of parameters that include anthropometric measures and the assay of serum proteins (Baxter et al., 1998). The proteins commonly measured include albumin, transferrin, prealbumin, and retinol binding protein. Transferrin is indicative of iron binding capability; retinol binding protein is indicative of vitamin A status and ability to transport vitamin A, prealbumin (considered by some to be best single marker of malnutrition due to its short half-life) is sensitive to protein malnutrition and zinc deficiency. The strength of these markers is that they provide insight into the nutritional status of the individual. Unfortunately, a number of non-nutritional factors can affect serum levels independent of dietary adequacy. For example, prealbumin levels fall with inflammation, albumin levels are affected by hydration state and oral contraceptive use, transferrin levels decline in response to protein malnutrition and with chronic illness and inflammatory states and liver disease. In contrast, IGF-I appears to be a more responsive and selective biomarker of energy status due to its rapid response to depletion and repletion (Baxter et al., 1998). The 2- to 4-hour half-life of IGF-I provides a distinct advantage versus other traditional serum protein biomarkers (prealbumin, ~ 2 days; albumin, 20 days; transferrin, 20 days).

In a study examining endocrine and metabolic recovery responses, Nindl and colleagues (1997) measured IGF-I, transferrin, ferritin, and prealbumin before and at the end of the U.S. Army Ranger Training Course and after 5 weeks of recovery. The 5-week recovery period produced a rebound effect such that body mass was significantly higher than measured before starting the course. Body composition analysis revealed a 1.1-kg increase in fat-free mass and a 4.1-kg increase in fat mass above precourse values. IGF-I fell ~ 50 percent during the course and was 30 percent above baseline values after 5 weeks of recovery. Transferrin levels did not significantly change during Ranger training or during recovery. Prealbumin levels declined 21 percent during the course (26.8–21.3 mg/dL) and returned to baseline levels during the recovery period, but the levels at the end of the course (despite accruing an 11 percent body-mass loss) were well above values indicative of malnutrition (< 15 mg/dL). Thus, in this study, IGF-I appeared more sensitive to changes in energy balance and body composition changes than the other markers of nutritional status.

Short-Term Military-Sustained Operations

To study the acute responses to energy and nutrient restriction, Nindl and colleagues (2003a) recently measured the circulating IGF-I and IGF binding proteins pattern of response to 4 days of near-continuous physical work, energy restriction, and sleep disruption. The participants had morning fasted blood drawn on days 1, 3, and 4 during a control week that contained physical performance testing but no sustained physical activity, caloric restriction, or sleep deprivation. They also had blood samples drawn on days 1, 3, and 4 of the experimental period that included the physical performance tests, near-continuous physical activity (energy expenditure ~ 4,500 kcal/day), energy restriction (~ 1,600 kcal/day), and sleep deprivation (6.2 ± 1.1 hours over an 84-hour course). Blood was assayed for concentrations of total IGF-I, free IGF-I, IGFBPs 1, 3, and 6, and the acid-labile subunit. Additionally, in order to gain further insight into whether this type of stress altered the partitioning of IGF-I among its various molecular complexes, IGF-I and IGFBP-3 were measured before and after immunoaffinity depletion of acid-labile subunit complex (i.e., ternary complex removal), thus yielding estimates of ternary (high-molecular weight complexes) versus nonternary (low-molecular weight complexes) IGF-I (Khosravi et al., 2000). Two days of military operational stress significantly lowered circulating total and free IGF-I values, and they remained low with continued operational stress (Nindl et al., 2003a). Accompanying the IGF-I reductions were small reductions in IGFBP-3 and large increases in IGFBP-1. These changes in circulating IGFBP levels, however, were not associated with a measurable shift in the quantity of IGF-I circulating in ternary, binary, or free forms (Nindl et al., 2003a). The importance of these data for metabolic monitoring is that they show the speed with which the IGF-I system responds to energy and/or nutritional restriction. They also illustrate a potential method for investigating changes in the bioavailable IGF-I in response to nutritional stress.

Influence of Dietary Protein Content of Circulating IGF-I During Military Training

Both energy restriction and protein-energy malnutrition are known to suppress circulating IGF-I. There are many logistical challenges to sustaining adequate nourishment for soldiers during military field training (e.g., food preparation, storage, and delivery, and meals that provide adequate levels of calories and macro- and micronutrients). With increased operational tempo of current military maneuvers, space allocation for food is often sacrificed for weapons, ammunition, and other necessary field gear. It would therefore seem essential that the nutrients that are provided during military operational stress consist of an optimal macronutrient mix that may protect against the decline in circulating anabolic and growth factors (Friedl, 1999). The Recommended Dietary Allowance (RDA) for protein is 0.8 g/kg body mass. Current recommendations for physically active populations are 1.2 to 1.5 g protein/kg body mass (Fielding and Parkington, 2002; Rand et al., 2003). It is common for infantry type units to subsist on one to two Meals Ready-to-Eat (MRE) per day during field operations. The MRE is a 1,300-kcal ration comprising of 24 menus. Protein content of the ration ranges from 26 to 60 g with a mean value of 44 g. Thus, if soldiers are limited to one MRE per day, their diet is low in both energy and protein content. Even consuming two MREs per day, soldiers may still not meet the minimal RDA for protein.

To examine the hypothesis that dietary protein supplementation during military operational stress would attenuate the decline in IGF-I observed when units were fed insufficient energy and protein, we recently conducted a study during which dietary protein was manipulated, while controlling both carbohydrate and energy intake. Thirty-five Marines were randomly divided into either a group receiving a low energy-low protein diet (1,600 kcal/day and 0.5 g protein/kg body mass/day) or a group receiving a similar amount of energy but with sufficient added protein to receive approximately 1.0 g protein/kg body mass/day. The group was participating in an 8-day field exercise consisting of sustained physical activity (total daily energy expenditure measured in previous iterations has ranged from 17–25 MJ/day) and sleep deprivation. Morning fasted blood was obtained before, midway, and at the end of the course. Preliminary results show trends suggesting that protein supplementation may have attenuated the decline in IGF-I during the course. If a more thorough examination of the data supports this conclusion, these data would provide further support for the merit of monitoring IGF-I as a biomarker for metabolic status. Another observation from this study was that IGF-I displayed a different temporal pattern in response to the course than other conventional nutritional status indicators (e.g. ferritin, prealbumin, transferrin, and retinol binding protein). Transferrin and ferritin initially increased during the course but reversed towards baseline values during the latter half of the course, whereas retinol binding protein and prealbumin declined over the course, but more abruptly during the latter half. Thus, while both IGF-I and the conventional markers responded to the training stress, their differential response suggests that they each provide a different index of nutritional status.

Measurement of IGF-I with a Filter Paper Blood Spot Assay

If IGF-I is to be used as a metabolic status indicator during military operational stress, field-expedient methods for collection and measurement must be established. Field environments present unique logistical challenges compared with the laboratory. There is more likelihood of sample contamination, and since it is difficult and sometimes impossible to bring the laboratory equipment to remote field environments, sample collection, processing, and transportation become significant logistical hurdles.

A technique that has been used successfully to study malnutrition in underdeveloped countries is chemical analysis of dried blood spots (Diamandi et al., 1998; Mitchell et al., 1987). The technique requires minimal amounts of blood, minimal field processing, and no refrigeration during shipping. Mitchell and colleagues (1987) originally described measurement of IGF-I from blood spots using a conventional radioimmunoassay. More recently, Diamandi and colleagues (1998) described the extraction and measurement of IGF-I and IGFBP-3 from dried blood spots using an enzyme-linked immunoabsorbent assay.

To study whether the dried blood spot methodology could track IGF-I responses to military operational stress, both blood spots and conventional blood samples were collected in a recent field study that manipulated dietary protein intake (described above). We found that IGF-I measured from blood spots declined during the 8-day course and the magnitude of decline was similar to the decline measured using serum samples (Figure D-11) (Nindl et al., 2003b). Overall, the blood spot IGF-I and serum IGF-I significantly ($p < 0.05$) correlated ($r = 0.92$), but the blood spot values were on average 61 percent lower than serum (Nindl et al., 2003b). Diamandi and colleagues (1998) also reported lower (20–25 percent) IGF-I values from blood spots when compared with plasma samples. Several possible factors could have contributed to the differences in IGF-I using the two sampling techniques. First, in order to reduce preanalytical variance and ensure maximal extraction, it is essential that complete dryness of the blood spot is maintained until the sample is analyzed. In both our study and that of Diamandi and colleagues (1998), the blood spots were stored in plastic bags without addition of desiccant. Work by others suggests that moisture can produce a glassing effect whereby hygroscopic blood proteins impede elution. Assaying dried blood spots also assumes that an absolute and consistent blood volume is distributed onto each punch. If the volume of blood on filter paper was consistently overestimated, it may have contributed to the bias between the two sampling methods as IGF-I was purposefully measured using different assays. Regardless of the reason for the bias, the outcomes of this study reveal that the blood spot on filter paper technique can be applied for measurement of IGF-I

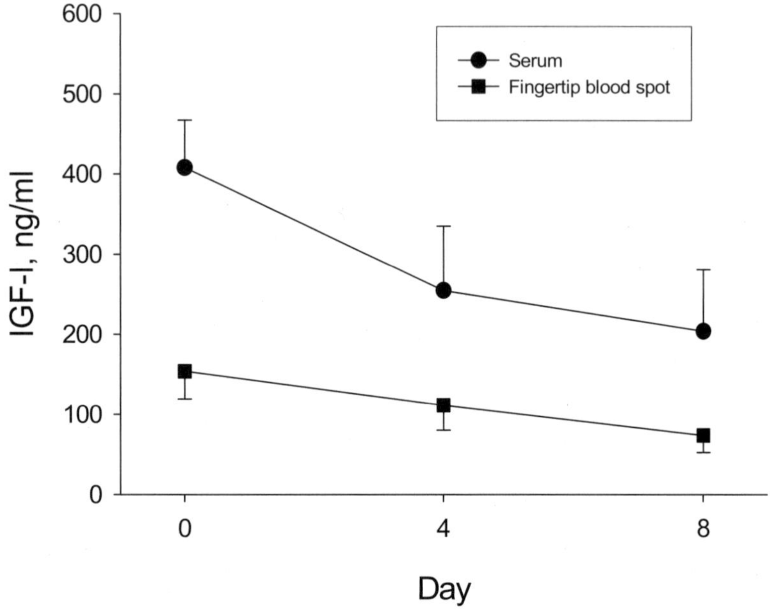

FIGURE D-11 Comparison between serum and filter paper blood spot IGF-I concentration during days 0, 4, and 8 of military operational stress. For both methods, a progressive decline over time was observed (day 0 > day 4 > day 8). Serum IGF-I was greater than filter paper blood spot IGF-I at each respective time point.
SOURCE: Reprinted, with permission Nindl et al. (2003b).

responses to military operational stress. The technique requires minimal blood and minimal equipment assets for sample collection, processing, and shipment. The filter paper blood spot method for IGF-I detected reductions accompanying nutritional stress and may be of potential value for characterizing the IGF-I response when conventional blood sampling methods are not feasible.

Future Directions and Enablers for the Objective Force Warrior

The data collected on the physiological responses to military operational stress support the potential utility of IGF-I as a metabolic sensor of energy status. IGF-I declines rapidly to energy restriction and remains a viable indicator of an altered energy state until the stressor is removed. IGF-I is sensitive to

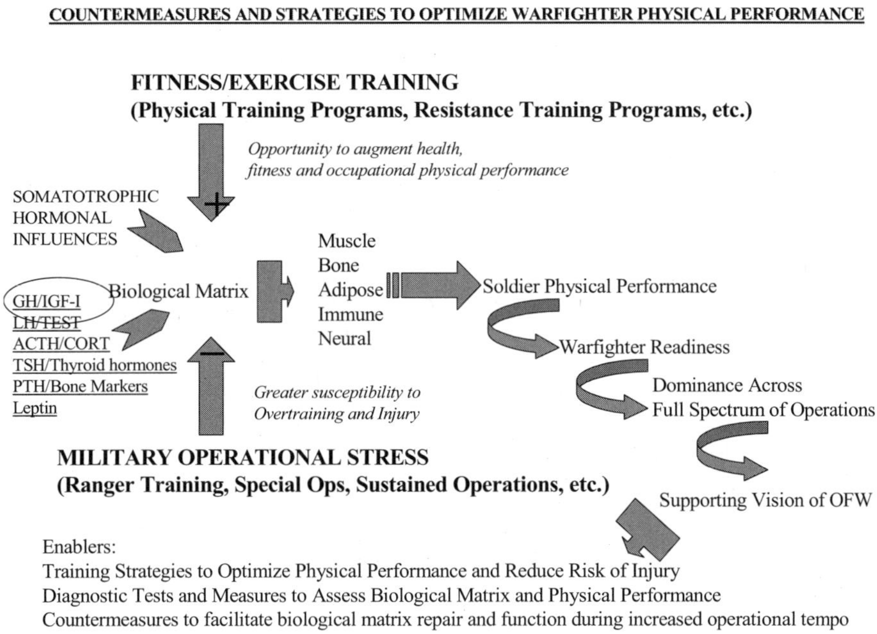

FIGURE D-12 A conceptual model depicting how a better understanding of somatotropic hormonal mediators may benefit soldier physical performance and support the vision of the Objective Force Warrior (OFW). Soldiers are exposed to rigorous physical training and military operational stress. These influences can either positively or negatively affect the body's biological matrix. Changes in the biological matrix can affect soldier physical performance (e.g., declines in muscle mass will inhibit strength and power). Soldier physical performance directly contributes to warfighter readiness and dominance across the full spectrum of operations. Monitoring insulin-like growth factor-I (IGF-I) may have great utility for assessing physical training, evaluating recovery strategies, and sustaining performance during operational stress.

dietary changes and can be used to evaluate adequacy of protein intake independent of energy intake. Future work, however, must establish whether IGF-I alone or in combination with other biological indices can provide useful information to preserve the health and performance of military personnel during operational stress (Friedl, 2003). In addition, sampling and processing techniques must be established that are safe and reliable that require minimal logistical support and, most important, provide rapid feedback to personnel tracking physiological status.

While this review has exclusively focused on the use of IGF-I measurement during military operational stress, IGF-I may also have merit as a biomarker during fitness and exercise training. Continued scientific efforts should focus on further elucidating the link between alterations in the biological matrix (e.g., muscle, bone, adipose, immune, and neural cells) and ensuing influences on soldier physical performance. A provocative hypothesis is that any changes in the biological matrix are mediated by somatotropic hormonal responses that act in both systemic and local mechanisms (Nindl et al., 2001, 2002). A greater understanding of the somatotropic influences mediating muscle repair and bone remodeling after the microtrauma of physical exertion and viable countermeasures that modulate muscle repair and tissue regeneration after microdamage is essential toward the transformation of the modern Army through Objective Force Warrior (see Figure D-12). To maintain dominance across the full spectrum of military operations, the twenty-first century warfighter must posses an optimal level of physical readiness and be able to recover quickly from fatigue and overexertion. IGF-I is emerging as a truly important regulator that is important to health and fitness. IGF-I is a promising outcome measure during altered energy states for military studies on the refinement of medical fitness standards, as well as on physical training and nutrition policies.

REFERENCES

Baxter RC. 2000. Insulin-like growth factor (IGF)-binding proteins: Interactions with IGFs and intrinsic bioactivities. *Am J Physiol Endocrinol Metab* 278:E967–E976.

Baxter RC, Hawker FH, To C, Stewart PM, Holman SR. 1998. Thirty-day monitoring of insulin-like growth factors and their binding proteins in intensive care unit patients. *Growth Horm IGF Res* 8:455–463.

Diamandi A, Khosravi MJ, Mistry J, Martinez V, Guevara-Aguirre J. 1998. Filter paper blood spot assay of human insulin-like growth factor I (IGF-I) and IGF-binding protein-3 and preliminary application in the evaluation of growth hormone status. *J Clin Endocrinol Metab* 83:2296–2301.

Fielding RA, Parkington J. 2002. What are the dietary protein requirements of physically active individuals? New evidence on the effects of exercise on protein utilization during post-exercise recovery. *Nutr Clin Care* 5:191–196.

Florini JR, Ewton DZ, Coolican SA. 1996. Growth hormone and the insulin-like growth factor system in myogenesis. *Endocr Rev* 17:481–517.

Friedl KE. 1999. Protein and amino acids: Physiological optimization for current and future military operational scenarios. In: *The Role of Protein and Amino Acids in Sustaining and Enhancing Performance.* Washington, DC: National Academy Press. Pp. 85–91.

Friedl KE. 2003. Insulin-like growth factor-I—A metabolic marker representing quality of life? *Diabetes Technol Ther* 5:463–465.

Friedl KE, Moore RJ, Martinez-Lopez LE, Vogel JA, Askew EW, Marchitelli LJ, Hoyt RW, Gordon CC. 1994. Lower limit of body fat in healthy active men. *J Appl Physiol* 77:933–940.

Friedl KE, Moore RJ, Hoyt RW, Marchitelli LJ, Martinez-Lopez LE, Askew EW. 2000. Endocrine markers of semistarvation in healthy lean men in a multistressor environment. *J Appl Physiol* 88:1820–1830.

Frystyk J, Delhanty PJD, Skjaerbaek C, Baxter RC. 1999. Changes in the circulating IGF system during short-term fasting and refeeding in rats. *Am J Physiol* 277:E245–E252.

Jones JI, Clemmons DR. 1995. Insulin-like growth factors and their binding proteins: Biological actions. *Endocrine Rev* 16:3–34.

Khosravi MJ, Diamandi A, Mistry J. 2000. Non-ternary complex IGF-I, IGF-II, and IGFBP-3 in normal, growth hormone deficient (GHD) and acromegalic subjects. In: *Program and Abstracts Book*. The Endocrine Society 82nd Annual Meeting. Chevy Chase, MD: The Endocrine Society. P. 483.

Mitchell ML, Hermos RJ, Moses AC. 1987. Radioimmunoassay of somatomedin-C in filter paper discs containing dried blood spots. *Clin Chem* 33:536–538.

Nindl BC, Friedl KE, Frykman PN, Marchitelli LJ, Shippee RL, Patton JF. 1997. Physical performance and metabolic recovery among lean, healthy men following a prolonged energy deficit. *Int J Sports Med* 18:317–324.

Nindl BC, Kraemer WJ, Marx JO, Arciero PJ, Dohi K, Kellogg MD, Loomis GA. 2001. Overnight responses of the circulating IGF-I system after acute, heavy-resistance exercise. *J Appl Physiol* 90:1319–1326.

Nindl BC, Leone CD, Tharion WJ, Johnson RF, Castellani JW, Patton JF, Montain SJ. 2002. Physical performance responses during 72 hrs of military operational stress. *Med Sci Sports Exerc* 34:1814–1822.

Nindl BC, Castellani JW, Young AJ, Patton JF, Khosravi MJ, Diamandi A, Montain SJ. 2003a. Differential responses of IGF-I molecular complexes to military operational field training. *J Appl Physiol* 95:1083–1089.

Nindl BC, Kellog MD, Khosravi MJ, Diamandi A, Alemany JA, Pietila DM, Young AJ, Montain SJ. 2003b. Measurement of insulin-like growth factor-I during military operational stress via a filter paper blood spot assay. *Diabetes Technol Ther* 5:455–461.

Rajaram S, Baylink DJ, Mohan S. 1997. Insulin-like growth factor-binding proteins in serum and other biological fluids: Regulation and functions. *Endocr Rev* 18:801–831.

Rand WM, Pellet PL, Young VR. 2003. Meta-analysis of nitrogen balance studies for estimating protein requirements in healthy adults. *Am J Clin Nutr* 77:109–127.

Rosen C. 1999. Serum insulin-like growth factors and insulin-like growth factor-binding proteins: Clinical implications. *Clin Chem* 45:1384–1390.

Rosendal L, Langberg H, Flyvbjerg A, Frystyk J, Orskov H, Kjaer M. 2002. Physical capacity influences the response of insulin-like growth factor and its binding proteins to training. *J Appl Physiol* 93:1669–1675.

Sara VR, Hall K. 1990. Insulin-like growth factors and their binding proteins. *Physiol Rev* 70:591–614.

Thissen J, Davenport ML, Pucilowska JB, Miles MB, Underwood LE. 1992. Increased serum clearance and degradation of ^{125}I-labeled IGF-I in protein-restricted rats. *Am J Physiol* 262:E406–E411.

Thissen JP, Underwood LE, Ketelslegers JM. 1999. Regulation of insulin-like growth factor-I in starvation and injury. *Nutr Rev* 57:167–176.

THE USE OF PORTABLE ACCELEROMETERS IN PREDICTING ACTIVITY ENERGY EXPENDITURE

Kong Y. Chen, Vanderbilt University

"*A soldier's level of physical fitness has a direct impact on his combat readiness*" (U.S. Army, 1998). The balance of energy intake (EI) and energy expenditure (EE) can significantly affect soldiers' physical fitness, conditioning, and overall health. The predominant contributor to the variations of EE is physical activity. Unlike most civilian populations, soldiers are often subjected to negative energy balance (EE significantly exceeds EI) (Friedl and Hoyt, 1997). For optimum designs of food rations and physical training, accurate and detailed measurements of EE are crucial. However, our current techniques in assessing physical activity are limited, such that possible associations between physical activity and the related EE (EE_{ACT}) with respect to the health and performance in military personnel have not been well determined.

Daily EE can be categorized into three major components: basal or resting EE (also called basal metabolic rate), thermic effect of food (or food-induced thermogenesis), and EE_{ACT}. Resting EE is the rate of EE measured in postabsorptive, well-rested, and thermoneutral conditions. In sedentary subjects, resting EE is the major component of EE (Flatt, 1978). Inter-individual variations in resting EE of normal humans can be explained by differences in fat-free mass (the primary contributor), age, sex, familial traits, and fat mass (Ravussin and Bogardus, 1989; Ravussin et al., 1986). Thermic effect of food represents the increase in EE following meal ingestion for absorbing, processing, and storing the nutrients. There are two recognized subcomponents, obligatory and facultative thermogenesis, which combine to represent a small component to total EE (< 8–10 percent) (Jéquier and Schutz, 1988; Welle et al., 1981) under normal conditions. EE_{ACT} is the largest variability to total EE in humans. Moderate walking can increase EE by three times, while a more vigorous activity such as running can elevate EE by ten times. Compared with civilians who generally have more sedentary lifestyles, EE_{ACT} is particularly important in soldiers' nutritional and physiological state, affecting performance and overall health (Burstein et al., 1996; DeLany et al., 1989).

MATERIAL AND METHODS

Measuring Energy Expenditure

Doubly Labeled Water (DLW) is considered as the "gold standard" for measuring EE in the field or free-living conditions. It determines the net disappearance of hydrogen (through water) and oxygen (through water and carbon dioxide) by stable isotope labeling, that is, $^{2}H_2{}^{18}O$ (Schoeller and Hlinicka, 1996; Schoeller et al., 1982). The major advantage of the DLW method is its noninvasiveness and nonintrusiveness. It has been used to assess EE of soldiers in the field and the impact of different rations (DeLany et al., 1989), climates (Burstein et al., 1996), and other training conditions (Forbes-Ewan et al., 1989). However, the main limitation of the DLW method is that it measures total EE during a period of 7 to 14 days without being able to detect the type, duration, and intensity of physical activity, or to trace variations in physical activity and related EE within certain periods. Furthermore, the high cost and relative limited availability of ^{18}O make this method difficult to apply.

Indirect calorimetry is the gold standard method of EE measurement under laboratory environments. It uses a facemask, a ventilated hood, or a respiratory chamber (Sun et al., 1994) to measure oxygen consumption and carbon dioxide production continuously and noninvasively. Major advantages of indirect calorimetry are the immediate and detailed measurements of the rates of EE during different activities and the macronutrient oxidations. The major disadvantage is the limited application under free-living conditions.

Methods of Assessing Physical Activity

Studying the relationship between physical activity and health in humans is complicated by the highly variable nature of physical activity. A particularly challenging area has been the development and application of accurate, valid, and cost-effective techniques to quantify physical activity under field conditions (Paffenbarger et al., 1993; Washburn and Montoye, 1986; Wilson et al., 1986). Numerous methods have been utilized to measure EE during physical activities. They vary greatly in their usefulness in different study populations and designs (Shultz et al., 2001). They can generally be categorized as subjective and objective methods.

Subjective Methods

Subjective methods include the use of direct observations, physical activity records, surveys and recall questionnaires. These techniques are used for various time periods and settings. Although inexpensive and easy to implement, their accuracies are greatly limited by the recording, recall, interviewer, and other biases. Predictions of EE_{ACT} using these methods could be further flawed by interpretation and translation errors. Results from most subjective monitoring methods are thus difficult to quantify and to compare interindividually.

Objective Methods

Objective methods for current measurements of physical activity mainly consist of mechanical/electronic devices. Since walking and running are the most common types of physical activities, step counters are often used to estimate overall activity levels. Several types of step counters exist, including pedometers that use a mechanical movement counter (Bassey et al., 1987; Washburn et al., 1980), mercury switches (Cauley et al., 1987), and electronic load transducers and foot contact monitors inserted into the heels of shoes that sense loads held, lifted, or carried, and walking activity (Barber et al., 1973; Dion et al., 1982; Hoyt et al., 1994; Weyand et al., 2001). These are generally simple, small, and relatively inexpensive devices that are based on the principle that EE_{ACT} is correlated with individual step frequency and foot contact times (Kram and Taylor, 1990). The main limitation is that the sensitivity and accuracy of step counting may vary significantly among activity types, inter- and intraindividually. Furthermore, stride lengths, a crucial element of the velocity and distance traveled, can only be estimated.

Researchers have recently focused on an array of new activity monitors based on accelerometers, which directly measure body movements in terms of acceleration. The most currently used are the piezoelectric sensors that detect accelerations in one (typically vertical direction) or in three orthogonal planes (anterior-posterior, lateral, and vertical). Results can be recorded in a microcomputer. Most monitors are usually placed on the hip or waist (for its closeness to the center of body mass), although ankle or wrist monitors are also used. Caltrac, Tritrac-R3D (both by Hemokinetics, Madison, Wisconsin), RT3 (Stayhealthy, Monrovia, California), Computer Science and Application (CSA, Shalimar, Florida), Tracmor (Maastricht, The Netherlands), and ActiWatch (Minimitter, Sunriver, Oregon) are just a few examples of marketed systems. In several validation studies using these monitors, correlation values ranged from 0.65 to 0.92 between EE measured by indirect calorimetry and accelerometer readings during various activities (Bouten et al., 1994; Bray et al., 1994; Chen and Sun, 1997; Freedson et al., 1998), where level walking showed the highest correlation with the hip-worn triaxial accelerometers. The advantages of the accelerometry devices include their small size, noninvasiveness, and minimal intrusiveness to normal subject movements during daily activities. Additionally, they are easy to use for subjects and testers, sensitive to relative intensity, frequency, and duration detections, and have extended measuring periods (minute-by-minute data for up to 28 days), thus making free-living monitoring more feasible. The major limitations include their inability to detect activity types (for

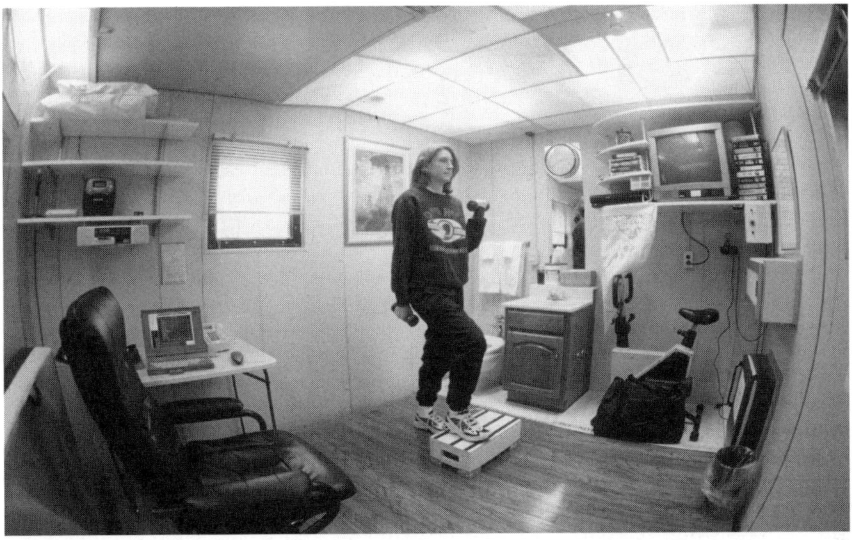

FIGURE D-13 The whole-room indirect calorimeter at Vanderbilt University.

which the associations between measured acceleration and EE_{ACT} are dependent upon), single-site monitoring that is unable to detect movements from various body segments, limited prediction algorithms to estimate EE_{ACT} across a wide range, and inability to differentiate EE due to postural changes and other low-intensity physical activities (Chen and Sun, 1997). To compensate for these errors, a combination of using accelerometry devices and inclinometers or mercury switches was used to detect postural changes and motions were reported (Levine et al., 2001; Walker et al., 1997). Recently, several research labs have tested the feasibility of using accelerometer arrays that were positioned at different body segments, mainly the chest, trunk, and thighs, to monitor the types of activities by postural identifications (Bussmann et al., 2001; Fahrenberg et al., 1997; Foerster and Fahrenberg, 2000; Zhang et al., 2003). However, EE_{ACT} predictions from these monitors have yet to be carefully validated.

Works from the Vanderbilt Energy Balance Lab

Equipped with the state-of-the-art whole-room indirect calorimeter at Vanderbilt, we are in a unique and ideal environment to develop and validate portable activity monitors for EE_{ACT} predictions. The room calorimeter is a small, airtight environmental room (2.6 × 3.3 × 2.3 m^3, 19,500 L in net volume), equipped with a desk, chair, outside window, toilet, sink, telephone, TV/VCR, audio system/alarm clock, and fold-down mattress to simulate free-living conditions (Figure D-13). Oxygen consumption and carbon dioxide production are calculated by measuring the changes of oxygen and carbon dioxide concentrations of the air inside the calorimeter and the flow rate of the purged air in an open-circuit design. A special multichannel air sampling system was designed to ensure an even sampling of the gas expired by the subject. Temperature, barometric pressure, and humidity of the room are precisely controlled and monitored. With the optimized controls and precision measurements, the minute-by-minute EE is calculated with the highest precision reported (> 90 percent with each minute and > 99 percent over 24 hours) (Sun et al., 1994).

RESULTS

In a previous study (Chen and Sun, 1997), we used a hip-worn triaxial accelerometer monitor, the Tritrac-R3D Research Ergometer (Hemokinetics, Inc. Madison, Wisconsin), to detect body motion during physical activities. A heterogeneous group of healthy adult volunteers (85 women and 40 men) each spent two separate 24-hour periods (one day with nonintensive walking and stepping exercises and the other day without), that respectively denoted the exercise and normal days in our room calorimeter and where each subject's minute-by-minute EE and body movements were measured simultaneously. The Tritrac-R3D's simple linear prediction model, using the combined signal from all three axes, significantly underestimated EE_{ACT} (by 33 percent and 49 percent) and total EE (by 17 percent and 26 percent) for normal and exercise days, respectively (Figure D-14, parts A and B). Using the EE and acceleration data measured during the exercise day, body acceleration components (A) measured by the Tritrac-R3D were fitted into a nonlinear two-parameter model:

$$EE_{ACT} = a \times A_{horizontal}^{p1} + b \times A_{vertical}^{p2}$$

where coefficients *a, b, p1,* and *p2* were determined by optimization with the least sum-squared error for each individual. Results showed significant improvements (all $P < 0.001$) in modeling total EE (Figure D-14, part C), standard error estimation parameters, and correlation coefficients. We then cross-validated these models by applying them to the acceleration recorded during the second 24-hour period (normal day) and demonstrated that the predicted total EE was now comparable to the measured values (Figure D-14, part D). Furthermore, we showed that a generalized model, using subject's gender, weight, height, and age to replace the individualized coefficients (*a, b, p1,* and *p2* from the equation above, shown in Figure D-14, parts C and D), was also significantly more accurate compared with the one-parameter-linear model by Tritrac-R3D.

However, this model underestimated the EE_{ACT} during low intensities, potentially due to inadequate movement detections of the upper body motion. In a recent study (unpublished), we used a similar study design and measured EE during a 24-hour period in the room calorimeter in 60 healthy volunteers. Body movements were simultaneously measured using the same Tritrac-R3D triaxial

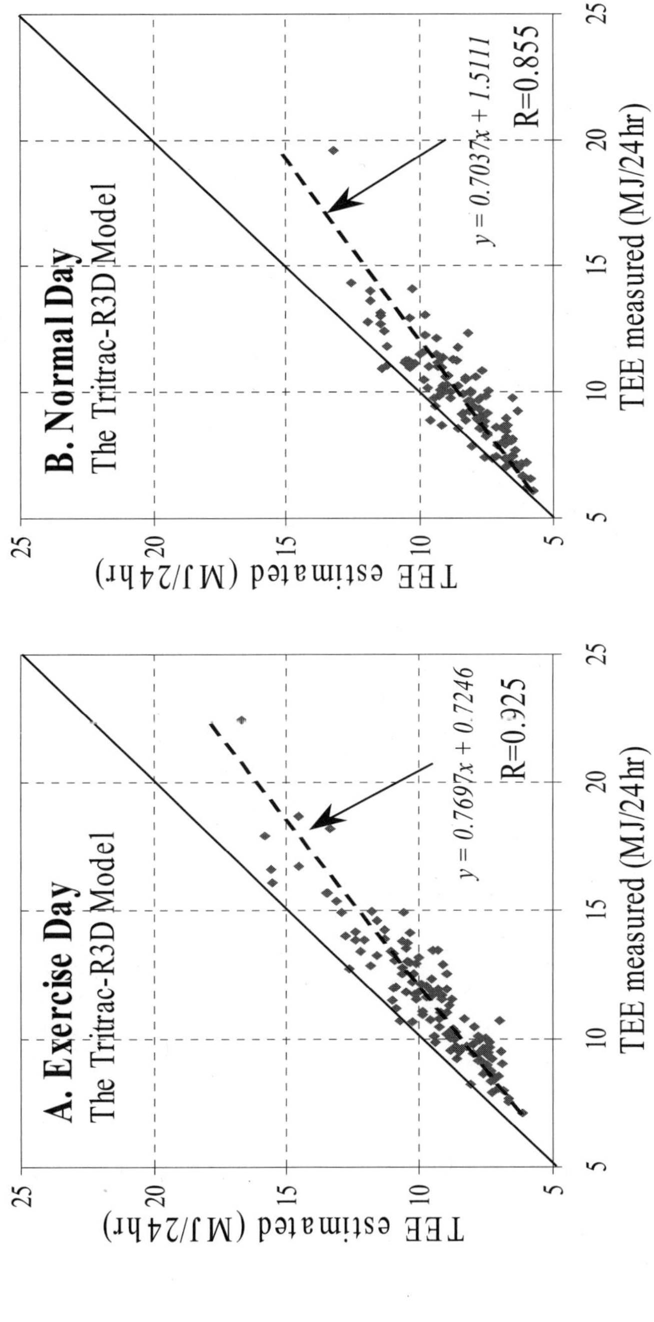
A. Exercise Day
The Tritrac-R3D Model
y = 0.7697x + 0.7246
R=0.925
TEE estimated (MJ/24hr)
TEE measured (MJ/24hr)
5
10
15
20
25
B. Normal Day
The Tritrac-R3D Model
y = 0.7037x + 1.5111
R=0.855
TEE estimated (MJ/24hr)
TEE measured (MJ/24hr)

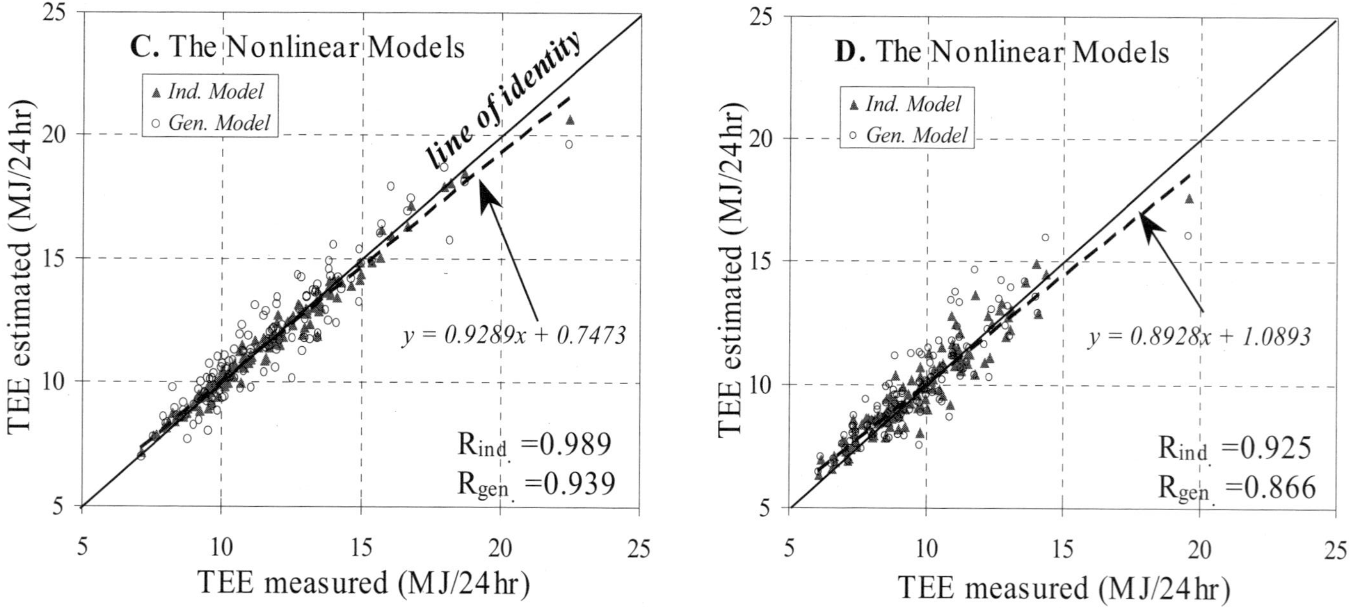

FIGURE D-14 Total daily energy expenditure (TEE) estimated by the Tritrac-R3D model (A., exercise day; B., normal day) in 85 healthy women and 40 men, and by the two-component nonlinear models (C., exercise day; D., normal day; shown on next page) versus TEE measured by the calorimeter. The line of identity signifies a perfect match between the estimated and the measured values in the room calorimeter. In C and D, individual (Ind.) model represents the parameters fitted for each volunteer and general (Gen.) model represents the model using only the subject's gender, weight, height, and age to replace the individualized coefficients.

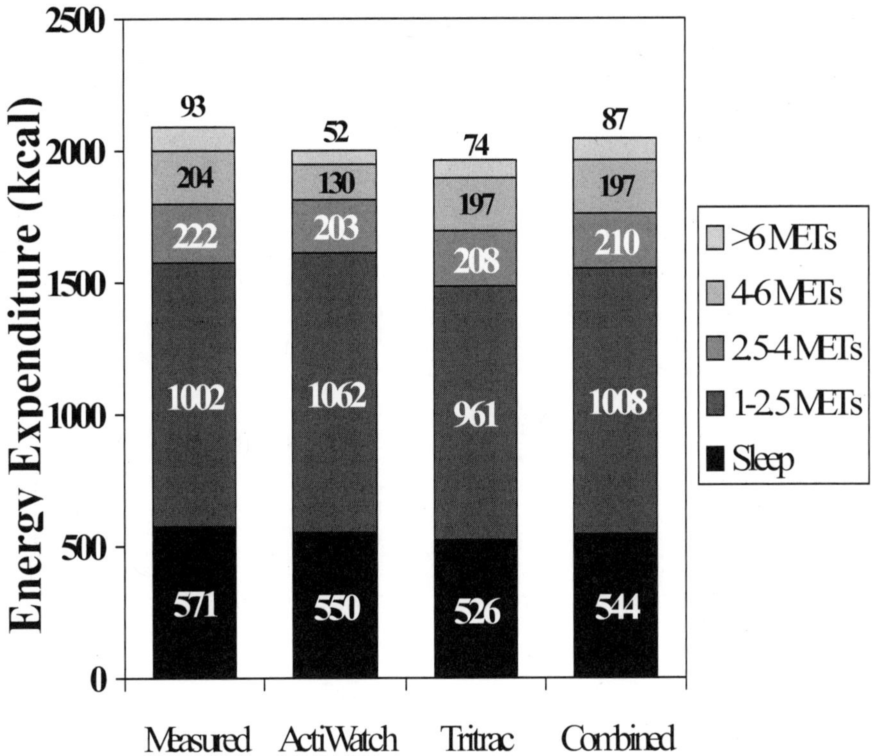

FIGURE D-15 Averaged energy expenditure (EE) in separate intensity categories of one 24-hour period in 60 healthy sedentary women (age, 35.4 ± 9.0 y, body mass index, 30.0 ± 5.9 kg/m^2). Comparison between EE measured in the whole-room indirect calorimeter, estimated by the ActiWatch, the Tritrac-R3D, and the ActiWatch and Tritrac-R3D monitors combined. METs = metabolic equivalents, calculated as ratio of individual energy expenditure and resting energy expenditure. (*$P < 0.05$ compared with the measured values).

accelerometer (worn at the hip). We added a wrist accelerometer (ActiWatch64, Minimitter, Sunriver, Oregon) on the dominant arm for upper body movement measurements. The nonlinear power-fitting model was then expanded to include the arm accelerations:

$$EE_{ACT} = a \times A_{hip,\ horizontal}{}^{p1} + b \times A_{hip,\ vertical}{}^{p2} + c \times A_{arm}{}^{p3}$$

We found that the Tritrac-R3D and the ActiWatch combined model accurately estimated EE_{ACT} in all intensity categories compared with measured

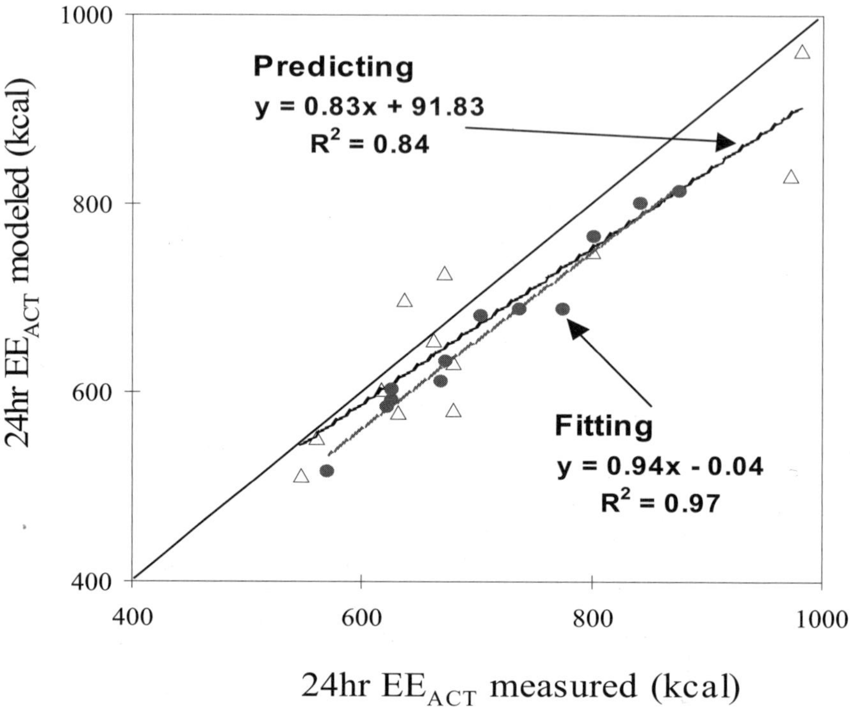

FIGURE D-16 Total energy expenditure of physical activity (EE_{ACT}) in 12 healthy women during two 24-hour periods (identical protocol) measured in the room calorimeter, compared with the estimated from the activity monitors. One day was randomly selected for fitting with combinations of ActiWatch on the wrist of the dominant hand and Tritrac-R3D at the waist, and the second day was used as the prediction validation.

EE_{ACT} by the calorimeter (Figure D-15). The particular improvements were in the measurement of lower-intensity physical activities, in which sedentary individuals tend to spend most of their time. A second 24-hour study was repeated in a subgroup of 12 volunteers and showed accurate EE_{ACT} prediction compared with measured values (Figure D-16).

DISCUSSION AND CONCLUSIONS

In view of the number of current field techniques for measuring detailed physical activity, accelerometers have been shown to be valid and useful. However, the applications of portable monitors to accurately predict energy demands in military personnel during training and field operations are unique. Compared with the more sedentary civilian populations, for whom most current activity monitors are designed, soldiers participate in routine training regimens that are often subject to increased physical demands. Marching and running with significant added loads (> 10 kg), crawling, jumping, climbing, and many other lifting or pulling activities are just a few of the activity types that present challenges to existing technologies. Furthermore, many trainings and operations are conducted in extreme external environmental conditions, such as hot or cold climates (Burstein et al., 1996), dry desert or humid jungles (Forbes-Ewan, 1989), and high altitude (Hoyt et al., 1994), while the internal stress from the imbalance of high total energy demands versus low energy intake, sleep deprivation, fatigue, and psychological stress (Nindl et al., 2002; Troumbley et al., 1990) may further exacerbate the complexity of the physical activity and EE_{ACT} estimations. Thus, we need to develop and optimize more specific portable methods for the measurements of the various activity types, intensities, durations, and frequencies. Two general areas of improvement are sensor designs and model development.

Currently marketed accelerometry activity monitors primarily use the piezoresistive sensors, either stand-alone or built-in (surface-mounted or integrated) chips. Although mostly unpublished, the ranges of acceleration are generally 0.05 to 1.0 g, with resolution of 0.02 or worse and sampling rates are 32 Hz or lower. Although this may be sufficient for monitoring the majority of physical movements of the center of mass (e.g., for the hip-worn monitors), movements of upper extremities contain higher frequency components in short bursts that may exceed the maximum range. These limitations would introduce inaccuracies in measurements. Most current activity monitors only use the dynamic component (or the AC component) of the raw signals from the sensors, partially to minimize the drifts from the baseline (or the static or DC component) due to temperature and directional changes. However, if the sensors are positioned at the proper locations, such as the chest, it may be useful to access such baseline change with respect to sensor direction for assessing body postures, which may indicate the type of activities. The dynamic signal from the sensor is generally filtered (corrected for baseline drifts), digitized, full-wave rectified (turn the negative values to positive), and integrated to 15-second epoch or longer to yield the output of activity counts. Although most of the current accelerometry monitors are packaged for easy operations for field researchers, almost all do not allow the user to change key parameters such as sampling rate or to allow raw signal collections, which are crucial to enable fundamental improvements in sensor designs.

Since currently available sensors have limited ability to detect wide ranges of physical activity types and intensities, the modeling of the acceleration output to predict EE_{ACT} is an area that needs much more development. We have demonstrated that the acceleration components recorded in the separate directions can be weighed differently to enhance EE_{ACT} prediction, since body movements in the vertical axis normally demand more energy due to the increased work against gravity, such as in the cases of weight-bearing activities like walking, running, and stepping (Haymes and Byrnes, 1993; Wong et al., 1981). Furthermore, the linear relationship between the acceleration and EE_{ACT} may not be the pertinent model for all activity types and intensities. Thus, we have systematically developed and cross-validated a relatively simple multicomponent power prediction model that significantly improved the EE_{ACT} estimation.

The placement of the monitor is also important. Previous studies have confirmed that the center of mass is the ideal site for monitoring, particularly for weight-bearing activities that contribute to the largest dynamic changes in energy cost. From our unpublished data, we have also seen that minute-to-minute EE during a 24-hour period correlated significantly better with raw measurements of physical activity with a hip-worn triaxial accelerometer ($R = 0.825 \pm 0.046$) than with a wrist-worn uniaxial accelerometer (0.646 ± 0.093, $P < 0.001$, $N = 60$). However, previous studies also illustrated that a single hip-worn monitor would be inadequate in measuring various physical activity types and intensities. Therefore, combination models that combine signals from multiple body segments need to be explored for improved accuracy in predicting EE_{ACT}.

In addition, other assessment techniques that involve physiological measurements may also be incorporated with simultaneous accelerometry monitoring to further improve EE_{ACT} modeling. An example is the use of heart-rate monitors, a simple and objective method for the estimation of EE during certain levels of physical activity and exercise (Spurr et al., 1988). Moreover, heart rate monitoring may facilitate the measurements of fatigue, state of hydration, body temperature changes, and emotional state (stress) that could affect the energy metabolism (Nielsen et al., 1993; Yoshida et al., 1994). Other physiological parameters, such as core body temperature (Gass and Gass, 1998; van Marken Lichtenbelt et al., 2001), galvanic skin conductance (estimating heat loss through sweating), and surface electromyography (measures of muscular activity), may also be explored to reveal their potentials to facilitate the prediction of EE_{ACT}.

In summary, to enhance our abilities to assess the energy demands of soldiers in the field, future research in technologies should focus on small and wireless sensors that can be positioned noninvasively and nonintrusively to measure body movements and physiological responses. Accelerometers are suitable for many aspects of the physical activity monitoring; however, much can be improved to increase their sensitivity and further reduce their size. The complex characteristics of the human physical activity, large inter- and intraindividual differences in energetic efficiencies, and inherent limitations of the sensors dictate that the development of advanced models to accurately predict EE_{ACT} should integrate more unique features of the signals from the sensors, rather than simple averaged signal outputs. This requires that we collect the raw signals from sensors while measuring EE_{ACT} simultaneously. Moreover, advanced pattern recognition and automated classification modeling techniques, such as artificial neural networks that can incorporate multiple input parameters and output feedbacks for nonlinear and adaptive modeling, need to be explored. The ideal development processes of such portable activity monitors should include the use of a respiratory chamber for sensor and model explorations under laboratory conditions, portable indirect calorimetry units for short-term field evaluations, and DLW for overall validations. Furthermore, we should optimize such monitoring systems to the specific applications through modeling, such as weather conditions and external loads, while broadening the general applications to benefit civilian medical research.

REFERENCES

Barber C, Evans D, Fentem PH, Wilson MA. 1973. A simple load transducer suitable for long-term recording of activity patterns in human subjects. *J Physiol* 231:94P–95P.

Bassey EJ, Dallosso HM, Fentem PH, Irving JM, Patrick JM. 1987. Validation of a simple estimation of walking activity. *Eur J Appl Physiol* 56:323–330.

Bouten CV, Westerterp KR, Verduin M, Janssen JD. 1994. Assessment of energy expenditure for physical activity using a triaxial accelerometer. *Med Sci Sports Exerc* 12:1516–1523.

Bray MS, Wong WW, Morrow JR, Butte NF, Pivarnik JM. 1994. Caltrac versus calorimeter determination of 24-hour energy expenditure in female children and adolescents. *Med Sci Sports Exerc* 26:1524–1530.

Burstein R, Coward AW, Askew WE, Carmel K, Irving C, Shpilberg O, Moran D, Pikarsky A, Ginot G, Sawyer M, Golan R, Epstein Y. 1996. Energy expenditure variations in soldiers performing military activities under cold and hot climate conditions. *Mil Med* 161:750–754.

Bussmann JBJ, Martens WLJ, Tulen JHM, Schasfoort FC, van den Berg-Emons HJ, Stam HJ. 2001. Measuring daily behavior using ambulatory accelerometry: The activity monitor. *Behav Res Methods Instrum Comput* 33:349–356.

Cauley JA, LaPorte RE, Black-Sandler R, Schramm MM, Kriska AM. 1987. Comparison of methods to measure physical activity in postmenopausal women. *Am J Clin Nutr* 45:1422.

Chen KY, Sun M. 1997. Improving energy expenditure estimation by using a triaxial accelerometer. *J Appl Physiol* 83:2112–2122.

DeLany JP, Schoeller DA, Hoyt RW, Askew EW, Sharp MA. 1989. Field use of $D_2{}^{18}O$ to measure energy expenditure of soldiers at different energy intake. *J Appl Physiol* 67:1922–1929.

Dion JL, Foufllot JP, Leblanc A. 1982. Ambulatory monitoring of walking using a thin capacitive force transducer. In: Scott FD, Raftery EB, Clement DL, Wright SL, eds. *Proceedings of the 4th International Symposium on Ambulatory Monitoring, and the Second Gent Workshop on Blood Pressure Variability*. London: Academic Press. Pp. 420–425.

Fahrenberg J, Foerster F, Mueller W, Smeja M. 1997. Assessment of posture and motion by multi-channel piezoresistive accelerometer recordings. *Psychophysiology* 34:607–612.

Flatt JP. 1978. The biochemistry of energy expenditure. In: Gray GS, ed. *Recent Advances in Obesity II*. London: Newmann. Pp. 211–228.

Foerster F, Fahrenberg J. 2000. Motion pattern and posture: Correctly assessed by calibrated accelerometers. *Behav Res Methods Instrum Comput* 32:450–457.

Forbes-Ewan CH, Morrissey BL, Gregg GC, Waters DR. 1989. Use of doubly labeled water technique in soldiers training for jungle warfare. *J Appl Physiol* 67:14–18.

Freedson PS, Melanson E, Sirard J. 1998. Calibration of the Computer Science and Applications, Inc. accelerometer. *Med Sci Sports Exerc* 30:777–781.

Friedl KE, Hoyt RW. 1997. Development and biomedical testing of military operation rations. *Annu Rev Nutr* 17:51–75.

Gass EM, Gass GC. 1998. Rectal and esophageal temperatures during upper and lower body exercise. *Eur J Appl Physiol* 78:38–42.

Haymes EM, Byrnes WC. 1993. Walking and running energy expenditure estimated by Caltrac and indirect calorimetry. *Med Sci Sports Exerc* 25:1365–1369.

Hoyt RW, Knapik JJ, Lanza JF, Jones BH, Staab JS. 1994. Ambulatory foot contact monitor to estimate metabolic cost of human locomotion. *J Appl Physiol* 76:1818–1822.

Jéquier E, Schutz Y. 1988. Energy expenditure in obesity and diabetes. *Diabetes Metab Rev* 4:583–593.

Kram R, Taylor CR. 1990. Energetics of running: A new prospective. *Nature* 346:265–267.

Levine JA, Melanson EL, Westerterp KR, Hill JO. 2001. Measurement of the components of nonexercise activity thermogenesis. *Am J Physiol Endocrinol Metab* 281:670–675.

Nielsen B, Astrup A, Samuelsen P, Wengholt H, Christensen NJ. 1993. Effect of physical training on thermogenic response to cold and ephedrine in obesity. *Intern J Obes Relat Metab Disord* 17:383–390.

Nindl BC, Leone CD, Tharion WJ, Johnson RF, Castellani JW, Patton JF, Montain SJ. 2002. Physical performance responses during 72 h of military operational stress. *Med Sci Sports Exerc* 34:1814–1822.

Paffenbarger RS, Blair SN, Lee IM, Hyde RT. 1993. Measurement of physical activity to assess health effect in free-living populations. *Med Sci Sports Exerc* 25:60–70.

Ravussin E, Bogardus C. 1989. Relationship of genetics, age, and physical fitness to daily energy expenditure and fuel utilization. *Am J Clin Nutr* 49:968–975.

Ravussin E, Lillioja S, Anderson TE, Christin L, Bogardus C. 1986. Determinants of 24-hour energy expenditure in man: Methods and results using a respiratory chamber. *J Clin Invest* 78:1568–1578.

Schoeller DA, Hlinicka JM. 1996. Reliability of the doubly labeled water method for the measurement of total daily energy expenditure in free living subjects. *J Nutr* 126:348S–354S.

Schoeller DA, Ravussin E, Schutz Y, Acheson P, Baertschi P, Jéquier E. 1982. Energy expenditure by doubly labeled water: Validation and proposed calculation. *Am J Physiol* 250:R823–R830.

Shultz Y, Weinsier RL, Hunter GR. 2001. Assessment of free-living physical activity in humans: An overview of current available and proposed new measures. *Obes Res* 9:368–379.

Spurr GB, Prentice AM, Murgatroyd PR, Goldberg GR, Reina JC, Christman NT. 1988. Energy expenditure from minute-by-minute heart rate recording: Comparison with indirect calorimetry. *Am J Clin Nutr* 48:552–559.

Sun M, Reed GW, Hill JO. 1994. Modification of a whole-room calorimeter for measurement of rapid changes in energy expenditure. *J Appl Physiol* 76:2686–2691.

Troumbley PF, Rinkle WJ, Burman KD, Lenz ER. 1990. A comparison of the health risk, health status, self-motivation, psychological symptomatic distress, and physical fitness of overweight and normal-weight soldiers. *Mil Med* 155:424–429.

U.S. Army. 1998. *Physical Fitness Training*. FM21-20. October 1. Washington, D.C.: U.S. Army Headquarters. P. 1.

van Marken Lichtenbelt WD, Westerterp-Plantenga MS, van Haydonek P. 2001. Individual variation in the relation between body temperature and energy expenditure in response to elevated ambient temperature. *Physiol Behav* 73:235–242.

Walker DJ, Heslop PS, Plummer CJ, Essex T, Chandler S. 1997. A continuous patient activity monitor: Validation and relation to disability. *Physiol Meas* 18:49–59.

Washburn RA, Montoye HJ. 1986. The assessment of physical activity by questionnaire. *Am J Epidemiol* 125:563–576.

Washburn R, Chin MK, Montoye HJ. 1980. Accuracy of pedometer in walking and running. *Res Q Exerc Sport* 51:695–702.

Welle S, Lilavivat U, Campbell RG. 1981. Thermic effect of feeding in man: Increased norepinephrine levels following glucose but not protein or fat consumption. *Metabolism* 30:953–958.

Weyand PG, Kelly M, Blackadar T, Darley JC, Oliver SR, Ohlenbusch NE, Joffe SW, Hoyt RW. 2001. Ambulatory estimates of maximal aerobic power from foot-ground contact times and heart rates in running humans. *J Appl Physiol* 91:451–458.

Wilson PWF, Paffenbarger RS, Morris JN, Havlik RJ. 1986. Assessment methods for physical activity and physical fitness in population studies. *Am Heart J* 11:1177–1192.

Wong TC, Webster JG, Montoye HJ, Washburn R. 1981. Portable accelerometer device for measuring human energy expenditure. *IEEE Trans Biomed Eng* 28:467–471.

Yoshida T, Sakane N, Umekawa T, Kondo M. 1994. Relationship between basal metabolic rate, thermogenic response to caffeine, and body weight loss fol-

lowing combined low calorie and exercise treatment in obese women. *Int J Obes Relat Metab Disord* 18:345–350.
Zhang K, Werner P, Sun M, Pi-Sunyer FX, Boozer C. 2003. Measurement of human daily physical activity. *Obes Res* 11:33–40.

ENERGY TRANSFORMATIONS AND METABOLISM DURING HUMAN LOCOMOTION: SENSING OPPORTUNITIES IN A CONSERVATIVE WORLD

Peter G. Weyand, Rice University

ENERGY CONVERSIONS: IDENTIFYING, MEASURING AND GAUGING THE TRANSFORMATIONS

Newton (1687) originally recognized that energy is neither created nor destroyed, merely transformed from one state to another. This late seventeenth-century idea provides the contemporary understanding that the energy transformations occurring in our environment proceed without any net loss in the total energy present. We take this for granted in the transformation of the chemical energy in fossil fuels into the heat energy to warm buildings or the mechanical energy to power automobiles. Indeed, Newton's breakthrough has enabled us to describe many of the energy transformations in the physical world in precise quantitative detail. However, in spite of the wide appreciation of the universal nature of Newton's conservation law, we are unable to fully quantify some of the energy transformations that affect us most directly. This is particularly true of the energy transformations occurring in skeletal muscle during walking and running. The energy sources and end products for skeletal muscles are similar to those of a gasoline engine. Both transform chemical energy into heat and mechanical work (Hill, 1950). Yet, for skeletal muscle during locomotion, the relative yields of heat and work are not fully known (Alexander, 1992; Taylor, 1994; van Ingen Schenau, 1998).

Despite ongoing uncertainty about the relative quantities of heat and work produced by muscle metabolism during locomotion, the total chemical energy transformed can be accurately measured. The stoichiometry of the reactions that liberate chemical energy from foodstuffs to fuel muscular contractions is well known. This knowledge allows the chemical energy released by the body's metabolism to be determined from the oxygen taken up and carbon dioxide given off by the process of respiration. The ease, utility, and accuracy of measurements of gas exchange have made this the method of choice for quantifying chemical energy transformations in the body for more than a century (Blaxter, 1989; Fedak et al., 1981; Zuntz, 1897).

Because energy transformations are an integral part of movement, quantitative descriptions of these transfers can be used to characterize the performance status of humans, automobiles, or other bodies in motion. The conventional descriptors for automobiles: horsepower, fuel available, fuel economy, and engine temperature, are fully familiar. Some of these are displayed on our dashboards in real time so that we can continuously monitor the energy status of our cars. Because the energy transformations in the human body involve similar conversions, equivalent descriptors of performance capabilities exist: metabolic power, fuel reserves, locomotor economy, fuel mixtures, and core body temperatures are all quantifiable biological entities. In some cases, such as the core temperature of the body, the sensor technology needed for continuous monitoring in the field is currently in use. In other cases, the biological knowledge needed to direct sensor research and development is incomplete. Advancing the understanding of the energy transformations that occur during human locomotion should identify the most productive avenues for future sensor development.

CHEMICAL ENERGY TRANSFORMED BY MUSCLE: HEAT AND WORK

Early formal ideas regarding the fate of the chemical energy humans and other animals transform during locomotion postulated that humans behave much like today's automobiles. Scientists considering the question believed humans produce forward movement by transforming chemical energy into the mechanical energy necessary to perform the work involved in locomotion (Fenn, 1930; Gray, 1968; Hill, 1950). Just as automobiles perform mechanical work to overcome inertia and wind resistance, human muscles were thought to convert chemical energy into the mechanical energy and work necessary to repeatedly lift and accelerate the body's center of mass and limbs during each stride.

However, two important distinctions differentiate human locomotion produced by muscular contractions from that of an automobile powered by a gasoline engine. These differences are most easily conceptualized under steady-speed conditions on level ground. First, automobiles must transform fuel into the mechanical energy necessary to overcome the frictional resistance offered by both air and internal components. This is not true for humans because they typically do not move at sufficient speeds to encounter appreciable resistance from air, and frictional forces within the body are negligible. Thus, the net requirement for mechanical energy during human locomotion under these conditions is nearly zero. Second, in contrast to the passive support provided by the frame of the automobile, humans rely on muscles to support the weight of the body against gravity. Muscles, unlike rigid car frames, expend chemical energy in order to provide the force necessary to support the body's weight. A car

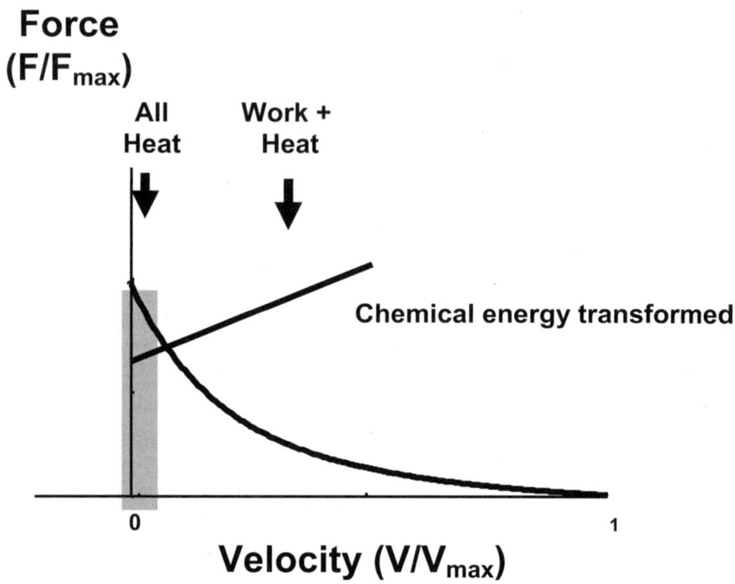

FIGURE D-17 Muscle force in relation to the velocity of shortening in an isolated muscle. The total energy transformed from chemical sources within muscle increases with the velocity of shortening during a contraction. During contractions with no length change, all of the chemical energy utilized by muscle is converted into heat. During contractions at 0.2 to 0.3 of maximal shortening velocity, 25 percent of the chemical energy fueling contraction is converted to mechanical work and the remaining 75 percent is converted into heat.

obviously does not require fuel to remain upright, but a person does, and the chemical energy transformed during motionless standing is appreciable (Margaria, 1976).

Although significant uncertainties remain about the relative yields of heat and work derived from the chemical energy transformed by muscles during locomotion, this is not the case for muscles observed in isolated preparations. Because force, shortening velocity, and heat production can be accurately measured under the latter conditions, the relationship between the mechanics of muscular contraction and the relative yields of heat and mechanical work in single muscles has been well established for more than half a century (Fenn, 1924; Hill, 1950). The maximum isometric force produced by different skeletal muscles is virtually invariant when expressed in relation to cross-sectional area (Figure D-17). Isometric contractions produce large forces that transform relatively little chemical energy. However, because no shortening occurs, and mechanical work by definition involves moving a force through a distance, isometric contractions produce no mechanical work, and hence provide no mechanical energy. Under isometric conditions, the chemical energy that fuels force production is converted entirely into heat. When muscles shorten while active, the largest yields of mechanical work are provided by contractions that occur at one-fifth to one-third of the muscles maximum shortening velocity (V_{max}). However, performing mechanical work at these shortening velocities compromises force production. At the relative shortening velocities that maximize the work performed, the force produced is reduced to roughly one-half that of an isometric contraction. Additionally, muscle performs this work with marginal efficiency: most muscles convert a maximum of only 25 percent of the total transformed chemical energy into mechanical work. This upper efficiency limit, similar to that of an automobile engine, results in 75 percent of the total chemical energy transformed being released as heat.

Although the relative energy yields of heat and work are well established from experiments on isolated skeletal muscle preparations, equivalent information about the energy transformations that occur in the body during locomotion is not available. To date, simultaneous measurements of muscle forces, shortening velocities, and heat from the many muscles active in the body during locomotion have not been possible. Yet, the absence of this data does not preclude further consideration of these issues. Sound conclusions can be drawn from the large bodies of experimental information available on both the mechanics and chemical energy transformations involved in human locomotion.

LOCOMOTOR ENERGETICS AND MECHANICS: ALL HEAT, NO WORK?

Typical rates and quantities of the metabolic or chemical energy transformed during walking and running are illustrated in Figure D-18. With increases in speed, the rates at which the body's chemical energy stores are transformed increase curvilinearly during walking and linearly during running (Figure D-18A, Margaria et al., 1963). These metabolic rates can be divided by speed to obtain the energy transformed per unit distance, or the metabolic cost of transport (Figure D-18B). Walking transport costs are minimized at the intermediate speeds people prefer to use and are relatively greater at both slower and faster speeds within this gait. Running transport costs are virtually constant across the range of speeds at which values can be obtained from measurements of gas exchange. In the process of covering a kilometer at self-selected speeds, a typical 70 kg person will transform approximately 270 and 420 kJ of chemical energy in these respective gaits.

Although the chemical energy transformed during walking and running has been established for many decades, the proportion converted into mechanical work is not known. Uncertainty regarding the completeness of mechanical energy transfers within each stride has precluded accurate quantification of the relative portions provided from stored mechanical versus stored chemical energy

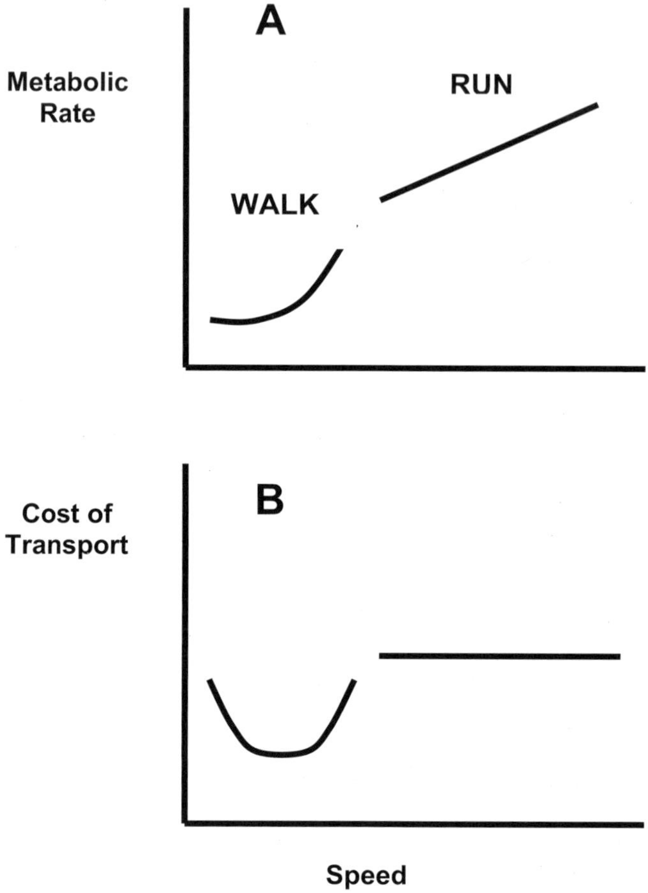

FIGURE D-18 The rate at which metabolic energy is transformed in relation to speed during steady-state human walking and running (A). Dividing metabolic rate by speed provides the energy expended per unit distance (B).
SOURCE: Reprinted, with permission Margaria et al. *JAP* (1963).

sources (Taylor, 1994; van Ingen Schenau, 1998). Mechanical energy is clearly required to repeatedly lift and accelerate the body's mass and limbs during each stride. This energy might be provided, either wholly or in part, by the transformation of chemical energy stores in the body. Early experimentalists started with the assumption that the energy source of all of the mechanical work required for each stride was chemical. This assumption provided them with a seemingly logical explanation for the chemical energy transformations that had been well-documented by gas exchange. Dozens of investigations, both past and recent, have attempted to establish a consistent relationship between the mechanical work performed and the chemical energy transformed during each locomotor stride (Heglund et al., 1982; Kaneko, 1990; Williams and Cavanagh, 1987). To date, these approaches have yielded neither consistent quantitative explanations, nor successful independent predictions of the quantities of chemical energy known to be transformed.

The alternative possibility, that the chemical energy transformed during human locomotion is not converted into mechanical work, but almost fully into heat, enjoys support from a growing body of experimental evidence. This evidence suggests that the mechanical energy needed for walking and running is continuously recycled from one stride to the next once a person is up to a constant speed. During walking, the musculoskeletal system transfers mechanical energy between gravitational potential energy and horizontal kinetic energy using a mechanism that has been likened to an inverted pendulum (Cavagna et al., 1976). The forward velocity of the body's center of mass slows as it gains height and gravitational potential energy while approaching its highest point in midstance. Once past this apex, the body accelerates down and forward by converting the gravitational potential energy gained earlier in the stride into forward kinetic energy (Figure D-19A). During running, the body stores elastic potential energy in springy tendons during the downward movement of the center of mass that occurs during the first half of the stance phase. The height and speed the body loses early in stance is then restored via an elastic recoil that lifts and reaccelerates the body during the latter portion of the stance phase (Cavagna et al., 1964, 1977; Figure D-19B).

The exact quantities of energy transferred back and forth between various mechanical forms during each walking and running stride are not fully known, but are undoubtedly considerable. Estimates for walkers indicate that up 70 percent of the total fluctuations in the horizontal kinetic and gravitational potential energy of the body can be accomplished via pendulum-like transfers (Cavagna et al., 1977). These transfers are most complete at those intermediate speeds at which transport costs are minimized and less are complete at the faster and slower speeds that incur greater metabolic transport costs. Estimates for runners indicate that well over half (Cavagna et al., 1964; Ker et al., 1987; Roberts et al., 1997), and perhaps nearly all (Taylor, 1994) of the mechanical energy fluctuations involved might be accomplished via elastic and other transfer mechanisms. Regardless of exactly how complete these energy transfers are, the possibility of nearly complete conservation of mechanical energy raises a counterintuitive possibility: humans traveling at steady speeds on level ground may not require little to no input of mechanical energy and therefore may not transform any appreciable chemical energy into mechanical work.

From a conceptual standpoint, the muscle mechanics and energy transformations taking place in humans traveling under their own power may not differ appreciably from those that occur while standing still. In both cases, there is essentially no net requirement for mechanical work to be performed, but a large

A

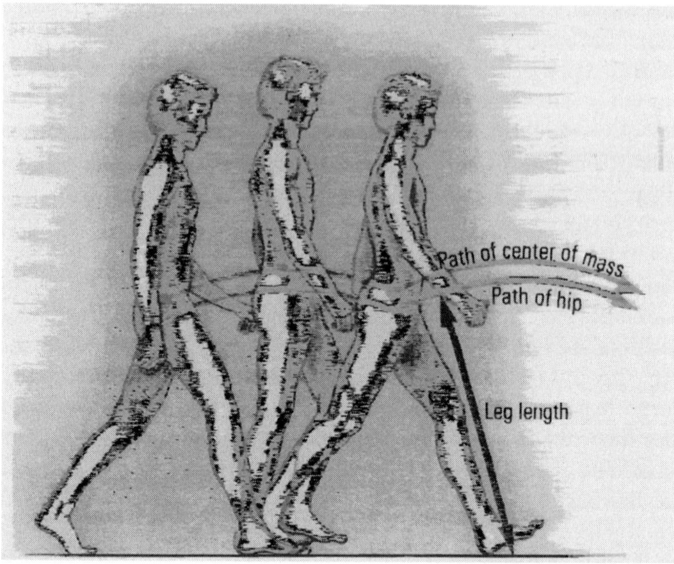

B

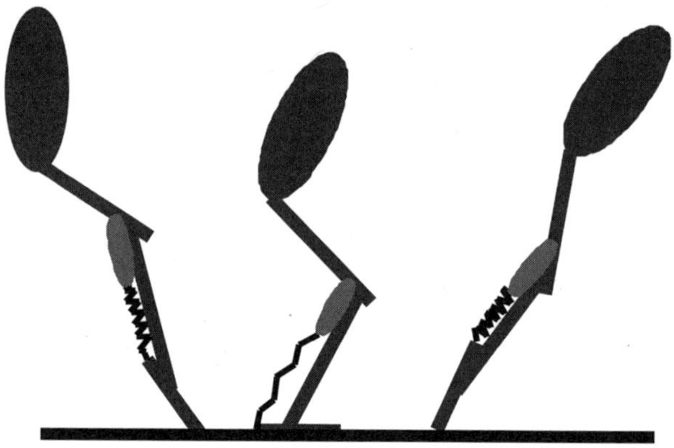

FIGURE D-19 Mechanisms by which mechanical energy is conserved during human locomotion. During walking, the mechanical energy of the body is conserved by a pendulum-like transfer between forward horizontal and gravitational potential energy (A, from Alexander, 1992 illustration from EXPLORING BIOMECHANICS: Animals in Motion by R. McNeil Alexander. Copyright © 1992 by Scientific American Library. Reprinted by permission of Henry Holt and Company, LLC), while during running, the gravitational and elastic potential energy are transferred by passive stretch and recoil of tendon springs (B).

requirement for muscles to generate the support forces that the skeleton ultimately applies to the ground. The mechanical and metabolic properties of muscle indicate that these requirements would be best satisfied by contractions during which muscle undergoes little to no change in length. For example, isometric muscle contractions would maximize the force produced per unit volume of muscle active, minimize the energy drawn from the body's chemical stores, and eliminate the mechanical work that is theoretically unnecessary. Although counterintuitive, the empirical evidence available (Fukunaga et al., 2001; Roberts et al., 1997; Taylor, 1994) supports the general validity of this idea.

RUNNING: SPRINGING FORWARD

However close to 100 percent perfection mechanical energy transfers might be, they do not influence the earth's gravitational field. Accordingly, there is no disagreement that muscles need to be active to support the body's weight during locomotion. This allows support forces to be regarded as a minimum mechanical requirement for human locomotion. When the force of gravity on the mass of an average human body is considered, the magnitude of the force that must be applied to the ground in order to travel on foot is readily apparent. Peak ground reaction forces typically exceed the force of the body's weight during walking and are at least twice as great during running (Margaria, 1976). The orientation of the ground reaction force vector in relation to the leg joints indicates that the muscle forces required for human locomotion generally exceed the ground forces by a factor of two (Biewener, personal communication; Wright and Weyand, 2001). Accordingly, the muscles of a 70 kg human must generate peak forces of approximately 1,400 to 2,800 N simply to oppose gravity during normal walking and running.

The large ground and muscle forces involved in locomotion led C. Richard Taylor and colleagues (Kram and Taylor, 1990; Roberts et al., 1998; Taylor, 1994) to hypothesize that the energy muscles require for force production is the predominant factor in determining the quantities of chemical energy transformed during locomotion. These investigators recognized that the time-averaged vertical force applied to the ground over the course of the stride must equal the body's weight, and that this force can only be applied during the period of foot-ground contact (t_c). These investigators observed a constant relationship between the metabolic rates of running or hopping animals and the rates at which they applied ground support forces (Kram and Taylor, 1990, Figure D-20). Two well-known properties of muscle helped these investigators explain this result. First, the rates at which chemical energy is transformed into heat while producing force is known to be proportional to the maximal shortening speed of the fibers generating the force (Barany, 1967). Second, during locomotion, muscle fibers are recruited in ascending order of their shortening speeds (Henneman et al., 1965; Walmsley et al., 1978). Using this information, Kram and Taylor proposed that the rates at which runners and hoppers apply force to the ground ($1/t_c$)

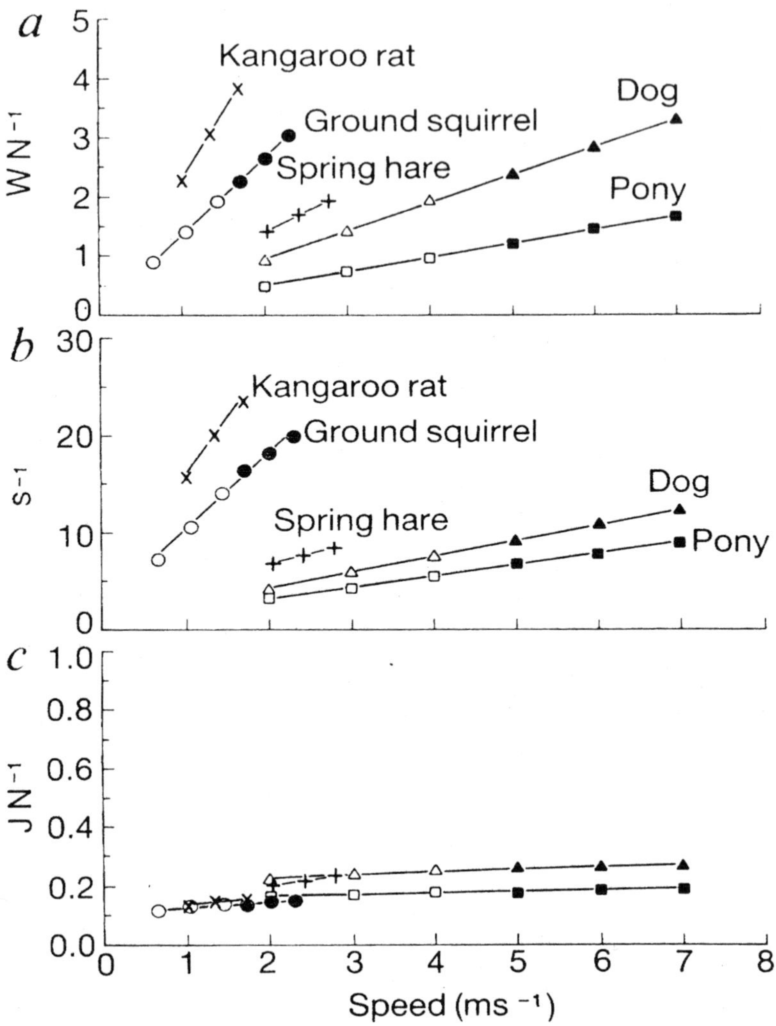

FIGURE D-20 The metabolic rates (a), during inverse periods of foot-ground contact, and (b) in different sized running and hopping animals over a range of speeds. The ratio of metabolic rates to the inverse periods of foot-ground contact (c) is a constant. This constant, the cost coefficient, represents the metabolic energy transformed in applying the ground force necessary to support the body's weight against gravity.

SOURCE: Reprinted by permission from Nature Kram and Taylor (1990) Macmillan Publishers Ltd.

dictates the speed of the muscle fibers recruited to support their body weight and, therefore, also the rate of chemical energy transformation in the body. They expressed this relationship as:

$$\dot{E}_{metab} = F_{Wb} \times 1/t_c \times C \quad (1)$$

Where $\dot{E}_{metab}$ is metabolic rate, F_{Wb} is the force required to support the weight of the body, $1/t_c$ is the inverse period of foot-ground contact used to estimated that rate of ground force application, and C is a cost coefficient representing the chemical energy expended per unit of force applied to the ground to support the body's weight. In accordance with convention for weight-bearing exercise, equation 1 can be rearranged to express metabolic rates on a mass-specific basis as:

$$\dot{E}_{metab}/F_{Wb} = 1/t_c \times C \quad (2)$$

The original relationship has since been found to apply to human locomotion with added weight or reduced weight (Kram, 2000), on skis (Bellizzi et al., 1998), with only ski poles (Bellizzi et al., 1998), while running on one's hands (Glasheen and McMahon, 1995), or even backwards (Wright and Weyand, 2001).

These results offer a consistent quantitative explanation for the chemical energy transformed during locomotion that has not come forth in the many previous investigations into the possible importance of mechanical work. The assumption of complete conservation of mechanical energy allowed Taylor and colleagues to establish a link between the chemical energy transformed during locomotion and whole-body mechanics that had been previously lacking. Taylor's hypothesis applied across a 4,500-fold range in the body sizes of running and hopping animals, a 10-fold range of speeds, and to several different gaits. Just as standing humans are recognized to be transforming chemical energy into force to support themselves against gravity, growing evidence supports Taylor's idea that running humans and animals do largely the same thing: humans and terrestrial animals simply convert chemical energy into the force necessary to support the body's weight while releasing this energy as heat in the process.

WALKING ENERGETICS: THE SCOOP ON SUPPORT FORCE?

Some have argued the Taylor's force hypothesis does not provide the correct explanation for the relationship reported between chemical energy transformation in the body and the mechanics of ground force application during running (Alexander, 1991; Minetti et al., 1994; Steudel, 1990). However, the empirical information available from walking is also consistent with the original ideas put forth by the force hypothesis. If support mechanics do determine the quantities of chemical energy transformed during human locomotion, several expectations for metabolic consequences can be inferred from the pendulum-like gait dynamics involved in walking. Metabolic energy requirements should be minimized when the transfer of mechanical energy by the pendulum is most complete. The greater the share of the mechanical energy provided conservatively by the pendulum, the smaller the demand on skeletal muscle to convert chemical energy into mechanical work during each stride. This idea can be evaluated by considering two metabolic variables introduced previously: the metabolic energy transformed per unit distance, and the metabolic energy transformed per unit of force applied to the ground (i.e., the cost coefficient; C in Figure D-21).

Several investigators (Cavagna et al., 1977; Griffin et al., 1999; Griffin et al., 2003; Heglund et al., 1982) have reported that the maximum possible energy savings from pendulum-like energy transfers occurs at intermediate walking speeds. With either positive or negative deviations from the intermediate speeds that people prefer to use, the proportions of the total mechanical energy of the body's center of mass conserved by pendulum-like exchange become progressively smaller (Cavagna et al., 1977). When the metabolic energy transformed at different walking speeds is expressed per unit distance, a minimum occurs at those intermediate speeds of maximum possible pendulum transfer (Figure D-22). At the slower and faster speeds at which mechanical energy transfers become less possible, the measured metabolic cost of transport is greater. A similar pattern is observed for the metabolic energy transformed per unit of force applied to the ground, or the cost coefficient (Griffin et al., 2003; Figure D-21C). Walking cost-coefficient values are minimized at the intermediate walking speeds at which mechanical energy transfer is most complete and are greater at both the faster and slower speeds at which walking dynamics limit pendulum-like transfers.

Simultaneous measurements of the chemical energy transformed and the heat given off by the body at different walking speeds have been obtained using a novel suit calorimeter developed by Paul Webb (Webb et al., 1988). These data, unique to human walking, also show a pattern across speed that supports the belief that ground force application determines the chemical energy transformations occurring in the body. Webb and colleagues reported that the largest fractions of the total chemical energy transformed, as determined from gas exchange, were given off as heat at those intermediate walking speeds at which the greatest fraction of the body's mechanical energy fluctuations can occur conservatively by pendulum-like exchange.

The fundamental importance of applying ground force to support the body's weight in determining the energy transformed in human locomotion prompted Reed Hoyt and colleagues to use this basic relationship to develop ambulatory sensing technologies. Hoyt recognized that if rates of ground force application, as estimated from foot-ground contact times (i.e., $1/t_c$), dictate the rates at which chemical energy is transformed in the human body, then accurate sensing of these periods should provide valid field estimates of the chemical energy

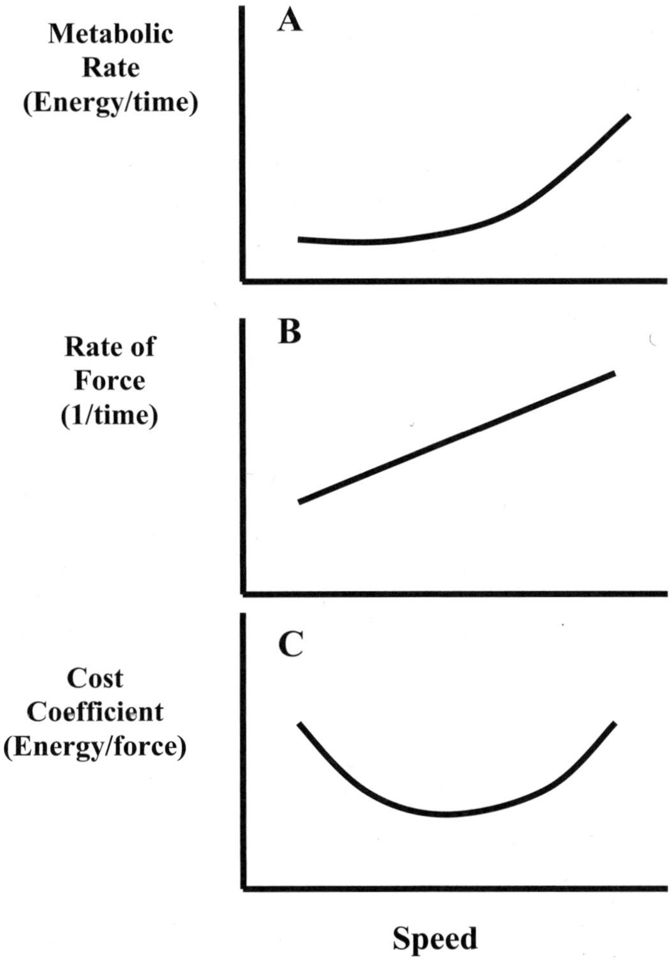

FIGURE D-21 Metabolic rate (A), inverse periods of foot-ground contact (B), and the cost coefficient (C) in relation to walking speed.
SOURCE: Reprinted, with permission adapted from Griffin et al. *JAP* (2003).

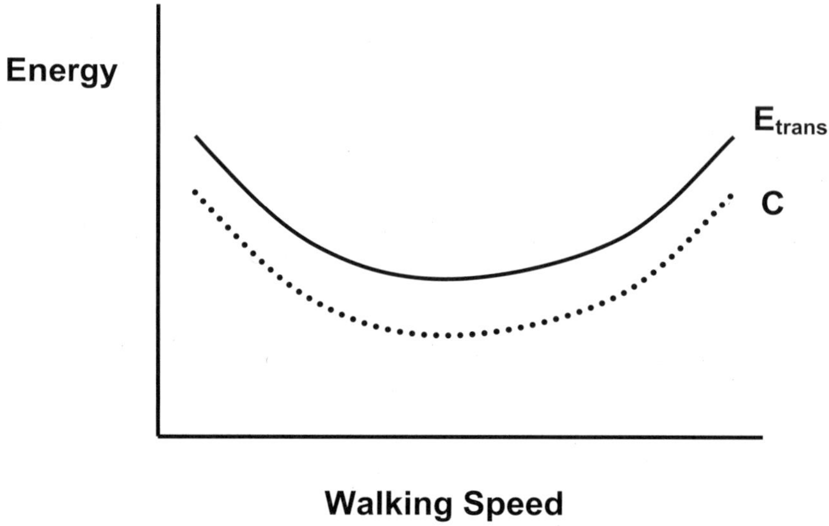

FIGURE D-22 The metabolic energy expended per unit distance (E_{trans}) and per unit force applied to the ground (C) to support the body's weight in relation to walking speed.

transformed. Successful sensing would allow the metabolic energy transformed during locomotion to be monitored during the daily lives of soldiers, hikers, medical patients, and others. Hoyt's idea proved to be both scientifically correct and practical, and thereby provided significant contributions toward the establishment of a human "energy status dashboard."

SENSING PERFECTION: ESTIMATING FOOT-GROUND CONTACT TIMES ON THE RUN

In their initial effort, Hoyt and colleagues (1994) succeeded in obtaining measurements of foot-ground contact times from pressure sensitive resistors embedded in shoe insoles. Their sensor measurements of foot-ground contact times provided highly accurate estimates of the metabolic energy released during both human walking and running (Figure D-23). For running, this was not a complete surprise given the results reported originally by Kram and Taylor (1990) and later by others (Roberts et al., 1998; Wright and Weyand, 2001). However, the estimates the sensors provided during walking were equally accurate even though direct walking tests of the relationship had been previously absent.

Although the initial impetus for the development of foot-ground contact monitors was obtaining ambulatory estimates of the metabolic energy released

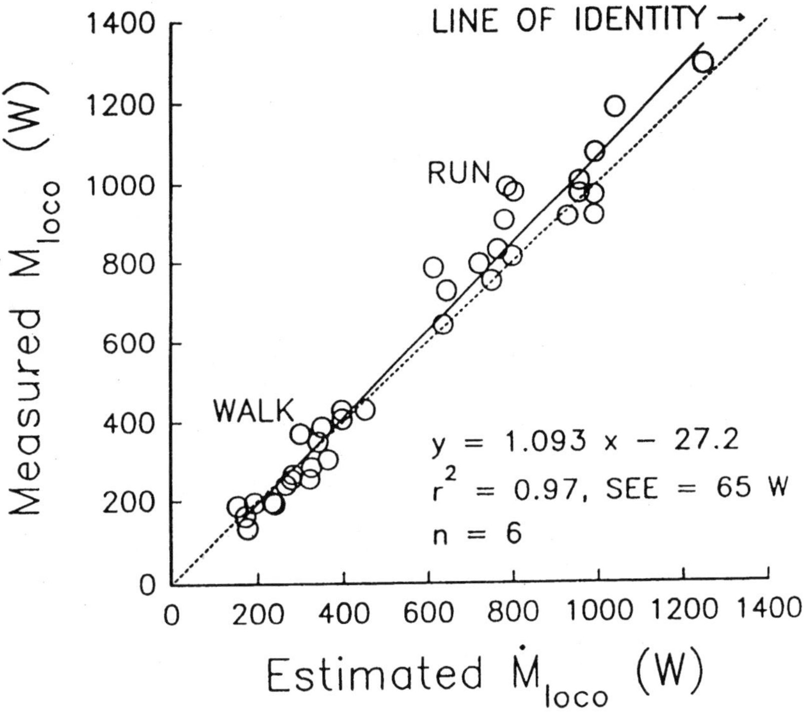

FIGURE D-23 Rates of chemical energy transformation in the body estimated by foot-ground contact time monitors and those measured directly using indirect calorimetry. SOURCE: Reprinted, with permission Hoyt et al. *JAP* (1994).

during locomotion, the monitoring capabilities that arose were not limited to sensing metabolism. The consistent support mechanics humans use to support the weight of their bodies against gravity results in highly reproducible rates of ground force application at any given speed. In fact, this relationship is sufficiently consistent that foot-ground contact times, once established in relation to speed for an individual, provide precise estimates of speed. The commercial t_c monitors spawned by this line of research (FitSense Incorporated, Southboro, Massachusetts) are able to estimate speeds and distances in field settings to within 2 percent or less (Weyand et al., 2001; Figure D-24).

The precision of these foot-ground contact monitors is greater, and the efficacy of the general approach is more apparent under conditions that are more controlled than those that typically exist in the field. In one application, the accelerometric method of estimating foot-ground contact times was used to monitor the world record holder in the 400 meter run during sprint competitions in

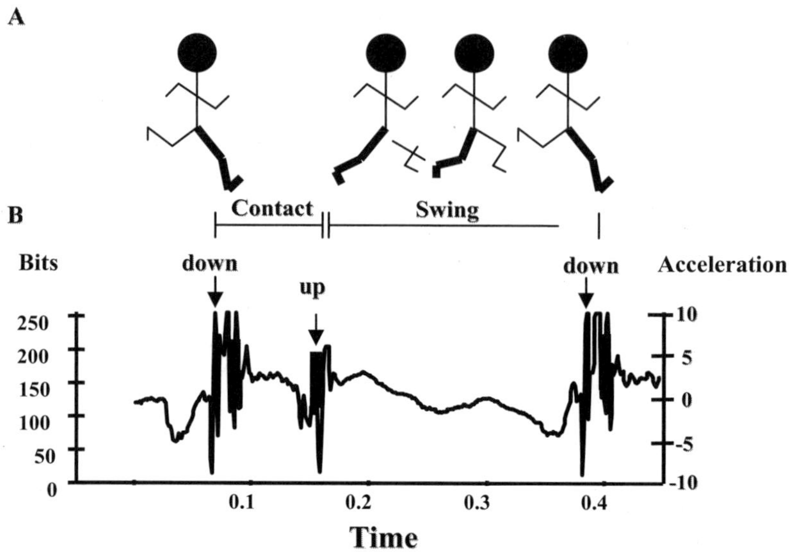

FIGURE D-24 The contact and swing phases of a single limb during a running stride (A) and the corresponding signal from a shoe-mounted accelerometer (B). The accelerometer signal allows both the instant the foot first contacts, and subsequently leaves, the surface to be identified. This allows this sensor to quantify periods of foot-ground contact (t_c) which can be used to estimate the rates at which force is applied to the ground to support the body's weight during walking and running.
SOURCE: Reprinted, with permission Weyand et al. *JAP* (2001).

the spring of 2000. In these instances, the foot-ground contact times of Michael Johnson were obtained from accelerometers fastened to the lateral aspect of both ankles. On the flat, consistent surface of 400 meter tracks, the speed estimates from the accelerometers agreed with the officially-timed speeds to within a fraction of a single percent. These estimates were so precise that accurate values for Michael Johnson's instantaneous speeds, stride frequencies, and lengths were available for every step of the races monitored (Figure D-25).

More recently, the commercial version of the foot-ground contact monitors were used in combination with heart rate monitors to obtain estimates of the body's maximal rate of chemical energy transformation from aerobic metabolism, or VO_{2max} (Weyand et al., 2001). In this case, the combination of newer and older sensor technologies provided a practical and accurate method that can be used in field settings to estimate maximal aerobic power, thereby contributing an ambulatory horsepower gauge to the human energy dashboard.

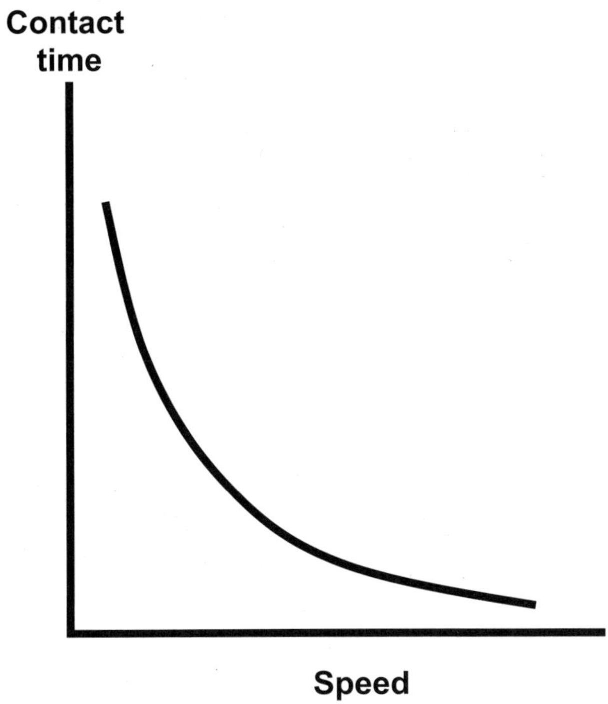

FIGURE D-25 Schematic illustration of the typical relationship between running speed and foot-ground time. The specific relationship for Michael Johnson was used to obtain his step-by-step speeds, stride lengths, and frequencies during competition in the spring of 2000. The accuracy provided by foot-ground contact sensors was equivalent to that of timing devices or video analysis.

FURTHER SENSING ADVANCES

The energy transfers involved in human locomotion considered here have focused on steady-state conditions on level ground. Scientific information, understanding, and the evolution of sensor technology warranted this focus. However, the conditions for locomotion in the natural world often deviate from these conditions. Hills and substrate quality can alter the mechanics of locomotion, the activity of the skeletal muscles, and the quantities of chemical energy transformed. Under these and other circumstances, significant challenges to biological understanding and sensor development remain. Nonetheless, experimental avenues that will provide further advances toward a human energy dashboard are clearly available. For example, the ability to assess maximal aerobic power from lightweight sensors on the body offers the possibility of obtaining reasonably accurate field estimates of the fuel mixtures that are transformed during human locomotion. Because the mixture of fat and carbohydrate oxidized is closely related to fraction of maximal aerobic power at which individuals operate during locomotion (Roberts et al., 1995; Sahlin, 1986), available techniques should predict fuel mixtures with reasonable accuracy.

CONCLUSIONS

Although significant work remains before metabolic monitoring technologies provide an energy dashboard for the human body equivalently comprehensive to that of the modern automobile, there is cause for optimism. The progress made thus far in the ability to monitor speed, distance, metabolic rate, and maximum aerobic power from sensors in field settings would have been difficult to imagine a decade ago. The foundation for this monitoring progress was the experimental work that differentiated the passive and active mechanical aspects of human locomotion. Because the mechanics of steady-state walking and running allow the large majority of the mechanical energy exchanges to be recycled from one stride to the next, the remaining requirement for the musculoskeletal system is simply supporting the body's weight against gravity. The avenues of further biological work and sensor development that are now available should provide for equally rapid progress in the coming decade.

While Newton's principles of perfect energy conservation are known to apply ubiquitously, some particulars of energy transfer during human locomotion remain to be characterized more fully. The possibility of 100 percent transfer that has been raised here under ideal, steady-state conditions is certainly simplified to some small degree. Regardless, the empirical support for the predominant importance of support force in human locomotion is difficult to dispute. The sensor development spawned by the ideas regarding the fundamental importance of support mechanics makes a more convincing case still. The existence, utility, and remarkable accuracy of the sensor measurements under consistent conditions strongly attest to the validity of the original support force ideas. The energy transfers in the world of human locomotion may not be completely perfect, but the biological reality is certainly close enough for us to sense it.

REFERENCES

Alexander RM. 1991. Energy-saving mechanisms in walking and running. *J Exp Biol* 160:55–69.

Alexander RM. 1992. *Exploring Biomechanics. Animals in Motion*. New York: Scientific American Library.

Barany M. 1967. ATPase activity of myosin correlated with speed of muscle shortening. *J Gen Physiol* 50:197–218.

Bellizzi MJ, King KAD, Cushman SK, Weyand PG. 1998. Does the application of ground force set the energetic cost of cross-country skiing? *J Appl Physiol* 85:1736–1743.

Blaxter K. 1989. *Energy Metabolism in Animals and Man*. Cambridge: Cambridge University Press.

Cavagna GA, Sabiene FP, Margaria R. 1964. Mechanical work in running. *J Appl Physiol* 19:249–256.

Cavagna GA, Thys H, Zamboni A. 1976. The sources of external work in level walking and running. *J Physiol* 262:639–657.

Cavagna GA, Heglund NC, Taylor CR. 1977. Mechanical work in terrestrial locomotion: Two basic mechanisms for minimizing energy expenditure. *Am J Physiol* 233:R243–R261.

Fedak MA, Rome L, Seeherman HJ. 1981. One-step N2-dilution technique for calibrating open-circuit VO_2 measuring systems. *J Appl Physiol* 51:772–776.

Fenn WO. 1924. The relation between the work performed and energy liberated in muscular contraction. *J Physiol* 58:373–395.

Fenn WO. 1930. Frictional and kinetic factors in the work of sprint running. *Am J Physiol* 92:583–611.

Fukunaga T, Kubo K, Kawakami Y, Fukashiro S, Kanehisa H, Maganaris CN. 2001. In vivo behaviour of human muscle tendon during walking. *Proc R Soc Lond B Biol Sci* 268:229–233.

Glasheen JW, McMahon TA. 1995. Arms are different from legs: Mechanics and energetics of human hand-running. *J Appl Physiol* 78:1280–1287.

Gray J. 1968. *Animal Locomotion*. London: Weidenfeld and Nicolson.

Griffin T, Tolani NA, Kram R. 1999. Walking in simulated reduced gravity: Mechanical energy fluctuations and exchange. *J Appl Physiol* 86:383–390.

Griffin T, Roberts TJ, Kram R. 2003. Metabolic cost of generating muscular force in human walking: insights from load carrying and speed experiments. *J Appl Physiol* 95:172–183.

Heglund NC, Fedak MA, Taylor CR, Cavagna GA. 1982. Energetics and mechanics of terrestrial locomotion. IV. Total mechanical energy changes as a function of speeds and body size in birds and mammals. *J Exp Biol* 79:57–66.

Henneman E, Somjen G, Carpentar D. 1965. Excitability and inhibility of motoneurons of different sizes. *J Neurobiol* 28:599–620.

Hill AV. 1950. The dimensions of animals and their muscular dynamics. *Sci Prog* 38:209–230.

Hoyt RW, Kanpik JJ, Lanza JF, Jones BH, Staab JS. 1994. Ambulatory foot contact monitor to estimate metabolic cost of human locomotion. *J Appl Physiol* 76:1818–1822.

Kaneko M. 1990. Mechanics and energetics in running with special reference to efficiency. *J Biomech* 23:57–63.

Ker RF, Bennett MB, Bibby SR, Kester RC, Alexander RM. 1987. The spring in the arch of the human foot. *Nature* 325:147–149.

Kram R. 2000. Muscular force or work: What determines the metabolic energy cost of running? *Exerc Sport Sci Rev* 28:138–142.

Kram R, Taylor CR. 1990. The energetics of running: A new perspective. *Nature* 346:2265–2267.

Margaria R. 1976. *Biomechanics and Energetics of Muscular Exercise*. Oxford: Clarendon.

Margaria R, Cerretelli P, Aghemo P, Sassi G. 1963. Energy cost of running. *J Appl Physiol* 56:367–370.

Minetti AE, Ardigò LP, Saibene F. 1994. Mechanical determinants of the minimum energy cost of gradient running in humans. *J Exp Biol* 195:211–225.

Newton I. 1687. *Philosophae Naturalis Principia Mathematica I–III (The Royal Society, London)*. Translated by Motte A, 1729. Revised and edited by Cajori F, University of California Press, Berkeley, 1934.

Roberts T, Weber J-M, Hoppeler H, Weibel E, Taylor C. 1995. Design of the oxygen and substrate pathways: II. Defining upper limits of carbohydrate and fat oxidation. *Resp Physiol* 199:1651–1658.

Roberts TJ, Marsh RL, Weyand PG, Taylor CR. 1997. Muscular force in running turkeys: The economy of minimizing work. *Science* 275:1113–1115.

Roberts TJ, Kram R, Weyand PG, Taylor CR. 1998. Energetics of bipedal running. I. Metabolic cost of generating force. *J Exp Biol* 201:2745–2751.

Sahlin K. 1986. Metabolic changes limiting muscle performance. In: Saltin B, ed. *Biochemistry of Exercise. VI. International Series on Sports Sciences*. vol. 16. Champaign, IL: Human Kinetics. Pp. 323–344.

Steudel K. 1990. The work and energetic cost of locomotion. I. The effects of limb mass distribution in quadrupeds. *J Exp Biol* 154:273–285.

Taylor CR. 1994. Relating mechanics and energetics during exercise. In: Jones J, ed. *Comparative Vertebrate Exercise Physiology: Unifying Physiological Principles*. San Diego: Academic. Pp. 181–215.

van Ingen Schenau G. 1998. Positive work and its efficiency are at their deadend: Comments on a recent discussion. *J Biomech* 31:195–197.

Walmsley B, Hodgson J, Burke R. 1978. Forces produced by medial gastrocnemius and soleus muscles during locomotion in freely moving cats. *J Neurophysiol* 41:1203–1216.

Webb P, Saris WH, Schoffelen PF, van Ingen Schenau GJ, Ten Hoor F. 1988. The work of walking: A calorimetric study. *Med Sci Sports Exerc* 20:331–337.

Weyand P, Kelly M, Darley J, Oliver S, Ohlenbusch N, Joffe S, Blackadar T, Hoyt R. 2001. Ambulatory estimates of maximal aerobic power from foot-ground contact times and heart rates in running humans. *J Appl Physiol* 91:451–458.

Williams K, Cavanagh P. 1987. Relationship between distance running mechanics, running economy, and performance. *J Appl Physiol* 63:1236–1245.

Wright S, Weyand P. 2001. The application of ground force determines the energetic cost of running backward and forward. *J Exp Biol* 204:1805–1815.

Zuntz N. 1897. Ueber den stoffvenbrauch des hundes bei muskelarbeit. *Arch Ges Physiol* 68:191–211.

BIOMARKERS FOR CHANGE IN PROTEIN TURNOVER OF MUSCLE

Robert Wolfe, Elisabet Børsheim, University of Texas Medical Branch

The net gain or loss of muscle protein represents the balance between the rates of synthesis and breakdown. Consequently, when considering potential markers for changes in protein turnover in muscle, it is necessary to evaluate potential candidates in terms of the ability to reflect changes in the net balance between synthesis and breakdown.

The fundamental processes that control the balance between muscle protein synthesis and breakdown are shown in Figure D-26. Amino acids that can potentially be used for incorporation into protein (i.e., synthesis) can be derived from transport from the plasma, breakdown, or in the case of certain (nonessential) amino acids, from de novo synthesis. In turn, the amino acids in the precursor pool for synthesis can also be transported back to the plasma and carried away by venous blood.

There is interplay between all of these factors in the context of normal daily activity, including exercise and eating. Since amino acids provide a readily measurable component of the system, it is worthwhile to consider in depth the possible utility of measures of blood amino acid concentrations as indices of the status of the overall system, in particular the balance between synthesis and breakdown. In that regard, it is pertinent to first consider the role of muscle in the overall regulation of whole-body protein metabolism.

Many tissues of the body, such as the skin, heart, brain and liver, have a constant demand for amino acids. Protein breakdown is always occurring in these tissues, and without a sufficient rate of synthesis to balance the rate of breakdown, the amount of protein would quickly diminish. Since these tissues and organs do not have significant reserves of protein, even transient periods of net catabolism might have significant physiological consequences. Therefore, these tissues are normally able to extract sufficient amino acids from the blood to maintain synthesis at a rate sufficient to match the rate of breakdown, thereby avoiding a net loss of protein. Muscle, on the other hand, serves as a reservoir for amino acids. At least 15 percent of muscle mass can be lost without physiological consequences. Thus, muscle catabolism serves to provide plasma amino acids when none are available from absorption of dietary intake. In other words, there is a net negative protein balance in muscle in the postabsorptive or fasted state in order to provide the amino acids needed by other tissue organs in which the maintenance of protein mass is more essential for survival. Consequently, when amino acids are being absorbed, the muscle protein pool is the principal

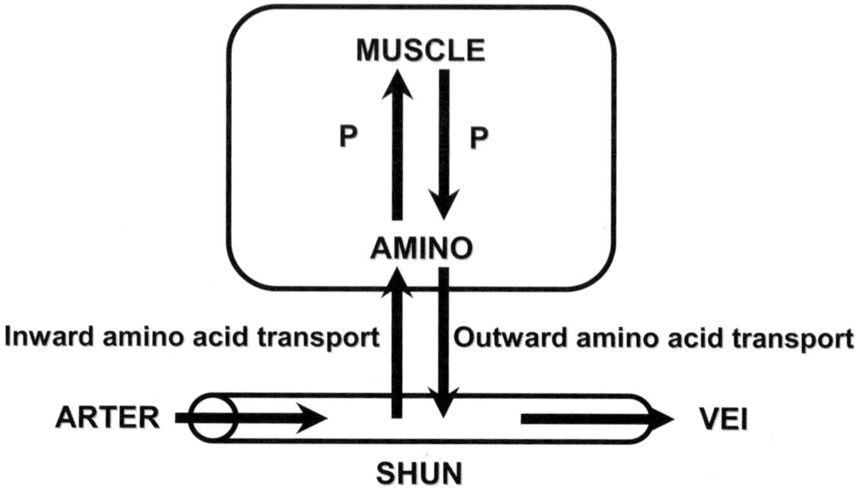

FIGURE D-26 Interaction between amino acids and protein kinetics.

target of repletion since other tissues received adequate amino acids via the blood to maintain protein balance in the absence of intake. Thus, muscle can be considered as a reservoir for amino acids that functions to keep amino acids available, via the plasma, for protein synthesis throughout the body.

The muscle performs its role as a reservoir quite efficiently. Even after 50 to 60 days of fasting in obese individuals, plasma essential and nonessential amino acids are maintained constant (Drenick et al., 1964). Further, intracellular concentrations of essential amino acids are regulated so as to remain constant unless there is a major perturbation in one or more of the factors controlling those concentrations (i.e., synthesis, breakdown, or transport). For example, when extracellular concentrations of amino acid were increased 40 percent by a primed-constant infusion, the intracellular essential amino acid concentrations remained constant, even though synthesis was stimulated (Bohe et al., In press). Further, when plasma amino acid concentrations were doubled by intravenous infusion, intracellular essential amino acid concentrations actually fell slightly, but significantly (Bohe et al., 2003). Only when the rate of infusion of amino acids increased sufficiently to exceed the capacity of synthesis to increase proportionately did the intracellular concentration of amino acids increase (Bohe et al., 2003). In an analogous response, when plasma amino acids were artificially lowered 40 percent below the basal level by hemodialysis, intracellular essential amino acid concentrations were unchanged (Kobayashi et al., 2003). Thus, under normal physiological conditions, changes in concentrations of essential amino acids cannot provide insight into the rates of muscle protein synthesis, breakdown, or the balance between them.

In severe stress, the stimulus for net protein catabolism provides the extra amino acids required for processes such as wound healing, immune function, and synthesis of acute phase proteins in the liver. In severe stress, such as burn injury, the signal for breakdown may exceed the increased requirement for amino acids, such that intracellular, and sometimes plasma concentrations, of essential amino acids increase. For example, intracellular concentrations of phenylalanine, leucine, and lysine are all elevated in burn patients (Biolo et al., 2000), although all may not be elevated in plasma. Interpretation of individual essential amino acids may be complicated by specific aspects of its metabolism. For example, phenylalanine is generally elevated in critically ill patients, but the plasma phenylalanine is clouded by the fact that its clearance not only reflects the uptake for the process of synthesis, but the liver clears phenylalanine and metabolizes it to tyrosine. Thus, in critically ill patients, an isolated increase in phenylalanine may reflect liver failure as much as net muscle protein breakdown.

The nonessential amino acids alanine and glutamine are the principal means by which nitrogen is transferred from muscle to the liver for eventual excretion as urea. Thus, when net muscle breakdown is accelerated, an increased production of alanine and/or glutamine would be expected. In fact, alanine release from muscle may be elevated by several-fold in severely burned patients (Jahoor et al., 1986); even after exercise alanine release is accelerated (Wolfe et al., 1979). However, plasma concentrations of alanine are not elevated when flux rates are elevated several-fold, probably due to the concurrent stimulation of gluconeogenesis that occurs in response to stress (Wolfe et al., 1979). In fact, alanine concentration may actually fall in severe sepsis (Gore and Wolfe, 2003). Consequently, alanine does not provide useful information about net muscle protein breakdown.

Depletion of the intramuscular glutamine pool occurs in stress states. Normally, the intramuscular concentration of glutamine is greater than the sum of all other amino acids. In severe stress, the intracellular concentration may fall by as much as 90 percent (Mittendorfer et al., 1999), but plasma concentrations are generally maintained or even fall. Thus, whereas plasma (and interstitial) concentrations of glutamine provide little insight into the net muscle protein balance, monitoring of the intracellular concentration of glutamine could likely provide reasonable insight as to whether the individual was under significant physiological stress. Current technology requires muscle biopsy to accomplish this measurement.

Muscle myofibrillar protein breakdown has been estimated using indirect measures such as 3-methylhistidine (3-MH) excretion (Young et al., 1973). 3-MH is produced by the posttranslational methylation (by protein-histidine N-methyltransferase) of specific histidine residues in the actin of all muscle fibers and in the myosin of type II fibers. It is released during protein breakdown and is not reutilized for protein synthesis or metabolized in man, but is excreted in urine. The skeletal muscle mass comprises the largest fraction of tissue-bound 3-MH in the body. Thus, urinary excretion of 3-MH in its free and acetylated form

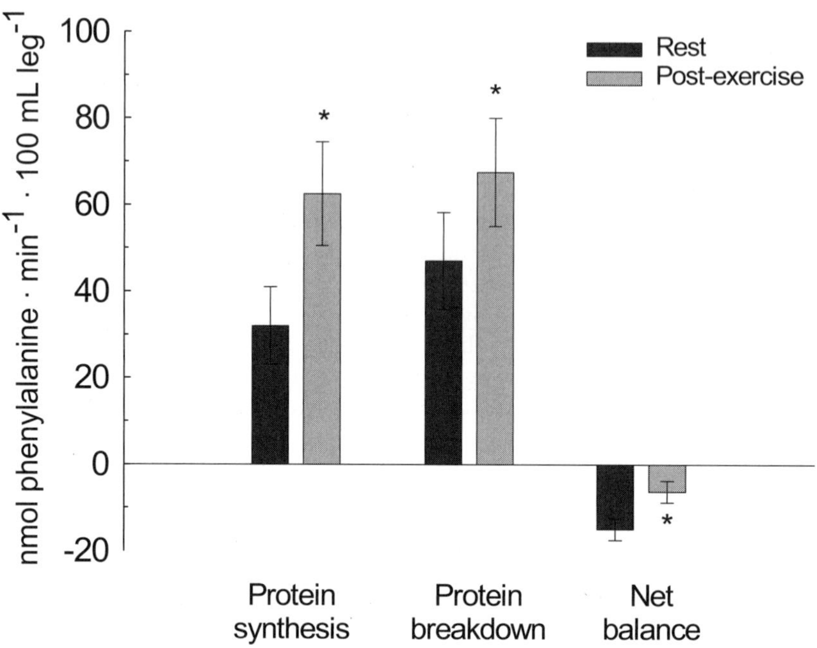

FIGURE D-27 Muscle protein synthesis, breakdown, and net protein balance at rest (black bars) and ~ 3 h after a heavy resistance exercise bout (gray bars) in untrained male volunteers. Values are mean ± standard error. Asterisk (*) indicates significant difference ($p < 0.05$) postexercise versus rest.
SOURCE: Reprinted, with permission Biolo et al. *AJP* (1995b).

has been used as a measure of the rate of muscle myofibrillar protein breakdown. Concerns about the validity of 3-MH excretion as an indicator of muscle protein breakdown relate to the contribution of nonmuscle sources to urinary 3-MH (e.g., gut smooth muscle and skin). Also, dietary protein intake can contribute to urinary 3-MH. Thus, urinary excretion of 3-MH may be problematic to use as a measure of skeletal muscle protein turnover. Determination of arterial-venous differences of 3-MH across muscle may be more useful in that regard. Nonetheless, even if it were to provide a precise measure of the rate of muscle protein breakdown, it would not be useful as an indicator of net muscle balance. When a large body of literature is considered, it is clear that changes in breakdown and synthesis normally occur in the same direction, and the magnitude of the individual responses (i.e., synthesis and breakdown) determines the nature of any change in net balance.

The best example of the lack of an obligatory relation between breakdown and net balance, particularly with relation to potential military applications, can be seen in Figure D-27. Resistance exercise caused an improvement in net muscle protein balance (i.e., reduced the fasting rate of muscle catabolism). However, the rate of breakdown actually increased—the improvement in net balance was due to an even greater increase in synthesis (Biolo et al., 1995b). Thus, whereas monitoring 3-MH could potentially give some indication of the rate of muscle protein breakdown, it is the balance between synthesis and breakdown that determines gain or loss of muscle mass; knowledge of breakdown alone provides little insight into the net balance.

Taken together, this discussion lends to the conclusion that measurement of plasma (or urinary) levels of amino acids or other potential markers of synthesis or breakdown cannot be expected to be reliable indicators of the balance between muscle protein kinetics or breakdown. Increasing levels of invasiveness enable more detailed information to be obtained.

With oral ingestion of a ^{15}N-alanine bolus and collection and analysis of urinary ammonia enrichment, it is possible to calculate whole body protein turnover. Coupled with ingestion of labeled 3-MH and measurement of the decay in enrichment, it is possible to distinguish the contribution of changes in muscle protein breakdown to the overall change in whole body protein turnover. In many, but not all, circumstances, changes in whole-body turnover reflect changes in muscle-protein turnover.

With increasing levels of invasiveness, it is possible to more directly obtain quantitative information. With the use of isotopically labeled tracer infusion and muscle biopsies and peripheral venous blood samples it is possible to quantify rates of muscle protein synthesis, and if arterial samples are added, breakdown can also be measured (Zhang et al., 1996). When arterial-venous sampling across the leg is coupled with biopsies, all of the factors shown in Figure D-27 can be quantified (Biolo et al., 1995a). Unfortunately, these invasive procedures are necessary because more readily accessible means of estimating muscle protein metabolism are unreliable.

SUMMARY

Changes in muscle mass occur because of an imbalance between the rates of protein synthesis and breakdown. Thus, the complication in finding a pertinent marker is that it must reflect the balance between two distinct processes. Consequently, the only reliable means of estimating changes in muscle protein turnover in a physiologically relevant manner is with the use of stable isotope tracers. Further, use of these tracers must be coupled with invasive procedures such as muscle biopsies and/or arterial and deep venous catheterizations to gain information about changes in muscle protein metabolism.

REFERENCES

Biolo G, Fleming RY, Maggi SP, Wolfe RR. 1995a. Transmembrane transport and intracellular kinetics of amino acids in human skeletal muscle. *Am J Physiol* 268:E75–E84.

Biolo G, Maggi SP, Williams BD, Tipton KD, Wolfe RR. 1995b. Increased rates of muscle protein turnover and amino acid transport after resistance exercise in humans. *Am J Physiol* 268:E514–E520.

Biolo G, Fleming RYD, Maggi SP, Nguyen TT, Herndon DN, Wolfe RR. 2000. Inhibition of muscle glutamine formation in hypercatabolic patients. *Clin Sci (Lond)* 100:299–301.

Bohe J, Low A, Wolfe RR, Rennie MJ. 2003. Human muscle protein synthesis is modulated by extracellular not intramuscular amino acid availability: A dose response study. *J Physiol* 552:315–324.

Drenick EJ, Swenseirl ME, Blahd WH, Tuttle SG. 1964. Prolonged starvation as treatment for severe obesity. *J Am Med Assoc* 187:100–105.

Gore D, Wolfe RR. 2003. Metabolic response of muscle to alanine, glutamine, and valine supplementation during severe illness. *J Parenter Enteral Nutr* 27:307–314.

Jahoor F, Herndon DN, Wolfe RR. 1986. Role of insulin and glucagon in the response of glucose and alanine kinetics in burn-injured patients. *J Clin Invest* 78:807–814.

Kobayashi H, Borsheim E, Anthony TG, Traber DL, Badalamenti J, Kimball SR, Jefferson LS, Wolfe RR. 2003. Reduced amino acid availability inhibits muscle protein synthesis and decreases activity of initiation factor eIF2B. *Am J Physiol Endocrinol Metab* 284:E488–E498.

Mittendorfer B, Gore DC, Herndon DN, Wolfe RR. 1999. Accelerated glutamine synthesis in critically ill patients cannot maintain normal intracellular free glutamine concentration. *J Parenter Enteral Nutr* 23:243–250.

Wolfe RR, Durkot MJ, Allsop JR, Burke JF. 1979. Glucose metabolism in severely burned patients. *Metabolism* 28:1031–1039.

Wolfe RR, Wolfe MH, Nadel ER, Shaw JH. 1984. Isotopic determination of amino acid-urea interactions in exercise in humans. *J Appl Physiol* 56:221–229.

Young VR, Havenbert LN, Bilamazes C, Munro HN. 1973. Potential use of 3-methylhistidine excretion as an index of progressive reduction in muscle protein catabolism during starvation. *Metabolism* 23:1429–1436.

Zhang X-J, Chinkes DL, Sakurai Y, Wolfe RR. 1996. An isotopic method for measurement of muscle protein fractional breakdown rate in vivo. *Am J Physiol* 270:E759–E767.

AMINO ACIDS AS BIOMARKERS FOR FATIGUE

T.P. Stein, University of Medicine and Dentistry of New Jersey

Muscle fatigue limits physical activity. Fatigue can be defined as the inability to maintain power output, and its causes are not known. The etiology can be of either local or central origin. Local fatigue originates within the muscle, whereas central fatigue is secondary to alterations within the brain. It is postulated that in central mechanisms, exercising muscle releases factors that act systemically and impact the central nervous system. In the context of military performance, systemic effects are likely to be of greater significance because of their potential to impact both physical and mental performance.

Muscle fatigue is not the same as muscle soreness. Muscle soreness is the pain that occurs about a day after exercise and peaks 2 to 3 days postexercise (Clarkson et al., 1992). The underlying mechanisms for delayed-onset muscle fatigue and fatigue are different. Soreness is believed to be due to a localized inflammatory response (Smith, 1991), and so the appropriate markers are markers for an inflammatory response. The onset of pain is also not considered to be a marker for muscle fatigue. Pain by itself is performance limiting and therefore is not a "predictor."

The majority of studies of muscle fatigue have assumed that the fatigue is the result of events localized within skeletal muscle (Davies and White, 1981; Edwards, 1981). Prior studies of muscle fatigue have focused on the relationship of a putative marker to the underlying biochemical or histological changes. This review has a somewhat different focus: the use of those markers as predictors for the onset of fatigue—specifically markers of protein origin.

For a marker to be of practical use, certain conditions must be met (Banister et al., 1985). The marker must apply to all subjects; a statistical relationship is inadequate when applied to the individual (Barron et al., 1985). In addition, the measurement must be technically feasible on a large number of subjects without costing too much. These criteria limit the assays to "spot" blood and urine measurements. In-line sensors in a selected muscle are not likely to be of much use. An isolated muscle may not reflect the whole musculoskeletal system and the muscle selected may not be one of the muscles that are becoming fatigued.

LOCAL FACTORS

Protein Turnover

Proteins are the machinery of the body. All of the work and all of metabolic functions in the body; movement, ion pumping, cell division, obtaining energy from foodstuffs, and host defense mechanisms are all affected by proteins. The health of the body protein pool is maintained by proteins being in a dynamic state; proteins are continually being made and broken down (protein turnover). A dynamic state of protein turnover allows a rapid response when a new mix of proteins is required. For example, with injury or infection, defense proteins need to be mobilized, any damaged proteins need to be removed, and protein levels need to be altered. Clearly, if the machinery begins to malfunction, performance will decrease.

Unfortunately, there is no simple means of assessing the status of protein turnover. The classical marker for protein breakdown is 3-methyl histidine (3-MeH) production. Monitoring the urinary 3-MeH is a standard assay for assessing myofibrillar protein breakdown; its limitations are well known (Long et al., 1981; Munro and Young, 1978; Rathmacher et al., 1995; Rennie and Millward, 1983). To obtain interpretable 3-MeH data, subjects should be on a meat-free diet. Placing combat troops on a meat free diet, or even attempting to control meat intake, is not a realistic option and thus monitoring of 3-MeH production is not feasible even if it were shown to somehow correlate with fatigue.

The other side of protein turnover is protein synthesis. There is no nonisotopic method for measuring human protein synthesis. Clinically, the classic method for assessing protein status (and still the most sensitive), and hence indirectly protein turnover, is nitrogen balance. The problem with the nitrogen balance method is that it is fraught with errors; the errors tend to be unidirectional towards over-estimating nitrogen retention.

Knowing that there has been a major change in nitrogen balance would be enough to cause concern. Classically, nitrogen balance is done by measuring input (food) and output (urine, sweat, feces, and any increase in blood urea nitrogen). To measure all of these parameters accurately is difficult in a clinical research center environment; to do so noninvasively in the field is not possible. There are no potential markers for protein turnover.

NUTRITIONAL FACTORS

Plasma Amino Acids

While not directly correlated with protein synthesis, plasma and tissue-free amino acid concentrations and distribution patterns provide useful information on protein metabolism. An important study by Kingsbury and colleagues (1998) compared fasting plasma amino acid patterns in elite athletes from the 1996 British Olympics team during training. Athletes were divided into three groups: group A, no lasting fatigue after training; group B, heavy fatigue at night but recovered after an overnight rest; and group C, chronic fatigue with full recovery taking a week or more. The results are summarized in Table D-5.

Plasma amino acid concentrations were lower in the two groups subject to fatigue (Table D-5). There were significant relationships between the fatigue and some of the changes in individual amino acids. Figure D-28 shows the distribution of plasma glutamine and histidine. There is virtually no overlap

TABLE D-5 Fasting Plasma Amino Acid Levels of Athlete Groups During Training (μmol/L^{-1})

Amino Acid	Normal Range	A (n = 21)	B (n = 12)	C (n = 18)
Glutamine	480–800	554 (25.2)	356 (16.0)[c]	383 (13.6)[c]
Histidine	30–150	79 (6.1)	32 (1.2)[c]	50 (2.9)[c]
Alanine	150–450	422 (24.7)	352 (20.4)[a]	344 (17.1)[a]
Threonine	70–220	121 (8.7)	72 (4.7)[c]	91 (4.6)[b]
Serine	90–290	104 (5.3)	109 (5.3)	88 (5.1)[a]
Lysine	100–300	161 (8.5)	89 (6.1)[c]	124 (8.2)[b]
Tryptophan	30–80	67 (3.5)	44 (3.7)[c]	55 (2.9)[a]
Tyrosine	30–120	62 (3.8)	43 (3.2)[c]	55 (4.3)
Valine	90–300	219 (11.4)	151 (8.8)	188 (10.4)
Leucine	65–220	146 (3.9)	127 (5.7)[a]	137 (9.5)
Isoleucine	26–100	77 (5.3)	59 (2.9)[b]	69 (4.6)
Arginine	40–120	82 (6.2)	57 (3.6)[b]	71 (4.9)
Proline	85–290	232 (12.1)	196 (13.8)	188 (18.7)
Ornithine	25–120	59 (3.9)	58 (5.3)	60 (5.5)
Methionine	10–60	35 (2.5)	26 (1.5)[a]	30 (1.3)
Glutamic acid	25–130	55 (6.3)	102 (4.9)[c]	56 (8.7)
Glycine	100–330	227 (10.3)	316 (20.4)[c]	199 (9.9)
Phenylalanine	35–100	71 (2.5)	88 (2.9)[c]	70 (4.1)
Total amino acids		2,839 (92.1)	2,396 (90.1)	2,307 (71.6)

NOTE: Mean with standard error of the mean in parentheses. Subjects were divided into three groups depending on level of fatigue: group A, no lasting fatigue; group B, heavy fatigue at night but with full recovery by the next day; and group C, chronic fatigue and poor performance.

[a] $p < 0.05$ vs. group A.

[b] $p < 0.01$ vs. .group A.

[c] $p < 0.001$ vs. group A.

SOURCE: Adapted from Kingsbury et al. (1998), *British Journal of Sports Medicine*, 32, 25–33, with permission from the BMJ Publishing Group.

between the fatigue groups and the controls with glutamine. What is important about the findings is the very high discriminatory power of the measurements for identify the subjects prone to fatigue. The study is promising, but not definitive because the subjects were not matched by athletic event and no dietary data was collected. An observational, nonrandomized follow-up study of increasing protein intake appeared to be of benefit to the subjects with low glutamine and histidine concentrations. Plasma glutamine and histidine concentrations were increased, as was performance (Kingsbury et al., 1998).

These observations may be indicative of early substrate depletion for the maintenance of protein synthesis. More likely they reflect limitations in energy generation by the tricarboxylic acid (TCA) cycle. Amino acids provide precursor substrates for the TCA cycle (Young and Marchini, 1990). If energy expenditure is increased, the need for the replenishment of amino acids is also increased (Wagenmakers, 1998).

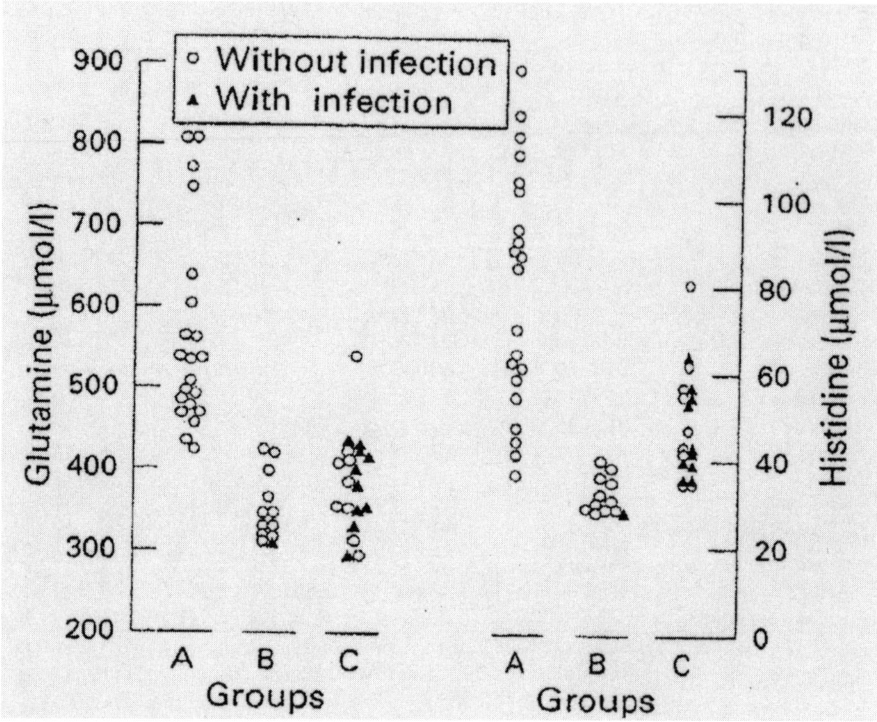

FIGURE D-28 Fasting plasma glutamine and histidine levels of athlete groups during training. Units are μmol/L^{-1}. Subjects were divided into three groups depending level of fatigue: group A (n = 21), no lasting fatigue; group B (n = 12), heavy fatigue at night but with full recovery by the next day; and group C (n = 18), chronic fatigue and poor performance.
SOURCE: Kingsbury et al. (1998), *British Journal of Sports Medicine*, 32, 25–33, with permission from the BMJ Publishing Group.

Assuming that the above results can be validated under more controlled conditions, it would appear that measurement of the fasting plasma aminogram has the potential for early identification of subjects prone to fatigue.

Energy

Troops in field situations may suffer from energy deficits either because of limited food availability or very high workloads. Indeed, rigorous military field training can induce energy deficits as high as 1,000 kcal/day (Friedl and Hoyt,

1997; Kramer et al., 1997). Such energy deficits lead to weight loss and some loss of lean body mass. Even so, nutrition is not likely to be the cause of fatigue. Glycogen depletion is a natural process, and after muscle glycogen has been used, muscle uses fat.

Humans have extensive energy reserves. The average male has enough endogenous fat to withstand starvation for up to 70 days. A controlled study by Zachwieja and colleagues (2001) found that moderate, short-term deficits (2 weeks, 750 kcal/day) in food intake does not impact performance in otherwise healthy individuals. Adequately fed humans have sufficient endogenous energy reserves to function normally for extended periods. With extreme depletion or nutritional deprivation, the situation will be different, but by that time fatigue will be of minor consequence in the health status of the soldier.

Alterations in fuel metabolism can be detected from reduced fuel availability in the plasma (fuels include energy substrates as well as oxygen) or from end products of fuel metabolism (e.g., lactate). However, since the fuel supply to the muscle is not likely to be limiting, monitoring dietary status as a potential predictor for the onset of fatigue is unlikely to be productive.

Other Nutritionally Related Factors

Several plausible mechanisms have been proposed to serve as biomarkers for fatigue. These include limited or decreased availability of energy fuels, glycogen depletion, depletion of phosphocreatine, proton accumulation, failure of neuromuscular transmission, and actual muscle damage (Davis, 1995). With the exception of proton accumulation (lactate production) and actual muscle damage, there is little supportive experimental evidence.

Monitoring specific fuels and metabolites within muscle (e.g., glycogen, phosphocreatine) is not likely to have the necessary reliability and sensitivity to serve as a biomarker for fatigue. There is no certainty that the muscle selected for monitoring is going to be one of the muscles causing the fatigue. Furthermore, such measurements are likely to be technically difficult.

MUSCLE DAMAGE

Excessive work leads to actual damage to muscle. Numerous studies have explored the use of plasma levels of muscle-derived proteins as indices of muscle damage. The principal markers that have been used are: aspartate amino transferase, lactate dehydrogenase, creatine kinase, myoglobin, fatty-acid binding proteins, carbonic anhydrase isoenzyme III, and myocyte contractile proteins such as troponins and myosin heavy chains (Janssen et al., 1989; Sorichter et al., 1999). In rodent studies it has been the clearly shown that the degree of damage estimated from plasma enzyme levels is greater than that found by histological examination. The reason is that plasma enzyme levels reflect a combination of actual muscle damage and transient changes in membrane permeability (Van der

Meulen et al., 1991). The most frequently used marker for muscle damage has been creatinine kinase.

A direct connection between muscle injury and muscle fatigue has not been proven. A little damage in one or two muscles is enough to increase plasma levels of muscle proteins, but a small degree of damage does not appear to impact performance, although if the muscle damage is severe enough, it should ultimately lead to impaired performance.

The problem with the use of proteins released from damaged muscle is that they are markers for damaged muscle—not fatigue. Subtle changes in muscle ultra structure may lead to decreased strength and fatigue, but such changes will not necessarily be reflected by increased leakage of muscle proteins into the plasma compartment (Behm et al., 2001). Muscle proteins can indicate damage, but they cannot predict fatigue in humans because the correlation between damage and fatigue is weak.

THE OVER-TRAINING SYNDROME

Related to muscle fatigue is the over-training syndrome. Over-training is a term that is used to describe the process where the training is excessive and results in a condition of staleness or burnout (Barron et al., 1985; Hooper et al., 1995). Staleness is characterized by chronic fatigue, poor performance, and delayed recovery (Fry et al., 1991; Kuipers and Keizer, 1988; Verde et al., 1992). The major symptom is underperformance (Budgett, 1998).

At present there are no objective markers for overtraining other than outcome. Parameters that have been investigated include heart rate, blood pressure, enzyme blood levels, hormones, and leukocyte numbers. In general, correlations have been observed, but they are weak and of no predictive potential. For example, a study by Hooper and colleagues (1995) investigated potential markers for overtraining in Olympic-caliber Australian swimmers. The only correlations between fatigue (as recorded by the subjects), staleness (failure to improve during training), and blood markers was higher levels of catecholamines ($r^2 = 0.33$) and leukocytes ($r^2 = -0.16$) with fatigue. Both of these parameters are also markers for stress (Hooper et al., 1995). Elsewhere, Budgett (1998) concluded that "there is no diagnostic test available."

CENTRAL FATIGUE

Little is known about the mechanisms for central fatigue as it has not been a very active area for research. But fatigue of central origin it is of potentially great significance to the Army because it could not only affect physical activity, but mental performance as well. Two viable hypotheses have been published: the ammonia hypothesis and the tryptophan hypothesis (Davis, 1995). In both cases, the theory is plausible; there is some experimental supporting evidence, but is suggestive at best. The tryptophan hypothesis has attracted the most interest.

The Tryptophan Hypothesis

Newsholme and colleagues proposed that exercise-induced change in the plasma amino acid distribution could induce central fatigue by influencing the synthesis, concentration, and release of neurotransmitters, particularly 5-hydroxy tryptamine (5-HT) within the brain (Blomstrand, 2001; Castell et al., 1999). Brain 5-HT is in involved in the control of arousal, sleepiness, and mood, so it is therefore conceivable that brain 5-HT levels could lead to fatigue during and after vigorous physical activity (Blomstrand, 2001). Indeed, there is a considerable amount of evidence from rodent studies showing that inhibiting the action of 5-HT improves endurance (Blomstrand, 2001).

Plasma tryptophan is the precursor for brain 5-HT. The rate limiting step in the synthesis of 5-HT is the transport of tryptophan across the blood-brain barrier into the brain (Fernstrom, 1990). The tryptophan transporter system also transports the other large neutral amino acids, specifically the three branched-chain amino acids (BCAAs). The hypothesis proposes that competition for the transport between tryptophan and BCAAs occurs. Thus, the rate of entry of tryptophan into the brain will depend on the amount of free tryptophan in the blood compared with the amount of competitive amino acids. During prolonged exercise there is a decrease in the concentration of most amino acids. Most of the tryptophan in the plasma is bound to albumin, and free fatty acids compete for the tryptophan binding sites on albumin. Thus, as exercise progresses, fatty acid mobilization occurs and the increased plasma free fatty acid levels displace bound tryptophan from albumin, leading to an increase in free tryptophan in the plasma. At the same time, the concentration of BCAAs decreases with prolonged exercise. The net effect is that the ratio of free tryptophan to BCAA increases several-fold and more tryptophan is taken up into the brain. At rest, only about 10 percent of blood tryptophan is in the free form. Whether the ratio tryptophan to BCAA increases with exercise depends on the type and duration of the exercise.

The tryptophan:BCAA theory predicts that increasing the plasma BCAA concentration should decrease tryptophan uptake into the brain, thereby decreasing 5-HT synthesis and the delaying fatigue. A number of studies have sought to test this prediction. Results have been ambiguous, with some studies reporting positive results and others no effects from BCAA supplementation (Blomstrand, 2001). Ingestion of carbohydrates can also lead to lower free tryptophan during exercise. Carbohydrates depress fat mobilization, thereby increasing the proportion of the blood tryptophan bound to albumin. One report found improved mental agility of psychological tests during sustained competitive exercise when the subjects were given both BCAA and carbohydrate (Hassmen et al., 1994).

The potential markers are plasma tryptophan, plasma BCAAs, plasma albumin together with determination of the amounts of free fatty acids bound to the albumin, and the plasma free fatty acid concentration. These are potential markers for the prediction of the onset of fatigue, and so should be considered as "real-time markers" rather than as predictors of future fatigue (e.g., amino acids). Overall the evidence is not very strong, but the hypothesis may be worth a definitive experiment. Part of the reason for favoring further investigation of the tryptophan hypothesis is that the hypothesis leads to a countermeasure: giving supplemental BCAAs. This would be feasible in a field situation.

The Ammonia Hypothesis

All tissues produce ammonia; high concentrations of ammonia in the brain are neurotoxic. With exercise, muscle ammonia production increases (Banister et al., 1985; Eriksson et al., 1985; Yuan and Chan, 2000). There is not, however, a direct correlation between exercise, blood ammonia levels, and the concentration of ammonia in the brain.

The major sources of the increased ammonia production in muscle are the purine nucleotide cycle in which adenosine monophosphate is deaminated to inosine monophosphate by adenylate deaminase, and the catabolism of BCAAs. Ammonia production through both pathways increases with duration and intensity of exercise.

Increasing the plasma ammonia levels with exercise leads to an increase in the tissues and a parallel increase within the brain (Meyer et al., 1980). The mechanisms for the increased brain ammonia are not known; both increased uptake and decreased export have been proposed (Banister et al., 1985; Yuan and Chan, 2000). Within the brain, ammonia participates in numerous reactions that could lead to neurotoxicity. The levels produced with exercise are comparable with neurotoxic levels (Banister et al., 1985), but exercise-induced increases are transient—they resolve soon after the termination of exercise. In the case of clinically induced hyperammonemia, reducing the ammonia load has been of benefit.

A potential marker for fatigue is the blood ammonia level. However, although this hypothesis is viable, there is little actual experimental evidence.

SUMMARY

The only amino acid-derived parameter with the potential for predicting future fatigue is measurement of the fasting plasma aminogram during a period of strenuous training (Kingsbury et al., 1998). If the findings on Olympic athletes can be reproduced with soldiers, measurement of the fasting plasma aminogram during training could have the potential for early identification of subjects prone to early fatigue. The measurement appears to have both the specificity and technical simplicity needed to be used in a real-life situation (Kingsbury et al., 1998). Moreover, Kingsbury and colleagues (1998) reported that in a small subset of their cohort with low plasma amino acid levels, increasing dietary intake did lead to improved performance. Thus, there is also the possibility of treatment. Replicating Kingsbury's results in the population of interest to the Army would be important.

The potential gain for the Army in following up Kingsbury's observations is great, the risks negligible, and the cost small. The results are scientifically plausible. Indeed, the Army suspected that amino acids intake might be a key factor in improving performance and in 1999 commissioned the Committee on Military Nutrition to investigate the role of amino acids in improving performance. The British study was published after the committee completed their report. One wonders what would the committee have concluded had it seen Kingsbury's data?

REFERENCES

Banister EW, Rajendra W, Mutch BJ. 1985. Ammonia as an indicator of exercise stress: Implications of recent findings to sports medicine. *Sports Med* 2:34–46.

Barron JL, Noakes TD, Levy W, Smith C, Millar RP. 1985. Hypothalamic dysfunction in overtrained athletes. *J Clin Endocrinol Metab* 60:803–806.

Behm DG, Baker KM, Kelland R, Lomond J. 2001. The effect of muscle damage on strength and fatigue deficits. *J Strength Cond Res* 15:255–263.

Blomstrand E. 2001. Amino acids and central fatigue. *Amino Acids* 20:25–34.

Budgett R. 1998. Fatigue and underperformance in athletes: The overtraining syndrome. *Br J Sports Med* 32:107–110.

Castell LM, Yamamoto T, Phoenix J, Newsholme EA. 1999. The role of tryptophan in fatigue in different conditions of stress. *Adv Exp Med Biol* 467:697–704.

Clarkson PM, Nosaka K, Braun B. 1992. Muscle function after exercise-induced muscle damage and rapid adaptation. *Med Sci Sports Exerc* 24:512–520.

Davies CT, White MJ. 1981. Muscle weakness following eccentric work in man. *Pflugers Arch* 392:168–171.

Davis JM. 1995. Central and peripheral factors in fatigue. *J Sports Sci* 13:S49–S53.

Edwards RHT. 1981. Human muscle function and fatigue: Physiological mechanisms. In: Porter R, Whelan WJ, eds. *CIBA Foundation Symposia*. London: Pitman Medical. Pp. 1–18.

Eriksson LS, Broberg S, Bjorkman O, Wahren J. 1985. Ammonia metabolism during exercise in man. *Clin Physiol* 5:325–336.

Fernstrom JD. 1990. Aromatic amino acids and monoamine synthesis in the CNS. Influence of diet. *J Nutr Biochem* 10:508–517.

Friedl KE, Hoyt RW. 1997. Development and biomedical testing of military operational rations. *Annu Rev Nutr* 17:51–75.

Fry RW, Morton AR, Keast D. 1991. Overtraining in athletes. An update. *Sports Med* 12:32–65.

Hassmen P, Blomstrand E, Ekblom B, Newsholme EA. 1994. Branched-chain amino acid supplementation during 30-km competitive run: Mood and cognitive performance. *Nutrition* 10:405–410.

Hooper SL, Mackinnon LT, Howard A, Gordon RD, Bachmann AW. 1995. Markers for monitoring overtraining and recovery. *Med Sci Sports Exerc* 27:106–112.

Janssen GM, Kuipers H, Willems GM, Does RJ, Janssen MP, Geurten P. 1989. Plasma activity of muscle enzymes: Quantification of skeletal muscle damage and relationship with metabolic variables. *Int J Sports Med* 10:S160–S168.

Kingsbury KJ, Kay L, Hjelm M. 1998. Contrasting plasma free amino acid patterns in elite athletes: Association with fatigue and infection. *Br J Sports Med* 32:25–32.

Kramer TR, Moore RJ, Shippee RL, Friedl KE, Martinez-Lopez L, Chan MM, Askew EW. 1997. Effects of food restriction in military training on T-lymphocyte responses. *Int J Sports Med* 18:S84–S90.

Kuipers H, Keizer HA. 1988. Overtraining in elite athletes. Review and directions for the future. *Sports Med* 6:79–92.

Long CL, Birkhahn RH, Geiger JW, Betts JE, Schiller WR, Blakemore WS. 1981. Urinary excretion of 3-methylhistidine: An assessment of muscle protein catabolism in adult normal subjects and during malnutrition, sepsis, and skeletal trauma. *Metabolism* 30:765–776.

Meyer RA, Dudley GA, Terjung RL. 1980. Ammonia and IMP in different skeletal muscle fibers after exercise in rats. *J Appl Physiol* 49:1037–1041.

Munro HN, Young VR. 1978. Urinary excretion of N gamma-methylihistidine (3-methylihistidine): A tool to study metabolic responses in relation to nutrient and hormonal status in health and disease of man. *Am J Clin Nutr* 31:1608–1614.

Rathmacher JA, Flakoll PJ, Nissen SL. 1995. A compartmental model of 3-methylhistidine metabolism in humans. *Am J Physiol* 269:E193–E198.

Rennie MJ, Millward DJ. 1983. 3-Methylhistidine excretion and the urinary 3-methylhistidine/creatinine ratio are poor indicators of skeletal muscle protein breakdown. *Clin Sci* 65:217–225.

Smith LL. 1991. Acute inflammation: The underlying mechanism in delayed onset muscle soreness? *Med Sci Sports Exerc* 23:542–551.

Sorichter S, Puschendorf B, Mair J. 1999. Skeletal muscle injury induced by eccentric muscle action: Muscle proteins as markers of muscle fiber injury. *Exerc Immunol Rev* 5:5–21.

Van der Meulen JH, Kuipers H, Drukker J. 1991. Relationship between exercise-induced muscle damage and enzyme release in rats. *J Appl Physiol* 71:999–1004.

Verde T, Thomas S, Shephard RJ. 1992. Potential markers of heavy training in highly trained distance runners. *Br J Sports Med* 26:167–175.

Wagenmakers AJ. 1998. Protein and amino acid metabolism in human muscle. *Adv Exp Med Biol* 441:307–319.

Young VR, Marchini JS. 1990. Mechanisms and nutritional significance of metabolic responses to altered intakes of protein and amino acids, with reference to nutritional adaptation in humans. *Am J Clin Nutr* 51:270–289.

Yuan Y, Chan KM. 2000. A review of the literature on the application of blood ammonia measurement in sports science. *Res Q Exerc Sport* 71:145–151.

Zachwieja JJ, Ezell DM, Cline AD, Ricketts JC, Vicknair PC, Schorle SM, Ryan DH. 2001. Short-term dietary energy restriction reduces lean body mass but not performance in physically active men and women. *Int J Sports Med* 22:310–316.

BIOMARKERS OF BONE AND MUSCLE TURNOVER: EFFECTS OF EXERCISE

Clifford J. Rosen, Wesley G. Beamer, Leah Rae Donahue, The Jackson Laboratory

Bone is a hard tissue with multiple components that provide mammals with a structural framework and a never-ending source of calcium for most homeostatic processes. Traditionally, the skeleton has been classified into trabecular and cortical elements. As such, the cortical shell has been classically viewed as protective with relatively slow remodeling rates, whereas the trabecular skeleton has been considered metabolically active due to its proximity to marrow elements and its large surface area. This, however, is a relatively simplistic model for the skeleton since it is clear that there are other major differences for these two components, both in respect to cell constitution and vascular supply. In addition, the regulation of bone growth, modeling, and acquisition differs in time, sequence, and outcome between cortical and trabecular sites. Thus, as growth occurs, modeling of the skeleton takes place at the growth plate and at periosteal sites along long bones. Muscle insertion also occurs on the periosteum, and repetitive stresses strongly influence periosteal expansion and turnover.

The process of remodeling and subsequent bone acquisition represents a complex consolidative process occurring at the endosteal surface as well as the periosteum, ultimately resulting in attainment of peak bone mass. For the trabecular skeleton, that point occurs around the time of linear growth cessation, whereas cortical bone continues to consolidate until people reach their early thirties. The control over growth and remodeling, as well as skeletal maintenance, has been the subject of intense investigation over the last two decades. However, less attention has been paid to the differential compartments as they relate to growth and remodeling. Recent evidence from our laboratory and others have provided significant insight into the role of periosteal growth and remodeling in the acquisition of bone mass and the potential role of the periosteum in modulating exercise-induced skeletal changes. This paper discusses one marker of bone and muscle turnover, IGF-I, insulin-like growth factor-I, and its role in the process of cortical peak acquisition and skeletal homeostasis.

THE PERIOSTEUM AND ENDOSTEUM

The periosteum is a highly specialized surface overlying the cortical envelop of all long bones. Although it contains all the necessary cells for bone remodeling (i.e., osteoclasts, osteoblasts, and osteocytes), the origin of these cells remains in doubt. Because of the prominent vascular supply to the periosteum and its role in fracture healing, it seems likely that these osteoblasts are, at the least, unique in respect to their signaling and origin from primitive cells outside the bone marrow. Indeed, there is some suggestion that periosteal osteoblasts may be derived from pericytes in the blood vessels of the outer cortical shell. Regardless of their site of origin, it is apparent that periosteal function changes with various stages of life, and that certain periosteal osteoblasts may work in opposition to their counterparts on the endosteum. In fact, there is likely to be differential regulation of these two compartments, and this in turn becomes important for targeting approaches aimed at strengthening bone or preventing stress fractures.

Several recent lines of evidence support differential regulation of periosteal and endosteal bone turnover. First, our group was the first to report that among inbred strains of mice, there are strong genetic differences in peak bone acquisition (Beamer et al., 1996). Initially due to the level of resolution of our scanning devices in mice, we hypothesized that the differences among inbred strains was purely genetic and not confined to a single skeletal compartment. However, recently we reported that although one inbred strain, C3H/HeJ, had much higher cortical bone mass than did another strain, C57BL6, that difference was reversed when we examined trabecular bone mass by uCT analysis (Beamer et al., 2001). Hence, within a given strain, one can find both high and low bone mass depending on the compartment being measured. Moreover, we had assumed that all bone mass was acquired in the mouse by 16 weeks of age (Beamer et al., 1996). This also proved incorrect! Cortical bone density reached peak at 4 months of age, but trabecular bone mineral density is more rapidly acquired and maintained by 6 weeks of age (Beamer et al., 1996; Bouxsein, personal communication). These findings confirm that there is dual regulation of skeletal compartments in mice.

More emerging evidence supports this thesis. A recent abstract from a group in Sweden confirmed that in humans, these two skeletal compartments work in opposite directions (Ahlborg et al., 2002). The authors followed more than 100 postmenopausal women for 19 years using single energy X-ray absorptiometry of the distal radius. They noted about a 1.7 percent/year rate of bone loss, principally from the endosteal surface, in these women over the two decades. By contrast, periosteal circumference increased 0.6 percent/year and hence expanded by nearly 12 percent over the two decades of observation. This expansion is associated with an improvement in the cross-sectional moment of inertia, and almost certainly results in modest, but not complete, structural protection against rapid bone loss. The third line of evidence is derived from unloading experiments in C3H animals with high cortical bone mass. Despite significant endosteal bone loss after sciatic neurectomy, cortical expansion becomes a major compensatory pathway that preserves bone strength, at least in the short run.

Very recently, Kim and colleagues (2003) examined the differential regulation of the periosteum and endosteum in growing rats of both genders. To begin with, they reported that male rats tend to have nearly 25 percent greater bone width than females, and this is associated with greater bone strength. They noted that growth hormone (GH) and androgens in males independently stimulate expansion of bone, but that GH deficiency alone does not significantly reduce bone fragility because of the androgen-mediated effects on periosteal growth. By contrast, in females, GH stimulates periosteal expansion, but estrogen inhibits such growth. Hence, gonadectomy in females results in trabecular bone loss, but periosteal expansion as the inhibitor of such activity is removed. As such, it is clear that under certain hormonal manipulations, as well as with mechanical influences, changes in the periosteal envelope differ considerably from that in the endosteum.

What controls periosteal and endosteal remodeling and growth? Since the origin of periosteal osteoblasts is not known, many questions remain about the control mechanisms involved in periosteal expansion during growth and with aging. Utilizing inbred strains of mice, our group has defined the importance of genetic determinants in periosteal and endosteal expansion. It is also clear that there are at least two principal regulators of the periosteum: skeletal muscle with its insertion into bone, and systemic hormones that likely make their way through the vascular network in the periosteum to alter the behavior of specific bone cells. As noted above, the sex steroids certainly are considered within this latter category, although many investigators would maintain that both types of regulators work through a single common pathway, the IGF regulatory system.

THE REGULATION OF THE PERIOSTEUM: A ROLE FOR IGF-I?

Several lines of evidence support a major role for circulating IGF-I in determining bone size. These data are principally derived from in vivo manipulations using genetic engineering and inbred strains of mice. IGF-I is a ubiquitous polypeptide that is expressed in most tissues and also circulates in very large concentrations bound to a series of IGF-specific binding proteins. Bone is a major site of IGF-I production, principally from early and mature osteoblasts. It is stored within the skeletal matrix bound to IGFBP-5 and IGFBP-2 and released during osteoclast-mediated bone resorption. Because the marrow bathes trabecular elements, it is not surprising that the relative content of IGF-I in sites such as the vertebrae is quite substantial. As such, the principal source of IGF-I in these areas is likely to be local synthesis. On the other hand, although the periosteum is rich in osteoblasts, IGF-I content in this region appears to be a function of both circulatory and local synthesis. Impressive in vivo data supporting this contention have recently been published by our group and others.

Technology that permits selective knockout or knockdown of ligands and receptors in mice has opened an exciting era for testing functional correlates of peptide growth factors and their signals. Yakar and colleagues (2002) recently demonstrated that with selective knockout of the IGF-I gene in liver, there are significant skeletal changes. The LID mice were generated by using an albumin promoter tied to Cre-recombinase and mating those mice with another group of mice carrying a floxed IGF-I gene. The resultant animals had normal expression of IGF-I in all other tissues besides the liver, including the skeleton, but a 75 percent reduction in serum IGF-I. Despite growth curves that were not markedly abnormal, the long bones of the LID mice were shorter and had markedly reduced bone volume despite normal skeletal IGF-I expression. All the skeletal changes were in the cortical component and reflected a reduction in periosteal circumference as well as cortical thickness. Trabecular bone was entirely normal. These data suggest that alterations in circulating IGF-I affect skeleton modeling and principally the cortical component. Similarly, recent work from Tom Clemens and from our laboratory have shown that knockout of the IGF-I Type I receptor in mature osteoblasts using an osteocalcin-specific promoter and Cre lox P recombinase resulted in a dramatic skeletal phenotype of reduced trabecular bone density and slow bone mineralization, but no change in the cortical envelop, periosteal circumference, or femur length (Zhang et al., 2002). These data are remarkably similar to over-expression studies of IGF-I in bone, in which the animals have significantly enhanced bone density but no change in size, volume, or length of their bones (Zhao et al., 2000). Finally, our laboratory has confirmed that in a spontaneous mutant mouse, *little,* which does not make growth hormone and has low serum IGF-I, periosteal size and circumference are markedly reduced (as is femur length), but that trabecular bone mass is not altered, nor is skeletal expression of IGF-I. In sum, it appears that circulating, but not skeletal, IGF-I controls periosteal growth and modeling, whereas local IGF-I almost certainly plays an important role in trabecular mineralization and acquisition.

Further support for that tenet comes from work with congenic mice at The Jackson Laboratory. Bouxsein and colleagues (2002) created a congenic mouse that has a knockdown in serum IGF-I of approximately 20 to 25 percent. This is associated with no change in skeletal IGF-I expression, but a significant reduction in periosteal circumference, femoral length, and cortical osteocyte apoptosis. This congenic (6-T) also has reduced free levels of IGF-I compared with parental C57BL6 controls, suggesting that alterations in the circulating concentration of IGF-I can have a significant impact on bone growth and consolidation.

WHAT IS THE ROLE OF EXERCISE, LEAN MASS, AND MUSCLE IN PERIOSTEAL GROWTH?

Particular animal models have allowed us to dissect the regulation of individual skeletal compartments by careful phenotyping. Another approach is to define how the second major regulator of cortical bone, skeletal muscle, affects periosteal growth and expansion. Once again, we can turn to animal models. Currently, at The Jackson Laboratory, a major endeavor is underway to completely characterize a number of phenotypes related to body composition and bone mass in 40 different strains of mice. Not surprising, there are major differences not only in bone mass, but also in IGF-I and body composition among these strains. The "Phenome Project" will provide tremendous insight into the role of muscle and lean mass, as well as adiposity in periosteal and endosteal growth. Several strains have been identified that have similar lean body mass but major differences in bone mineral content. Experimental manipulation of these mice, followed by public dissemination of this information, will allow investigators to dissect how muscle mass, or repetitive muscle action, affects peak cortical and trabecular bone mass on various genetic backgrounds. Other approaches are likely to include repetitive exercise and muscle stimulation studies to define how muscle determines the structure of bone envelopes. In the meantime, more studies are needed to define how circulating IGF-I may predict risk for failure of the cortical skeleton, principally in respect to stress fractures. Randomized controlled trials are needed with periosteal changes as an important end point to define how particular interventions may improve both mineral and structure, thereby optimizing bone strength. Serum IGF-I is regulated by genetic factors, nutritional determinants, age of the individual, growth hormone secretion, insulin status, and systemic cytokine elaboration. As such, this test may prove to be extremely useful as an integrative measure of physiological homeostasis, as well as an indirect indicator of periosteal status.

REFERENCES

Ahlborg HG, Johnel O, Turner CH, Karlsson MK. 2002. Decreased postmenopausal bone strength due to bone loss is compensated by increased bone size, and a strength index including both bone mass and size, predict future fractures. *J Bone Miner Res* 17:S163.

Beamer WG, Donahue LR, Rosen CJ, Baylink DJ. 1996. Genetic differences in peak bone mass in mice. *Bone* 18:397–405.

Beamer WG, Shultz KL, Donahue LR, Churchill GA, Sen S, Wergedal JR, Baylink DJ, Rosen CJ. 2001. Quantitative trait loci for femoral and lumbar vertebral bone density in B6 and C3H inbred strains of mice. *J Bone Miner Res* 16:1195–1206.

Bouxsein ML, Rosen CJ, Turner CH, Ackert CL, Shultz KL, Donahue LR, Churchill G, Adamo ML, Powell DR, Turner RT, Muller R, Beamer WG. 2002. Generation of a new congenic mouse strain to test the relationship among serum IGF-I, bone mineral density and skeletal morphology in vivo. *J Bone Miner Res* 17:570–579.

Kim BT, Mosekilde L, Duan Y, Zhang XZ, Tornvig L, Thomsen JS, Seeman E. 2003. The structural and hormonal basis of sex differences in peak appendicular bone strength in rats. *J Bone Miner Res* 18:150–155.

Yakar S, Rosen C, Beamer WG, Ackert C, Wu Y, Liu JL, Ooi GT, Setser J, Frystyk J, Boisclair YR, LeRoith D. 2002. Circulating levels of IGF-I directly regulate bone growth and density. *J Clin Invest* 110:771–781.

Zhang M, Xuan S, Bouxsein ML, Stechow D, Akeno N, Guagere M, Maulluche H, Zhao G, Rosen CJ, Efstriatiadis A, Clemens TL. 2002. Osteoblast specific knockout of the IGF receptor gene reveals an essential role of IGF signaling in bone matrix mineralization. *J Biol Chem* 277:44005–44012.

Zhao G, Monier-Faugere MC, Langub MC, Geng Z, Nakayama T, Pike JW, Chernausek SD, Rosen CJ, Donahue LR, Malluche H, Fagin JA, Clemens TL. 2000. Targeted overexpression of IGF-I to osteoblasts of transgenic mice increases trabecular bone volume. *Endocrinology* 141:2674–2682.

BIOMARKERS FOR MONITORING BONE TURNOVER AND PREDICTING BONE STRESS

Michael Kleerekoper, Wayne State University

BONE TURNOVER (REMODELING)

Bone is a structural tissue that, in common with all structural materials, is subject to fatigue damage and fracture if left unprepared. As living tissue, one has the unique potential for self-repair of fatigue damage via a process termed bone turnover or bone remodeling. This process is continuous throughout life and is governed by a variety of systemic hormonal and nutritional factors, local factors (cytokines), and local mechanical stress. During intrauterine and early postnatal life, remodeling is very rapid as the cartilaginous "scaffolding" is removed and replaced with early bone elements. This rapid phase in early infancy results in positive skeletal balance as bone is modeled into its adult shape. During childhood, the process slows dramatically but remains in slight positive balance, only to accelerate again coincident with the pubertal growth spurt, again maintaining positive balance. Once peak adult bone mass and maturity is reached in the third or fourth decade, the balance between removal of older, "damaged" bone (resorption) and replacement with new bone at the same site (formation) is in equilibrium with no net gain or loss of bone. Beginning late in the fifth decade or early in the sixth decade, this balance is upset. For unknown reasons, resorption exceeds formation with net negative skeletal balance such

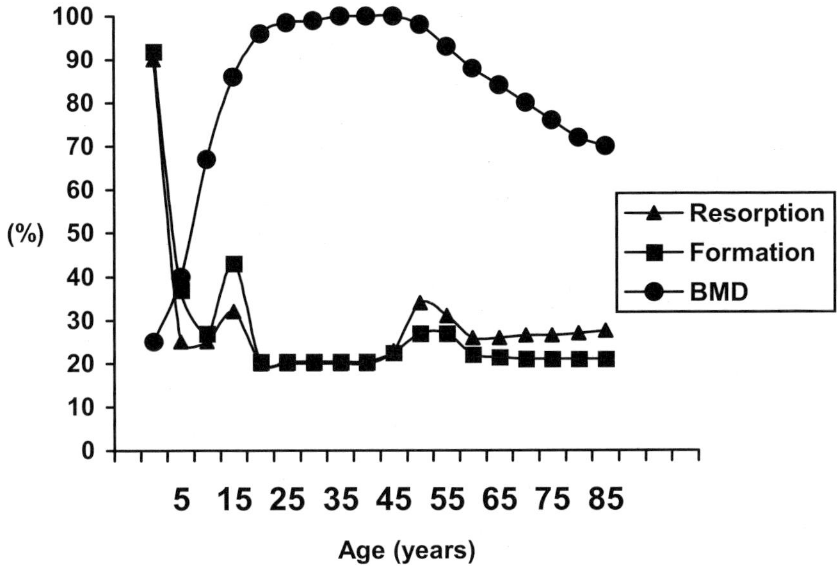

FIGURE D-29 Relative changes in bone mineral density (BMD), bone resorption, and bone formation as a function of age.

that bone loss is a universal phenomenon in human aging. The natural menopause in women results in a decline in estrogen levels to a point that local cytokine production is stimulated and bone remodeling rate increases again, but to nowhere near the levels seen during early skeletal development. This process is reversed by replacement of estrogen, by administration of antibodies to the local cytokines, or by administration of pharmacological agents that inhibit bone resorption. The rapid bone loss of the early menopause is short-lived (5–7 years), again via unknown mechanisms since estrogen levels remain low in the untreated state, but age-related bone loss continues as seen in Figure D-29.

The cells involved in bone remodeling are osteoclasts (responsible for bone resorption), osteoblasts (responsible for bone formation), and osteocytes (responsible for bone nutrition, channels for transport of nutrients and chemicals, and possibly also as local stretch or stress receptors). A number of metabolic diseases and pharmacological agents have direct effects on the bone remodeling process resulting in accelerated negative skeletal bone balance. Menopausal and age-related negative skeletal balance results in osteoporosis.

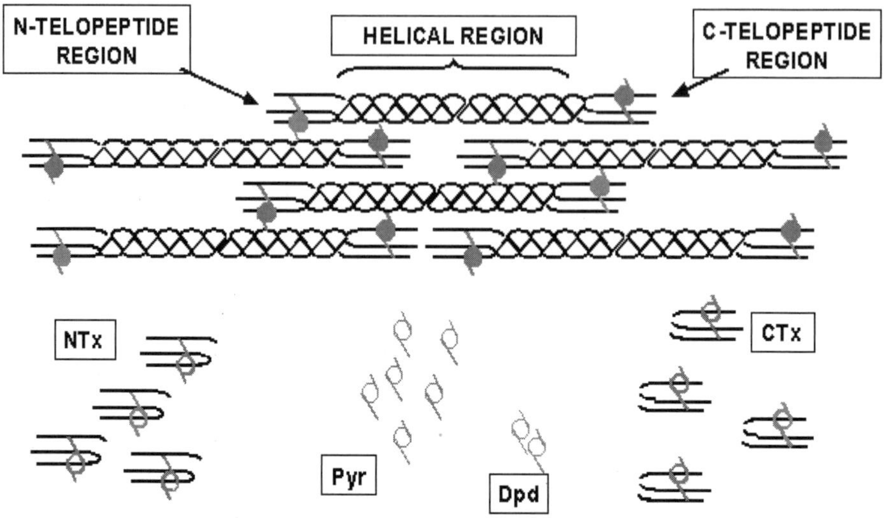

FIGURE D-30 A cartoon depicting the cross-linking between molecules of type I collagen and the breakdown products.
SOURCE: Reprinted, with permission Watts (1999), American Association for Clinical Chemistry.

BIOCHEMICAL MARKERS OF BONE TURNOVER

As osteoclasts breakdown, the skeleton to begin the process of turnover. There is removal of bone mineral (mainly calcium) and bone matrix (mainly type I collagen), and these breakdown products enter the circulation and are subsequently excreted in the urine, largely unchanged. The rise in serum calcium resulting from bone resorption is imperceptible in most circumstances because of rapid renal clearance. While urine calcium increases, it is a very nonspecific marker of the bone turnover process. The breakdown of type I collagen begins with cleavage of pyridinium cross-links between adjacent collagen molecules. Collagen is a triple helix consisting of two α1 chains and one α2 chain. At each end of the helix is a straight portion known as telopeptides with one at the amino terminal (NTX) and one at the carboxy terminal (CTX). The cross-links are between the telopeptide of one collagen molecule and the helical portion of the adjacent molecule. There are two main cross-links, pyridinoline (PYR), which is the more abundant moiety but less specific for type I collagen, and deoxypyridinoline (DPD), which is less abundant but more specific for type I collagen. These breakdown products of bone resorption may be excreted as free moieties or bound to the telopeptides. Thus NTX, CTX, PYR, and DPD constitute the main biomarkers of bone resorption. The cross-linking and breakdown products are depicted in Figure D-30. Tartrate-resistant acid phosphatase (TRAP),

TABLE D-6 Biochemical Markers of Bone Turnover

Stage	Location	Biochemical Marker
Resorption	Serum	Amino-terminal telopeptide of collagen cross-links
		Carboxy-terminal telopeptide of collagen cross-links
		Tartrate-resistant acid phosphatase
		Carboxy-terminal telopeptide of type I collagen
	Urine	Amino-terminal telopeptide of collagen cross-links
		Carboxy-terminal telopeptide of collagen cross-links
		Deoxypyridinoline
		Pyridinilone
Formation	Serum	Bone specific alkaline phosphatase
		Carboxy-terminal fragment of type 1 procollagen
		Amino-terminal fragment of type I procollagen
Turnover	Serum	Osteocalcin
		Osteoprotegerin
		Bone sialoprotein

particularly the 5b epitope (TRAP 5b), are specific gene products of the osteoclast and can also be measured as an assessment of bone resorption.

Type I collagen is a secretory product of the osteoblast. It leaves the cell as a larger procollagen molecule from which an amino terminal and a carboxy terminal propeptide are cleaved before incorporation into the bone matrix. These extension peptides remain in the circulation where they can be measured (P1NP and P1CP) as markers of osteoblastic activity. Alkaline phosphatase (AP) is an enzyme secreted by the osteoblast and is involved in bone mineralization. There are many isoenzymes of AP that differ in post-translational glycosylation. While total AP is a useful marker when levels are quite elevated, the bone-specific isoenzyme has better sensitivity and specificity. Osteocalcin (OCN) is also a secretory product of the osteoblast and is incorporated into the bone matrix as a noncollagenous protein. While this could qualify OCN as a marker of formation, as part of the bone matrix it is also released during bone resorption so is really a marker of "turnover," with some resultant loss of sensitivity. A summary of the biochemical markers of bone turnover is presented in Table D-6.

CLINICAL UTILITY OF BONE MARKERS

In those conditions where a specific disease process directly alters bone turnover (e.g., Paget's disease of bone, osteomalacia, rickets), the level of biochemical markers is usually quite elevated, and changes in these levels can be used to monitor progression or regression of the disease in individual patients. In contrast, in diseases that result from a primary abnormality in the remodeling balance, most notably osteoporosis, the markers have lesser sensitivity and specificity for monitoring progression or regression of disease in individual patients. Population studies do suggest that the higher the turnover, the greater the

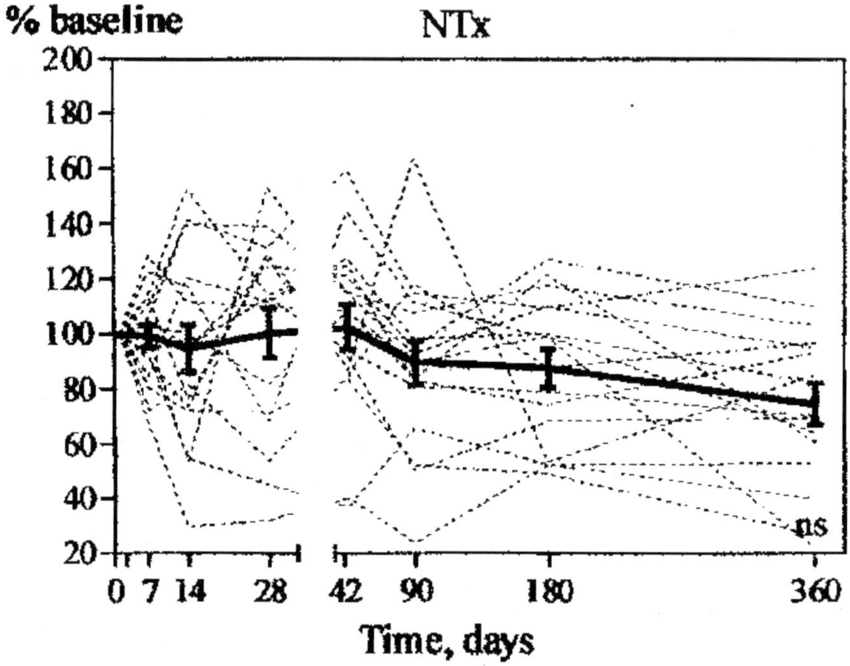

FIGURE D-31 Serial changes in urine amino-terminal telopeptide of collagen cross-links (NTX) following ankle fracture.
SOURCE: Osteoporosis International, Ingle et al. (1999a), with permission from Springer-Verlag.

anticipated rate of bone loss, but there are only weak correlations between baseline levels of markers and prospectively measured changes in bone mineral density (BMD). Similarly, population-based studies in the elderly have demonstrated that high levels of markers can predict hip fracture risk almost as well as can hip BMD, but here too that is of limited sensitivity and specificity in individual patients. Patients with osteoporosis who are treated with drugs that inhibit bone resorption generally have low levels of markers while compliant with therapy. A high level of marker on therapy in a compliant patient suggests that another metabolic bone disease might have supervened on the osteoporosis. With the recent introduction of teriparatide (synthetic amino-terminal parathyroid hormone) as a therapy to directly stimulate bone formation, there are likely to be expanded roles for markers in selecting patients for specific therapies and in monitoring the therapeutic response (Watts, 1999).

BONE TURNOVER MARKERS AND FRACTURES

An acute fracture is a potent stimulus to bone repair, and there are resultant changes in markers of bone turnover. However, this has been surprisingly little studied and those few studies that have been reported have yielded disappointing results. This is not really a surprise as fracture repair is a local process and the markers of bone turnover reflect global skeletal remodeling.

The most extensive work has come from two back-to-back articles by Ingle and colleagues (1999a, 1999b). The first followed serial changes after distal forearm fracture and the second after ankle fracture (see Figure D-31). The forearm fracture study followed 20 women, mean age 63 years, for 52 weeks following the fracture. In individual subjects there were marked changes in some of the markers studied, but not in any consistent pattern. Overall there was minimal serial change in the studied markers.

BONE TURNOVER AND STRESS FRACTURES

Only one group has studied changes in bone markers before and after the development of stress fractures in athletes (Bennell et al., 1998). There were no differences in baseline levels of markers between those who did or did not sustain a stress fracture. The serial data demonstrated no change in markers from before to after fracture during a total of 12 months of follow-up.

SUMMARY AND CONCLUSIONS

Bone turnover is an efficient mechanism for ongoing repair of microdamage to the skeleton. Stress fractures occur when the rate of accumulation and propagation of microdamage exceeds the capacity of the repair process. Several biochemical markers are available to monitor the global rate of bone turnover and have proven useful in monitoring progression or regression of systemic metabolic diseases resulting in abnormal turnover or resulting from abnormalities in the remodeling cycle. Changes in these markers undoubtedly occur during the repair phases following acute traumatic fracture, but the extent of skeleton involved is too small to be reflected in these markers of global skeletal activity. It is likely that changes in markers occur during the development and repair of stress fractures. However, here too the extent of skeleton involved is too small to be reflected in these markers of global skeletal activity.

THE FUTURE?

It is extremely unlikely that a marker of bone turnover with sufficient sensitivity to detect change when only small area of the skeleton is damaged will be developed in the foreseeable future. Functional imaging studies (magnetic resonance imaging, positron emission tomography, regional bone scintigraphy) are far more likely to detect changes in local skeletal remodeling that precede stress fractures, even in the asymptomatic state. Whether it will ever be economically feasible to apply these technologies to asymptomatic recruits in the hopes of predicting stress fracture will require extensive and expensive prospective studies. Whether such early prefracture detection will decrease the "down-time" for recruits recovering from stress fractures is questionable.

REFERENCES

Bennell KL, Malcolm SA, Brukner PD, Green RM, Hopper JL, Wark JD, Ebeling PR. 1998. A 12-month prospective study of the relationship between stress fractures and bone turnover in athletes. *Calcif Tissue Int* 63:80–85.

Ingle BM, Hay SM, Bottjer HM, Eastell R. 1999a. Changes in bone mass and bone turnover following ankle fracture. *Osteoporos Int* 10:408–415.

Ingle BM, Hay SM, Bottjer HM, Eastell R. 1999b. Changes in bone mass and bone turnover following distal forearm fracture. *Osteoporos Int* 10:399–407.

Watts NB. 1999. Clinical utility of biochemical markers of bone remodeling. *Clin Chem* 45:1359–1368.

BIOMARKERS TO PREDICT THE OCCURRENCE OF BONE STRESS AND MATRIX ABNORMALITIES DUE TO SUSTAINED AND INTENSIVE PHYSICAL ACTIVITY

Wendy M. Kohrt, Catherine M. Jankowski,
University of Colorado Health Sciences Center

There are two major competing hypotheses for the pathogenesis of stress fractures that occur as a result of high-intensity repetitive mechanical loading, such as in basic training for the military. The first hypothesis is that it is mechanical stress, per se, that causes bone to fail. The second hypothesis is that mechanical loading triggers an increase in bone remodeling activity that causes a transient reduction in bone mass, thereby increasing the vulnerability of bone to damage if mechanical loading continues. This brief review will focus on the concept that the initiation of vigorous exercise training could trigger an increase in bone resorption through three general pathways: (1) a normal, mechanical stress-induced increase in bone remodeling, (2) an increase in bone resorption to repair microdamage caused by mechanical stress, and (3) the effects of exercise training on other physiological factors that influence bone resorption or forma-

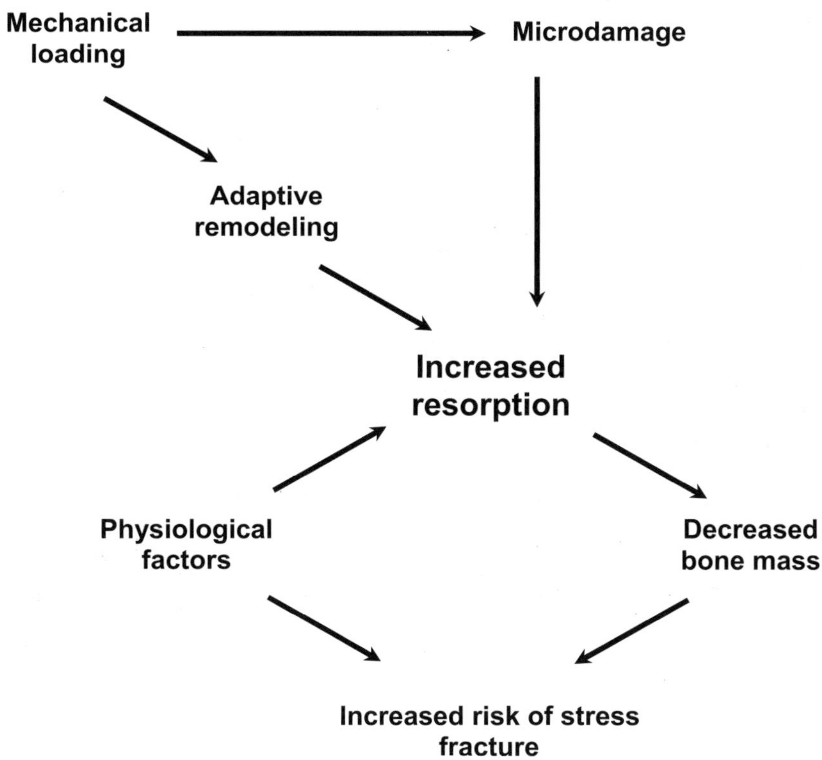

FIGURE D-32 Theoretical model for an increase in bone resorption in response to (a) loading-induced remodeling activity, (b) microdamage that occurs as a result of mechanical loading, and (c) exercise-induced changes in physiological factors that increase bone resorption. The "hyper-resorptive" state would result in a transient reduction in bone mass, increasing the vulnerability of bone to stress fracture. Physiological factors may also exacerbate risk of stress fracture through other mechanisms (e.g., reduced calcium absorption consequent to increased cortisol excretion).

tion (see Figure D-32). Finally, biomarkers thought to be potential predictors of risk for stress fracture will be identified.

EPIDEMIOLOGY OF STRESS FRACTURES

Stress fractures are nontraumatic fractures that are due to repeated loading of the skeleton (Burr, 1997). They typically occur in physically active individuals, including soldiers, runners, and dancers. The most common fracture sites are the tibia (soldiers, runners), metatarsals (dancers), and calcaneus. In military recruits, incidence rates of stress fracture are elevated within 2 to 3 weeks of the onset of training, and peak rates occur after 5 to 8 weeks (Burr, 1997).

In a recent study of 3,758 female U.S. military recruits, the incidence of stress fracture was 8.5 percent during 8 weeks of basic training (Lappe et al., 2001). Women who fractured, compared with those who did not, were: older, more likely to use depo-medroxyprogesterone acetate, had a lower adult body weight, and were more likely to report current or past smoking, alcohol consumption of more than 10 drinks per week, and use of corticosteroids. A history of regular exercise was protective. Such findings suggest that risk for stress fracture is influenced by a number of physiological and behavioral factors.

DEVELOPMENT OF STRESS FRACTURES—MECHANICAL LOADING FACTORS

There is a wealth of evidence from a variety of animal models that repetitive mechanical loading results in bone damage (Burr, 1997; Burr et al., 1997). Furthermore, the rate of development of lesions is consistent with the observation in humans that stress fractures develop in a matter of weeks in response to an abrupt increase in mechanical stress (Burr et al., 1990). Based on theoretical modeling and empirical data from studies of animals, very high levels of bone strain (e.g., 8,000 microstrain) will cause bone to fail after only 10^3 to 10^4 loading cycles. However, in humans, peak shear strains of the tibia measured during walking and running under a variety of conditions (e.g., uphill, downhill, zigzag, while carrying extra weight) are typically less than 2,000 microstrain. At this level of strain, it has been estimated that bone can withstand at least 10^6 loading cycles, or roughly 1,100 miles of running (Burr, 1997).

Although these observations suggest that mechanical stress, per se, is not likely to be the sole cause of stress fractures that occur after only a few weeks of basic training, definitive evidence to rule this out is lacking. It is possible that bone strain is increased under certain conditions, such as when muscles are fatigued (Christina et al., 2001), or that brief periods of mechanical stress in excess of 2,000 microstrain induce damage. Although higher degrees of strain may not occur during planned activities (Milgrom et al., 2000), they may occur during unplanned movements. For example, in patients with hip prostheses outfitted with telemetrically monitored force sensors, the highest forces were recorded during unexpected movements, such as stumbling (Bergmann et al., 1993, 1995). However, even when all these factors are considered, it seems unlikely that the development of stress fractures after only a few weeks of intensive physical activity is attributable solely to mechanical stress. In an animal model, more than 30,000 loading cycles applied to a limb over a 3-week period resulted in bone damage, whereas applying the same number of loading cycles in 1 day did not (Burr, 1993). The temporal factor suggests that physiological responses to the mechanical stress contribute to the propensity for fracture.

DEVELOPMENT OF STRESS FRACTURES—BONE REMODELING FACTORS

Mechanical stress is thought to trigger an increase in bone remodeling activity that begins with an increase in bone resorption, leading to a transient decrease in bone mass, followed by an increase in bone formation. The transient reduction in bone mass would increase the vulnerability of bone to damage if mechanical loading continues during this period because forces of the same magnitude would now represent a greater relative stress. This hypothesis is consistent with theoretical models and empirical data on the time course of remodeling and of the development of stress fractures (Burr, 1997). The recruitment of osteoclasts, the bone resorbing cells, typically occurs in a few days. The period of bone resorption lasts about 3 to 4 weeks, with subsequent activation of bone formation activity.

If the induction of bone resorption and consequent decrease in bone mass does, indeed, increase the susceptibility of bone to stress fracture, it could be postulated that use of an antiresorptive agent would diminish this risk. However, it is likely that mechanical loading results in microdamage to bone, and that an increase in remodeling activity is an obligatory step in the repair of microdamage. In this scenario, use of antiresorptive agents could result in an accumulation of microdamage and an increased, rather than a decreased, risk of stress fracture.

The temporal nature of the response of bone to severe mechanical stress was evaluated by Bentolila and colleagues (1998). In their experiment, the right ulnae of rats was loaded to fatigue on day 1 and the left ulnae underwent the same fatigue loading on day 10; both bones were harvested immediately after the second loading session. Microcrack density was significantly higher in the acutely loaded ulnae than in the ulnae that had been stressed 10 days earlier, suggesting that some healing had occurred in the intervening period. However, bone resorption activity was evident only in the bones that had been stressed 10 days earlier and tended to be concentrated in regions of microcracks. Three-quarters of all microcracks were associated with resorption spaces, but resorption spaces were also visualized in regions of bone in which there was no detectable matrix damage. This suggests that resorptive activity was initiated as part of the normal remodeling response to mechanical stress (in undamaged regions) and also to repair areas of microdamage. Thus, it seems plausible that the degree of activation of bone resorption and the extent of transient bone loss depends on the severity of the mechanical stress and the extent of damage that it causes.

The notion that inhibiting bone remodeling could lead to an accumulation of microdamage and increased bone fragility has been studied in animals using bisphosphonate therapy (Hirano et al., 2000; Mashiba et al., 2001a, 2001b). One year of etidronate therapy at a dose 100 times higher than the recommended clinical dose in humans resulted in increased osteoid volume and a high incidence of spontaneous fractures. At a dose 10 times the clinical dose, there was evidence of microdamage accumulation, but no significant increase in spontaneous fractures. The relevance of these findings to the concept of using antiresorptive therapy to prevent stress fractures remains uncertain. It will be important to determine the effects of lower doses of bisphosphonates and other antiresorptive agents and to specifically evaluate the effects on bone microdamage and fragility under conditions of increased mechanical stress.

DEVELOPMENT OF STRESS FRACTURES—OTHER PHYSIOLOGICAL FACTORS

The fact that stress fractures develop in only a few weeks in response to an increase in mechanical loading is temporally consistent with the hypothesis that an increase in bone resorption triggers a decrease in bone mass that transiently increases the vulnerability of bone to fracture. In this context, other physiological factors that may further exaggerate bone resorption or impair the coupling with subsequent bone formation activity should be considered. The following discussion is not meant to be an exhaustive list of possible factors, but rather an overview of a few factors that can be influenced by vigorous exercise training and are known to affect bone metabolism.

Sex Hormones

Both estradiol and testosterone have potent effects on bone metabolism (Riggs et al., 2002), and levels of these sex hormones have been reported to be decreased in highly trained athletes (Laughlin et al., 1998; Roberts et al., 1993). There is emerging evidence that it is low energy availability during vigorous training, rather than the exercise per se, that causes this hormonal dysregulation, at least in women (Loucks, 2001; Loucks and Thuma, 2003). Whatever the cause, if estradiol levels decrease during vigorous exercise training, this would be expected to stimulate an increase in bone resorption, because even normal fluctuations in estradiol across the menstrual cycle are inversely associated with bone resorption rate (Chiu et al., 1999). There have been few studies of bone metabolism and testosterone levels in young male athletes, but the suppression of androgens in men results in a dramatic increase in the rate of bone resorption (Stoch et al., 2001). Because estradiol appears to play a more important role than testosterone in maintaining bone mass in men, it is important to note that reductions in serum testosterone in men will be accompanied by reductions in estradiol because the primary source of estradiol in men is the aromatization of testosterone (Riggs et al., 2002).

Sex hormones have independent effects on bone metabolism, but they may also influence risk for stress fracture through other mechanisms. Recent studies have found an increase in apoptosis of rat (Tomkinson et al., 1998) and human (Tomkinson et al., 1997) osteocytes in response to estrogen withdrawal. The investigators suggested that, because the capacity of bone to repair microdamage and to modulate the effects of mechanical strain may be dependent on osteocyte viability, this could be a mechanism by which estrogen deficiency leads to bone fragility. It has also been demonstrated that estrogen receptor alpha is involved in generating the bone response to mechanical stress (Cheng et al., 2002; Damien et al., 2000), and that the combined effects of estradiol and mechanical stress on bone formation activity are additive or synergistic (Cheng et al., 1997; Kohrt et al., 1995). Thus, the effectiveness of mechanical loading to favorably affect bone metabolism may be diminished in the estrogen-deficient state or when estrogen receptor function is alerted.

Glucocorticoids

The physical and psychological stresses of basic training and survival training can increase the secretion of stress hormones, including cortisol (Hellhammer et al., 1997; Morgan et al., 2002), which has a potent, negative effect on bone. With respect to direct actions on bone metabolism, cortisol both increases bone resorption, by stimulating osteoclastogenesis and inhibits bone formation, by inhibiting osteoblastic cell replication and differentiation and increasing apoptosis of mature osteoblasts (Canalis and Delany, 2002). Cortisol may also influence bone metabolism through indirect actions (Manelli and Giustina, 2000). Glucocorticoids have been found to decrease calcium absorption, modify vitamin D metabolism, and inhibit activity of both the gonadotropic and the somatotropic axis.

Growth Hormone and IGF-1

Growth hormone and growth factors such as IGF-1 have potent and complex effects on bone metabolism (Rosen and Donahue, 1998). The effects of physical stress to suppress the somatotropic axis and the potential adverse consequences on bone metabolism were presented by other participants in the workshop (Nindl and Rosen, respectively) and are reviewed elsewhere in this publication.

Use of Nonsteroidal Anti-inflammatory Drugs

The use of nonsteroidal anti-inflammatory drugs (NSAIDs) is known to impair fracture healing (Simon et al., 2002). In animal models, NSAIDs also impair the bone formation response to mechanical loading (Cheng et al., 1997; Chow and Chambers, 1994). The likely mechanism of this action is the inhibition by NSAIDs of cyclooxygenase activity, which catalyzes the conversion of arachidonate to prostanoids. Prostaglandin E_2 has been identified as an important signaling factor in mechanotransduction in bone (Chow, 2000) and has been found to increase in response to mechanical loading in humans (Thorsen et al., 1996). Currently, there are no controlled studies of the potential adverse effects of NSAIDs on the bone formation response to mechanical stress in humans. However, the compelling findings from animal studies suggest that attention should be directed to this issue, particularly since NSAID use is likely to be increased during periods of vigorous physical activity.

POTENTIAL BIOMARKERS FOR THE DEVELOPMENT OF STRESS FRACTURES

Based on the discussion above, potential biomarkers to predict the development of stress fractures could fall within three general categories: mechanical stress, bone metabolism, and physiological factors.

Biomarkers of Mechanical Stress

Although it is unlikely that stress fractures develop solely as a result of mechanical loading, the extent of mechanical stress may influence other predictors of stress fracture. The number of loading cycles is thought to be of less importance than the stress magnitude, which could potentially be monitored by load sensors in the shoes. However, of even greater importance would be the ability to monitor the bone response to mechanical stress, that is, strain. Strain gauges positioned on regions of bone prone to stress fracture (e.g., anterior tibia) could potentially measure strain magnitude and strain rate, since both are important determinants of the bone remodeling response. Because bone is weaker in shear than in compression, it may be particularly important to monitor shear strain. A more futuristic goal would be the early detection of microdamage in bone. The development of such methodologies as vibration analysis, ultrasound, or peripheral quantitative computed tomography for this purpose should be considered.

Biomarkers of Bone Metabolism

If the concept put forth above is correct, that an exaggerated increase in bone resorption in response to multiple stimuli increases the vulnerability of bone to fracture, it will be very important to monitor markers of bone resorption and formation. However, the methodologies currently available measure these markers in serum or urine, which reflect whole-body bone metabolism and are not likely to be useful in identifying the targeted changes in bone remodeling that occur in response to localized strain and microdamage. Methodologies to measure local changes in markers of resorption and formation are not currently available.

Other Physiological Factors as Biomarkers

The identification of appropriate physiological factors that predict the development of stress fractures will depend on extending the current state of knowledge of the mechanisms for the pathogenesis of stress fractures in humans. Candidate markers that are likely to be important include those that change in response to vigorous physical training and have potent effects on bone metabolism, such as estradiol and cortisol.

Currently, the signaling pathway by which mechanical stress generates the appropriate cellular responses in bone remains poorly defined. It will be important to promote research directed toward furthering our understanding of the cellular mechanisms of mechanotransduction. However, it will be equally important to support clinical research that evaluates these mechanisms in humans using applied, integrative approaches to determine the relative importance in maintaining bone health. For example, prostaglandin E_2 has been found to play a critical role in the bone formation response to mechanical stress in both isolated cell and in vivo animal models, and the response is abrogated by NSAIDs. Despite the widespread use of NSAIDs by humans, particularly in conjunction with exercise training, there is no knowledge of the potential adverse effects on bone metabolism. Because it is likely that risk for stress fractures is multifactorial, involving both localized parameters of strain and bone metabolism and systemic hormonal modulators of bone metabolism, understanding the pathophysiology of stress fracture development in humans will likely require collaborative research that considers these factors in an integrative fashion.

The authors are supported by National Institutes of Health research awards AG18198 and AG18857 and U.S. Army Medical Research and Materiel Command award DAMD17-01-1-0805.

REFERENCES

Bentolila V, Boyce TM, Fyhrie DP, Drumb R, Skerry TM, Schaffler MB. 1998. Intracortical remodeling in adult rat long bones after fatigue loading. *Bone* 23:275–281.

Bergmann G, Graichen F, Rohlmann A. 1993. Hip joint loading during walking and running, measured in two patients. *J Biomech* 26:969–990.

Bergmann G, Graichen F, Rohlmann A. 1995. Is staircase walking a risk for the fixation of hip implants? *J Biomech* 28:535–553.

Burr DB. 1993. Remodeling and the repair of fatigue damage. *Calcif Tissue Int* 53:S75–S80.

Burr DB. 1997. Bone, exercise, and stress fractures. *Exerc Sport Sci Rev* 25:171–194.

Burr DB, Milgrom C, Boyd RD, Higgins WL, Robin G, Radin EL. 1990. Experimental stress fractures of the tibia. Biological and mechanical aetiology in rabbits. *J Bone Joint Surg Br* 72:370–375.

Burr DB, Forwood MR, Fyhrie DP, Martin RB, Schaffler MB, Turner CH. 1997. Bone microdamage and skeletal fragility in osteoporotic and stress fractures. *J Bone Miner Res* 12:6–15.

Canalis E, Delany AM. 2002. Mechanisms of glucocorticoid action in bone. *Ann N Y Acad Sci* 966:73–81.

Cheng MZ, Zaman G, Rawlinson SC, Pitsillides AA, Suswillo RF, Lanyon LE. 1997. Enhancement by sex hormones of the osteoregulatory effects of mechanical loading and prostaglandins in explants of rat ulnae. *J Bone Miner Res*12:1424–1430.

Cheng MZ, Rawlinson SC, Pitsillides AA, Zaman G, Mohan S, Baylink DJ, Lanyon LE. 2002. Human osteoblasts' proliferative responses to strain and 17beta-estradiol are mediated by the estrogen receptor and the receptor for insulin-like growth factor I. *J Bone Miner Res* 17:593–602.

Chiu KM, Ju J, Mayes D, Bacchetti P, Weitz S, Arnaud CD. 1999. Changes in bone resorption during the menstrual cycle. *J Bone Miner Res* 14:609–615.

Chow JW. 2000. Role of nitric oxide and prostaglandins in the bone formation response to mechanical loading. *Exerc Sports Sci Rev* 28:185–188.

Chow JW, Chambers TJ. 1994. Indomethacin has distinct early and late actions on bone formation induced by mechanical stimulation. *Am J Physiol* 267:E287–E292.

Christina KA, White SC, Gilchrist LA. 2001. Effect of localized muscle fatigue on vertical ground reaction forces and ankle joint motion during running. *Hum Mov Sci* 20:257–276.

Damien E, Price JS, Lanyon LE. 2000. Mechanical strain stimulates osteoblast proliferation through the estrogen receptor in males as well as females. *J Bone Miner Res* 15:2169–2177.

Hellhammer DH, Buchtal J, Gutberlet I, Kirschbaum C. 1997. Social hierarchy and adrenocortical stress reactivity in men. *Psychoneuroendocrinology* 22:643–650.

Hirano T, Turner CH, Forwood MR, Johnston CC, Burr DB. 2000. Does suppression of bone turnover impair mechanical properties by allowing microdamage accumulation? *Bone* 27:13–20.

Kohrt WM, Snead DB, Slatopolsky E, Birge SJ Jr. 1995. Additive effects of weight-bearing exercise and estrogen on bone mineral density in older women. *J Bone Miner Res* 10:1303–1311.

Lappe JM, Stegman MR, Recker RR. 2001. The impact of lifestyle factors on stress fractures in female Army recruits. *Osteoporos Int* 12:35–42.

Laughlin GA, Dominguez CE, Yen SS. 1998. Nutritional and endocrine-metabolic aberrations in women with functional hypothalamic amenorrhea. *J Clin Endocrinol Metab* 83:25–32.

Loucks AB. 2001. Physical health of the female athlete: Observations, effects, and causes of reproductive disorders. *Can J Appl Physiol* 26 :S176–S185.

Loucks AB, Thuma JR. 2003. Luteinizing hormone pulsatility is disrupted at a threshold of energy availability in regularly menstruating women. *J Clin Endocrinol Metab* 88:297–311.

Manelli F, Giustina A. 2000. Glucocorticoid-induced osteoporosis. *Trends Endocrinol Metab* 11:79–85.

Mashiba T, Turner CH, Hirano T, Forwood MR, Jacob DS, Johnston CC, Burr DB. 2001a. Effects of high-dose etidronate treatment on microdamage accumulation and biomechanical properties in beagle bone before occurrence of spontaneous fractures. *Bone* 29:271–278.

Mashiba T, Turner CH, Hirano T, Forwood MR, Johnston CC, Burr DB. 2001b. Effects of suppressed bone turnover by bisphosphonates on microdamage accumulation and biomechanical properties in clinically relevant skeletal sites in beagles. *Bone* 28:524–531.

Milgrom C, Finestone A, Levi Y, Simkin A, Ekenman I, Mendelson S, Millgram M, Nyska M, Benjuya N, Burr D. 2000. Do high impact exercises produce higher tibial strains than running? *Br J Sports Med* 34:195–199.

Morgan CA III, Rasmusson AM, Wang S, Hoyt G, Hauger RL, Hazlett G. 2002. Neuropeptide-Y, cortisol, and subjective distress in humans exposed to acute stress: Replication and extension of previous report. *Biol Psychiatry* 52:136–142.

Riggs BL, Khosla S, Melton LJ III. 2002. Sex steroids and the construction and conservation of the adult skeleton. *Endocr Rev* 23:279–302.

Roberts AC, McClure RD, Weiner RI, Brooks GA. 1993. Overtraining affects male reproductive status. *Fertil Steril* 60:686–692.

Rosen CJ, Donahue LR. 1998. Insulin-like growth factors and bone: The osteoporosis connection revisited. *Soc Exp Biol Med* 219:7.

Simon AM, Manigrasso MB, O'Connor JP. 2002. Cyclo-oxygenase 2 function is essential for bone fracture healing. *J Bone Miner Res* 17:963–976.

Stoch SA, Parker RA, Chen L, Bubley G, Koy J, Vincelette A, Greenspan SL. 2001. Bone loss in men with prostate cancer treated with gonadotropin-releasing hormone agonists. *J Clin Endocrinol Metab* 86:2787–2791.

Thorsen K, Kristoffersson AO, Lerner UH, Lorentzon RP. 1996. In situ microdialysis in bone tissue. Stimulation of prostaglandin E2 release by weight-bearing mechanical loading. *J Clin Invest* 98:2446–2449.

Tomkinson A, Reeve J, Shaw RW, Noble BS. 1997. The death of osteocytes via apoptosis accompanies estrogen withdrawal in human bone. *J Clin Endocrinol Metab* 82:3128–3135.

Tomkinson A, Gevers EF, Wit JM, Reeve J, Noble BS. 1998. The role of estrogen in the control of rat osteocyte apoptosis. *J Bone Miner Res* 13:1243–1250.

AUTONOMIC NERVOUS SYSTEM ACTIVITY AND ITS RELATIONSHIP TO ATTENTION AND WORKING MEMORY

Julian F. Thayer, National Institute on Aging; Bjorn Helge Johnsen, University of Bergen

In this paper we describe a model of neurovisceral integration in which a set of neural structures involved in cognitive, affective, and autonomic regulation are related to heart rate variability (HRV) and cognitive performance. Neural network studies in humans have reported increased activity in the prefrontal cortex during tasks involving executive function and working memory (Goldman-Rakic, 1998). Compte and colleagues (2000) have proposed that the prefrontal cortex holds sensory information temporarily online through sustained activity. This continued activation of a neural network is essential for the linking of "input" with "output" to achieve flexible responding to changing environments. As such, optimal prefrontal functioning is necessary for the formation of associations and the representation of acquired relationships between disparate pieces of information, including information separated in time (Miller, 2000). In addition, these cortical regions are implicated in inhibitory functions that are known to be critical for the performance of executive function tasks. Relatedly, performance on working memory tasks have been reported to be significantly related to general intelligence as indexed by standard intelligence quotient tests. Direct and indirect pathways by which the frontal cortex modulates parasympathetic activity via subcortical inputs have been identified (Ter Horst, 1999; Ter Horst and Postema, 1997). A number of researchers have hypothesized inhibitory cortical-subcortical circuits (Benarroch, 1993, 1997; Masterman and Cummings, 1997; Mayberg et al., 1999; Spyer, 1989). However, Thayer and Lane (2000) have been the first to tie these circuits to HRV.

We will provide an overview of the neural structures linking the central nervous system to HRV. Next, we will review a number of studies from our group showing that individual differences in HRV are related to performance on tasks associated with executive function and prefrontal cortical activity. We propose that these findings have important implications for the development of biomarkers related to performance in modern warfighters.

THE CENTRAL AUTONOMIC NETWORK

Investigators have identified functional units within the central nervous system (CNS) that support goal-directed behavior and adaptability. One such entity is the central autonomic network (CAN; Benarroch, 1993, 1997). Functionally, this network is an integrated component of an internal regulation system through which the brain controls visceromotor, neuroendocrine, and behavioral responses that are critical for goal-directed behavior, adaptability, and health.

Structurally, the CAN includes the anterior cingulate, insular, orbitofrontal, and ventromedial prefrontal cortices, the central nucleus of the amygdala, the paraventricular and related nuclei of the hypothalamus, the periaquaductal gray matter, the parabrachial nucleus, the nucleus of the solitary tract, the nucleus ambiguus, the ventrolateral medulla, the ventromedial medulla, and the medullary tegmental field. These components are reciprocally interconnected such that information flows bidirectionally between lower and higher levels of the CNS. The primary output of CAN is mediated through preganglionic sympathetic and parasympathetic neurons that innervate the heart via the stellate ganglia and vagus nerve, respectively. The interplay of these inputs to the cardiac sinoatrial node produces complex variability that characterizes the heart-rate time series (Saul, 1990). Thus, the output of CAN is directly linked to HRV. Notably, vagal influences dominate cardiac chronotropic control (Levy, 1990). In addition, sensory information from peripheral end organs such as the heart and the immune system are fed back to the CAN. As such, HRV is an indicator of central-peripheral neural feedback and CNS-autonomic nervous system integration.

Other functional units within the CNS serving executive, social, affective, attentional, and motivated behavior in humans and animals have been identified (Damasio, 1998; Devinsky et al., 1995; Masterman and Cummings, 1997; Spyer, 1989). One such network has been termed the anterior executive region (AER; Devinsky et al., 1995). The AER and its projections regulate behavior by monitoring the motivational quality of internal and external stimuli. The AER network has been called the "rostral limbic system" and includes the anterior, insular, and orbitofrontal cortices, amygdala, periaquaductal gray, ventral striatum, and autonomic brainstem motor nuclei. Damasio (1998) has recognized a similar neural "emotion circuit," for which there is considerable structural overlap with CAN and AER (Thayer and Lane, 2000).

We propose that CAN, the AER network, Damasio's "emotion circuit", and related systems (Masterman and Cummings, 1997; Spyer, 1989) represent a common central functional network recognized by different researchers from diverse approaches. This CNS network is associated with the processes of response organization and selection and serves to control psychophysiological resources in attention and emotion (Friedman and Thayer, 1998a, 1998b; Thayer and Friedman, 1997). Additional structures are flexibly recruited to manage specific behavioral adaptations. This sparsely interconnected neural complex allows for maximal organism flexibility in accommodating rapidly changing environmental demands. When this network is either rigidly coupled or completely uncoupled, the ability to recruit and utilize appropriate neural support to meet a particular demand is hampered and the organism is thus less adaptive.

It has been proposed that the prefrontal cortex is taken "off-line" during emotional stress to let automatic, prepotent processes regulate behavior (Arnsten and Goldman-Rakic, 1998). This selective prefrontal inactivation may be adaptive by facilitating predominantly nonvolitional behaviors associated with subcortical neural structures (e.g., the amygdala) to organize responses without delay from the more deliberative and consciously guided prefrontal cortex. In modern society, however, inhibition, delayed response, and cognitive flexibility are vital for successful adjustment and self-regulation, and prolonged prefrontal inactivity can lead to hypervigilance, defensiveness, and preservation.

ATTENTIONAL REGULATION AND EXECUTIVE FUNCTION

Attentional regulation and the ability to inhibit prepotent but inappropriate responses is also important for health and optimal performance in a complex environment. Many tasks important for survival in today's world involve cognitive functions such as working memory, sustained attention, behavioral inhibition, and general mental flexibility. These tasks are all associated with prefrontal cortex activity (Arnsten and Goldman-Rakic, 1998). Deficits in these cognitive functions tend to accompany aging and are also present in negative affective states and dispositions such as depression and anxiety. Stress can also impair cognitive function and may contribute to the cognitive deficits observed in various mental disorders and in extreme environments. It is also possible that autonomic dysregulation contributes to deficits in attention and cognitive performance. A series of experiments in our lab have been conducted to examine this issue and are described below.

In a recent experiment, Johnsen and colleagues (2003) examined inhibitory responses in an emotional Stroop paradigm. Dental phobics were first exposed to recorded scenes of dental procedures and then administered the emotional Stroop test. In addition to the traditional color congruent and color incongruent words, phobic subjects also were asked to respond to neutral words and dental-related words (e.g., drill and cavity) that were threatening to them. All subjects exhibited longer reaction times to the incongruent color words and the dental-related threat words and, thus, displayed a difficulty in inhibiting prepotent responses. However, greater HRV was associated with faster reaction times to these words, consistent with the link among vagally mediated HRV, inhibitory ability, and frontal lobe function. These results support the idea that vagally mediated HRV is associated with efficient attentional regulation and greater ability to inhibit prepotent but inappropriate responses.

Subsequent studies further examined executive function and working memory in healthy individuals in a military context. In the first experiment, subjects performed a number of tasks involving continuous performance, including a simple reaction-time task, a choice reaction-time task, and three tasks that involved delayed responding and working memory (Hansen et al., 2003; Johnsen et al., 2002). The California Computerized Assessment Package Abbreviated version, (CalCAP; Norland Software, Los Angeles, California; Miller, 1999) was chosen as a continuous performance task. CalCAP is recognized as a test of sustained attention and consists of four subtests, two with nonexecutive components (simple reaction time and response latencies to specific stimuli components) and two with executive components (detection of identical stimuli and a simple addition task). The test was self-explanatory and needed only minimal supervision by the investigator. In addition, a modified version of a working memory test developed by Hugdahl and colleagues (2000), based on Baddeley and Hitch's research (1974), was chosen. This test consisted of a continuous flow of digits and subjects were to detect identical digits to the one presented two trials previously. The stimuli were numbers from one to nine. These latter three tasks involved aspects of delayed responding and working memory and have been shown to be associated with prefrontal activity (Goldman-Rakic, 1998). HRV and cortisol responses were recorded, and subjects were grouped into low- and high-HRV groups.

Performance on tasks involving simple and choice reaction times did not differ between these groups. However, on tasks associated with prefrontal activity, subjects in the low-HRV group performed more poorly in terms of reaction time, number of errors, and number of correct responses than those in the high-HRV group. In addition, the groups did not differ in baseline, morning, or evening cortisol, but the low-HRV group showed larger cortisol responses to cognitive tasks that lasted into the post-task recovery period. Stress is associated with an increased cortisol release, and cortisol plays a major role in immune function through its association with proinflammatory cytokines (Kiecolt-Glaser et al., 2002). Cortisol is also known to impair function on cognitive tasks associated with the prefrontal cortex (Lupien et al., 1999). Thus, the low-HRV group was less stress tolerant as indexed by cortisol responses and more impaired cognitively than the high-HRV group.

In another study in the series, military subjects performed the same tasks as above, but half did so under threat of electric shock (Hansen et al., 2002). Again, subjects were divided into two groups based on resting HRV levels. In the shock threat condition, task performance involving delayed responding and prefrontal activity was significantly impaired in the low-HRV group. Thus, persons with high HRV were more stress tolerant and less affected by the threat compared with those with low HRV. In yet another study, HRV was manipulated by having half of the subjects in a physically active group undergo mild detraining for four weeks. Aerobic capacity and HRV were significantly reduced in this group compared with those that maintained their fitness and HRV levels. All subjects again performed the above cognitive tasks: once before the four-week detraining period and once after. The detrained, low-HRV group failed to show the expected learning effect associated with repeated performance of the cognitive tasks and, thus, did not reap the typical benefit of previous task exposure.

CONCLUSIONS

Taken together, these results support the use of HRV to index efficient allocation of attentional and cognitive resources needed for efficient functioning in a challenging environment in which delayed responding and behavioral inhibition are key. In addition, these data show that low HRV marks increased risk to stress exposure. Significantly, these results provide a connection among stress-related cognitive deficits, high negative affect, and negative health consequences via the common mechanism of autonomic imbalance and low parasympathetic activity.

REFERENCES

Arnsten AFT, Goldman-Rakic PS. 1998. Noise stress impairs prefrontal cortical cognitive function in monkeys: Evidence for a hyperdopaminergic mechanism. *Arch Gen Psychiatry* 55:362–368.

Baddeley AD, Hitch G. 1974. Working memory. In: Bower GA, ed. *The Psychology of Learning and Motivation.* vol. 8. New York: Academic Press. Pp. 47–89.

Benarroch EE. 1993. The central autonomic network: Functional organization, dysfunction, and perspective. *Mayo Clin Proc* 68:988–1001.

Benarroch EE. 1997. The central autonomic network. In: Low PA, ed. *Clinical Autonomic Disorders.* 2nd ed. Philadelphia: Lippincott-Raven. Pp. 17–23.

Compte A, Brunel N, Goldman-Rakic PS, Wang XJ. 2000. Synaptic mechanisms and network dynamics underlying spatial working memory in a cortical network model. *Cereb Cortex* 10:910–923.

Damasio AR. 1998. Emotion in the perspective of an integrated nervous system. *Brain Res Rev* 26:83–86.

Devinsky O, Morrell MJ, Vogt BA. 1995. Contributions of anterior cingulate cortex to behavior. *Brain* 18:279–306.

Friedman BH, Thayer JF. 1998a. Anxiety and autonomic flexibility: A cardiovascular approach. *Biol Psychol* 49:303–323.

Friedman BH, Thayer JF. 1998b. Autonomic balance revisited: Panic anxiety and heart rate variability. *J Psychosom Res* 44:133–151.

Goldman-Rakic PS. 1998. The prefrontal landscape: Implications of functional architecture for understanding human mentation and the entral executive. In: Roberts AC, Robbins TW, Weiskrantz L, eds. *The Prefrontal Cortex: Executive and Cognitive Function.* Oxford: Oxford University Press. Pp. 87–102.

Hansen AL, Johnsen BH, Sollers JJ, Thayer JF. 2002. Neural control of the heart modulates cognitive processing during stress. *Clin Auton Res* 12:167.

Hansen AL, Johnsen BH, Thayer JF. 2003. Vagal influence on working memory and attention. *Int J Psychophysiol* 48:263–274.

Hugdahl K, Thomsen T, Landrø NI, Ersland L, Smievoll AI, Lundervold A, Barndon R, Sundberg H, Iversen JK, Roscher B. 2000. Separating mental arithmetic from working memory: A fMRI-study. *Neuroimage* 11:384.

Johnsen BH, Hansen AL, Sollers JJ, Murison R, Thayer JF. 2002. Heart rate variability is inversely associated with cortisol reactivity. *Psychosom Med* 64:128.

Johnsen BH, Thayer JF, Laberg JC, Wormnes B, Raadal M, Skaret E, Kvale G, Berg E. 2003. Attentional and physiological characteristics of patients with dental anxiety. *J Anxiety Disord* 17:75–87.

Kiecolt-Glaser JK, McGuire L, Robles TF, Glaser R. 2002. Emotions, morbidity, and mortality: New perspectives from psychoneuroimmunology. *Ann Rev Psychol* 53:83–107.

Levy MN. 1990. Autonomic interactions in cardiac control. *Annals N Y Acad Sci* 601:209–221.

Lupien SJ, Gillin CJ, Hauger RL. 1999. Working memory is more sensitive than declarative memory to the acute effects of corticosteroids: A dose-response study in humans. *Behav Neurosci* 113:420–430.

Masterman DL, Cummings JL. 1997. Frontal-subcortical circuits: The anatomical basis of executive, social and motivated behaviors. *J Psychopharmacol* 11:107–114.

Mayberg HS, Liotti M, Brannan SK, McGinnis S, Mahurin RK, Jerabek PA, Silva JA, Tekell JL, Martin CC, Lancaster JL, Fox PT. 1999. Reciprocal limbic-cortical function and negative mood: Converging PET findings in depression and normal sadness. *Am J Psychiatry* 156:675–682.

Miller EK. 2000. The prefrontal cortex and cognitive control. *Nature Rev* 1:59–65.

Miller EN. 1999. *CalCAP. California Computerized Assessment Package Manual.* 2nd ed. Los Angeles: Norland Software.

Saul JP. 1990. Beat-to-beat variations of heart rate reflect modulation of cardiac autonomic outflow. *News Physiol Sci* 5:32–37.

Spyer KM. 1989. Neural mechanisms involved in cardiovascular control during affective behavior. *Trends Neurosci* 12:506–513.

Ter Horst GJ. 1999. Central autonomic control of the heart, angina, and pathogenic mechanisms of post-myocardial infarction depression. *Eur J Morphol* 37:257–266.

Ter Horst GJ, Postema F. 1997. Forebrain parasympathetic control of heart activity: Retrograde transneuronal viral labeling in rats. *Am J Physiol* 273:H2926–H2930.

Thayer JF, Friedman BH. 1997. The heart of anxiety: A dynamical systems approach. In: Vingerhoets A, ed. *The (Non)Expression of Emotions in Health and Disease*. Amsterdam: Springer Verlag.

Thayer JF, Lane RD. 2000. A model of neurovisceral integration in emotion regulation and dysregulation. *J Affect Disord* 61:201–216.

SWEAT PATCH AS A NOVEL APPROACH TO MONITOR THE LEVEL OF ACTIVITY OF THE STRESS SYSTEM: POTENTIAL APPLICATION FOR STUDIES CONDUCTED IN THE FIELD

Giovanni Cizza, National Institute of Mental Health; Farideh Eskandari, National Institute of Mental Health; Terry Phillips, National Institutes of Health; Esther M. Sternberg, National Institute of Mental Health

THE STRESS SYSTEM: GENERAL CHARACTERISTICS

The stress system has evolved to maintain homeostasis in response to disruptive internal or external stimuli (Chrousos et al., 1995). A highly conserved system, the stress system is represented in lower species and has a central as well as a peripheral component. The central component involves several areas in the central nervous system, including the paraventricular nucleus of the hypothalamus, the main source of corticotrophin-releasing-hormone (CRH); the locus coeruleus, the main source of catecholamines; and the prefrontal cortex, the cortical coordinating center. The afferent limbs of the stress system include the pituitary-adrenal axis with its main effector molecule, cortisol, and the sympathoadrenal system with its two main effectors, the catecholamines norepinephrine and epinephrine, produced by the sympathetic terminal nerves and by the adrenal medullary gland, respectively.

These effectors of the stress system regulate a highly coordinated response aimed at mobilizing energy, increasing arousal, and restoration of homeostasis in the face of threatening stimuli. Other endocrine systems, including the growth hormone/insulin-like growth factor-1 (GH/IGF-1) and the reproductive and the thyroid hormone axes are inhibited by the stress. During acute and chronic stress, complex alterations of the immune system also take place, which result in a switching from a cellular immune pattern of response to a humoral response (T-helper 1 to T-helper 2) (Chrousos and Elenkov, 2000). Such a coordinated series of responses is essential to survival. A complex network of inhibitory feed-back loops within and among the above components of the stress system has evolved to ensure that the stress response is effective, but contained.

The Stress Response: Specific or Nonspecific?

Initially, the stress response was thought to be homogeneous in response and independent of the nature of the perturbatory challenge, a concept originally formulated by Hans Selye and known as the doctrine of the nonspecificity of the stress response. More recently, it is being recognized that different stressful stimuli may elicit different patterns of stress responses. In addition, there is growing evidence suggesting that genetic variability, as well as differences in experiences during the first years of life, or even during intrauterine life, may "imprint" the stress responsivity of any given individual in a stable fashion. A corollary of the specificity of the stress response is that different stressful stimuli, if protracted and/or severe enough, are associated with different diseases.

The Stress System: Theoretical and Practical Challenges in Monitoring Its Activity in Vivo

There are several challenges to measuring the levels of activity of the stress system (Eskandari and Cizza, 2002): (a) the complexity of the system and the multiplicity of the effector molecules to be measured, (b) the methodology used to measure the activity of the stress system must not perturb the system, (c) the intrinsic variability of several hormones due to their circadian rhythmicity, (d) the importance of measuring stress reactivity, as well as baseline stress response measures, and (e) for studies conducted in the field, the feasibility of collecting integrated measures without using large volumes of blood or other biological samples.

The approaches currently used to measure the activity of the stress system in field studies originally evolved from the approaches used to measure the activity of the hypothalamic-pituitary-adrenal axis in selected categories of patients, including patients with hyperactivity of the stress system such as those with Cushing's disease, with a major depression, or with a rare tumor of the adrenal gland, the pheochromocytoma (Cizza and Chrousos, 1997). The clinical methods used in these cases involve measurements of the relevant circulating hormones during both basal and stimulated conditions, and often, given the diurnal rhythmicity of these hormones, around the clock measurements. Biological fluids collected in clinical settings include blood and sometimes cerebrospinal fluid or hypophysial portal blood for specific research purposes; more frequently, in an outpatient setting urine or saliva are collected. However, in the field it would be necessary to collect biological fluids in a noninvasive manner with a nonbulky collection apparatus, minimal discomfort, and cooperation from the subject. The purpose of this paper is to provide support for the sweat patch method (in which sweat collected by means of a commercially available, cutaneously applied patch) as a viable option for monitoring indices of stress system activity in the field.

Biology of the Stress Response and Bone Mass

An example of a serious medical consequence resulting from chronic stress is osteoporosis. Bone loss and fractures are often observed as a consequence of hypercortisolism resulting from endogenous Cushing's syndrome or the chronic use of steroids (Cizza et al., 1996). It is becoming more evident that subjects suffering from major depression also exhibit bone loss likely due to

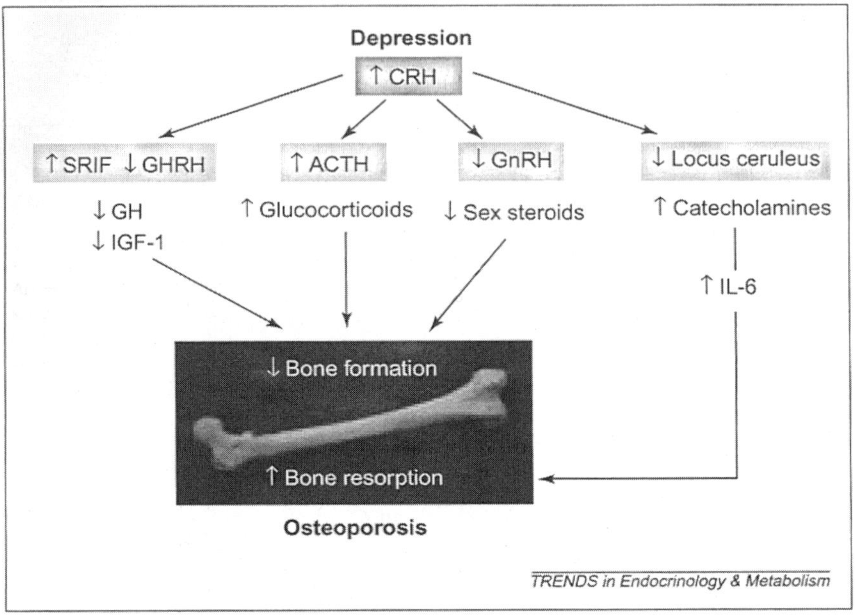

FIGURE D-33 The proposed endocrine mechanisms contributing to bone loss in subjects suffering from depression.
SOURCE: Reprinted from Cizza et al. (2001), with permission from Elsevier.

hypercortisolism (Figure D-33) (Cizza et al., 2001). CRH hypersecretion and hypercortisolism in turn lead to the inhibition of the reproductive axis and hypogonadism. The latter is an established risk factor for bone loss in both genders. CRH hypersecretion and hypercortisolism also decrease the activity of the GH-IGF-1 axis, an important enhancer of bone formation. In depression, a dysregulation of several inflammatory mediators, including interleukin-6, has also been reported. Interleukin-6, a major mediator of bone resorption, is elevated in depressed subjects, especially at an older age. Increased sympathetic activity, often observed in depressed subjects, also is associated with increased interleukin-6 secretion. This cytokine may be implicated in some of the other medical consequences of major depression, such as cardiovascular disease and insulin resistance.

Stress fractures are often observed in young military recruits of both genders during intense military training or operations (Imeida et al., 1999). In addition to the obvious physical component of mechanical overload associated with marching for a long period time with heavy loads, it is reasonable to hypothesize that some of the endocrine responses associated with the psychological stress may accelerate bone resorption and decrease bone formation. Specifically, an increase in cortisol and a decrease in IGF-1 (an important contributor to skeletal integrity) may, with mechanical overload, synergistically decrease bone mass at specific skeletal sites below the threshold for fractures (Munoz-Torres et al., 2001). Stress fractures are a common problem in young people who engage in vigorous physical activity, especially endurance training. For example, stress fractures during basic training occur in approximately 7 percent of male and 14 percent of female recruits. It is therefore important to identify subjects at greater risk; known risk factors include low level of physical fitness, current or past history of smoking, more than ten alcoholic beverages per week, use of corticosteroids, and low body weight. In women, additional factors include amenorrhea, delayed menarche, and use of depo-medroxyprogesterone acetate. In young men, low levels of testosterone, a hormone with an anabolic effect on bone, in a hypogonadal range are reported during intense training. To the best of our knowledge, there are no studies addressing the potential association between patterns of the individual stress response and subsequent risk of stress fractures, most likely because of the lack of a feasible method to measure the stress response in the field in an integrated fashion.

SWEAT: BACKGROUND AND PHYSIOLOGY

Summarized below is information supporting the notion that sweat may represent a biological fluid from which it is feasible to measure endogenous substances released during stress in ambulatory or field situations (Guyton, 2000). In humans, three types of sweat glands are present. Apocrine sweat glands are largely confined to the axillary and perineal regions and their ducts open directly into hair follicles. The apoeccrine sweat glands are present in adult axillae. They develop from eccrine-like precursor glands and their ducts open directly onto the skin surface. The eccrine sweat glands are distributed over the entire body. Generalized eccrine sweating is the physiological response to an increased body temperature. This is the most effective means by which humans regulate their body temperature through evaporative heat loss.

The eccrine sweat glands develop from the epidermal ridge as a cord of epithelial cells growing downward. These glands are stimulated by the cholinergic sympathetic nervous system. The preoptic hypothalamic area plays an essential role in regulating body temperature. Efferent nerve fibers originating from the hypothalamic preoptic sweat center descend through the ipsilateral brain stem and synapse in the intermediolateral cell columns of the spinal cord without crossing. The myelinated axons rising from the intermediolateral horn of the spinal cord (preganglionic fibers) pass through the anterior roots to reach the sympathetic chain and synapse. Unmyelinated, postganglionic sympathetic class C fibers arising from sympathetic ganglions join the major peripheral nerves and end around the sweat glands. The major neurotransmitter released from the periglandular nerve endings is acetylcholine. In addition, adenosine triphosphate, catecholamine, vasoactive intestinal peptide, natriuretic peptide, calcitonin gene-related peptide, and galanin have been localized in the periglandular nerves.

The eccrine sweat gland consists of two segments: a secretory coil and a duct. The secretory coil secretes an ultrafiltrate of plasma-like fluid called the primary secretion. The concentration of sodium is about 142 mmol/L and chloride about 104 mmol/L, with much smaller concentrations of the other solutes of plasma. In addition, sweat glands excrete heavy metals, organic compounds, and macromolecules. As this precursor solution flows through the duct portion of the gland, it is modified by reabsorption of most of the sodium and chloride ions. This reduces the osmotic pressure of the sweat fluid to such a low level that most of the water is then also reabsorbed. The degree of this reabsorption depends on the rate of sweating. When the sweat glands are stimulated only slightly, the primary secretion passes through the duct slowly and essentially all the sodium and chloride ions are reabsorbed. The concentration of each of these falls to as low as 5 mmol/L, followed by reabsorption of water, which concentrates most of the other constituents. Conversely, when the sweat glands are strongly stimulated by the sympathetic nervous system, large amounts of primary secretions are formed and the concentrations of the sodium and chloride ions are then at a maximum of about 50 to 60 mmol/L and little of the water is reabsorbed.

Content of Human Sweat in Hormones or Cytokines

Several studies have been reported using skin biopsy specimens or sweat specimens collected over an oil barrier on a plastic film or in a polypropylene sack. Traditionally, sweat is collected after exercise or exposure to intense heat. Interleukin (IL)-1 and IL-1β, IL-6, IL-8, and tumor necrosis factor have been identified in human sweat. Interestingly, to the best of our knowledge, there are no published reports on the presence of cortisol or catecholamines in sweat in humans.

Why the Sweat Patch?

We propose to use a cutaneous patch as a convenient and noninvasive technique that may overcome several of the limitations intrinsic to blood and urine collection. Such a technique would have the advantage of being noninvasive, of being easily applied at any time of the day, and of being worn for an extended period of time with minimal discomfort. A series of biochemical markers of bone turnover, cytokines, and neurohormones may be measured in microliters of specimen, using state-of-the art technologies, such as recycling immunoaffinity chromatography and cytokine chip technology. These techniques require a minimum amount of biological sample, thus overcoming the need for collection of large volumes of blood. Once validated, the cutaneous patch, in conjunction with an ultramicro analytical immunochemistry method, should substantially expand our ability to examine and understand the interactions between the endocrine, immune, and nervous systems and their role in stressful conditions in the field.

Current Clinical Application of the Cutaneous Patch in Diagnostic Testing

A cutaneous patch is approved by the Food and Drug Administration for qualitative detection of a variety of drugs and their metabolites, including opioids, benzodiazepines, and methamphetamines. It can also be used to measure methadone, caffeine, and nicotine. This device is commercially available under the trade name of Osteopatch and has been used for determinations of free pyridinoline cross-links in sweat. It has been validated in healthy subjects and in subjects affected by metabolic bone disease, including postmenopausal osteoporosis, and hyperparathyroidism. The Osteopatch has been used in subjects treated with estrogen replacement therapy and treated with alendronate. Sweat determinations of pyridinoline reflected true changes in bone resorption due to metabolic disease and antiresorptive treatments, indicating that these measurements were valid and accurate (Sarno et al., 1999, 2001). In addition, as pyridinoline in sweat arises from plasma, measurements of pyridinoline in this biological fluid reflect true bone resorption more closely than urine measurements.

To correct for sweat volume, determinations of potassium are performed. Potassium is consistently recovered from the patch and its secretion is reasonably well correlated with sweat volume. In contrast to sweat sodium and chloride, potassium is relatively insensitive to subject age, diet, and methods of fluid replacement (i.e., intake of water only as compared with glucose-electrolyte solution) in situations of extreme heat. The latter characteristics make this test potentially valuable for field studies.

In order to validate the reliability and sensitivity of use of the Osteopatch for collection of stress, neuroendocrine, and immune biomarkers in sweat, it is necessary to: (1) determine the range of stress, neuroendocrine, and immune biomarkers that can be measured in sweat and the stability of these biomarkers under various collection conditions, and (2) determine the degree to which these sweat biomarkers reflect their concentrations in other biological fluids, including blood, urine, and saliva.

METHODS

Description of the Sweat Patch: Advantages and Pitfalls

The transdermal diagnostic skin patch is a device that provides easy, noninvasive, reliable and relatively nonvariable access to body sweat. The patch is a nonocclusive sweat collection device. It consists of an adhesive layer on a thin transparent film of surgical dressing with a cellulose-absorbent pad attached. The patch passively collects and concentrates nonaqueous components of sweat.

The outside surface of the patch forms a barrier for substances in the environment. The potential disadvantage of the nonocclusive design is that the volume of the secreted sweat is not measurable and, thus, the concentrations of analytes cannot be normalized to sweat volume. This limitation may be overcome by normalizing against potassium measurements. The patch can be worn over an extended period of time (usually a few days) and is reported by the manufacturer as being well tolerated. However, we propose to limit its application to a period of time not longer than 24 hours. In our limited experience we have observed no adverse reaction with the exception of one subject, a 36-year-old female normal volunteer who, 6 months after the application of a patch, had an area of discoloration on the abdomen in the area in which the adhesive part of the patch had been applied.

Analytical Procedures

Two major challenges are encountered from an analytical perspective when measuring biological analytes in sweat: (1) the available assays are not sufficiently sensitive to detect some analytes, and (2) there may not be sufficient volume to perform all the measurements needed. The application of newer technologies, including recycling immunoaffinity chromatography and the cytokine chip technology, described below, should address both challenges (Brown et al., 2000; Phillips et al., 1997).

Recycling Immunoaffinity Chromatography

Specimens can be analyzed for cytokines, hormones, biochemical markers of bone turn-over, or any other substance of interest using a 25-μL sample injected into a modified liquid chromatography system, equipped with a panel of 25 to 30 immunoaffinity columns packed with antibody-coated glass beads. The specimen passes through the columns in a serpentine fashion, each column extracting a single analyte, while allowing the nonreactive materials to pass to the next column. The bound analytes are measured by sequential acid elution of each column, followed by laser-induced fluorescence detection. Concentrations of each recovered analyte is calculated by comparing them with standard curves constructed by running known amounts of pure analyte through identical conditions.

Cytokine Chip Technology

Glass chips are constructed by covalently immobilizing 200 nL spots of avidin to the glass surface via a robotics system. The chips are heat annealed, washed in 0.01 M phosphate buffer, pH 7.4, and blocked with 0.1 percent bovine albumin. The chips are then rewashed in phosphate buffer, dried, and stored under nitrogen at –70°C. Biotinylated antibodies, directed against the analytes of

TABLE D-7 Substances Detected in Sweat Collected by the Osteopatch

Type	Substance
Cytokines	Tumor necrosis factor α, interleukin (IL)-1α[a], IL-1 β, IL-6, IL-8
Hormones	Cortisol, substance P, calcitonin gene-related peptide, neuropeptide Y, β endorphin, prolactin[a], vasoactive intestinal peptide, angiotensin, insulin-like growth factor (IGF)-1[a], growth hormone
Miscellaneous compounds	Pituitary adenyl cyclase-activating peptide[a], neurotrophin-3[a], transforming growth factor ß, leukemia inhibitory factor[a], gamma interferon-inducible protein 10[a], epidermal growth factor, ciliary neutrophic factor, nerve growth factor, ß fibroblast growth factor[a], macrophage inflammatory protein α[a]

[a] Substance that can be detected in sweat only after a 12-min walking-running test.

interest, are spotted in appropriate patterns onto rehydrated chips and incubated in a moist chamber for 60 minutes at 37°C. The chips are then incubated with fluorescent-labeled specimens for 60 minutes at 37°C, washed in phosphate buffer, and read in a laboratory-built, laser-induced fluorescence reader (Instrument Development Resource, Division of Bioengineering and Physical Science, Office of Research Services, National Institutes of Health). The concentration of each analyte is calculated from calibration curves constructed by subjecting known standards to the same analytical procedure.

RESULTS

Table D-7 lists analytes that can be detected either under baseline conditions or after a brief bout of exercise in sweat collected by the means of the patch. The panel of substances that can be measured in sweat includes inflammatory cytokines such as IL-1, tumor necrosis factor-alpha, IL-6, and IL-8; neuropeptides stimulated by pain such as substance P; hormones increased during the stress response, such as cortisol or prolactin; IGF-1, an important factor for bone regeneration; and several chemokines. In addition, this device is already marketed for the measurements of several markers of bone turnover.

SUMMARY

In summary, we have collected sweat at baseline conditions and after a short course of exercise from which we measured several biomarkers, including stress hormones, neuropeptides, and cytokines, by applying ultrasensitive techniques requiring minute amounts of biological samples. Many of the analytes that we have detected in sweat have never been described in this biological fluid. As the endocrine and immune responses to stress are highly interconnected, the ability to measure many of the molecules involved in these responses in the same sample greatly enhances the ability to more precisely define those complex interactions at an individual level. Since the Osteopatch is designed and approved for measurements of biomarkers of bone turn-over, the integration of these bone measures in sweat, together with stress hormone and immune cytokine measures that contribute to bone loss, should provide a sensitive method for detection of predictive conditions leading to deleterious effects.

In conclusion, the sweat patch provides the opportunity to conduct naturalistic studies outside of the laboratory on a very large number of subjects. Once validated in a reference population, this technique would allow for the early identification of subjects who, because of their individual physiological responses to stress, may be at greater risk during intense training of stress fractures, acute infections, or other stress-related accidents.

Conflict of Interest: None of the authors has any commercial interest in the development of the device described in this paper or in any other similar device.

REFERENCES

Brown SA, Mayberry AJ, Mathy JA, Phillips TM, Klitzman B, Levin LS. 2000. The effect of muscle flap transposition to the fracture site on TNFalpha levels during fracture healing. *Plast Reconstr Surg* 105:991–998.

Chrousos GP, Elenkov IJ. 2000. Interactions of the endocrine and immune system. In: De Groot L, Jameson JL, eds. *Endocrinology*. Philadelphia: WB Saunders. Pp. 571–586.

Chrousos GP, McCarty R, Pacak K, Cizza G, Sternberg E, Gold PW, Kvetnansky R, eds. 1995. Stress: Basic mechanism and clinical implications. *Ann N Y Acad Sci* 771.

Cizza G, Chrousos GP. 1997. ACTH-dependent Cushing syndrome: Clinical presentation, differential diagnosis, treatment and potential pathophysiological implications. In: Arnold A, ed. *Endocrine Neoplasms Treatment and Research Series*. Boston: Kluwer Academic. Pp. 25–40.

Cizza G, Nieman L, Doppman J, Czerwiek F, Passaro MD, Chrousos GP, Cutler GB. 1996. Factitious Cushing syndrome. *J Clin Endocrinol Metab* 81:3573–3577.

Cizza G, Ravn P, Chrousos GP, Gold PW. 2001. Depression: A major unrecognized risk factor for osteoporosis. *Trend Endocrinol Metab* 5:198–203.

Eskandari F, Cizza G. 2002. Cortisol, DHEA, the Holy Grail and the Fountain of Youth. *J Endocrinol Invest* 25:753.

Guyton AC. 2000. Body temperature, temperature regulation, and fever. In: Hall G, ed. *Textbook of Medical Physiology*. Philadelphia: WB Saunders. Pp. 822–823.

Imeida SA, Williams KM, Shaffer RA, Brodine SK. 1999. Epidemiological patterns of musculoskeletal injuries and physical training. *Med Sci Sports Exerc* 31:1176–1182.

Munoz-Torres M, Mezquita-Raya P, Lopez-Rodriguez F, Torres-Vela E, de Dios Luna J, Escobar-Jimenez F. 2001. The contribution of IGF-I to skeletal integrity in postmenopausal women. *Clin Endocrinol* 55:759–766.

Phillips TM, Kennedy LM, De Fabo EC. 1997. Microdialysis-immunoaffinity capillary electrophoresis studies on neuropeptide-induced lymphocyte secretion. *J Chromatogr Biomed Sci Appl B* 697:101–109.

Sarno M, Powell H, Tjersland G, Schoendorfer D, Harris H, Adams K, Ogata P, Warnick GR. 1999. A collection method and high-sensitivity enzyme immunoassay for sweat pyridinoline and deoxypyridinoline cross-links. *Clin Chem* 45:1501–1509.

Sarno M, Sarno L, Baylink D, Drinkwater B, Farley S, Kleerekoper M, Lang R, Lappe J, Licata A, McClung M, Miller P, Nattrass S, Recker R, Schwartz EN, Tucci JR, Wolf S, Powell H, Tjersland G, Warnick GR. 2001. Excretion of sweat and urine pyridinoline crosslinks in healthy controls and subjects with established metabolic bone disease. *Clin Chem Lab Med* 39:223–228.

BIOMARKERS FOR BRAIN HYPOMETABOLISM DUE TO SLEEP DEPRIVATION

Nancy Wesensten, Walter Reed Army Institute of Research

Both acute and chronic sleep deprivation (roughly surge and sustained operations, respectively) degrade cognitive performance (Belenky et al., 2003). The neurobiological basis of this cognitive performance degradation appears to be a global decrease in brain energy metabolism, with the greatest decreases occurring in the prefrontal cortex (Thomas et al., 2000). The prefrontal cortex governs the highest-order cognitive processes, including anticipation, planning, situational awareness, and common mental models; the ability to envision the desired end state; and the paths to achieving it. In military operations, these functions translate into the ability to adapt at all levels of command and control to take advantage of tactical, operational, and strategic opportunities in real time.

Surge operations and sustained operations differ in their effects on performance and thus presumably on underlying neurobiology. During surge operations (less than 4 hours of sleep per 24 hours), performance degrades in a linear fashion, while brain metabolism declines over the first 24 hours and then stabilizes at this lower level (Thomas et al., 2000). Because recovery from surge operations is rapid and generally complete within 24 to 48 hours with adequate (8 hours per night) recovery sleep, it is assumed that brain metabolism also recovers completely. The effects of sustained operations (more than 4 but less than 7 hours of sleep per 24 hours) on performance has received far less attention, and therefore are less well understood—however, results from a recently completed study by our group indicate that with less than 8 hours of sleep per night, performance degrades over the first few days and then stabilizes at a lower submaximum level of performance (Balkin et al., 2000; Belenky et al., 2003). Unlike surge operations, recovery from sustained operations can take days or weeks (Belenky et al., 2003). The effects of sustained operations on brain metabolism are not known, but our performance data suggest that sustained operations are associated with a more enduring down-regulation of brain metabolic capacity.

As both military and civilian industrial endeavors become increasingly continuous (24 hours per day) operations, the potential for sleepiness-related incidents—ranging from operational inefficiencies to errors resulting in serious accidents—is increasing. The task of determining how, or what, to measure to predict human performance degradation is difficult and complex. Because brain hypometabolism is assumed to underlie performance deficits, the former would be the "gold standard" biological signal to monitor. Biomarkers of brain metabolism changes during sleep deprivation include blood flow (Braun et al., 1997) and glucose metabolism (Thomas et al., 2000). Clearly, however, these markers are not fieldable—and to date evidence indicating that they are *predictive* of performance degradation is lacking. Since in most operational settings changes in actual performance are of concern, the question could be rephrased as, "Are measures of actual performance as good as (or perhaps better than) measures of brain hypometabolism?" If the answer to the latter is positive, the question then becomes, "What constitutes a promising metric of general sleep-related performance capacity for use in the operational environment?" To this end, we tested, compared, and judged several candidate measures across seven consecutive days in which subjects were allowed 9, 7, 5, or 3 hours in bed per night. This design constituted an in-laboratory simulation of sustained operations (as defined above).

MATERIALS AND METHODS

General Design and Procedures

A complete description of the study subjects, design, and procedures can be found in Balkin and colleagues (2000). Briefly, 66 commercial motor vehicle-licensed drivers (16 women, 50 men; age range 24–62 years) participated. They spent 14 days in the laboratory. The first 2 days were adaptation/training (T1, T2) and the third served as baseline (B). Subjects were allowed 8 hours in bed (TIB) from 2300 to 0700 on the nights prior to T2 and B. Beginning on the fourth day and continuing for a total of 7 days (E1–E7) subjects were assigned to one of four sleep conditions: 9 hours TIB (2200–0700); 7 hours TIB (2400–0700); 5 hours TIB (0200–0700); or 3 hours TIB (0400–0700). On the eleventh day and continuing for a total of 3 "recovery" days (R1–R3), subjects were again allowed to sleep from 2300 to 0700 (8 hours TIB). Data from these recovery days are not reported here.

Cognitive/Psychomotor Tests

Subjects performed a series of cognitive and alertness tests daily, including psychomotor vigilance (PVT) (Dinges and Powell, 1985); synthetic work (Elsmore, 1994); simulated driving (StiSim) (Balkin et al., 2000); running memory; grammatical (logical) reasoning; Stroop color naming; serial addition/subtraction; 10-choice reaction time (RT); time estimation or "interval reproduction"; code substitution; subjective sleepiness via the Stanford Sleepiness Scale (SSS) (Hoddes et al., 1973); objective sleepiness via a sleep latency test (SLT) (Carskadon et al., 1986); 4-choice RT (Thorne et al., 1985); and an oculomotor function test (FIT). A detailed description of these tests can be found in Balkin and colleagues (2000).

Data Analyses

Analysis of Variance

Data were first analyzed using conventional analysis of variance (ANOVA; Kirk, 1995) techniques: a mixed ANOVA for sleep group (between subjects) × day (within subjects) was applied to all data, with additional factors for time of day as appropriate. Greenhouse-Geisser corrections (Kirk, 1995) were applied to repeated measures effects. Significant sleep group × day interactions were followed by simple effects analyses for sleep group at each day. Significant sleep-group simple effects were then analyzed using post-hoc Tukey honestly significant difference (HSD) comparisons (Kirk, 1995) among all possible pairs of sleep groups (maximum of six comparisons: 3 hr vs. 5 hr, 7 hr, and 9 hr; 5 hr vs. 7 hr and 9 hr; 7 hr vs. 9 hr). All performance data were normalized by converting to percent baseline.

Effect Size Analysis

Data were also explored by generating an effect size estimate (also known as a *d* statistic) for the relationship between nightly sleep time and each task/dependent variable listed above independent of sleep group assignment (Balkin et al., submitted). Variability of the effect size was estimated using a bootstrap procedure to determine whether the effect size differed from zero. The bootstrap procedure also provided estimates of confidence intervals.

RESULTS

Analysis of Variance

ANOVA revealed that nightly total sleep time (TST) increased significantly in the 9-hour group and decreased significantly in the 3-, 5-, and 7-hour groups across the sleep restriction/augmentation phase (E1–E7) compared with baseline (B) (group × night, $p < 0.05$). TST significantly differed among all sleep groups on nights E1 through E7 (Tukey HSD, $ps < 0.05$).

Table D-8 summarizes the number of significant post-hoc comparisons among sleep groups for each task and dependent variable baseline (B) through experimental day 7 (E7) for which both the sleep group × day interaction and significant simple effects of sleep group at each day were significant. The tasks/dependent variables are rank-ordered by total number of significant post-hoc contrasts summed across baseline and E1 through E7. As indicated in Table D-8, by this criterion PVT relative speed was most sensitive.

Effect Size Analyses

Figure D-34 shows results of the effect size analysis (Balkin et al., submitted). Using this technique, SLT accounted for the largest percentage of variance in nocturnal sleep during the experimental phase (45 percent), followed by PVT speed (21 percent), StiSim lane deviations (19 percent) 4-choice RT speed (13 percent), and SSS (10 percent); the effect sizes for these tasks/dependent measures were statistically significant ($ps < 0.05$). Note that although StiSim accidents showed a relatively large effect size, the confidence intervals for this measure also were large; thus, the effect size was nonsignificant. On the other hand, effect sizes for StiSim lane position (7 percent), 10-choice RT number correct (7 percent), serial addition/subtraction speed (5 percent), and 4-choice RT correct (3 percent) were relatively small but significant since the confidence intervals were relatively narrow.

DISCUSSION AND CONCLUSIONS

Although it is assumed that biomarkers of brain hypometabolism (presumed to underlie performance deficits) would be the preferred biological signal to monitor to predict sleep deprivation-induced performance impairments, such markers are currently not fieldable. Therefore, the question of what constitutes a promising metric of general sleep-related performance capacity for use in the operational environment is addressed.

Of the various measures compared, the most sensitive (as reflected by the number of statistically significant post-hoc comparisons from the ANOVA) was PVT (Dinges and Powell, 1985). The most sensitive test as reflected by the effect size analysis was SLT. Although the rank ordering of tasks differed somewhat between ANOVA and effect size analysis, in general those tests found to be most sensitive by one technique also ranked highly using the other technique. Tasks in the top rankings for both included PVT, simulated driving lane deviations and lane position, SLT, SSS subjective sleepiness self-ratings, and serial addition/subtraction speed.

That SLT accounted for the most variance by the effect size technique is perhaps not surprising since it could be argued that SLT is the most "direct" measure of sleep loss in that it actually gauges sleep (onset) itself. However, under most circumstances the SLT is not practical—and more important, sleep latency does not necessarily predict performance. PVT speed most frequently mirrored the gradations in total sleep times—and, by inference, the differential levels of recuperation that result from spending 3, 5, 7, or 9 hours in bed over 7 consecutive nights. That PVT speed did not account for a greater proportion of variance in nocturnal sleep time (effect size analysis) may indicate that total sleep time, rather than PVT speed, is not a particularly sensitive index of recuperation processes. It may be that some other index of sleep-mediated recuperative processes, such as slow-wave activity, might better predict performance.

The present results suggested relatively poor sensitivity of FIT for detecting sleepiness. It is possible that sensitivity could have been increased by increasing FIT test duration. In its current configuration, FIT is a short (45 sec) test. Even extremely sleepy subjects can perform adequately for short periods of time, suggesting that *any* short-duration task will lack sensitivity. For example, had PVT been administered only for 45 seconds, it likely would have been relatively insensitive and, in fact, our analyses of PVT data across time on task indicate that decrements do not become evident until the third or fourth minute on task. SLT may also constitute a 20-minute vigilance task, the sensitivity of which would be decreased by shortening the test to 1 to 2 minutes.

In the near-term, progress in developing the means to measure and monitor the effects of sleep loss in the operational environment will require further, similar studies—systematic, head-to-head comparisons of the sensitivity and reliability of multiple measures (with consideration of the likelihood that these measures could be obtained in the operational environment of interest). At the core of these near-term (within 2–5 years) studies will be performance metrics, with a vision toward integration of newer, "high-risk/high-payoff" technologies, such as analyses of changes in gene expression across sleep deprivation/sleep restriction, and how such changes in gene expression relate to specific performance metrics. Also needed in the near-term are studies describing the exact relationship between sleep deprivation-induced brain hypometabolism and specific aspects of cognitive performance to determine whether there is actually a need for measuring hypometabolism directly. That is, does a marker of brain hypometabolism (blood flow, metabolism) confer some predictive advantage beyond that of performance measures? Do markers of brain hypometabolism better determine individual differences in response to sleep loss? Far-term (10–20 years out) studies will consist of aggregate measures of sleep/wake history over

TABLE D-8 Number of Significant Post-hoc Contrasts Among Sleep Groups for Each Task and Dependent Measure

Task[a]	Dependent Measure[b]	Number of Significant Post-hoc Contrasts Among Sleep Groups (max = 6/day)[c]									Actual Group n (max possible)					*	^
		B	EI	E2	E3	E4	E5	E6	E7	Total	3 (18)	5 (16)	7 (16)	9 (16)	Total (66)		
Total sleep time	Abs Min of sleep	NS	6	6	6	6	6	6	6	42	18	16	15	16	65		
PVT	Rel speed	NA	2	3	4	4	3	4	4	24	14	13	14	16	57		
PVT	Rel speed – 2 times of day	NA	2	3	4	4	4	4	3	24	16	15	15	16	62		
StiSim	Rel SD of lane tracking	NA	NS	4	2	2	3	2	3	16	10	13	13	12	48		
StiSim	Rel lane position	NA	1	2	3	2	2	2	2	14	10	13	13	12	48		
Stanford Sleepiness Scale	Rel sleepiness score	NA	NS	2	3	1	2	2	1	11	17	15	15	13	60		
Wilkinson 4-choice RT	Rel speed	NA	NS	1	2	2	2	1	3	11	14	15	15	10	54		
Running memory	Rel speed	NA	1	NS	1	0	3	2	3	10	17	14	15	14	60		

Modified MSLT	ABS latency to sleep (min)	NA	NS	4	0	NS	4	2	0	10	16	14	15	9	54
Stroop	Rel speed	NA	1	NS	NS	1	1	1	2	6	17	15	14	15	61
Serial addition/subtraction	Rel speed	NA	NS	NS	1	1	1	1	2	6	17	14	15	13	59
Running memory	Rel accuracy	NA	NS	NS	NS	NS	1	1	3	5	17	14	15	14	60
Serial addition/subtraction	Rel accuracy	NA	NS	NS	NS	NS	1	2	2	5	17	14	15	13	59
Grammatical reasoning	Rel accuracy	NA	0	0	NS	NS	NS	NS	NS	0	17	14	15	13	59
Time estimation	Rel CV	NA	NS	NS	NS	0	0	0	0	0	17	13	15	13	58
Wilkinson 4-choice RT	Rel accuracy	NA	NS	NS	0	NS	NS	0	0	0	14	15	15	10	54

(continued on next page)

TABLE D-8 Continued

Task[a]	Dependent Measure[b]	Number of Significant Post-hoc Contrasts Among Sleep Groups (max = 6/day)[c]									Actual Group n (max possible)					* ^
		B	EI	E2	E3	E4	E5	E6	E7	Total	3 (18)	5 (16)	7 (16)	9 (16)	Total (66)	
10-Choice RT	Rel speed (group x day, p = 0.0)	NA	NS	NS	0	1	0	3	2	6	17	13	15	13	58	
Stroop	Rel accuracy	NA	NS	NS	NS	NS	NS	NS	NS	0	17	15	14	15	61	*
Grammatical reasoning	Rel speed	NA	NS	NS	NS	NS	NS	NS	NS	0	17	14	15	13	59	*
10-Choice RT	Rel accuracy	NA	NS	NS	NS	NS	NS	NS	NS	0	17	13	15	13	58	*
SYNWORK	Rel composite score	NA	NS	NS	NS	NS	NS	NS	NS	0	17	15	11	15	58	*
Code substitution	Rel accuracy (IRE score)	NA	NS	NS	NS	NS	NS	NS	NS	0	16	13	13	8	50	*
StiSim	Abs number of accidents	NA	NS	NS	NS	NS	NS	NS	NS	0	13	14	13	13	53	*

FIT	Rel CA	NA	NS	NS	NS	NS	NS	NS	NS	0	13	8	10	11	42	*	^
FIT	Rel eye closure	NA	NS	NS	NS	NS	NS	NS	NS	0	13	8	10	11	42	*	^
FIT	Rel pupil diameter	NA	NS	NS	NS	NS	NS	NS	NS	0	13	8	10	11	42	*	^
FIT	Rel INDEX	NA	NS	NS	NS	NS	NS	NS	NS	0	13	8	10	11	42	*	^
FIT	Rel saccadic velocity	NA	NS	NS	NS	NS	NS	NS	NS	0	13	8	10	10	41	*	^

NOTE: Tasks are rank-ordered by the total number of significant post-hoc Tukey honestly significant difference contrasts found.
[a]PVT = psychomotor vigilance, StiSim = simulated driving. RT = reaction time, MSLT = multiple sleep latency test, SYNWORK = synthetic work, FIT = oculomotor function test.
[b]SD = standard deviation, CV = coefficient of variation.
[c]NS = not significant, NA = not applicable.

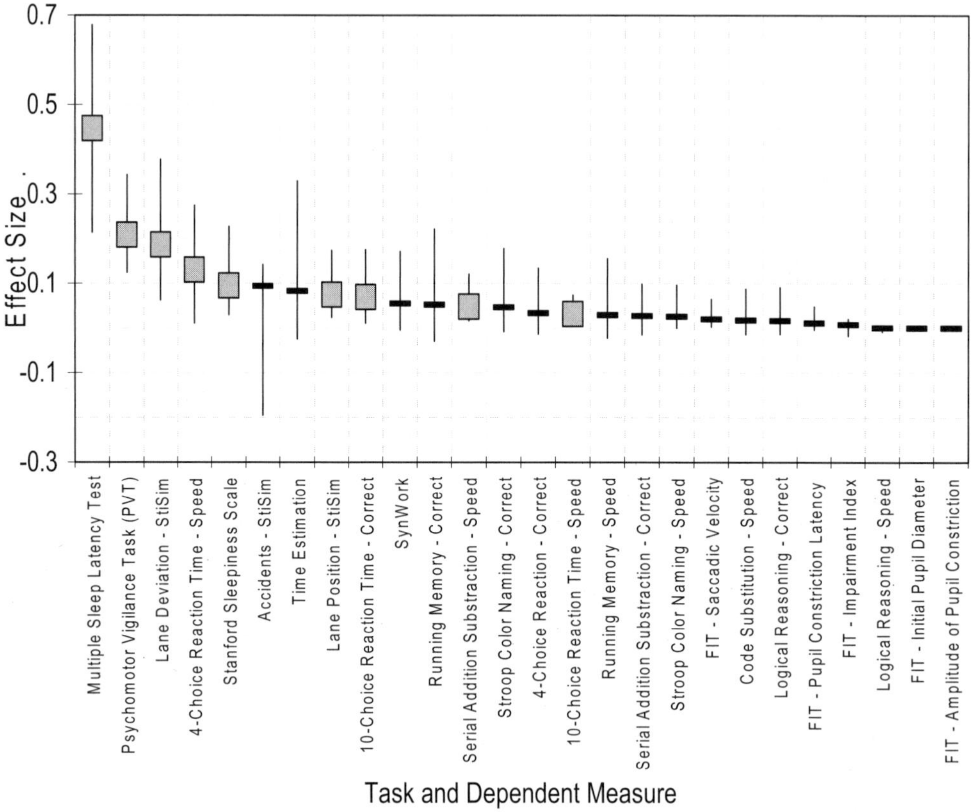

FIGURE D-34 Effect size for each task and dependent measure. Significant effect sizes are denoted by filled gray squares; nonsignificant effect sizes are denoted by a solid dash. Vertical lines indicate confidence intervals. StiSim = simulated driving, SynWork = synthetic work, FIT = oculomotor function test.

weeks, analogous to glycosylated hemoglobin as an index of blood glucose control over a period of weeks.

In both the near and far terms, investigations into the underlying neurobiology of sleep and wakefulness are critical; for example, no chemical has yet been identified in the blood that accumulates during sleep deprivation and causes performance impairments. The analogous state of affairs would be alcohol-induced impairment, where alcohol levels are measurable in exhaled air, and levels of alcohol have been correlated with degree of performance impairment. The latter is the end result of a long and complex (and still ongoing) process.

REFERENCES

Balkin T, Bliese P, Belenky G, Sing H, Thorne D, Thomas M, Redmond D, Russo M, Wesensten N. Submitted. Comparative utility of instruments for monitoring sleepiness-related performance decrements in the operational environment. *J Sleep Res*

Balkin T, Thorne D, Sing H, Thomas M, Redmond D, Wesensten N, Williams J, Hall S, Belenky G. 2000. Effects of sleep schedules on commercial driver performance. Report No. DOT-MC-00-133. Washington, DC: Federal Motor Carrier Safety Administration, U.S. Department of Transportation.

Belenky G, Wesensten NJ, Thorne DR, Thomas ML, Sing HC, Redmond DP, Russo MB, Balkin TJ. 2003. Patterns of performance degradation and restoration during sleep restriction and subsequent recovery: A sleep dose-response study. *J Sleep Res* 12:1–12.

Braun AR, Balkin TJ, Wesensten NJ, Carson RE, Varga M, Baldwin P, Selbie S, Belenky G, Herscovitch P. 1997. Regional cerebral blood flow throughout the sleep-wake cycle: An H215O positron emission tomography study. *Brain* 120:1173–1197.

Carskadon MA, Dement WC, Mitler MM, Roth T, Westbrook PR, Keenan S. 1986. Guidelines for the multiple sleep latency test (MSLT): A standard measure of sleepiness. *Sleep* 9:519–524.

Dinges DF, Powell JW. 1985. Microcomputer analyses of performance on a portable, simple visual RT task during sustained operations. *Behav Res Methods Instrum Comput* 17:652–655.

Elsmore TF. 1994. SYNWORK1: A PC-based tool for assessment of performance in a simulated work environment. *Behav Res Methods Instrum Comput* 26:421–426.

Hoddes E, Zarcone V, Smythe H, Phillips R, Dement WC. 1973. Quantification of sleepiness: A new approach. *Psychophysiology* 10:431–436.

Kirk RE. 1995. *Experimental Design: Procedures for the Behavioral Sciences.* 3rd ed. Monterey, CA: Brooks/Cole.

Thomas M, Sing H, Belenky G, Holcomb H, Mayberg H, Dannals R, Wagner H, Thorne D, Popp K, Rowland L, Welsh A, Balwinski S, Redmond D. 2000. Neural basis of alertness and cognitive performance impairments during sleepiness. I. Effects of 24 h of sleep deprivation on waking human regional brain activity. *J Sleep Res* 9:335–352.

Thorne DR, Genser SG, Sing HC, Hegge FW. 1985. The Walter Reed performance assessment battery. *Neurobehav Toxicol Teratol* 7:415–418.

ELECTROENCEPHALOGRAPHIC INDICATORS OF IMPAIRED AVIATOR STATUS DURING SLEEP DEPRIVATION

John A. Caldwell, Brooks Air Force Base

Monitoring the brain activity of aviators for indications of degraded cognitive/performance capacity is desirable for enhancing flight safety. Research has shown that degraded pilot status has caused serious mishaps. For instance, McCann and Schulze (1963) reported that a substantial number of fatal aviation accidents have resulted from pilot incapacitation due to hypoxia, hyperventilation, or blackout; Yacavone (1993) found that serious flight mishaps have been associated with inadequate crew coordination or decrements in the physical or mental status of pilots. Pilot fatigue is now recognized as a serious threat to aviation safety, especially in operations that involve sleep loss from circadian disruptions, extended duty periods without sleep, and episodes of night duty during which alertness is typically impaired due to circadian factors (Akerstedt, 1995). Aviator fatigue degrades response accuracy and speed, impairs the capacity to integrate information, and narrows attention (Perry, 1974). Fatigued pilots tend to decrease their physical activity, withdraw from social interactions, and lose the ability to effectively divide mental resources among different tasks. These effects are compounded by the fact that increased sleepiness in the cockpit is associated with less consistent performance and deteriorations in vigilance (Dinges, 1990).

Kirsh (1996) estimates that fatigue may be involved in 4 to 7 percent of civil aviation mishaps, and data from the U.S. Army suggest fatigue is involved in 4 percent of Army accidents (Caldwell and Gilreath, 2002). Furthermore, 25 percent of the Air Force's night tactical fighter Class A accidents were attributed to fatigue between 1974 and 1992, and 12.2 percent of the Navy's total Class A mishaps were thought to be the result of aircrew fatigue from 1977 to 1990 (Ramsey and McGlohn, 1997). Especially noteworthy mishaps in the commercial aviation sector include the crash of Korean Air flight 801 in which 228 people died (NTSB, 1999), the near crash of China Airlines flight 006 in which two people were severely injured while numerous other passengers were traumatized (Kostad, 1989), and the accident involving American Airlines flight 1420 in which 11 people died (Krause, 1999). In each of these cases, crew fatigue from insufficient sleep and/or circadian factors was implicated.

It is regrettable that a suitable metric has not been developed to determine the point at which aviator fatigue becomes a hazard to safe flight. In fact, neither the military nor the civilian aviation sector has identified a better fatigue countermeasure than the age-old strategy of flight-time or duty-time limitations. Unfortunately, this approach fails to account for the known effects of fatigue-inducing factors such as: (1) the quality of sleep prior to reporting for duty, (2) the deleterious impact of chronically restricted sleep periods, and (3) the hour-by-hour fluctuations in physiological alertness that stem from circadian rhythms. What is needed is a validated, objective measurement of aviator status that ultimately can be monitored continuously and in real time.

Since the electroencephalogram (EEG) is the most direct indication of central nervous system functioning (which presumably underlies all cognition and performance), this measure holds great promise for objectively and accurately monitoring the fatigue state of operators. The fact that EEG activity can be collected without interfering with the primary task of flying the aircraft (Caldwell et al., 2002) supports the feasibility of continuous, real-time monitoring. In addition, numerous ground-based studies have established the sensitivity of EEG activity to work-related stressors such as sleep deprivation. Several researchers have shown that slow-wave EEG activity (i.e., delta and/or theta) is significantly elevated by even moderate sleep loss (e.g., Caldwell et al., 1996; Comperatore et al., 1993; Lorenzo et al., 1995; Pigeau et al., 1987). Recently, Caldwell and Hall (2001) reported that both delta and theta are reliably accentuated after 23 to 26 hours of continuous wakefulness, approximately the same time that both mood and performance are adversely affected.

Although studies relating in-flight EEG data to the readiness level of aviators are virtually nonexistent, a few investigators have suggested a link. Sterman and colleagues (1987) demonstrated changes in EEG theta and alpha as a function of increased flying demands, as well as increased EEG asymmetries as a function of increased workload, and Wilson and Hankins (1994) found differences in EEG theta activity attributable to alterations in attention and cognitive demands in flight. With regard to the appearance of EEG indications of in-flight fatigue, several researchers have reported EEG microsleeps (bursts of slow-wave EEG) in aircrews during trips ranging from 8 to 15 hours in duration (Cabon et al., 1993; Rosekind et al., 1994; Samel et al., 1997; Wright and McGown, 2001). Since such events signal an impaired ability to respond to incoming stimuli (Belyavin and Wright, 1987; Ogilvie et al., 1989, 1991), these findings are relevant to aviation safety.

In this study, EEG data were systematically collected from sleep-deprived subjects in a specially-instrumented, rotary-wing aircraft to determine whether the typical increases in theta and reductions in alpha (recorded under controlled conditions in the laboratory) would occur in the in-flight environment, particularly while pilots were at the controls of the aircraft. The magnitude of differences at selected points during 29 hours of continuous wakefulness was examined. In addition, the extent to which EEG changes were associated with fatigue was assessed by collecting cognitive and mood data between flight times.

MATERIALS AND METHODS

Ten UH-60 current and qualified aviators served as subjects. The average age of the participants was 31.2 years (with a range of 26–46). Resting (eyes open/eyes closed) EEG evaluations were completed both in the laboratory and in the aircraft (while the safety pilot was on the controls). In addition, EEG evaluations were performed while the pilot was flying the aircraft. Performance and mood evaluations were conducted between flights in the laboratory.

In-flight EEG evaluations were conducted using a Cadwell Laboratory Airborne Spectrum 32, which transmitted data to a standard ground-based Cadwell Spectrum 32 for review and analysis. Laboratory EEG evaluations were made with a standard Cadwell Spectrum 32. The low filters were set at 0.53 Hz, the high filters were set at 100 Hz, and the 60 Hz notch filters were used. Grass E5SH electrodes were used to detect EEG.

Subjective mood evaluations were made in the laboratory using the Profile of Mood States (POMS) (McNair et al., 1981), a 65-item test that measures: (1) tension-anxiety, (2) depression-dejection, (3) anger-hostility, (4) vigor-activity, (5) fatigue-inertia, and (6) confusion-bewilderment. Subjective sleepiness/alertness was measured via the Visual Analog Scale (VAS). Several items were included, such as sleepy, alert, energetic, and talkative.

Basic cognitive abilities were examined in the laboratory with the Multi-Attribute Task Battery (MATB), a test that requires subjects to track a target and tune a communications radio while monitoring fuel levels and warning lights and dials.

The test schedule included three training sessions on the first day of participation. These were followed by three testing sessions that began on the second day of participation, continued during the night, and ended on the morning of the third day. On the training day, subjects arrived at the laboratory at approximately 1000 and were released by approximately 2200. On the following (testing) day, subjects awakened at 0700, reported to the laboratory at 1700, and remained in the laboratory (except for the flights) until approximately 1200 the next day (no sleep was permitted).

On the testing day, EEG electrodes were attached, and the subject proceeded to the first EEG test in the laboratory. The subject was instructed to sit quietly for 5 minutes with eyes open, followed by 5 minutes with eyes closed. Following EEG testing, the subject completed one VAS, one POMS, and performed the MATB for 30 minutes. Afterward, he completed another resting EEG, VAS, and POMS. Once laboratory testing for the session was complete, the subject was driven to an airfield for the first flight at 2300. After reaching altitude, with the safety pilot at the controls, the subject completed an eyes-open/eyes-closed EEG while the safety pilot was in control of the aircraft. Afterward, the subject flew several standard flight maneuvers. At the conclusion of the flight, the subject was driven back to the laboratory for the next test session (EEG, VAS, POMS, and MATB) at 0200. Afterward, the subject departed for the second flight (at approximately 0400). Following this flight, there was one final laboratory test session at 0700 and one final flight at 0900.

RESULTS

A variety of detailed analyses were conducted in this study. For the sake of brevity these will be summarized here, but a detailed account is available in Caldwell and colleagues (2002).

Electroencephalogram Laboratory Data

The analysis of variance (ANOVA) on delta activity included two factors: session (2045, 2140, 0145, 0240, 0645, and 0740) and eyes (eyes open and eyes closed). There were session main effects at Fz , Cz , and Pz; eyes main effects at Fz, Cz, and Pz; and session-by-eyes interactions at Cz and Pz ($p < 0.05$). Delta power increased from 2045 to 0740 and was greater under eyes closed than eyes open. The session-by-eyes interaction at Cz was due to the fact that there was a small increase in delta from eyes-open to eyes-closed early in the deprivation period (at 2045), followed by a much larger increase later in the deprivation period (at 0645). A similar pattern occurred at Pz. The analysis of theta activity revealed session main effects at Fz, Cz, and Pz primarily because of linear increases from the first to the last sessions of the deprivation cycle. Eyes main effects at all three electrodes were due to less theta at eyes-open than at eyes-closed. Session-by-eyes interactions at Fz, Cz, and Pz were all because of more theta under eyes-closed than eyes-open at various points in the deprivation cycle (particularly at 2045, 0145, 0645, and 0740), with the differences being more noticeable at certain times than at others. The ANOVA on alpha activity indicated session main effects and eyes main effects at Fz, Cz, and Pz. There were session-by-eyes interactions at Fz and Cz ($p < 0.05$). A decrease in alpha activity occurred from the first to the last part of the deprivation period at Fz and Cz, and an increase in alpha occurred under the eyes-closed versus the eyes-open condition at all three electrodes. The session-by-eyes interactions were the result of large differences between the eyes-open and eyes-closed conditions at 2045, 2140, 0145, and 0740, with smaller or more variable differences at 0240 and particularly at 0645. Beta activity revealed a session difference only at Pz ($p < 0.05$) which was the result of higher amounts of beta during the first part of the deprivation period (from 2045 to 0145) than at 0645, after which there was a rebound at 0740. Eyes main effects occurred at all three sites ($p < 0.05$) because of greater amounts of beta under eyes-closed than eyes-open. There were no significant interactions.

Electroencephalogram In-Flight Data

In the in-flight (aircraft) setting, EEG data were collected under a resting eyes-open condition (with the safety pilot on the controls) at the beginning of each flight and subsequently during each of the 15 maneuvers (with the participant on the controls). Only time-related effects will be reported here.

The ANOVA on delta activity for flight (2300, 0400, and 0900) and segment (resting, maneuver 1, maneuver 2, maneuver 3, … maneuver 15) indicated there was a flight- (or session) related difference only at Pz ($p < 0.05$). This was due to increased delta from the first two flights to the third. Theta power at Fz, Cz, and Pz increased from the first to the last flight, and theta at Pz showed a particularly striking increase by the time of the third flight. Alpha power at Fz, Cz, and Pz increased from the 2300 flight to the 0900 flight as well, but EEG beta activity did not change as a function of flight time.

Profile of Mood States

One-way ANOVAs of the scales from the POMS given at 2100, 2155, 0200, 0255, 0700, and 0755 revealed main effects on tension-anxiety, vigor-activity, fatigue-inertia, and confusion-bewilderment ($p < 0.05$). These occurred because mood deteriorated as the hours of continuous wakefulness increased.

Visual Analog Scale

The one-way ANOVAs on the VAS given after the POMS (at 2100, 2155, 0200, 0255, 0700, and 0755) indicated significant session differences on six of the eight subscales: alertness, energy, confidence, irritability, sleepiness, and talkativeness ($p < 0.05$). Once again, these were due to linear deteriorations in mood from the first to the last test sessions. Alertness, energy, confidence, and talkativeness declined generally from the beginning to the end of the deprivation period, whereas irritability and sleepiness increased.

Multiattribute Task Battery

There were statistically significant effects on the reaction times to warning lights and dials, the standard deviation of reaction times to the dials, and the root-mean-square (RMS) errors in the tracking task, due to a linear deterioration in performance from the 2105 session to the 0705 session in all four cases ($p < 0.05$). In addition, there were quadratic trends in the reaction times to lights, the standard deviation of reaction times to dials, and the tracking RMS errors due to more pronounced decrements towards the end of the deprivation period than the beginning.

DISCUSSION

There were EEG effects in both the laboratory and the in-flight testing situations, and theta activity was affected consistently across the two settings. Theta activity (3.0–8.0 Hz) progressively increased from the beginning to the end of the deprivation period, suggesting that fatigue from sleep deprivation was exerting a negative impact on the physiological alertness of the pilots. In addition, lower-frequency delta (1.5–3.0 Hz) activity also was accentuated as a function of sleep deprivation in both testing situations, but the effect was localized to Pz in the aircraft, whereas it was seen at all three recording sites in the laboratory. Increases in delta activity are primarily associated with sleep in normal adult subjects (Ray, 1990). Differences in alpha activity were not consistent from the laboratory to the aircraft, possibly because of environmental effects (the laboratory environment is more soporific than the noisier and less comfortable in-flight environment). However, the uniform effects in both delta and theta strongly suggest that: (1) participants were becoming more fatigued as the deprivation period progressed, and (2) this increase in fatigue was detectable via EEG recordings both in the more traditional laboratory setting and in the less-well-researched aircraft setting.

These EEG findings agree with the subjective mood data (from the POMS and the VAS), which indicated that the pilots were adversely affected by sleep deprivation. Ratings of fatigue, sleepiness, irritability, tension, and confusion all increased significantly as a function of prolonged wakefulness, whereas ratings of vigor, alertness, energy, confidence, and talkativeness decreased. These decrements no doubt contributed to the deterioration in basic cognitive abilities observed on MATB. Although less than half of MATB outcome measures apparently were sensitive to the effects of sleep loss and fatigue, the ones that did degrade seem particularly pertinent to aviator performance. Degradations in the reaction time to warning lights and out-of-bounds dial indications, along with more variable performance and increased tracking errors, became more pronounced as the amount of sleep deprivation progressed. Thus, not only were self-perceptions of alertness declining with increased hours awake, but objective measures of performance were deteriorating as well.

Overall, the findings from this study suggest that it is feasible to monitor increases in the fatigue levels of pilots via the real time acquisition of EEG activity from the in-flight environment. Thus, it is possible to gain insight into the functional status of aviators without disrupting performance on the primary task of flying the aircraft. However, future studies are needed to establish whether there are significant correlations between in-flight physiological changes and in-flight performance changes.

Acknowledgments: The author greatly appreciates the resources provided by the U.S. Army Medical Research and Materiel Command, which made this research effort possible.

REFERENCES

Akerstedt T. 1995. Work hours, sleepiness, and the underlying mechanisms. *J Sleep Res* 4:15–22.

Belyavin A, Wright NA. 1987. Changes in electrical activity of the brain with vigilance. *Electroencephalogr Clin Neurophysiol* 66:137–144.

Cabon PH, Coblentz A, Mollard R, Fouillot JP. 1993. Human vigilance in railway and long-haul flight operations. *Ergonomics* 36:1019–1033.

Caldwell JA, Gilreath SR. 2002. A survey of aircrew fatigue in a sample of Army aviation personnel. *Aviat Space Environ Med* 73:472–480.

Caldwell JA, Hall KK. 2001. The effects of 40 hours of continuous wakefulness on EEG power and flight performance. *Sleep* 24:A31.

Caldwell JA, Caldwell JL, Crowley JS. 1996. Sustaining helicopter pilot alertness with Dexedrine during sustained operations. *Proceedings of the Advisory Group for Aerospace Research and Development, Aerospace Medical Symposium on Neurological Limitations of Aircraft Operations: Human Performance Implications, CP -579*. Neuilly Sur Seine, France: North Atlantic Treaty Organization.

Caldwell JA, Hall KK, Erickson BS. 2002. EEG data collected from helicopter pilots in flight are sufficiently sensitive to detect increased fatigue from sleep deprivation. *Int J Aviat Psychol* 12:19–32.

Comperatore CA, Caldwell JA, Stephens RL, Mattingly A, Chiaramonte J, Trast ST. 1993. *The Use of Electrophysiological and Cognitive Variables in the Assessment of Degradation during Periods of Sustained Wakefulness*. USAARL Technical Report No. 93-5. Fort Rucker: U.S. Army Aeromedical Research Laboratory.

Dinges DF. 1990. The nature of subtle fatigue effects in long-haul crews. In: *Proceedings of the Flight Safety Foundation 43rd International Air Safety Seminar*. Arlington, VA: Flight Safety Foundation.

Lorenzo I, Ramos CA, Guevara MA, Corsi-Cabrera M. 1995. Effect of total sleep deprivation on reaction time and waking EEG activity in man. *Sleep* 18:346–354.

Kirsch AD. 1996. Report on the statistical methods employed by the U.S. FAA in its cost benefit analysis of the proposed "Flight Crewmember Duty Period Limitations, Flight Time Limitations and Rest Requirements," Docket No. 28081. *Comments of the Air Transport Association of America to FAA notice 95-18, FAA Docket No. 28081,* Appendix D. Washington, DC: Federal Aviation Administration. Pp. 1–36.

Kostad JL. 1989. National Transportation Safety Board safety recommendation. In: *Evaluation of U.S. Department of Transportation Efforts in the 1990s to Address Operator Fatigue, Appendix A*. Report No. NTSB/SR-99/01. Washington DC: National Transportation Safety Board. Pp. 30–37.

Krause KS. 1999. Little Rock aftermath. *Trafficworld* June:11–12.

McCann JP, Schulze VE. 1963. In-flight pilot incapacitation. *J Am Med Assoc* 183:1088–1090.

McNair DM, Lorr M, Droppleman LF. 1981. *Manual for the Profile of Mood States*. San Diego: Educational and Industrial Testing Service.

NTSB (National Transportation Safety Board). 1999. *Aircraft Accident Report: Controlled Flight into Terrain, Korean Air Flight 801, Boeing 747-300,*

HL7468, Nimitz Hill, Guam, August 6, 1997. Report No. NTSB/AAR-99-02. Washington DC: NTSB.

Ogilvie RD, Wilkinson RT, Allison S. 1989. The detection of sleep onset: Behavioral, physiological and subjective convergence. *Sleep* 12:458–474.

Ogilvie RD, Simons IA, Kuderian RH, MacDonald T, Rustenburg J. 1991. Behavioral, event-related potential and EEG/FFT changes at sleep onset. *Psychophysiology* 28:54–64.

Perry IC. 1974. *Helicopter Aircrew Fatigue*. AGARD-AR-69. Paris: Advisory Group for Aerospace Research and Development.

Pigeau RA, Heselegrave RJ, Angus RG. 1987. Psychophysiological measures of drowsiness as estimators of mental fatigue and performance degradation during sleep deprivation. In: *Electric and Magnetic Activity of the Central Nervous System: Research and Clinical Applications in Aerospace Medicine*. AGARD CP-432, 21-1/21-16. Neuilly Sur Seine, France: Advisory Group for Aerospace Research and Development.

Ramsey CS, McGlohn SE. 1997. Zolpidem as a fatigue countermeasure. *Aviat Space Environ Med* 68:926–931.

Ray W. 1990. The electrocortical system. In: Cacioppo T, Tassinary LG, eds. *Principles of Psychophysiology: Physical, Social, and Inferential Elements*. Cambridge: Cambridge University Press. Pp. 385–412.

Rosekind MR, Graeber RC, Dinges DF, Connell LJ, Rountree MS, Spinweber CL, Gillen KA. 1994. *Crew Factors in Flight Operations IX: Effects of Planned Cockpit Rest on Crew Performance and Alertness in Long-Haul Operations*. NASA Technical Memorandum no. 108839. Moffet Field, CA: Ames Research Center, National Aeronautics and Space Administration.

Samel A, Wegmann HM, Vejvoda M. 1997. Aircrew fatigue in long-haul operations. *Accid Anal Prev* 29:439–452.

Sterman MB, Schummer GJ, Dushenko TW, Smith JC. 1987. Electroencephalographic correlates of pilot performance: Simulation and in-flight studies. In: *Electrical and Magnetic Activity of the Central Nervous System: Research and Clinical Applications in Aerospace Medicine*, AGARD CP No. 432, 31-1/31-16. Neuilly Sur Seine, France: NATO.

Wilson GF, Hankins T. 1994. EEG and subjective measures of private pilot performance. In: *Proceedings of the Human Factors and Ergonomics Society 38th Annual Meeting*. Santa Monica, CA: Human Factors and Ergonomics Society. Pp. 1322–1325.

Wright N, McGown A. 2001. Vigilance on the civil flight deck: Incidence of sleepiness and sleep during long-haul flights and associated changes in physiological parameters. *Ergonomics* 44:82–106.

Yacavone DW. 1993. Mishap trends and causal factors in Naval aviation: A review of Naval Safety Center data, 1986–90. *Aviat Space Environ Med* 64:392–395.

CIRCULATING PLASMA MARKERS OF COGNITIVE STATUS

Harris R. Lieberman, Mark D. Kellogg, Gaston P. Bathalon,
U.S. Army Research Institute of Environmental Medicine

BACKGROUND

Basic scientists and clinicians have been searching for biochemical markers of cognitive state for many years. Unfortunately, little progress has been made with regard to identification of markers that, in normal individuals, relate metabolic status to cognitive function or assess general cognitive state. It would be a significant breakthrough for basic science and clinical practice to have reliable plasma markers of cognitive function. Many devastating diseases are either cognitive in nature or produce secondary cognitive deficits. Biochemical tests for the cognitive deficits associated with Alzheimer's disease, depression, or Attention Deficit Hyperactivity Disorder (ADHD) would be of extraordinary value to society. In addition, it would be very useful for understanding the biological basis of human behavior to have objective plasma markers of cognitive state. On the battlefield, such markers could also be of significant value. They could potentially be employed to optimize warfighter cognitive function and to prevent errors associated with the stress of combat and illnesses associated with combat, such as Post-Traumatic Stress Disorder (PTSD) or Gulf War Syndrome-like diseases.

Current State of the Field

Many peripheral metabolic diseases such as diabetes, hyperthyroid syndromes, and Cushing's disease (elevated cortisol), are associated with impaired cognitive function. Frequently, the metabolic markers of the disease are biochemical markers of cognitive state, and sometimes these indicators can provide information about cognitive status in healthy humans. For example, elevated plasma cortisol is an indicator of acute stress and is negatively correlated with various aspects of cognitive function. The adverse effects of elevated cortisol on cognitive function can be observed in various disease states and also when exogenous cortisol is administered to normal humans (for a review, see Jameison and Dinan, 2001). Unfortunately, cortisol and similar markers appear to provide little information about normal human cognitive function beyond serving as an index of stress-induced declines in cognition. Decrements in military operational performance can be stress-related, but in many instances are not (Johnson and Merullo, 2000). We will provide data that suggest that another endogenous glucocorticoid, dehydroepiandrosterone sulphate (DHEA-S) is, at least in a population we have recently studied, a better marker of normal cognitive status than cortisol.

Plasma glucose, as discussed in detail below, is also an indicator of impaired cognitive function in diseases such as diabetes. When it is artificially lowered to below physiological levels using the insulin clamp technique, cognitive deficits result. However, it often seems to provide little information about cognitive status in healthy individuals, in part because it is tightly regulated. We will provide data that suggest that other metabolic factors associated with energy and carbohydrate metabolism, in particular free fatty acids (FFA) and triglycerides, may, in healthy individuals, be better markers of cognitive state, and perhaps metabolic status, than glucose.

The Inherent Difficulty of Identifying Biochemical Markers for Cognitive State

Although there is great need for objective markers of cognitive state, there are a variety of reasons why it has been extremely difficult to define reliable markers for brain function in normal humans. The greatest difference in normal human cognitive states is between sleep and waking. Classical electrophysiological techniques (polysomnography), as well as functional measures (e.g., monitoring physical activity), can distinguish sleep from waking state. However, it is not possible to biochemically distinguish these states. The only biochemical measure that, under certain conditions, corresponds to sleep state is the hormone melatonin, but it is not a marker of sleep state. If states as disparate as sleep and waking—which exhibit the most extreme differences in human cognitive function—are not biochemically distinguishable, we cannot expect to easily find a marker for more subtle differences in human cognitive state, such as optimal alertness versus sleepiness.

The lack of markers for cognitive state is reflected by the fact that there are no biochemical markers for any common psychiatric or neurological disease. Diagnosis and assessment of most psychiatric and neurological disorders typically rely on labor-intensive, often subjective, clinical evaluations and self-reports. Common diseases such as depression, schizophrenia, ADHD, PTSD, narcolepsy, and Alzheimer's and Parkinson's diseases, cannot be diagnosed or their progression followed by a biochemical test. Progress has been made using scanning technologies to assess cognitive function, as well as to diagnose and follow the progression of certain central nervous system (CNS) diseases. However, it is difficult to conceive of how such technologies could be practically employed in military field operations to assess cognitive state until significant technological advances occur.

Why has there been so little progress in discovering biological markers of CNS function? It has been known for many years that specific neurotransmitter systems were involved in various CNS disorders, including depression, schizophrenia, and Parkinson's disease. However, no biochemical test has been developed to diagnose or follow the course of these diseases. Clearly, the development of biochemical tests to assess brain function and behavior has been hampered by the unique, protected status of the brain. The blood-brain-barrier

(BBB) isolates, and thereby protects, the brain by preventing the transfer of metabolites from the periphery into the brain. However, the BBB also isolates the periphery from brain metabolites. Therefore, when biochemical markers are assessed in the periphery, usually no direct information regarding central function is provided. Limited exceptions to this principle include hormones released by the brain into the periphery and a few substances that cross from the brain to the plasma.

Usually glucose is the major source of energy for the brain and, under certain limited conditions; plasma glucose is a predictor of cognitive state. When plasma glucose is reduced from normal euglycemic levels of about 5.0 $mmol/L^{-1}$ (90 mg/dL) to 2.6 $mmol/L^{-1}$ (47 mg/dL) in nondiabetic individuals and using a hyperinsulinemic clamp, cognitive function is impaired (Strachan et al., 2001). Although this nonphysiological paradigm demonstrates the importance of glucose to the brain, peripheral glucose is tightly regulated in healthy individuals and rarely reaches levels below 3.6 $mmol^{-1}$ (Wilson et al., 1998). Studies of sustained military training scenarios that simulate combat (e.g., Ranger Training) support these clinical observations. In Ranger trainees who are in a chronic state of semistarvation due to several months of severe undernutrition in harsh field conditions, plasma glucose levels fell to no lower then 3.8 $mmol/L^{-1}$ (Friedl et al., 2000; Moore et al., 1992).

In military as well as civilian populations, a consistent relationship between plasma glucose within the normal range and cognitive performance has never been demonstrated. Carbohydrate administration can clearly enhance physical performance when high levels of energy are being expended. However, the data relating cognitive performance, carbohydrate administration, and plasma glucose are not consistent. Both beneficial and adverse effects on cognition of increasing plasma glucose and providing carbohydrate have been reported (for a review, see Bellisle et al., 1998). Overall, while it is clear that carbohydrate supplementation can, in certain circumstances, alter cognitive function (Lieberman et al., 2002b); these effects are probably not associated in any simple manner with plasma glucose levels in healthy, nondiabetic individuals.

NEW MARKERS OF COGNITIVE STATE: STUDIES ON MILITARY POPULATIONS IN WHICH COGNITIVE AND BIOCHEMICAL FACTORS WERE ASSESSED

On several occasions, as part of field studies, we have examined the relationship between cognitive performance and plasma or saliva metabolites. Initially, neurotransmitter precursors like tryptophan and tyrosine were of interest as they are actively transported into the brain across the BBB. In an early study, the volunteers were soldiers participating in an evaluation of a lightweight ration and were modestly undernourished for several weeks (Askew et al., 1987). In that study, the ratio of plasma tryptophan to the other large neutral amino acids

(LNAA), which predicts the rate of transport of tryptophan across the BBB, was correlated with cognitive performance ($r = 0.40–0.44$, $p < 0.02$). We believe that the tryptophan/LNAA ratio was associated with cognitive performance because tryptophan is the precursor of a critical brain neurotransmitter, serotonin. Levels of other plasma amino acids were not related to cognitive performance (Lieberman et al., 1997). In a previous presentation to the Committee on Military Nutrition Research, we discussed these findings and addressed the overall importance of a variety of neurotransmitter precursors (Lieberman, 1999). In the last few years we have focused on hormones and metabolic factors that can be measured in saliva or that do not require assessment of multiple amino acids (all the LNAAs).

Study I: A Brief, Intense Training Exercise Conducted by an Operational Ranger Unit

Recently, we evaluated cognitive function and several biochemical markers of stress of soldiers engaged in a brief (52 h) high-intensity training operation. The exercise was conducted by U.S. Army Rangers and had been designed to evaluate junior leaders (Lieberman et al., 2002a). The scenario simulated combat-like conditions, specifically a high-intensity, light infantry operation in a hostile environment, by combining multiple stressors: near total sleep deprivation; continuous physical activity; substantial physiological, environmental, and psychological stress; and simulated combat-like activities. All volunteers (N = 31) were Ranger officers (mean age = 32 years) with the rank of Captain, and had served on average 9 years on active duty. The exercise was conducted in a hot, humid environment.

The exercise consisted of three phases: a garrison preparation phase, a field exercise, and a concluding garrison phase. Cognitive performance, mood, and body composition were assessed once during each phase. We used a battery of cognitive tests that were administered on notebook computers and took less than an hour to complete. The battery was designed to assess a wide range of militarily relevant cognitive functions. To assess mood we employed the most widely accepted measure of mood state, the Profile of Mood States (POMS), which has been used in hundreds of civilian and military studies (McNair et al., 1971). It is a standardized, validated self-report questionnaire consisting of 65 mood-related adjectives that are rated on a five-point scale in response to the question, "How are you feeling right now?" It takes less than 5 minutes to complete. The adjectives factor into six mood subscales: tension, depression, anger, vigor, fatigue, and confusion.

Carefully selected measures of mood state are excellent predictors of cognitive performance and sensitive indicators of functional capability. Depressed patients perform poorly, and drowsy normal subjects have impaired cognitive function. Drugs, environmental stress, foods, and dietary supplements that affect cognitive performance have repeatedly been shown to have analogous effects on related mood states. Compounds that enhance cognitive performance, such as amphetamine, caffeine, and tyrosine, improve corresponding moods, while treatments that degrade performance, such as benzodiazepines (e.g., valium), melatonin, and antihistamines, invariably impair mood (Dollins et al., 1993; Fine et al., 1994; Lieberman et al., 1986; Newhouse et al., 1989). Advantages of mood questionnaires include: the brief period of time required to administer even comprehensive versions of them and the fact that no equipment is needed for their administration. In situations like Marine basic training, where volunteers are available for only brief periods of time and a large number of subjects must be tested simultaneously, they are the only practical way of gathering frequent and detailed data on cognitive state.

At both the in-field and post-field testing sessions we observed very large decrements in cognitive performance, including changes in fundamental functions like vigilance ($p < 0.001$; Figure D-35) and choice reaction time ($p < 0.001$), as well as more complex abilities: learning ($p < 0.001$), memory ($p < 0.001$), and logical reasoning ($p < 0.001$; Figure D-35). All mood states assessed were adversely affected, including vigor ($p < 0.001$), fatigue ($p < 0.001$; Figure D-35) , confusion ($p < 0.001$; Figure D-35), tension ($p < 0.02$), depression ($p < 0.002$), and anger ($p < 0.01$) (Lieberman et al., 2002a). We also assessed cortisol, testosterone, and melatonin in saliva samples collected three times per day. As in previous short-duration studies conducted with soldiers exposed to multiple stressors (for example see Opstad, 1994), rather than an increase in cortisol or testosterone, we observed suppression in their circadian pattern of release. Patterns of melatonin release did not change. We did not observe any consistent relationship between hormone levels and impairments in cognitive performance over the course of the exercise, although pre-exercise cortisol did predict, in several instances, pre-exercise and subsequent cognitive performance. This association suggests Rangers who perceived the exercise as likely to be stressful, or who were already stressed when they reported for the exercise, performed worse than their peers. In this study, conducted with soldiers who were subjected to a variety of stressors, but not severe psychological stress, saliva cortisol, testosterone, and melatonin levels provided limited information on cognitive state.

Study II: Marine Basic Training Relationships Between Cognitive and Biochemical Changes in Female Trainees

Recently, our laboratory conducted a comprehensive study of a large group of female trainees enrolled in the 12-week Marine basic training course at Parris Island, South Carolina (Bathalon et al., In press). Every 4 weeks, on the same day, plasma was collected and a POMS mood state questionnaire was administered. A variety of other parameters was also regularly assessed. The mood questionnaire was administered in the morning and blood samples were obtained in the afternoon. Mood was assessed to provide information on the cognitive state of the volunteers as they progressed through training. We also attempted to

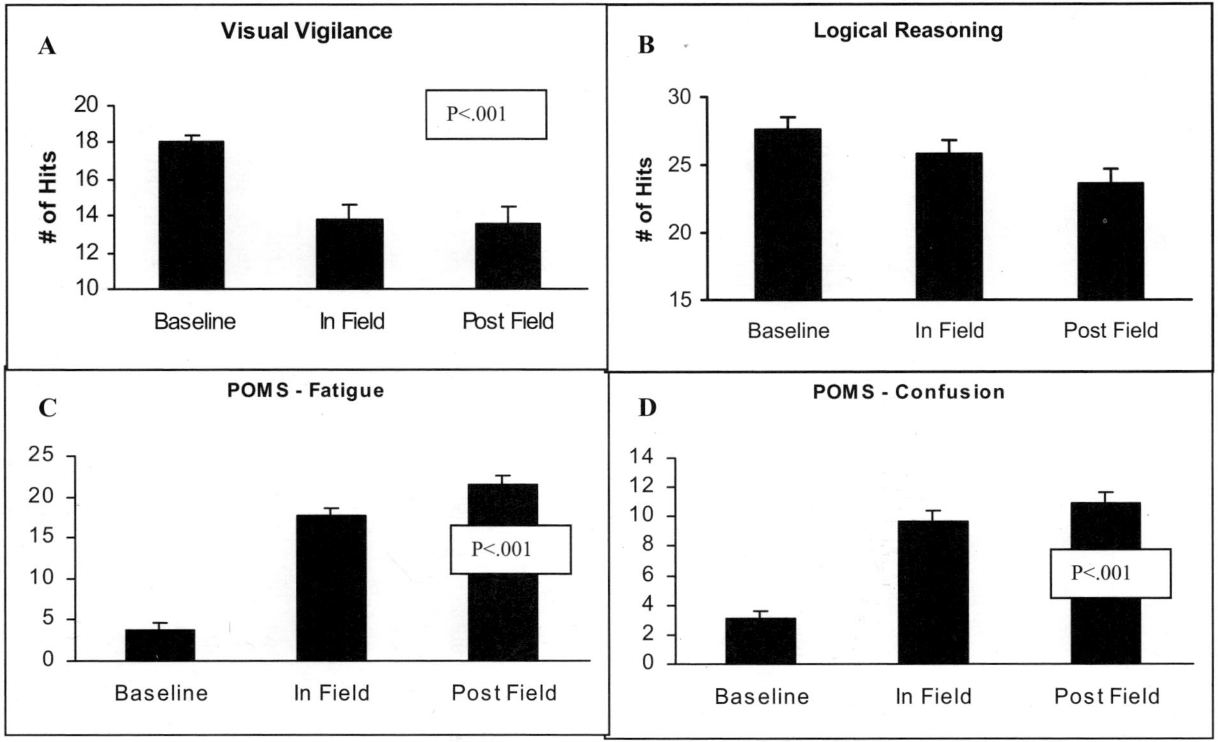

FIGURE D-35 Changes in cognitive performance and mood (mean + standard error of the mean) assessed before, during, and immediately after a brief, high intensity Ranger training exercise. Statistical significance over time, as determined by a within-subject analysis of variance, is provided. POMS = Profile of Mood States.
SOURCE: Lieberman et al. (2002a).

assess the relationship between mood state and biochemical markers of metabolic state, endocrine status, and inflammation.

All mood states assessed by the POMS in the female Marine basic trainees improved substantially over the course of basic training (Figure D-36). The trainees began basic training feeling worse than is typical of age-matched females, but by the time they had completed training their scores were better than the norm (McNair et al., 1971). During training there were also significant changes in a number of biochemical parameters, particularly FFAs, triglycerides, and DHEA-S (Figure D-37). Other biochemical markers such as glucose and cortisol were more stable (Figure D-37). The changes in FFA and triglycerides were consistent with the changing physiological and nutritional status of the trainees. Over the course of the study, the women lost substantial body mass overall (mean = 1.7 kg), especially fat (mean = 4.4 kg), but gained muscle mass (mean = 3.3 kg) as assessed by dual-energy X-ray absorptiometry. A gain in muscle mass would be expected given the rigorous nature of basic training. The trainees' diets also changed, with a significant reduction in total food intake and reduced fat in the diet, compared with their prerecruit diets. Levels of stress appeared elevated as indicated by chronically elevated levels of cortisol (near the upper limits of normal) and high levels of tension on the POMS, particularly during the earlier phases of training (Figures D-36 and D-37).

There were robust, highly significant correlations between mood and DHEA-S, substance P, FFA, and triglycerides (Table D-9) over the course of training. Plasma levels of fructosamine, which reflects average blood glucose levels for the last 17 to 21 days, thyroid-stimulating hormone, and substance P also were associated with mood states, but not as frequently or as robustly as DHEA-S, FFA, and triglycerides (Table D-9). When stepwise multiple linear regression analyses were performed, the most reliable predictor variables for mood were DHEA-S, FFA, and triglycerides. The extent of overall individual weight loss over the course of training was only associated with the mood state of vigor, with the greater weight loss associated with less vigor ($r = -0.20$, $p < 0.02$). Weight loss was often a statistically significant predictor variable in the multiple regression analyses, even though the correlations between weight loss and moods were modest ranging from ± 0.02 to 0.20. It also appeared that the predictive biochemical parameters were associated with a similar underlying factor, as they often were individually correlated. When these markers—FFA, triglycerides, fructosamine, and DHEA-S—were aggregated in multiple regression models with weight loss included as a predictor variable, ability to predict mood states was increased and r^2 values as high 0.40 were obtained, indicating the regression model could account for 40 percent of the overall variance associated with certain mood states.

The magnitude of the relationships we observed between mood states and these biochemical markers, both as individual correlations and within multiple regression models, was surprising. We are not aware of any combination of putative physiological markers for mood or cognitive state where such robust asso-

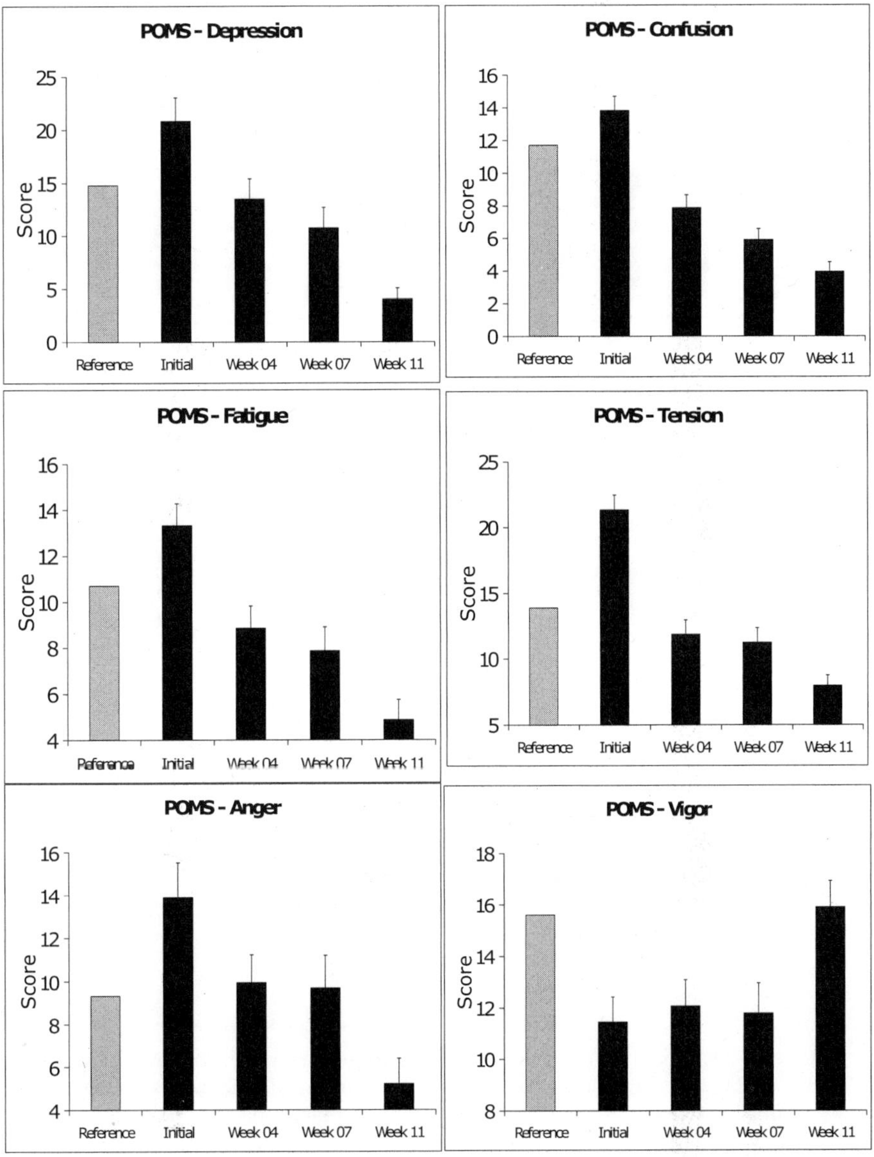

FIGURE D-36 Mean (+ standard error of the mean) changes in mood state in female trainees as assessed by the Profile of Mood States (POMS) over the course of Marine basic training. A reference value for female college students, of approximately the same age as the trainees, is provided for comparison (McNair et al., 1971). Statistical significance over time, as determined by a within-subject analysis of variance, is provided.

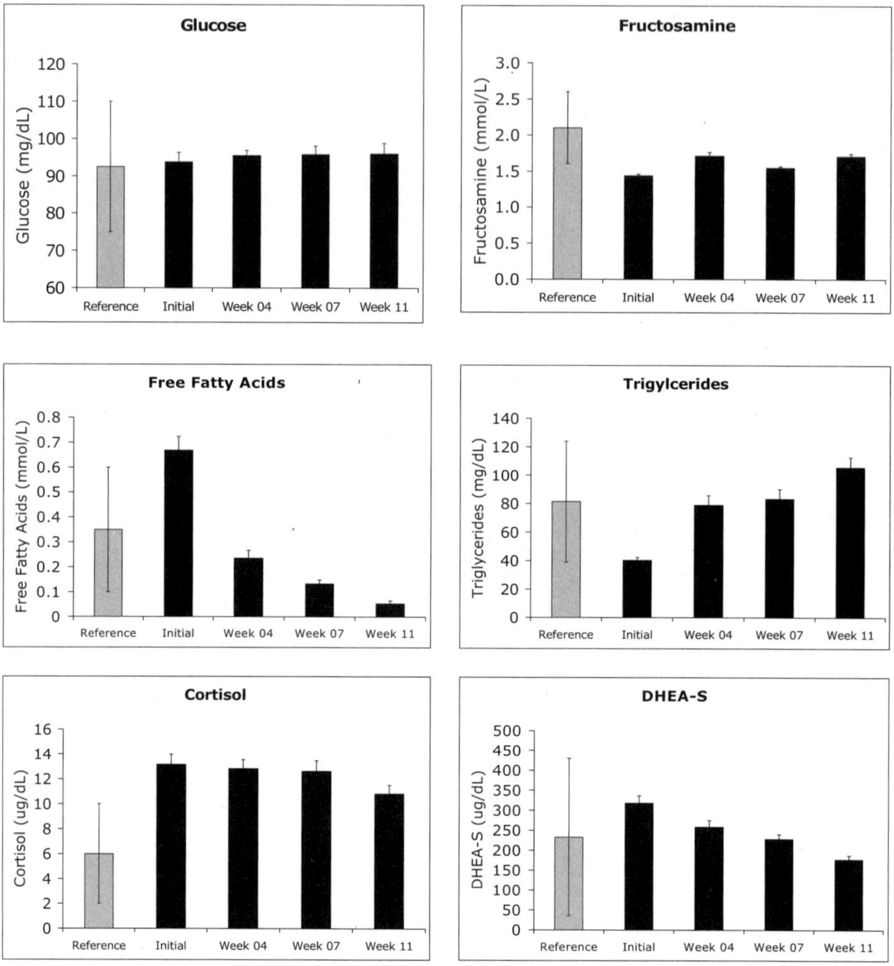

FIGURE D-37 Variation in mean (± standard error of the mean) plasma concentration of the indicated marker in female trainees over the course of Marine basic training. A reference value (± 2 standard deviations) is provided for comparison. Whenever the data were available, the reference value is for females of approximately the same age. Statistical significance over time, as determined by a within-subject analysis of variation, is provided.

ciations have been observed in healthy individuals. The magnitude of the individual relationships between plasma markers and mood (many *r* values were in the range of 0.3–0.45, as shown in Table D-9) should be placed in the context of firmly established, clinically significant relationships between other biochemical markers and functional outcomes. Widely accepted markers of disease generally have only modest associations with the underlying disease state they predict. For example, the association of "ratio of high density cholesterol to total cholesterol" with the extent of coronary occlusion in patients with cardiovascular disease is only $r = -0.20$ (Naito et al., 1980).

The associations we have observed between these peripheral metabolic markers and cognitive state during Marine basic training are of the same magnitude as those we had previously observed for the tryptophan/LNAA ratio in soldiers participating in the lightweight ration study discussed above. The tryptophan/LNAA ratio determines the rate of tryptophan transport across the BBB. Tryptophan, because it is a rate-limiting precursor of the neurotransmitter serotonin, serves a critical CNS need (Lieberman, 1999; Lieberman et al., 1997). It should be emphasized that many of the metabolites and hormones evaluated in the Marine basic training study, including glucose, corticotrophin-releasing factor, cortisol, and leptin which, based on their known associations with brain function, might have been expected to be associated with cognitive function, but were not (Table D-9).

CONCLUSIONS AND RECOMMENDATIONS

There are many obstacles associated with identifying biochemical markers of cognitive state. In the study we conducted with U.S. Army Rangers engaged in a brief, high-intensity field exercise, saliva cortisol, melatonin, and testosterone were not usually associated with performance and mood. However, the preliminary findings from the Marine basic trainee study we describe suggest that at least one endocrine factor (DHEA-S) and several metabolites associated with energy status are robust markers for cognitive state in female recruits during basic training. Of course, these associations may be unique to the gender of the volunteers or to the combination of physiological, nutritional, and psychological factors the basic trainees experienced. To determine if these relationships generalize to other populations, this study will have to be replicated and extended, including studies of males. Of particular interest will be whether cognitive performance, as well as mood, is associated with these biochemical markers. It will require a substantial effort to address these questions since it is more difficult to assess cognitive performance than mood state in large samples. Furthermore, the unique factors associated with basic training, especially the large changes in mood and biochemical state that occur, make attempts at replications in other populations of questionable validity. We believe that we observed these biochemical-behavioral relationships because we were evaluating individuals who had unusually robust changes in both metabolism and behavior. Rarely are

TABLE D-9 The Relationship Between Plasma Markers and Mood States During Marine Basic Training in Females

Plasma Marker	Fatigue	Confusion	Depression	Tension	Anger	Vigor
Hormones						
Adrenocorticotropic hormone	–0.22, 0.005	NS[a]	NS	NS	NS	0.19, 0.02
Cortisol	NS	NS	NS	NS	NS	NS
Corticotropin releasing factor	NS	NS	NS	NS	NS	NS
Dehydroepiandrosterone sulfate	**0.36, < 0.001**	**0.45, < 0.001**	**0.35, < 0.001**	**0.44, < 0.001**	**0.30, < 0.001**	NS
Follicle-stimulating hormone	NS	NS	NS	NS	NS	NS
Growth hormone	NS	NS	NS	NS	NS	NS
Leptin	NS	NS	NS	NS	NS	NS
Leutenizing hormone	NS	NS	NS	NS	NS	NS
Neuropeptide Y	NS	–0.18, 0.02	NS	NS	NS	0.23, 0.006
Progesterone	NS	NS	NS	NS	NS	NS
Substance P	**0.18, 0.03**	**0.23, 0.005**	**0.23, 0.007**	NS	**0.18, 0.03**	**–0.22, 0.01**
Testosterone	NS	NS	NS	NS	NS	NS
Thyroid stimulating hormone	NS	–0.15, 0.05	NS	–0.18, 0.02	–0.20, 0.009	NS
Free T3	NS	NS	NS	NS	NS	NS
T4	NS	0.22, 0.006	NS	0.18, 0.02	NS	NS
Metabolites						
Total cholesterol	NS	NS	NS	NS	NS	NS
Free fatty acids	**0.22, 0.005**	**0.46, < 0.001**	**0.24, 0.002**	**0.44, < 0.001**	**0.16, 0.05**	**–0.18, 0.02**
Fructosamine	NS	–0.23, 0.003	–0.23, 0.003	–0.31, < 0.001	–0.22, 0.005	NS
Glucose	NS	NS	NS	NS	NS	NS
Glycated hemoglobin	NS	NS	NS	NS	NS	NS
High-density lipoprotein	0.21, 0.007	NS	NS	NS	0.16, 0.04	NS
Low-density lipoprotein	NS	NS	NS	NS	NS	NS
Triglycerides	**–0.25, 0.001**	**–0.45, < 0.001**	**–0.35, < 0.001**	**–0.44, < 0.001**	**–0.29, < 0.001**	**0.19, 0.02**

Markers of inflammation						
C-Reactive protein	NS	NS	NS	NS	NS	NS
Interleukin-1	Undetectable	Undetectable	Undetectable	Undetectable	Undetectable	Undetectable
Interleukin-6	Undetectable	Undetectable	Undetectable	Undetectable	Undetectable	Undetectable
Tumor necrosis factor	Undetectable	Undetectable	Undetectable	Undetectable	Undetectable	Undetectable

NOTE: Pearson correlations, expressed as *r* values, between mood, assessed by the Profile of Mood States, and selected plasma hormones, metabolites, and markers of inflammation are presented. The subjects were 41 volunteers. If the association was significant ($p < 0.05$), a *p* value is presented. Markers that had five or more significant associations are in **bold**.

[a] NS = not significant.

metabolic and cognitive changes of this magnitude observed in healthy individuals.

Acknowledgments: This work was supported by the U.S. Army Medical Research and Materiel Command (USAMRMC). Approved for public release; distribution is unlimited. The views, opinions, and/or findings in this report are those of the authors, and should not be construed as an official Department of the Army position, policy, or decision, unless so designated by other official documentation. Human subjects participated in these studies after giving their free and informed voluntary consent. Investigators adhered to AR 70-25 and USAMRMC Regulation 70-25 on the use of volunteers in research. For the protection of human subjects, the investigators adhered to policies of applicable Federal Law CFR 46. Citation of commercial organization and trade names in this report do not constitute an official Department of the Army endorsement or approval of the products or services of these organizations.

REFERENCES

Askew EW, Munro I, Sharp MA, Siegel S, Popper R, Rose MS, Hoyt RW, Reynolds K, Lieberman HR, Engell D, Shaw CP. 1987. *Nutritional Status and Physical and Mental Performance of Soldiers Consuming the Ration, Lightweight or the Meal, Ready-to-Eat Military Field Ration During a 30 Day Field Training Exercise*. Natick, MA: U.S. Army Research Institute of Environmental Medicine.

Bathalon GP, McGraw SM, Falco CM, Georgelis JH, DeLany JP, Young AJ. In press. Total energy expenditure during strenuous U.S. Marine Corps recruit training. *Proceedings of the 51st Meeting of the American College of Sports Medicine*. June 2–5. Indianapolis, IN.

Bellisle F, Blundell JE, Dye L, Fantino M, Fern E, Fletcher RJ, Lambert J, Roberfroid M, Specter S, Westenhofer J, Westerterp-Plantenga MS. 1998. Functional food science and behavior and psychological functions. *Br J Nutr* 80:S173–S193.

Dollins AB, Lynch HJ, Wurtman RJ, Deng MH, Kischka KU, Gleason RE, Lieberman HR. 1993. Effect of pharmacological daytime doses of melatonin on human mood and performance. *Psychopharmacology* 112:490–496.

Fine BJ, Kobrick JL, Lieberman HR, Marlowe B, Riley RH, Tharion WJ. 1994. Effects of caffeine or diphenhydramine on visual vigilance. *Psychopharmacology* 114:233–238.

Friedl KE, Moore RJ, Hoyt RW, Marchitelli LJ, Marinez-Lopez LE, Askew EW. 2000. Endocrine markers of semistarvation in healthy lean men in a multistressor environment. *J Appl Physiol* 88:1820–1830.

Jameison K, Dinan TG. 2001. Glucocorticoids and cognitive function: From physiology to pathophysiology. *Hum Psychopharmacol Clin Exp* 16:293–302.

Johnson RF, Merullo DJ. 2000. Caffeine, gender, and sentry duty: Effects of a mild stimulant on vigilance and marksmanship. In: Friedl KE, Lieberman HR, Ryan DH, Bray GA, eds. *Pennington Center Nutrition Series, Volume 10: Countermeasures for Battlefield Stressors*. Baton Rouge, LA: Louisiana State University Press. Pp. 272–289.

Lieberman HR. 1999. Amino acid and protein requirements: Cognitive performance, stress, and brain function. In: *The Role of Protein and Amino Acids in Sustaining and Enhancing Performance*. Washington DC: National Academy Press. Pp. 289–307.

Lieberman HR, Spring B, Garfield GS. 1986. The behavioral effects of food constituents: Strategies used in studies of amino acids, protein, carbohydrate and caffeine. *Nutr Rev* 44:61–70.

Lieberman HR, Askew EW, Hoyt RW, Shukitt-Hale B, Sharp MA. 1997. Effects of 30 days of undernutrition on plasma neurotransmitter precursors, other amino acids, and behavior. *J Nutr Biochem* 8:119–126.

Lieberman HR, Bathalon GP, Falco CM, Georgelis JH, Morgan CA III, Niro P, Tharion WJ. 2002a. The "Fog Of War": Documenting cognitive decrements associated with the stress of combat. In: *Proceedings of the 23rd Army Science Conference*. Orlando, FL. December 2–5. Available at http://www.asc2002.com/manuscripts/I/IO-01.PDF.

Lieberman HR, Falco CM, Slade SS. 2002b. Carbohydrate administration during a day of sustained aerobic activity improves vigilance, assessed with a novel ambulatory monitoring device, and mood. *Am J Clin Nutr* 76:120–127.

McNair DM, Lorr M, Droppelman LE. 1971. *Edits Manual for the Profile of Mood States*. San Diego: Educational and Industrial Testing Service.

Moore RJ, Friedl KE, Dramer TR, Martinez-Lopez LE, Hoyt RW, Tulley RE, DeLany JP, Askew EW, Vogel JA. 1992. *Changes in Soldier Nutritional Status and Immune Function During the Ranger Training Course.* NTIS accession no. AD-A257 437. Natick, MA: U.S. Army Research Institute of Environmental Medicine.

Naito HK, Greenstreet RL, David JA, Sheldon WL, Shirey EK, Lewis RC, Proudfit WL, Gerrity RG. 1980. HDL-cholesterol concentration and severity of coronary atherosclerosis determined by cine-angiography. *Artery* 8:101–112.

Newhouse PA, Belenky G, Thomas M, Thorne D, Sing HC, Fertig J. 1989. The effects of d-amphetamine on arousal, cognition, and mood after prolonged total sleep deprivation. *Neuropsychopharmacol* 2:153–164.

Opstad PK. 1994. Circadian rhythm of hormones is extinguished during prolonged physical stress, sleep and energy deficiency in young men. *Eur J Endocrinol* 131:56–66.

Strachan MWJ, Deary IJ, Ewing FME, Ferguson SSC, Young MJ, Frier BM. 2001. Acute hypoglycemia impairs the functioning of the central but not peripheral nervous system. *Physiol Behav* 72:83–92.

Wilson JD, Foster DW, Kronenberg HM, Larsen PR, Williams WB, eds. 1998. *Textbook of Endocrinology*. 9th ed. Philadelphia: WB Saunders.

CIRCULATING PLASMA MARKERS OF COGNITIVE STATUS: ODORS AS BIOMARKERS

Gary K. Beauchamp, Monell Chemical Senses Center

Chemical signals (herein termed body odors or just odors) provide information on many characteristics of an organism and are involved in coordination and regulation of all aspects of behavior and physiology. Typically, body odors have been divided into two broad classes, those termed pheromones and all others. In the former category are included chemical signals that have evolved to convey very specific information, elicit specific behavioral and physiological responses, and are in principle rather simple chemically. Examples include odorants that elicit behavioral responses such as sexual attraction and aggression (often termed releaser pheromones) and those that elicit physiological responses such as estrus synchrony and sexual maturation (often termed primer pheromones). The other broad class (sometimes included in the pheromone category but at other times excluded) encompasses odors that signal information such as individual identity, age, emotional status, and health. However, both in practice and in principle, the distinctions between these two categories are often difficult to discern (Beauchamp et al., 1976; Wysocki and Preti, 1998). In the remainder of this paper, this distinction will be ignored.

Body odors have a number of inherent characteristics that should make them particularly useful for those interested in monitoring organic states of individual humans. First, many body odors evolved to communicate messages between individuals. As a consequence, these messages ought to be relatively unambiguous and difficult to falsify. Second, unlike many visual and auditory signals, odors often persist in the environment. Indeed, many species make use of this characteristic during territorial scent marking, such as dogs urinating on posts. Darwin noted that the odor on a handkerchief that he had rubbed on a scent gland of an animal persisted on the cloth for years in spite of repeated washings. Third, body odors often directly reflect physiological processes. For example, odors associated with stress have been suggested to arise from action of stress hormones on odor-producing body structures. Fourth, odors can be detected from a distance and hence noninvasively. It has often been noted that when a dog follows a scent of an individual person, it does not put its nose directly on the ground, but instead holds it above the presumed odor source. Finally, in principle, it ought to be relatively straight-forward to develop devices to detect and recognize specific chemical signatures indicative of particular physio-

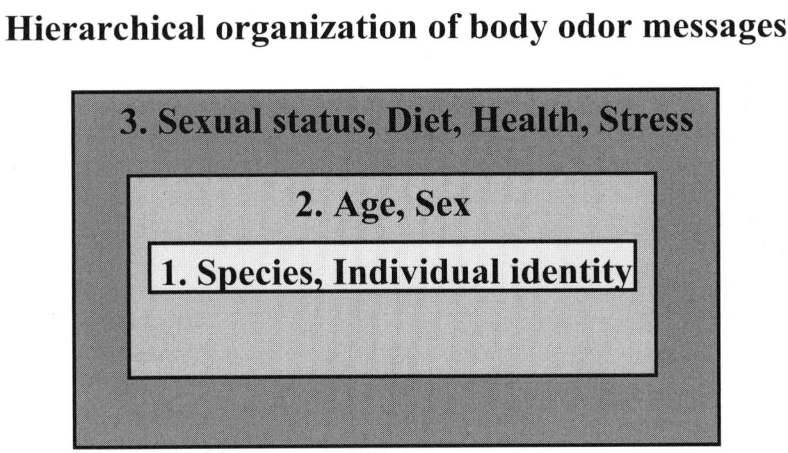

FIGURE D-38 Three levels of chemical signals derived from body odors illustrated by the mouse system. 1. Core messages largely innately determined and with little variation across the life span. 2. Messages that are relatively fixed but do vary in expression across the life span of the organism. 3. Messages that vary from time to time and may reflect short term physiological fluctuations.

logical states. In practice, however, this has remained a challenge as will be described below.

In the following brief paper, the kinds of information that exist in body secretions and excretions are discussed. Next, the possible use of body odor to identify messages signaling physiological states, such as stress, will be discussed. Finally, speculation on the future use of body volatiles in monitoring physiological status will be provided.

MESSAGES IN BODY ODOR

Work with body odors in nonhuman animals has clearly demonstrated that a variety of messages is transmitted and that these messages influence the behavior and physiology of the receiver. The categories of information are illustrated in Figure D-38.

Core Messages

Core messages (1. in Figure D-38) involve characteristics of the animal that are relatively fixed. Thus, animals are able to determine the species of the odor producer and its individual identity. For example, a large series of studies have demonstrated that the individual identity of a mouse is coded in part by the genes of the major histocompatibility complex, the same genes involved in self-nonself recognition within the context of the immune system (Penn and Potts, 1998; Yamazaki et al., 1999). Presumably an individual mouse's odor (and very likely an individual human's odor as well) is a fixed characteristic of that animal. Based on these ideas, we are now attempting to identify the odorous materials in mouse and human emanations with a long-range goal of developing sensors that could recognize individuals by their genetically determined characteristic body odors.

Life Span Messages

At a second level (2. in Figure D-38) there are a number of messages that are relatively stable yet do vary over the life span of an individual. Two of these are age and odor-expressed gender. Consider gender first. Although basic biological gender is fixed at conception, many data indicate that body odors reflecting this do change over the course on an individual's life. Most dramatic are odor changes that accompany sexual maturation. Indeed, in human males almost the first easily observable sign of male puberty is a change in body odor—this clearly precedes changes in body hair and voice. These changes clearly reflect changes in amounts of circulating sex hormones. As a practical example, it is well known that castration reduces male body odor in pigs, reducing "boar taint" in male pig meat.

In many species it has been speculated that information on the age of an animal may serve to modulate mate choice. Older males may be preferred mates due to the fact since they survived, they must possess "good" genes that are advantageous for the female to pass on to her offspring. Recently we (Osada et al., 2003) have identified some of the volatile chemicals in mouse urine that change with age and may underlie age-related discriminative odors. Several of these are plausibly linked to changes in immune function. This raises the possibility that immune system activity could be determined by sensors that detect body odors (see below).

Varying Messages

Finally, there is a series of odor-based messages that are quite variable (3. in Figure D-38). Included here is information on sexual receptivity or willingness to mate, incidence of disease, and emotional state. For example, many animal studies have documented changes in female odor as a function of estrus cycle, and there is some evidence that the body odors of women change over the menstrual cycle (independent of the odors associated with menses; Stern and McClintock, 1998). In nonhuman animals, female odors associated with sexual receptivity are often highly attractive to males.

That body odors can be indicative of disease has a long history in medical practice (Penn and Potts, 1998). Nevertheless, little systematic study of this topic has been conducted. For example, there are many anecdotes of dogs identifying the presence of cancers prior to formal diagnosis, but few experimental studies document this in a rigorous fashion.

As a first model system to investigate disease and body odor, we (Yamazaki et al., 2002) have recently reported on a model system: the mouse mammary tumor virus (MMTV). It is possible in this model to test for changes in odor profiles that arise prior to overt disease. Mouse mammary tumors are notably lacking in cachectic, metastatic, and other general systemic effects on the host that might be expected to alter body odor in a nonspecific manner. Our studies revealed that mice can be trained to discriminate female or male intact mice or their urine odors as a function of the presence of MMTV, either acquired through infection or genetically. Furthermore, odor distinction based on the presence of virus occurs in the absence of overt disease. We are currently investigating the chemical pattern change that occurs following infection and are attempting to identify biologically relevant odorants. More generally, however, these studies suggest that it may be possible to identify and diagnose certain diseases (e.g., viral diseases such as AIDS and smallpox) before they are otherwise obvious and via the relatively noninvasive route of body odors.

BODY ODORS INDICATIVE OF OTHER PHYSIOLOGICAL STATES

Very little experimental work has been conducted on odors indicative of emotion (e.g. fear, anger, happiness) or fatigue in humans. Nevertheless, there is a widespread belief that an individual's emotional state is reflected in changes in body odor and this belief is reinforced by the results of some animal studies. For example, there are a number of studies that indicate that stressed animals emit a distinctive odor. It has been suggested that these odors may function to warn others of danger; these odors often elicit avoidance.

Anecdotal evidence in humans is consistent with animal studies. It is said that when one is under stress, sweating increases and this in turn leads to increases in body odor. Whether this purported change in odor is qualitative (new odorants being produced specifically indicating stress) or quantitative is not known. There is a plausible mechanism for a change in odor production with stress, however, since it is well known that certain neurotransmitters, such as epinephrine, stimulate heightened sweat gland activity.

As far as can be determined, there are no studies on changes in body odor with fatigue. Also, there is very little research on body odor changes with other emotional variations, with two exceptions. Chen and Haviland-Jones (2000) have reported that arousal of the emotions of happiness and fear by film clips results in production of body odors that can be discriminated by human noses. Similarly, Ackerl and colleagues (2002) have also reported that women made "fearful" by watching a scary movie produce an axillary odor that can be discriminated (by other women) from axillary odors collected under nonfear conditions. These studies are admittedly tentative but in light of their implications, a number of investigators are following them up.

BODY ODORS AS SIGNALS: FUTURE PROSPECTS

Based on studies with nonhuman animals and much more limited work with humans, it is safe to say that body odor is a rich potential medium for monitoring physiological states. There are, however, a number of problems that make it difficult to put this potential into practice at the present time.

Production and Communication

The first problem is our current lack of definitive studies on what information human body odors contain. Such studies are difficult to conduct for a variety of reasons, but they are not impossible. It is encouraging that there is considerable interest now in the potential to identify individuals based on their body odors. Here it is assumed that there is a genetically based individual odor, but whether this can be reliably discriminated in spite of variation in such factors as diet, perfume use, and odors associated with home and work place remains a major question. Apparently dogs can discern the individual signature of a person in spite of these potential distracters indicating that, at least in principle, it should be possible for a device to do this as well.

Similar studies should be encouraged to determine further how odors reflect emotional states. The Chen and Haviland-Jones and Ackerl and colleagues work represent just the very beginning. Both of these investigations asked whether humans can make olfactory discriminations between samples of body odors based on the emotional state of the odor donor. Based on nonhuman animal work, it is highly likely that human stress induces specific odor changes, but this must be rigorously demonstrated before programs to try to identify specific odorants and to develop sensors are instituted. It is also important to recognize that for volatile signals indicative of emotional states to be useful for monitoring emotion, it is not necessary that human noses be able to detect these substances. More discriminative devices, be they other biological ones such as rats or dogs, or specialized nonbiological sensors (see below), may be able to detect these volatile signals and thereby serve as monitors, even if other people find these discriminations difficult or impossible.

Detection and Discrimination

A second major problem involves techniques to identify and monitor odorants. In nature the olfactory system has evolved to be astoundingly sensitive to small molecules. Recently, much progress has been made in our understanding of this system, although many mysteries remain. Briefly, it is now thought that mammals have about 1,000 different molecular receptors for odorants (however, about two-thirds of these are not functional in humans). Each receptor, located on an individual receptor cell that is actually a primary sensory neuron, is responsive to a variety of structurally similar odorants (Zhang and Firestein, 2002). It is thus the pattern of receptor activity that is monitored and that determines odor quality and intensity. Processing and fine-tuning this pattern occurs beginning at the first synapse in the olfactory bulbs, but how further central nervous system processing occurs remains mostly unknown.

One strategy is to develop devices that mimic or even use biological principles to detect specific body odors. Particularly attractive is the idea that one might be able to express olfactory receptors in a device that monitors their activity using, for example, fluorescence to express overall patterned activity. This is a promising approach, but it clearly needs much more research.

A very active research area involves using a variety of artificial sensors to develop so-called e-noses, or artificial odor sensing devices. Although success of these devices has been mixed (initial claims turned out to be highly exaggerated), there is no doubt that progress is being made in sensors and sensor-interpretation interfaces. It seems likely that for highly accurate sensors, a knowledge of the specific odorants of interest will be needed. Hence, detector device development must go hand in hand with studies on the biology and chemistry of odors of interest.

CONCLUSIONS AND PROSPECTUS

Nonhuman animal studies confirm that body odors are a rich source of information about an organism. Human studies are few; nevertheless it is highly likely that our odors serve communicative functions. Because these odors presumably evolved to communicate, the messages should be much more readily useful for monitoring physiological states than, for example, hormones or metabolites from body fluids. In this latter case, multiple extraneous factors can obviously interfere with what is measured since there have been no evolutionary constraints to insure a high signal-to-noise ratio. For an evolved signal like an odor, in contrast, the signal-to-noise ratio should be high and the information content buffered against disruption from environmental and physiological variables. Consequently, additional work aimed at investigating odors for monitoring various physiological states is a very promising line of inquiry. Future work should reveal what information is available in body odor and the chemical identity of the odorants. In parallel, devices to accurately and reliably monitor these odors will be developed.

REFERENCES

Ackerl K, Atzmueller M, Grammer K. 2002. The scent of fear. *Neuroeendocrinol Lett* 23:79–84.

Beauchamp GK, Doty RL, Moulton DG, Mugford R. 1976. The pheromone concept in mammalian chemical communication: A critique. In: Doty RL, ed. *Mammalian Olfaction, Reproductive Processes, and Behavior*. New York: Academic Press. Pp.144–160.

Chen D, Haviland-Jones J. 2000. Human olfactory communication of emotion. *Percept Mot Skills* 91:771–781.

Osada K, Yamazaki K, Curran M, Bard JA, Beauchamp GK. 2003. The scent of age. *Proc R Soc Lond B Biol Sci* 270:929–933.

Penn D, Potts WK. 1998. Chemical signals and parasite-mediated sexual selection. *Trends Ecol Evol* 13:391–396.

Stern K, McClintock MK. 1998. Regulation of human ovulation by pheromones. *Nature* 392:177–179.

Wysocki CJ, Preti G. 1998. Pheromonal influences. *Arch Sex Behav* 27:627–629.

Yamazaki K, Singer A, Beauchamp GK. 1999. Origin, functions and chemistry of H-2 regulated odorants. *Genetica* 104:235–240.

Yamazaki K, Boyse EA, Bard J, Curran M, Kim D, Ross SR, Beauchamp GK. 2002. Presence of mouse mammary tumor virus specifically alters the body odor of mice. *Proc Natl Acad Sci* 99:5612–5615.

Zhang X, Firestein S. 2002. The olfactory receptor superfamily of the mouse. *Nature Neurosci* 5:124–133.

MOLECULAR MARKERS OF MECHANICAL ACTIVITY/INACTIVITY INDUCED ANABOLIC AND CATABOLIC STATES IN STRIATED MUSCLE

Kenneth M. Baldwin, Fadia Haddad, Gregory R. Adams,
University of California, Irvine

BACKGROUND

Striated muscle is highly plastic in that the individual cells or myocytes comprising this complex system have the capacity to change their mass, metabolic capacity, and contractile properties in accordance with the chronic functional demands (or lack thereof) imposed on it (Baldwin and Haddad, 2001). In the last 30 years, considerable evidence has accumulated to suggest that several key processes involving gene expression are closely linked in the regulation of both the amount and types of protein that are expressed in the muscle cells, thereby enabling them to adapt to various environmental stimuli (Adams, 2002; Baldwin and Haddad, 2001; Booth and Baldwin, 1996). Therefore, the goal of this report is to determine if different activity/inactivity paradigms can induce altered expression/activity in certain molecular markers (studied in an acute setting) to predict long-term adaptations reflecting changes in either the phenotype and/or net protein balance (anabolic and catabolic states) in skeletal muscle.

Fundamental Concepts of Gene Expression

Figure D-39 presents a schematic of how the expression of a gene is typically regulated via collective molecular processes to produce a specific protein product. Through these processes as depicted for a single gene, it is now recognized that expression of a variety of genes could contribute collectively to the regulation of many fundamental processes occurring in the cell. These are illustrated by, but are not limited to, the following processes that are known to undergo dramatic alteration in their functional properties: (a) the contraction process (e.g., actin and myosin interaction); (b) aerobic and anaerobic energy transformations; (c) muscle growth regulation (growth factor expression); (d) protein synthetic pathways; and (e) protein degradation pathways. Also depicted are key steps in the cascade that interact to control the amount of protein that is expressed, depending on how each step in the cascade is regulated. These steps include transcription and pretranslational processes that combine to produce the message substrate (mature messenger ribonucleic acid [mRNA]) of the gene for producing the protein. The mRNA is then translated into protein, a process that is commonly referred to as protein synthesis. This process is known to be regulated by several important steps, the chief of which is at the "protein initiation" step. Also operating simultaneously are post-translational events, including the process whereby proteins become targeted for subsequent degradation. It should be noted that all proteins within the cell undergo turnover (synthesis and degradation). It is through this process of protein turnover that both the type and amount of protein expression in the muscle can be changed from one functional state to another.

Factors Defining Protein Balance in Muscle

Based on the above, it is apparent that the amount of the protein maintained in a given muscle cell is controlled by the balance of those processes that transcribe/translate a protein relative to those processes that regulate its degradation. When the muscle is in a stable steady state (e.g., neither growing nor atrophying), the synthetic processes are in balance with the degradation processes. However, when the muscle is exposed to stimuli that induce a net accumulation of protein (referred to herein as an anabolic state), the transcriptional/translational processes of the muscle must be greater than those operating on the degradation side. On the other hand, if the conditions are such that the transcript-

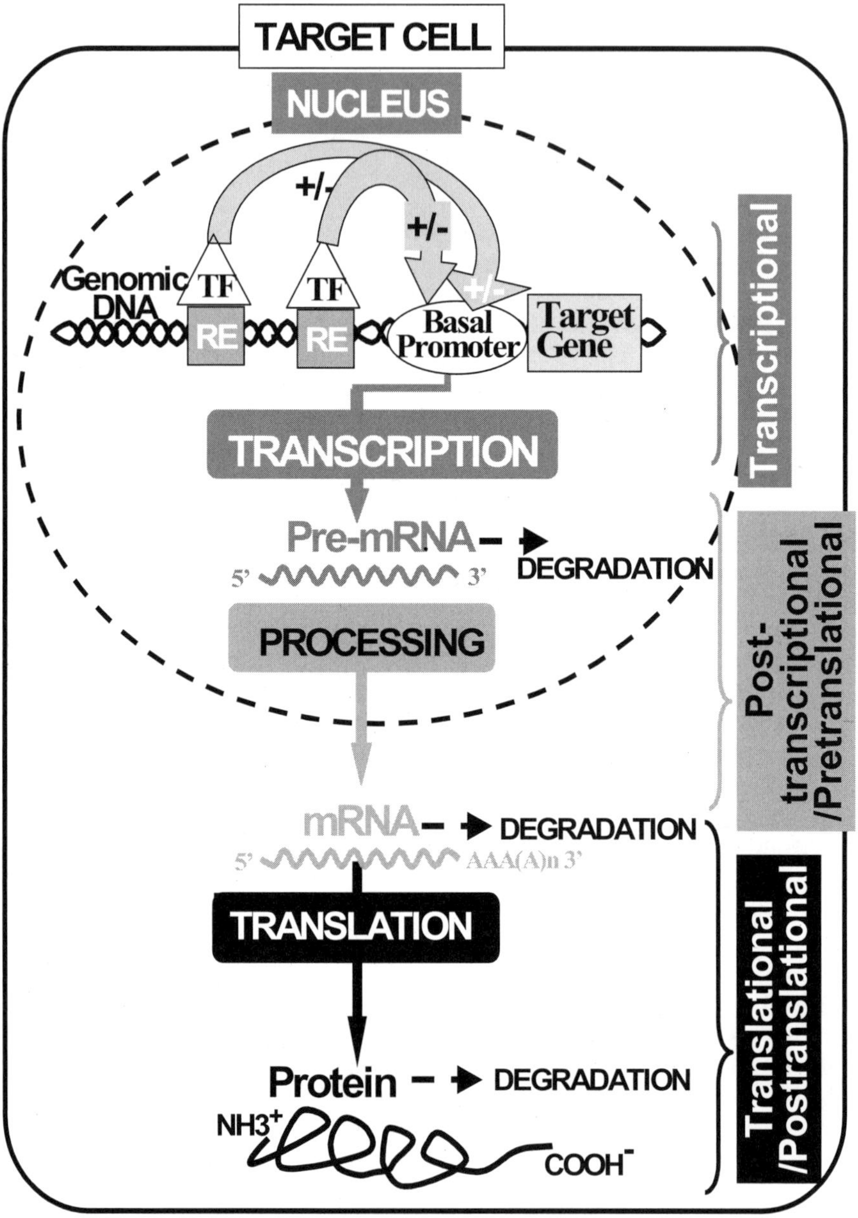

FIGURE D-39 Processes regulating gene function.

tional/translational processes cannot match those of degradation, then the muscle enters a state of catabolism, which results in net protein loss leading to its atrophy. Thus, it is important to note that all of the processes operating in the cascade can undergo altered rates of operation to thereby significantly influence the net protein balance in the muscle cell.

The Importance of Protein Isoforms

Coupled to this general scheme of gene/protein regulation is the fact that the genome of mammalian species contains a variety of multigene families. These consist of groups of very similar genes that encode slight variants of the protein product that have slightly different functional properties. An example of this is the myosin heavy chain (MHC) gene family, which collectively encode several different isoforms or species of myosin. Each isoform has distinct functional properties that ultimately dictate the intrinsic contraction properties (speed of contraction, fatigability) of the cells in which it is expressed. Depending on how this gene family is regulated in a given fiber, it is possible to repress one type of MHC gene and increase expression of another MHC type. This plasticity of gene expression enables the muscle to transform its intrinsic contractile properties. Thus, it is possible for the muscle to change both its size and its contraction phenotype depending on how the complex cascade in Figure D-39 is regulated from one functional state to another.

Signaling Pathways in Adaptive Processes

Presented in Figure D-40 is a complex array of processes/pathways that collectively operate to modulate those proteins/enzymes that coordinate the functional operation of the cascade depicted in Figure D-39. While it is beyond the scope of this short review to describe these signaling molecules and pathways in detail, it is important to emphasize that there are both upstream initiation factors (e.g., growth factors) and downstream effector proteins that regulate the integrated events governing transcription, translation, and degradation processes, thereby enabling the muscle cell to remodel its structure and functional properties. Importantly, this simplified scheme in no way reflects all of the signaling molecules and regulatory factors that control adaptive processes in striated muscle.

Activity Paradigms for Studying Adaptations in Skeletal Muscle: Animals Models

In this paper we will focus on three different activity/inactivity paradigms: (1) a model of chronic functional overload (FO) in which a smaller target muscle is continually overloaded due to the surgical removal of its larger synergist

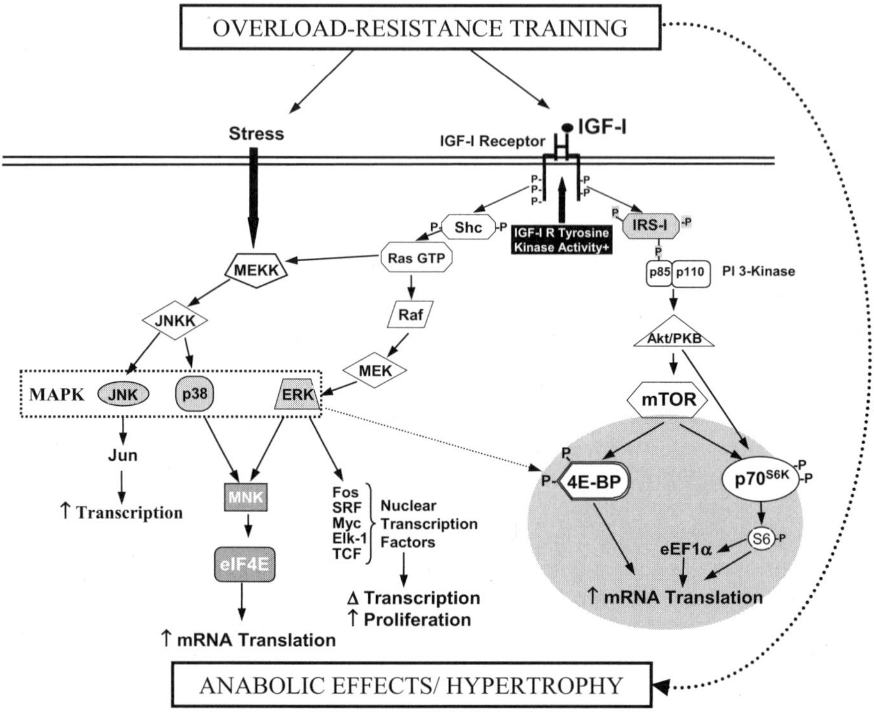

FIGURE D-40 Signaling pathways in adaptive processes.

(Adams et al., 2002); (2) intermittent resistance overload training (RT), in which the target muscle is trained with a specified contraction regimen spanning 1 or 2 training sessions (Haddad and Adams, 2002); and (3) the model of spinal isolation (SI) in which the target muscles are rendered almost completely inactive by midthoracic/sacral spinal cord transectioning that is coupled to a dorsal rhizotomy procedure. This procedure eliminates all sensory and higher center input to the motor unit pool of the lower extremity muscles, while keeping the muscle-nerve connections intact (Huey et al., 2001). This latter model, in essence, provides a "ground zero" catabolic reference state to which the anabolic mechanical overload paradigms can be compared.

METHODS AND MATERIALS

All the animal projects involved adult female rats. Functional overload and resistance training procedures were as described in detail elsewhere (Adams et al., 2002; Baldwin and Haddad, 2001; Haddad and Adams, 2002). The spinal isolation model involved surgical procedures as described by (Huey et al.,

2001). The biochemical/molecular analyses of marker protein phosphorylation, RNA concentration, and mRNA levels (via reverse transcriptase-polymerase chain reaction techniques) for specific genes were adapted from procedures described previously (Adams et al., 2002; Haddad and Adams, 2002). For comparative purposes, we report some initial findings (unpublished results) on humans that have undergone a combination of limb unloading plus resistance training in an attempt to ameliorate the atrophy that occurs in unloaded human skeletal muscle (Carrithers et al., In press).

RESULTS AND DISCUSSION

Early Events Leading to Net Protein Accumulation in Response to Mechanical Loading

Previous studies show that infusing physiological levels of insulin-like growth factor-1 directly into the muscle can induce significant hypertrophy within several days (Adams and McCue, 1998). The question is whether a mechanical stimulus, in and of itself, can induce rapid increases in muscle-derived IGF-1 expression in muscle thereby stimulating compensatory growth. If such a response occurs, it would suggest the involvement of an autocrine/paracrine process in the anabolic cascade following mechanical loading. As shown in Figure D-41, there is a rapid increase in mRNA expression for both IGF-1, and a variant isoform of IGF-1 (Adams et al., 1999, 2002) called mechanical growth factor in response to functional overload. This response occurs early in the adaptive response, and it is seen in both FO and isometric RT paradigms (Adams et al., 2002; Haddad and Adams, 2002; Huey et al., 2001) suggesting that growth factors are likely playing a key role in inducing anabolic responses in muscle under conditions that produce high mechanical stress on the muscle.

In addition to the response of growth factors, we also determined if there are rapid adaptive changes in the machinery that translates mature mRNA into protein (Figure D-39). Therefore, we examined levels of total RNA in skeletal muscle, since approximately 85 percent of the RNA pool exists as ribosomal RNA. Ribosomal RNA provides the scaffolding to which the mature mRNA is attached, providing the template for synthesizing the encoded protein. As shown in Figure D-42, there is a rapid increase in the concentration and content of total RNA in response to FO, suggesting that this is an important adaptive response to provide the machinery for producing more protein.

Based on the above observations, it is apparent that there are early events occurring to enable the muscle to enter into an anabolic state. Therefore, it was of interest to determine if adaptive changes occur in the pathways that are considered to be rate limiting steps in protein synthesis (e.g., the initiation steps in protein translation). We examined two different but complementary markers of this process. The first involves the phosphorylation of p70S6 kinase (pS6K). When this kinase is phosphorylated, it increases phosphorylation/activity levels of other proteins involved in the translation of mRNAs encoding proteins

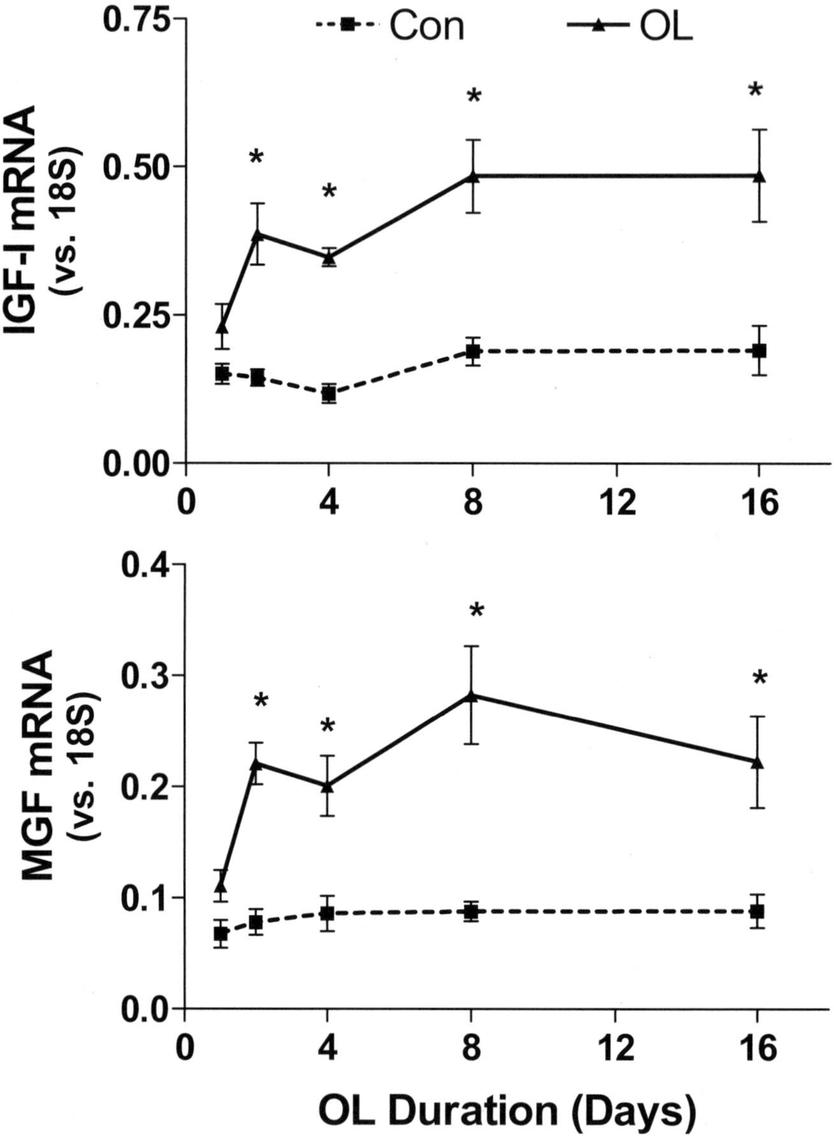

FIGURE D-41 Soleus insulin-like growth factor-1 (IGF-1) and mechanical growth factor (MGF) mRNA expression in response to overload.

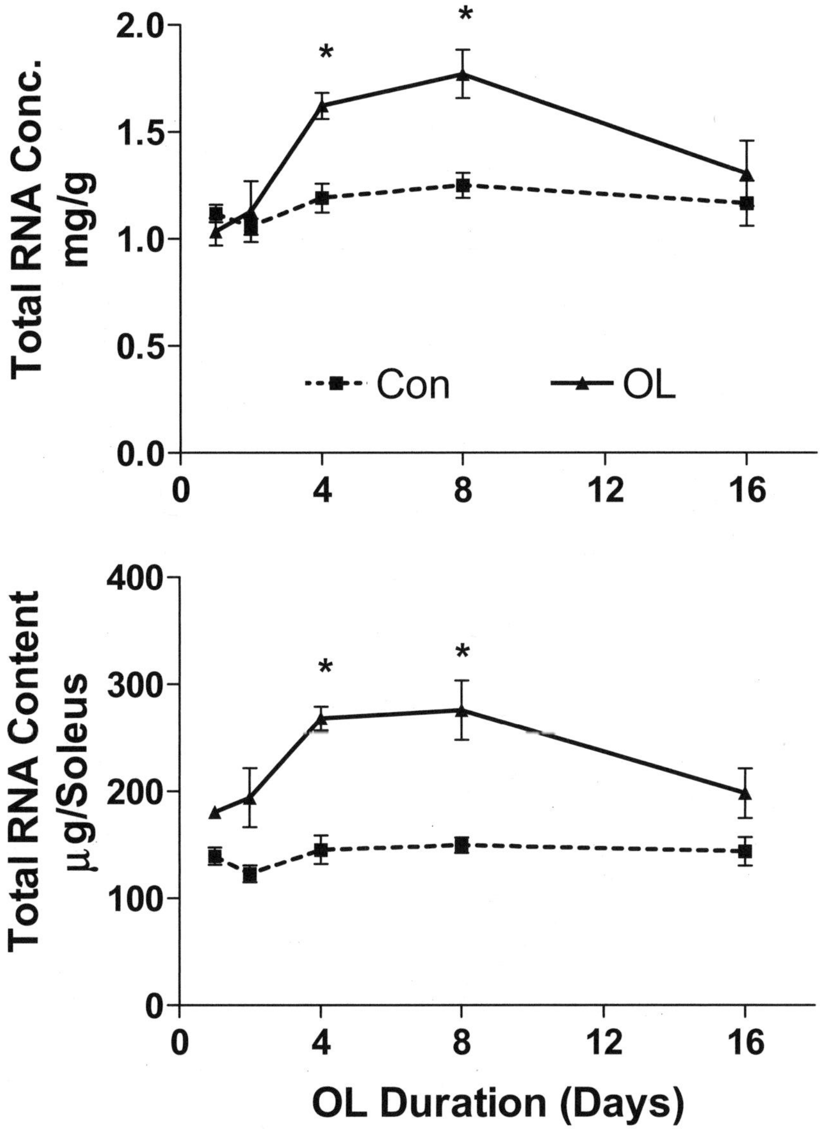

FIGURE D-42 Soleus total RNA concentration and content in response to overload.

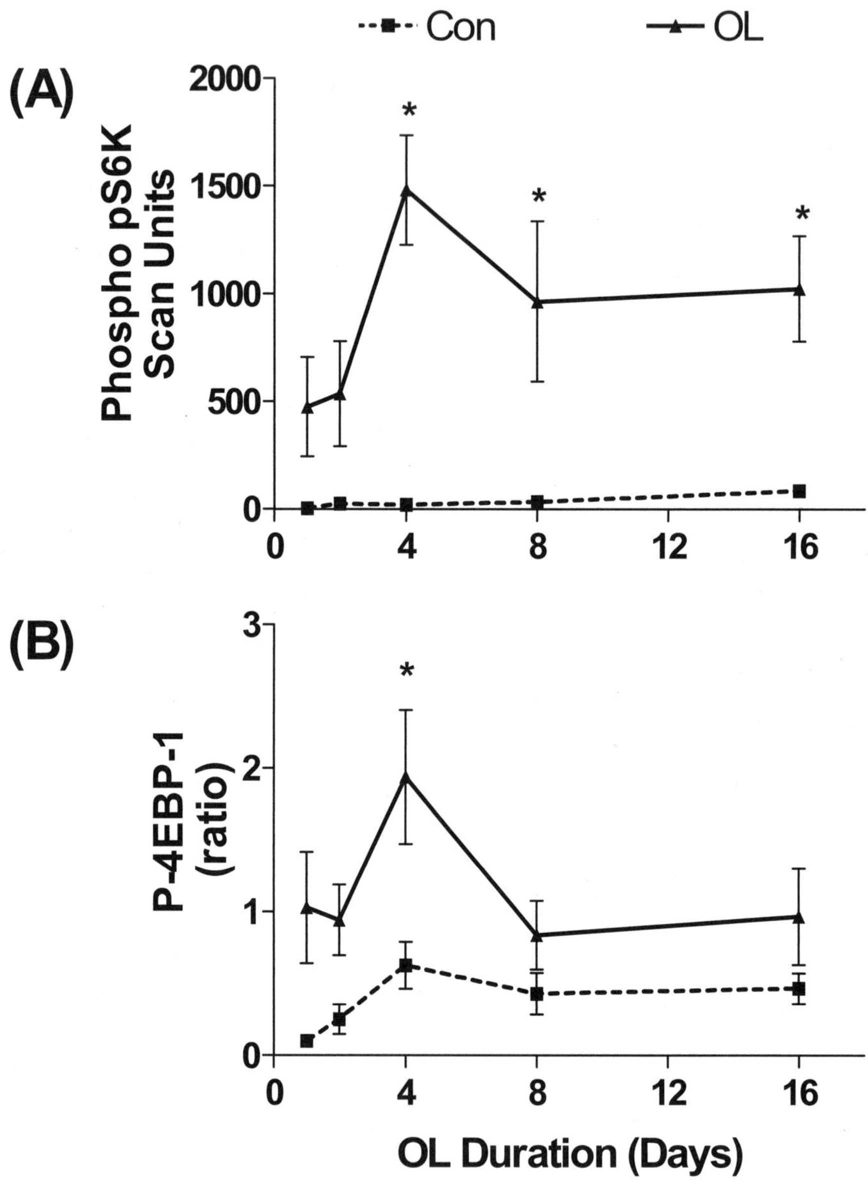

FIGURE D-43 Phosphorylation level of pS6K (A) and 4EBP-1 (B) in overloaded soleus.

comprising the ribosomal machinery. As shown in Figure D-43A, there was a marked increase in the phosphorylation state of pS6K indicative that this pathway was activated. This observation is also consistent with the increase in total RNA presented in Figure D-42. Also, we examined the phosphorylation state of another marker of protein initiation (e.g., eukaryotic initiation factor 4E bind-ing protein, or 4EBP-1). This factor normally functions as a negative regulator of the formation of the 43 kD pre-initiation complex that is essential for protein translation. However, when 4EBP-1 undergoes increased phosphorylation, it dissociates from the protein, eIF4E, a key protein subunit that is necessary for the 43S complex to form so that the initiation process can occur. As presented in Figure D-43B, 4EBP-1 also undergoes increased phophorylation at the early stages of mechanical loading, which is also indicative that protein initiation processes are being activated. Thus, we have demonstrated that there are several molecular markers that can serve as early-event signaling molecules to predict that the muscle is entering a state of positive protein balance. All of the markers that have been identified above to predict that an anabolic state is occurring in response to functional overload show similar adaptive responses when the mechanical stimulus is intermittent, rather than continuous. For example, when isometric resistant training paradigms are imposed on the muscle, the muscle responds in a way similar to that seen in the functional overload paradigm (Haddad and Adams, 2002).

Early Responses of Molecular Markers During Muscle Atrophy

In response to anabolic stimuli, do inactivity paradigms that induce marked degrees of muscle atrophy cause the opposite responses of those markers presented above? The answer to this question appears to be negative, since some of the markers (IGF-1, p6SK, 4EBP-1) that are highly responsive to mechanical loading either are maintained at normal levels or show some level of increased expression or increased activity when the target muscles undergo rapid atrophy in response to SI (Haddad et al., submitted). Instead, there appears to be a different set of molecular markers that are highly sensitive to the unloading state. First, at the onset of muscle unloading, there is a decrease in the transcriptional activity of key genes that encode important structural/functional proteins that comprise the sarcomere machinery, that is, the system that produces contraction (e.g., myosin heavy chain and actin). This is depicted in Figure D-44, which shows that transcriptional activity of actin as well as the slow type I MHC gene (which predominates in load-sensitive muscle cells) are significantly reduced. Second, there is a reduction in total RNA and specific mRNA expression for both actin and total MHC. These responses are indicative of a reduction in both the substrate and the machinery necessary for carrying out translation of key proteins. Third, genes encoding enzymes that are involved in the process of protein ubiquitination are up-regulated (Figure D-45). These enzymes define the process whereby specific proteins become targeted for degradation by the

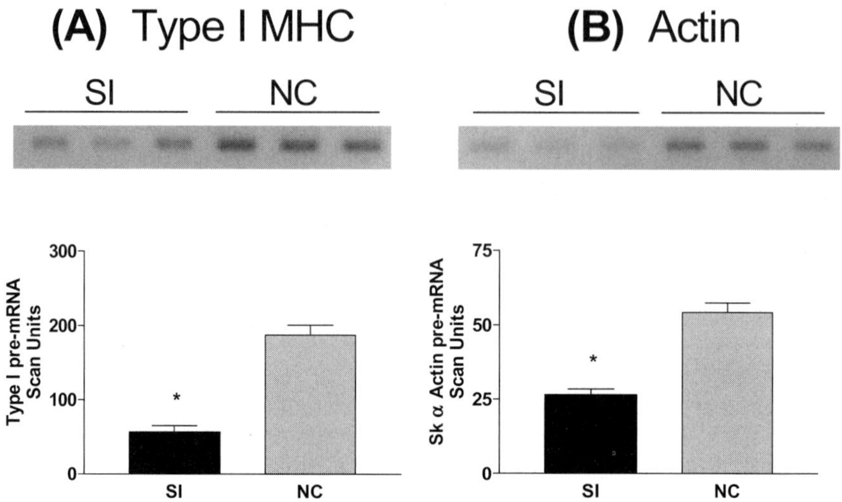

FIGURE D-44 Type I myocin heavy chain (MHC) (A) and actin (B) pre-mRNA expression in control and 8 days SI soleus muscle. Pre-mRNA is the nascent transcriptional product and changes in its expression represent changes in gene transcriptional activity.

proteasome system, which is the major pathway for protein degradation in muscle cells. These collective responses provide a mechanism to rapidly reduce muscle mass by decreasing the ability of the muscle to accumulate protein while increasing the processes for decreasing protein pools, thereby creating a catabolic state and net protein loss. Since those processes that regulate factors such as IGF-1 and the phosphorylation of pS6K and 4EBP-1 do not appear to be down-regulated, it is apparent that the loss of muscle protein is not necessarily the result of a "shutting down" of those processes that cause muscle cell enlargement. Thus, one must focus on a different set of molecular markers to distinguish a net catabolic state from that which defines a net anabolic state in predicting a protein balance profile of the muscle under different physiological conditions.

Do the Molecular Responses Seen in Animal Models Have Relevance to Adaptation in Human Muscle?

While there is abundant evidence that there are viable human models (e.g., resistance training, bed rest, and the unique model of unilateral limb suspension [ULLS] that can mimic, to a certain extent, the gross responses seen in animal models of hypertrophy and of atrophy), questions arise as to whether acute

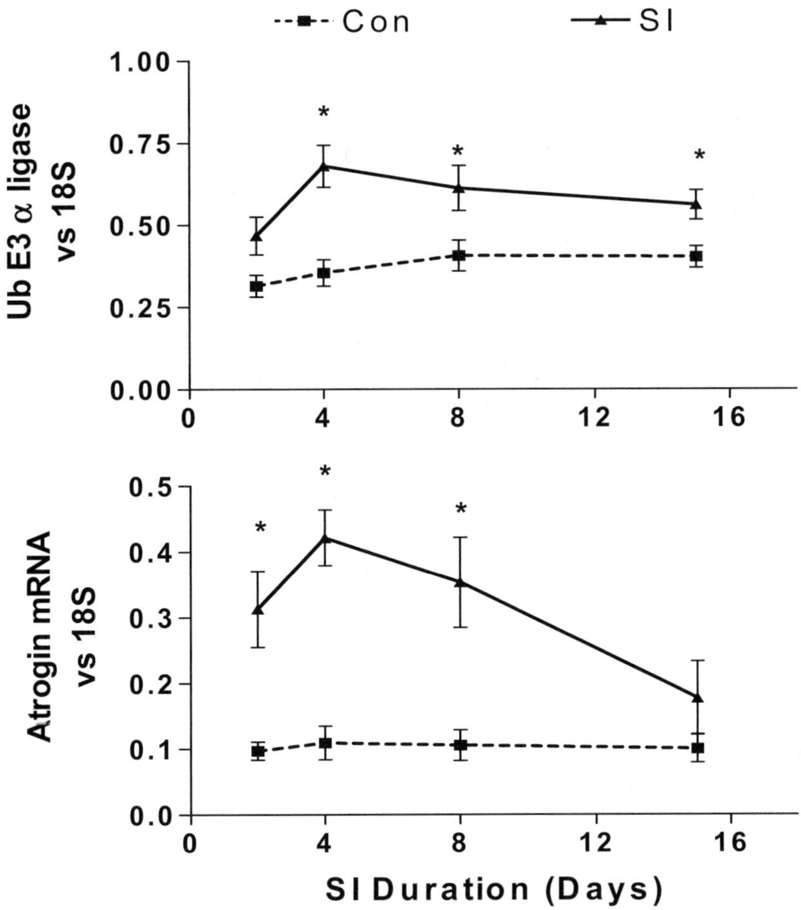

FIGURE D-45 Degradation marker mRNAs expression in soleus in response to SI.

changes in the mechanical stress imposed on human skeletal muscle induce the same type of responses as reported herein for rodent muscle. In an attempt to address this issue, we performed preliminary analyses in conjunction with Dr. Per Tesch at the Karolinska Institute in Stockholm (Carrithers et al., In press) on selected molecular markers in biopsy samples obtained from three groups of subjects (*n* = 8 each): (1) a group subjected to ULLS for 3 weeks (left limb unloaded, right limb ambulatory), (2) a group of subjects subjected to ULLS plus a resistance training paradigm (Carrithers et al., In press), and (3) a group

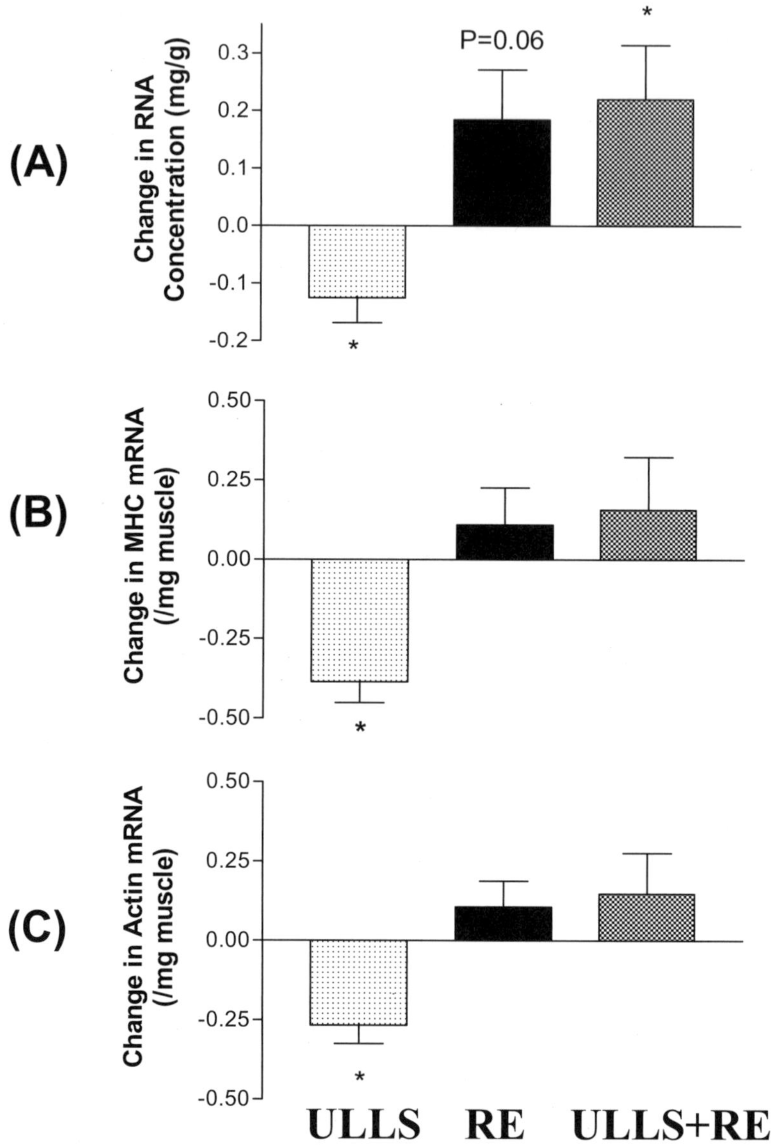

FIGURE D-46 Changes in total RNA concentration (A), total myocin heavy chain (MHC) (B) and actin (C) mRNA expression in human muscle when subjected to unilateral limb suspension (ULLS), resistance exercise (RE) or ULLS+RE.

as seen for ULLS-trained group. The results indicated that the ULLS caused a of fully ambulatory subjects that received the same resistance training paradigm reduction in strength and muscle mass in the suspended limb. This response was attenuated in the ULLS plus resistance-trained group. The resistance training of the ambulatory subjects did not significantly enhance muscle mass or muscle strength beyond that which was observed for the ULLS plus trained group. Biopsies were obtained on each subject at the beginning and end of the experimental protocol. As presented in Figure D-46A, there was a deficit in the pre- and post-change in muscle total RNA concentration for the ULLS versus the two resistance-trained groups. Also there were net deficits in both the MHC and actin mRNA responses in the ULLS group versus that seen for the two resistance trained groups (Figures D-46B and D-46C). Thus, we propose that the same general adaptive processes that operate in the muscles of animal models also are seen in human subjects when they are exposed to perturbations that alter the homeostasis of the skeletal muscles under different loading states.

SUMMARY AND CONCLUSION

In this report we have demonstrated that skeletal muscle of both animal and human subjects possess a high level of plasticity (ability to change in response to altered environment) of gene expression in response to altered states of loading and/or mechanical stress. This phenomenon makes it possible to establish molecular marker profiles based on adaptive responses to acute disruptions in muscle homeostasis that predict impending alterations in catabolic and anabolic states that affect outcomes in the net protein balance in muscle cells. This information paves the way for the eventual development of technologies with the capability of monitoring the muscle's molecular status for predicting outcomes to paradigms that may have either a positive or negative impact on the structure and function of the skeletal muscle system.

This research was supported by a grant from the National Space Biomedical Research Institute (NCC9-78-70) and National Institutes of Health grants AR 30346 (KMB) and AR 45594 (GRA).

REFERENCES

Adams GR. 2002. Autocrine/paracrine IGF-1 and skeletal muscle adaptation. *J Appl Physiol* 93:1159–1167.

Adams GR, McCue SA. 1998. Localized infusion of IGF-1 results in skeletal muscle hypertrophy in rats. *J Appl Physiol* 84:1716–1722.

Adams GR, Haddad F, Baldwin KM. 1999. The time course of changes in markers of myogenesis in overloaded rat skeletal muscles. *J Appl Physiol* 87:1705–1712.

Adams GR, Caiozzo VJ, Haddad F, Baldwin KM. 2002. Cellular and molecular responses to increased skeletal muscle loading following irradiation. *Am J Physiol Cell Physiol* 283:C1182–C1195.

Baldwin KM, Haddad F. 2001. The effects of different activity and inactivity paradigms on myosin heavy chain gene expression in striated muscle. *J Appl Physiol* 90:345–357.

Booth FW, Baldwin KM. 1996. Muscle plasticity: Energy demand/supply processes. In: Rowell LB, Shepherd JT, eds. *American Physiological Society Handbook of Physiology: Section 12. Exercise: Regulation and Integration of Multiple Systems.* New York: Oxford University Press. Pp. 1075–1123.

Carrithers JA, Tesch PA, Trieschmann J, Ekberg A, Trappe TA. In press. Skeletal muscle protein composition following 5 weeks of ULLS and resistance exercise countermeasures. *J Grav Physiol.*

Haddad F, Adams GR. 2002. Acute cellular and molecular responses to resistance exercise. *J Appl Physiol* 93:394–403.

Huey KA, Roy RR, Baldwin KM, Edgerton VR. 2001. Time dependent effects of inactivity on myosin heavy chain gene expression in antigravity skeletal muscles. *Muscle and Nerve* 24:517–527.

E

Biographical Sketches of Workshop Speakers

Kenneth M. Baldwin, Ph.D., is a professor in the Department of Physiology and Biophysics in the College of Medicine at the University of California, Irvine. His laboratory research focuses on the impact of activity patterns and exercise regimens on the biochemical and physiological properties of cardiac and skeletal muscle in mammals. Of primary interest is how the effects of these various activities are translated into biochemical events that lead to alterations in protein expression in muscle. As a corollary to these experiments, Dr. Baldwin's group, in conjunction with NASA (National Aeronautics and Space Administration), recently sent rats on a Space Shuttle mission to study the effects of weightlessness on skeletal muscle. Recently he received the NASA Public Service Medal and the American Physiological Society Edward Adolph Award. He received his Ph.D. from the University of Iowa in exercise physiology.

Gary K. Beauchamp, Ph.D., received his B.A. in biology from Carleton College in Northfield, Minnesota, in 1965 and his Ph.D. in biopsychology from the Pritzker School of Medicine of The University of Chicago in 1971. He then went to the newly established Monell Chemical Senses Center, a nonprofit, basic research institute loosely affiliated with the University of Pennsylvania, as a postdoctoral fellow. He has remained at Monell since that time and is currently director of the Center. He is also an adjunct professor of anatomy in the School of Veterinary Medicine and an adjunct professor of psychology in the School of Arts and Sciences of the University of Pennsylvania. His research interests include genetics of chemosensation, development and aging of taste and smell, taste interactions, and the role of smell and taste in food and beverage choice and acceptance. During his research career, he has authored or coauthored over 250 original research papers, book chapters, and review articles. Among his awards are the Claude Pepper Award of Excellence from the National Institute on Deafness and Other Communication Disorders (NIDCD), National Institutes of Health (NIH) (1990–1997) and the Outstanding Achievement in the Chemical Senses Award in 1999 from the Association for Chemoreception Sciences. He currently serves on numerous advisory bodies and is a member of the NIDCD Advisory Council and the Board of Directors of the American Institute of Wine and Food, The Ambrose Monell Foundation, and The G. Unger Vetlesen Foundation.

John A. Caldwell, Jr., Ph.D., is the principal research psychologist with the Warfighter Fatigue Countermeasures Program at the Air Force Research Laboratory, Brooks Air Force Base, Texas. He has published over 80 articles in peer-reviewed scientific journals and laboratory technical reports. He frequently lectures at safety briefings and scientific symposia, and he conducts operationally-focused workshops on fatigue countermeasures for aviators and industrial personnel. He is a member of the National Sleep Foundation's Speakers Bureau and Science Advisory Council, and he frequently consults with various organizations on the effects of fatigue on pilots and methods for overcoming the adverse impact of fatigue in the aviation environment. Dr. Caldwell received his Ph.D. in experimental psychology in 1984 from the University of Southern Mississippi. In 1983 he became the assistant director of the Behavioral Medicine Laboratory at Children's Hospital National Medical Center in Washington, D.C., where he spent 3 years. Afterwards, he spent 16 years with the U.S. Army Medical Research and Materiel Command (USAMRMC) conducting studies on methods of aviator status monitoring and on the effects of medications on aviator performance in specially-instrumented flight simulators and aircraft. In August 2002 he transferred to the Air Force Research Laboratory at Brooks. The focus of his research is to fully understand the effects of sleep deprivation on pilots and to develop monitoring methodologies and fatigue countermeasures for use in the operational aviation environment. Key accomplishments have included the first-ever controlled aviator flight-performance evaluations of the efficacy of dextroamphetamine and modafinil for sustaining performance and the completion of several unique protocols investigating the feasibility of real-time monitoring of aviator physiological activity in flight.

Kong Y. Chen, Ph.D., is a research assistant professor in the Department of Medicine of Vanderbilt University. He also serves as the director of the Energy Balance Core Laboratory. His areas of expertise include advanced designs and modeling techniques of biomedical engineering and developing new methods and improving existing techniques for measuring human energy metabolism, body composition, and physical activity. Dr. Chen is a member of the American Gastroenterology Association, the North American Association for the Study of Obesity, and the American College of Sports Medicine. He was the Young Investigator of the Year for the Vanderbilt Clinical Nutrition Research Center for two consecutive years (1999, 2000) and served as a reviewer for numerous journals. His research is funded by NIH, the Department of Defense, other government agencies, and private nonprofit foundations.

Giovanni Cizza, M.D., Ph.D., is an endocrinologist who works as a senior staff physician at the National Institute of Mental Health, Clinical Neuroendocrinology Branch, Mood and Anxiety Program. He is also an adjunct scientist at the National Institute of Child Health and Human Development, Bethesda, Maryland. Between 1996 and 1999, Dr. Cizza worked as associate director in clinical research, Department of Endocrinology and Metabolism, Merck Research Laboratories, in Rahway, New Jersey. An author and lecturer on the medical consequences of depression, including osteoporosis and metabolic alterations, neuroendocrinology of aging, the physiology of the hypothalamic-pituitary-adrenal axis and its relationships with the leptin axis, Dr. Cizza coedited the book *Stress: Basic Mechanisms and Clinical Implications*, and he authored several articles in medical journals, such as the *Annals of Internal Medicine*, *Journal of Clinical Investigation, Nature Medicine*, *Endocrinology,* and the *Journal of Clinical Endocrinology & Metabolism.* Awards include the Late Breaking Clinical Trial Symposium at the Endocrine Society in 1999, the Henry Christian Award from the American Federation for Clinical Research, the New Investigator Award for the Neurosciences from the American Geriatric Society, and two Trainee Investigator Awards at Clinical Research Meetings. Dr. Cizza is a member of the Endocrine Society, the American Society for Bone and Mineral Research, and the Society for Neurosciences. Dr. Cizza holds a medical degree from Pisa University School of Medicine, Italy, and a Ph.D. in experimental pathology from the same university. His training in clinical endocrinology was both at Pisa University School of Medicine and at the Interinstitute Endocrine Program of NIH. He also attended a 3-year postgraduate program in clinical pharmacology at the Mario Negri Institute for Pharmacological Research in Milano, Italy. Dr. Cizza's current research interests include the medical consequences of depression, the development of a novel pharmacological treatment, a CRH type-1 antagonist for depression and anxiety disorders, prevention and treatment of postmenopausal osteoporosis, glucocorticoid-induced osteoporosis, and related diseases of bone metabolism.

William J. Evans, Ph.D., is the director of the Nutrition, Metabolism, and Exercise Laboratory in the Donald Reynolds Department of Geriatrics at the University of Arkansas for Medical Sciences and a research scientist in the Geriatric Rehabilitation, Education, and Clinical Center at the VA Medical Center. He is a professor of geriatrics, physiology, and nutrition. From 1993 to 1997 he was the director of the Noll Physiological Research Center at the Pennsylvania State University, and from 1982 to 1993 he served as the chief of the Human Physiology Laboratory at the U.S. Department of Agriculture Human Nutrition Research Center on Aging at Tufts University. He is a fellow of the American College of Sports Medicine and the American College of Nutrition and an honorary member of the American Dietetic Association. Dr. Evans is the author or coauthor of more than 190 publications in scientific journals. Much of his research has examined the functional and metabolic consequences of physical activity in elderly people. Along with Irwin Rosenberg, M.D., he is the author of *Bio-*

markers: The Ten Determinants of Aging You Can Control and has recently authored *AstroFit*. He receives grant support from a variety of sources, including NIH, the Veterans Administration, NASA, and private industry. Ongoing research in the Nutrition, Metabolism, and Exercise Laboratory is examining the effects of a low protein diet and exercise on renal function, body composition, and functional capacity in elderly men and women with chronic renal failure, effects of exercise on fatigue in anemic cancer patients, effects of physical activity and diet on insulin action in elderly people, and the etiology of late life dysfunction. He has been an associate editor for *Medicine and Science in Sport and Exercise* and *Journal of Gerontology* and is a member of the editorial board of the *Journal of Clinical Endocrinology and Metabolism*. Dr. Evans serves as a reviewer for more than ten journals and has been a reviewer of grants for the American Federation for Aging Research, NIH, NASA, and the Veterans Administration.

Karl E. Friedl, Ph.D., is the research area manager for the Army Operational Medicine Research Program at USAMRMC, Fort Detrick, Maryland. Prior to this assignment, he was an Army research physiologist in the Occupational Physiology Division at the U.S. Army Research Institute of Environmental Medicine (USARIEM), where he specialized in physical and biochemical limits of prolonged, intensive military training. Previously, LTC Friedl worked in the Department of Clinical Investigation at Madigan Army Medical Center in Tacoma, Washington, performing studies in endocrine physiology. He received his Ph.D. in physiology in 1984 from the Institute of Environmental Stress at the University of California, Santa Barbara.

Reed W. Hoyt, Ph.D., is a research physiologist at USARIEM, Natick, Massachusetts. Dr. Hoyt received his Ph.D. in biomedical sciences from the University of New Mexico in 1981 and was a postdoctoral fellow and a research assistant professor at the University of Pennsylvania before joining USARIEM in 1986. He is a member of the American Physiological Society, Sigma Xi, the American Institute of Nutrition, and the American Society of Clinical Nutrition. He is a recipient of the American Physiological Society Caroline tum Suden Professional Opportunity Award for Meritorious Research on Exercise and Energy Metabolism and the Department of the Army Superior Civilian Service Award. He has served on the editorial board of the *Journal of Applied Physiology*, has published over 40 scientific articles, and holds five patents. He is interested in using new methods to understand the effects of exercise and environmental extremes on the metabolic and thermal status of soldiers in the field.

Michael Kleerekoper, M.D., received his medical training at the University of Sydney, Australia. After completing a fellowship in endocrinology and metabolism at Washington University-St. Louis, he joined the faculty at Henry Ford Hospital and began his research in the area of bone and endocrinology. In 1993 he joined Wayne State University in the endocrinology section of the Department of Internal Medicine. He serves as the director of research for the areas of bone and mineral metabolism and gerontology for the School of Medicine. Dr. Kleerekoper is a member of the Institute for Gerontology.

David C. Klonoff, M.D., F.A.C.P., is a practicing endocrinologist. He is interested in new technology for diabetes, including noninvasive glucose monitoring, drug delivery systems, medical economics of interventions, and pharmacology of diabetes drugs. Dr. Klonoff is a clinical professor of medicine at the University of California, San Francisco (UCSF) and editor-in-chief of the peer-reviewed journal, *Diabetes Technology & Therapeutics*. As medical director of the Dorothy L. and James E. Frank Diabetes Research Institute of Mills-Peninsula Health Services in San Mateo, California, he conducts clinical trials of drugs and devices. Dr. Klonoff has authored over 60 publications. He has chaired or served on grant review panels for NIH, the Centers for Disease Control and Prevention (CDC), NASA, the Juvenile Diabetes Research Foundation International (JDRFI), the U.S. Army, and the University of Michigan. Dr. Klonoff has given invited presentations at the Food and Drug Administration, NIH, CDC, and nine U.S. medical schools. He was named best endocrinologist in San Mateo County by Bay Area Consumer Checkbook. Dr. Klonoff is a graduate of University of California, Berkeley, where he was elected to Phi Beta Kappa in his junior year, and University of California, San Francisco (UCSF) Medical School, where he was elected to Alpha Omega Alpha in his junior year. He completed two years of postgraduate training at UCLA Hospital and three years at UCSF hospitals. Dr. Klonoff founded the annual Diabetes Technology Meeting in 2001. Dr. Klonoff chaired the JDRFI/NASA Bioartificial Pancreas Meeting and the NASA Smart Medicine/Clinical Studies Grant Review Panel. Dr. Klonoff is a member of the U.S. Army Technologies for Metabolic Monitoring (TMM) Steering Committee and was scientific chair of the TMM meeting in 2002 in Washington, D.C. and was on the Scientific Sessions Planning Committee for the American Diabetes Association 2003 meeting in New Orleans.

Wendy M. Kohrt, Ph.D., is a professor of medicine at the University of Colorado Health Sciences Center (UCHSC) in the Department of Internal Medicine, Division of Geriatric Medicine, in Denver. She also holds an adjunct appointment in the Department of Kinesiology and Applied Physiology, University of Colorado, Boulder. Dr. Kohrt's research interests include aging, exercise, regional adiposity, energy metabolism, and hormone replacement. She is a member of the NIH Geriatric and Rehabilitative Medicine study section; the American College of Sports Medicine (ACSM) Strategic Health Initiative for Women, Sport, and Physical Activity Committee; the UCHSC Hartford/Jahnigen Center of Excellence in Geriatrics Advisory Board; the Executive Committee, Center for Human Nutrition, UCHSC; and the editorial board of the *Journal of Applied Physiology*. Dr. Kohrt is the editor of the *Yearbook of Sports Medicine*. She received her M.S. and Ph.D. in the field of exercise physiology at Arizona State University, Tempe.

Harris R. Lieberman, Ph.D., is a research psychologist in the Military Nutrition Division of USARIEM in Natick, Massachusetts. Dr. Lieberman is an internationally recognized expert in the area of nutrition and behavior and has published over 100 original, full-length papers in scientific journals and edited books. He has been an invited lecturer at numerous national and international conferences, government research laboratories, and universities. He received his Ph.D. in physiological psychology from the University of Florida and then conducted postdoctoral research at the Department of Psychology and Brain Science at the Massachusetts Institute of Technology (MIT). From 1980 to 1990 he was on the research staff at MIT, where he examined the effects of food constituents and drugs on human behavior and brain function. In 1990 Dr. Lieberman joined the civilian research staff of USARIEM where he has continued his work in nutrition, behavior, and stress. From 1994 to 2000 he was chief or deputy chief of the Military Nutrition program at USARIEM. His recent research has addressed the effects of various nutritional factors, diets, and environmental stress on animal and human performance, brain function, and behavior. His work has focused on developing and applying a variety of emerging technologies in nutrition, neuroscience, and microelectronics to sustain and enhance human performance in stressful environments. He holds two patents for novel technologies to assess and enhance cognitive performance. Dr. Lieberman currently chairs an International Defense Panel on Cognitive and Ergogenic Aids.

Bradley C. Nindl, Ph.D., is a research physiologist in the Military Performance Division at USARIEM in Natick, MA. Dr. Nindl received a B.S. in biology from Clarkson University in 1989, an M.S. in physiology of exercise from Springfield College in 1993, and a Ph.D. in physiology from The Pennsylvania State University in 1999. Dr. Nindl served as a captain in the U.S. Army Medical Service Corps at USARIEM from 1999–2002. His lines of research are centered on endocrine, body composition, and physical performance responses to both exercise and military operational stress. Dr. Nindl's current work involves measuring the insulin-like growth factor-I system in response to longitudinal physical training as it relates to optimizing warfighter physical readiness for MRMR Science and Technology S: Physical Training Interventions to Enhance Military Task Performance and Reduce Musculoskeletal Injuries. Dr. Nindl is an author or coauthor of 70 journal articles, book chapters, and government technical reports. He is a member of ACSM, the American Physiological Society, The Endocrine Society, and the National Strength and Conditioning Association. He is on the editorial board of *Medicine and Science in Sports and Exercise* and *The Journal of Strength and Conditioning Research* and on the executive committee of the New England chapter of ACSM. Dr. Nindl was a recipient of the 2002 American College of Sports Medicine New Investigator Award.

Clifford J. Rosen, M.D., is the executive director at the Maine Center for Osteoporosis Research and Education at St. Joseph Hospital in Bangor, Maine; a staff scientist at the Jackson Laboratory in Bar Harbor, Maine; and a professor of nutrition at the University of Maine, Orono. He is currently the president of the American Society of Bone and Mineral Research, editor-in-chief of the *Journal of Clinical Densitometry*, and chairman of the NIH Study Section OBM-2. Dr. Rosen has published over 180 peer-reviewed journal articles and authored, coauthored, or edited over 20 books and chapters. He received his M.D. from the State University of New York at Syracuse, Upstate Medical Center.

Michael N. Sawka, Ph.D., is chief, Thermal and Mountain Medicine Division at USARIEM. He directs Department of Defense research programs in: cold stress physiology, heat stress physiology, high altitude physiology, environmental pathophysiology, and environmental genomics. He received a B.S. and an M.S. from East Stroudsburg University, and a Ph.D. from Southern Illinois University. Dr. Sawka's research interests are environmental and exercise physiology and rehabilitation medicine. He has published over 250 full-length scientific papers and a graduate textbook on environmental physiology. His research has been frequently cited by the national news media and he serves on numerous editorial boards, scientific review panels, and professional committees.

T. Peter Stein, Ph.D., is a professor of surgery and nutrition at the University of Medicine and Dentistry of New Jersey. His expertise is in the areas of clinical nutrition and protein and energy metabolism during space flight. Dr. Stein was a cowinner of the American Institute of Aviation and Astronautics Jeffries Medical Research Award in 1992 for his work on Spacelab Life Sciences-1. Memberships include the American Association for the Advancement of Science, the American Institute of Nutrition, the American Society for Clinical Nutrition, the American Physiological Society, the American Chemical Society, and the American Society for Gravitational Physiology. Dr. Stein received a B.Sc. from the Imperial College of Science and Technical University of London, an M.Sc. (biochemistry) from University College, University of London, and a Ph.D. (molecular biology/chemistry) from Cornell University.

Julian F. Thayer, Ph.D., received a B.A. in psychology from Indiana University and his Master's and Ph.D. from New York University. After academic positions at Penn State University and the University of Missouri, he joined the National Institute on Aging to initiate a program on emotions and quantitative psychophysiology. His research interests are biological and psychological adaptation and flexibility in the context of dynamical systems models with applications to psychopathology, pathophysiology, and health. This work utilizes indices of autonomic nervous system function derived from cardiac variability measures to probe whole organism systems.

Nancy J. Wesensten, Ph.D., is a research psychologist and deputy chief of the Department of Neurobiology and Behavior, Division of Neuropsychiatry, Walter Reed Army Institute of Research (WRAIR), Washington, D.C. She received her Ph.D. in experimental psychology from Bowling Green State University, specializing in electroencephalographic indices of decision-making and psychophysiological responsivity to external stimuli across sleep stages. At WRAIR, her focus has been on determining fieldability of sleep-inducing agents (via evaluation of their hypnotic and amnestic effects) (in collaboration with Lorex Pharmaceuticals), and whether fieldability can be improved by amelioration of hypnotic side effects using reversal agents. More recently, she conducted studies to evaluate the efficacy and fieldability of the novel synthetic stimulant modafinil on performance and alertness during sleep deprivation (in collaboration with Cephalon, Inc.) compared with caffeine. These lines of research are aimed at determining the role of various neurotransmitter systems in sleep/wake regulation in order to produce more effective countermeasures for military use. Dr. Wesensten was a coinvestigator on a recently completed, large-scale study funded by the Federal Highway Administration in which the chronic effects of different amounts of nighttime sleep on daytime performance (including simulated driving) were evaluated. Her other research efforts include an on-going collaborative effort with NIH investigating regional cerebral blood flow changes during the various stages of sleep and wakefulness and a collaborative effort with USARIEM, which investigated hypnotic efficacy of triazolam on sleep and degradation of electroencephalographic indices of cognitive capacities at simulated high altitude.

Peter G. Weyand, Ph.D., is physiologist and biomechanist who specializes in terrestrial locomotion. His primary research focus is the relationship between skeletal muscle function, metabolic energy expenditure, and performance. Dr. Weyand is currently an assistant professor of kinesiology at Rice University. He is also a research physiologist at Harvard University's Concord Field Station, a large-animal facility specializing in animal locomotion, and formerly served as a senior research fellow at USARIEM. Dr. Weyand combines his research and teaching interests by involving numerous undergraduate students in his research program. To date, student work has been published in *Nature*, the *Journal of Experimental Biology,* and the *Journal of Applied Physiology*. Past courses taught include Harvard biology classes entitled "Muscles, Metabolism and Movement" and "See Spot Run." In 1996, he received Harvard University's Joseph E. Levenson Award for excellence in undergraduate teaching. Dr. Weyand received his Ph.D. in exercise physiology from the University of Georgia.

Robert R. Wolfe, Ph.D., is a professor and chief of metabolism at the Shriners Hospital for Children-Galveston and The University of Texas Medical Branch, Galveston. His research focuses on the physiological regulation of metabolism. He has made extensive use of stable isotope methodology in his investigations of human subjects. He has served on numerous national and international committees, including NIH study sections and advising committees to NASA, the Federation of American Societies for Experimental Biology, and several research councils of foreign countries. Dr. Wolfe has published over 300 peer-reviewed papers and 90 review articles and text chapters.

Andrew J. Young, Ph.D., is a research physiologist and chief of the Military Nutrition Division at USARIEM in Natick, Massachusetts, and an adjunct associate professor in the Sargent College of Allied Health Professions at Boston University. He obtained his B.S. in biology and his commission in the U.S. Army at the Virginia Military Institute, and his Ph.D. in physiology at the North Carolina State University. Following graduate school, Dr. Young served six years on active duty in the U.S. Army with assignments at USARIEM (1977–1981) and at WRAIR (1981–1983). After leaving active duty, Dr. Young continued government service as a civilian scientist at USARIEM. Dr. Young's research has concerned the biological basis for, and strategies to mitigate, physical performance degradations in military personnel exposed to physiological stressors, such as intense physical exertion coupled with sleep restriction, nutritional deprivation, and exposure to extremes of heat, cold, and high altitude, all of which could be expected during continuous or sustained military operations. Dr. Young is a graduate of the Command and General Staff Officer's Course and has been awarded the Army Commendation Medal with Oak Leaf Cluster, the Department of the Army Achievement Medal for Civilian Service, and the Expert Field Medical Badge. He is a member of the American Physiological Society, a fellow of ACSM, and has published over 100 scientific papers in peer-reviewed professional journals, government technical reports, and other open literature.

F

Biographical Sketches of Committee Members

John E. Vanderveen, Ph.D. *(chair),* is a former director of the Food and Drug Administration's (FDA) Office of Plant and Dairy Foods and Beverages in Washington, D.C. His previous position at FDA was as director of the Division of Nutrition at the Center for Food Safety and Applied Nutrition. He also served in various capacities (both military and civilian) at the U.S. Air Force (USAF) School of Aerospace Medicine at Brooks Air Force Base, Texas. During his time in the Air Force, Dr. Vanderveen participated in the development of USAF body composition standards. He has received numerous accolades for service from both FDA and USAF. Dr. Vanderveen is a member of ASCN, the American Society for Nutritional Sciences (ASNS), the Aerospace Medical Association, the American Dairy Science Association, and the American Chemical Society. He is a fellow of the Institute of Food Technologists (IFT) and an honorary member of the American Dietetic Association (ADA). He has served as treasurer of the American Society for Clinical Nutrition (ASCN) and as a member of IFT's National Academy of Sciences Advisory Committee. Dr. Vanderveen holds a B.S. in agriculture from Rutgers University in New Jersey and a Ph.D. in chemistry from the University of New Hampshire.

Bruce R. Bistrian, M.D., M.P.H., Ph.D., is a professor of medicine at Harvard Medical School and chief of Clinical Nutrition, Beth Israel Deaconess Medical Center. Formerly he was codirector of Hyperalimentation Services, New England Deaconess Hospital, and a lecturer in the Department of Nutrition and Food Science, Massachusetts Institute of Technology (MIT). He earned his M.D. from Cornell University, his M.P.H. from Johns Hopkins University in Baltimore, and his Ph.D. in nutritional biochemistry and metabolism from MIT. Dr. Bistrian's primary research interests include nutritional assessment, metabolic effects of acute infections, nutritional support of hospitalized patients, and the pathophysiology of protein-calorie malnutrition. He is a fellow of the American College of Physicians and received an Award of Merit from Harvard University and the Army Commendation Medal for his services as a Captain in the Medical Corps of the U.S. Army 7th Special Forces Group. Dr. Bistrian was president of the American Society for Parenteral and Enteral Nutrition, vice-president and president of ASCN, and a member of the board of directors of the Federation of American Societies of Experimental Biology. He served on the editorial boards of numerous nutrition and medical journals and is the author or coauthor of over 400 articles in scientific publications.

John Caldwell, Jr., Ph.D., is the principal research psychologist with the Warfighter Fatigue Countermeasures Program at the Air Force Research Laboratory, Brooks Air Force Base, Texas. He has published over 80 articles in peer-reviewed scientific journals and laboratory technical reports. He frequently lectures at safety briefings and scientific symposia, and he conducts operationally focused workshops on fatigue countermeasures for aviators and industrial personnel. He is a member of the National Sleep Foundation's Speakers Bureau and Science Advisory Council, and he frequently consults with various organizations on the effects of fatigue on pilots and methods for overcoming the adverse impact of fatigue in the aviation environment. Dr. Caldwell received his Ph.D. in experimental psychology in 1984 from the University of Southern Mississippi. In 1983 he became the assistant director of the Behavioral Medicine Laboratory at Children's Hospital National Medical Center in Washington, D.C., where he spent 3 years. Afterward, he spent 16 years with the U.S. Army Medical Research and Materiel Command conducting studies on methods of aviator status monitoring and on the effects of medications on aviator performance in specially instrumented flight simulators and aircraft. In August 2002 he transferred to the Air Force Research Laboratory at Brooks. The focus of his research is to fully understand the effects of sleep deprivation on pilots and to develop monitoring methodologies and fatigue countermeasures for use in the operational aviation environment. Key accomplishments have included the first-ever controlled aviator flight-performance evaluations of the efficacy of dextroamphetamine and modafinil for sustaining performance and the completion of several unique protocols investigating the feasibility of real-time monitoring of aviator physiological activity in flight.

Johanna T. Dwyer, D.Sc., R.D., is director of the Frances Stern Nutrition Center at New England Medical Center and a professor in the Departments of Medicine and of Community Health at the Tufts Medical School and School of Nutrition Science and Policy in Boston. She is also a senior scientist at the Jean Mayer U.S. Department of Agriculture Human Nutrition Research Center on Aging at Tufts University. Dr. Dwyer's work centers on life-cycle related concerns, such as the prevention of diet-related disease in children and adolescents and maximization of quality of life and health in the elderly. She also has a long-standing interest in vegetarian and other alternative lifestyles. Dr. Dwyer is currently the editor of *Nutrition Today* and on the editorial boards of *Family Economics* and *Nutrition Reviews*. She received her D.Sc. and M.Sc. from the Harvard School of Public Health, an M.S. from the University of Wisconsin, and completed her undergraduate degree with distinction from Cornell University. She is a member of the Institute of Medicine, the Technical Advisory Committee of the Nutrition Screening Initiative, and a past president of ASNS, a past secretary of ASCN, and a past president of the Society for Nutrition Education.

John W. Erdman, Jr., Ph.D., is a professor of nutrition and food science in the Department of Food Science and Human Nutrition and a professor in the Department of Internal Medicine at the University of Illinois at Urbana-Champaign. His research interests include the effects of food processing upon nutrient retention, the metabolic roles of vitamin A and beta-carotene, and the bioavailability of minerals from foods. His research regarding soy protein has extended into studies on the impact of non-nutrient components of foods, such as phytoestrogens on chronic disease. Dr. Erdman has published over 110 peer-reviewed research papers. He has authored or edited six books and major symposia proceedings. In 1994 he received the Borden Award for "distinctive research on the nutritional significance of any food or food component" from ASNS. In 1998 he chaired a Gordon Conference on Carotenoids, was a Burroughs Wellcome Visiting Professor in Basic Medical Sciences at the University of Georgia, and the G. Malcolm Trout Visiting Scholar at Michigan State University. In 1999 he received the Babcock-Hart Award from IFT. Dr. Erdman has served on many editorial boards, including: *Journal of Food Science*, *Cereal Chemistry*, *Journal of Nutrition*, and *Plant Foods for Human Nutrition*. He has also served on many program and planning committees for ASNS, IFT, and the National Academy of Sciences. In 1992 he was elected a fellow of IFT. Dr. Erdman received his M.S. and Ph.D. in food science from Rutgers University.

Helen W. Lane, Ph.D., R.D., is the chief nutritionist for NASA (National Aeronautics and Space Administration), and chief scientist for the Johnson Space Center's Habitability, Environmental Factors, and Bioastronautics Office. She has also served as the assistant to the Director for Advanced Program Coordination and Research and branch chief for Biomedical Operations and Countermeasures. Dr. Lane was an associate professor of nutrition at the University of Texas Medical Center from 1977 to 1984 and a professor of nutrition at Auburn University from 1984 to 1989. At present she serves as an adjunct professor, Department of Preventive Medicine and Community Health, at the University of Texas Medical Branch in Galveston. She has led efforts to define nutritional requirements for healthy crew members during spaceflight. Dr. Lane has completed research on body composition and on nutritional requirements for energy, water, electrolytes, protein, calcium, and iron, as well as clinical and basic research on selenium and breast cancer. As a registered dietitian, she is active in the ADA. She is also a member of ASNS and ASCN.

Melinda M. Manore, Ph.D., R.D., is currently a professor and chair, Department of Nutrition, Oregon State University, and is a registered dietitian. Her research interests include the interaction of nutrition and exercise in health, exercise performance, disease prevention, and reduction of chronic disease across the life cycle. Dr. Manore's research also focuses on factors regulating energy balance (i.e., energy expenditure, eating behaviors, and body weight and composition), and the role of nutrition, exercise, and energy balance on the reproductive cycle. She is a fellow of the American College of Sports Medicine (ACSM), and a member of ADA, ASCN, ASNS, and the North American Association for the Study of Obesity. She is currently chair of the ADA Nutrition Research Practice Group and received the ADA's Sports, Cardiovascular and Wellness Nutritionists Excellence in Practice award in 2001. Dr. Manore currently serves as a member of the USA Gymnastics National Health Advisory Board, the Gatorade Sport Science Institute Nutrition Board, and the Arizona Osteoporosis Coalition Medical Advisory Board. She is associate editor for *Medicine and Science in Sports and Exercise* and ACSM's *Health and Fitness Journal* and is on the editorial boards of the *Journal of the American Dietetic Association* and the *International Journal of Sport Nutrition and Exercise Metabolism*. Dr. Manore obtained her M.S. in health education and community health from the University of Oregon and her Ph.D. in human nutrition from Oregon State University.

William P. Morgan, Ed.D., is a professor of kinesiology and director of the Exercise Psychology Laboratory at the University of Wisconsin-Madison. Formerly he was a professor of physical education and director of the Sport Psychology Laboratory at the University of Arizona in Tucson. Dr. Morgan also spent 2 years as a visiting research psychologist, U.S. Army Research Institute of Environmental Medicine in Natick, MA. He earned an M.A. in health and physical education from the University of Maryland and an Ed.D. in psychology and physical education from the University of Toledo. Dr. Morgan's primary research interests focus on the antidepressant and anxiolytic effects of vigorous physical activity and selected psychological states and traits for developing prediction models that could be used for predicting panic behavior (and thus survival) in individuals performing physical activity in extreme environments. He has received numerous awards, including the Service Award of the Wisconsin Association for Health, Physical Education and Recreation; the Citation Award of ACSM; corecipient (with Dr. Peter B. Raven) of the John M. White Award for best research on respiratory protection from the American Industrial Hygiene Association; and the Medal of the Swedish Society of Medicine. Dr. Morgan has served as vice-president of the North American Society for the Psychology of Sport and Physical Activity, vice-president of ACSM, and president of the Division of Psychological Hypnosis of the American Psychological Association. He has served on the editorial boards of a number of sports, exercise, and psychology journals and has authored or coauthored over 200 articles in scientific publications.

Patrick M. O'Neil, Ph.D., is a professor of psychiatry and behavioral sciences at the Medical University of South Carolina, where he is also director of the

Weight Management Center. Dr. O'Neil has been involved in the study of obesity and its management since 1977, including clinical trials, basic research, teaching, and public education. He has been the principal investigator on a number of clinical trials of weight-loss agents. He is the author of over 100 professional publications primarily concerning psychological, behavioral, and other clinical aspects of obesity and its management. Dr. O'Neil has served on the Education Committee of the North American Association for the Study of Obesity since 1994 and was a member of its Ad Hoc Committee for Development of the Practical Guidelines. He is also immediate past president of the South Carolina Academy of Professional Psychologists, former member and chair of the South Carolina Board of Examiners in Psychology, and former chair of the Obesity and Eating Disorders Special Interest Group of the Association for the Advancement of Behavior Therapy. Dr. O'Neil received his B.S. in economics from Louisiana State University and his M.S. and Ph.D. in clinical psychology from the University of Georgia.

Esther M. Sternberg, M.D., is chief of the Section on Neuroendocrine Immunology and Behavior and associate branch chief of the Clinical Neuroendocrinology Branch of the National Institute of Mental Health Intramural Research Program at the National Institutes of Health (NIH). Dr. Sternberg received her M.D. and trained in rheumatology at McGill University, Montreal, Canada. She did post doctoral training at Washington University, Barnes Hospital, St. Louis, in the Division of Allergy and Immunology. She was subsequently a Howard Hughes associate and instructor in medicine at Washington University and Barnes Hospital before joining NIH. Dr. Sternberg is internationally recognized for her ground-breaking discoveries in the area of central nervous system-immune system interactions. She received the Arthritis Foundation William R. Felts Award for Excellence in Rheumatology Research Publications, was awarded the Public Health Service Superior Service Award, and was elected to the American Society for Clinical Investigation in recognition of this work. Dr. Sternberg is also internationally recognized as a foremost authority on the L-Tryptophan Eosinophilia Myalgia Syndrome. She was the first to describe this syndrome in relation to a similar drug, L-5-hydroxytryptophan, and published this landmark work in the *New England Journal of Medicine* in 1980.

Beverly J. Tepper, Ph.D., is an associate professor of food science at Cook College, Rutgers University. Her primary areas of research are the sensory evaluation, perception, and preference for foods; food intake regulation; and the effects of genetics, disease, and dietary restraint on food ingestion and eating behavior. She has published extensively in these areas. Formerly, she was a postdoctoral fellow at the Monell Chemical Senses Center. Dr. Tepper earned her M.S. and Ph.D. in nutrition from Tufts University. She currently serves on the editorial board of the *Journal of Sensory Studies* and has served as a reviewer for the *American Journal of Clinical Nutrition, Appetite, Brain Research*

Bulletin, European Journal of Clinical Nutrition, Journal of Food Science, Nutrition Research, and *Physiology and Behavior*.

Julian Thayer, Ph.D., is head of the Program on Emotions and Quantitative Psychophysiology, which he initiated, at the National Institute on Aging (NIA) of NIH. Prior to joining NIA, he held academic positions at Penn State University and the University of Missouri. His research interests concern biological and psychological adaptation and flexibility in the context of dynamic systems models with applications to psychopathology, pathophysiology, and health. This work utilizes indices of autonomic nervous system function derived from cardiac variability measures to probe whole organism systems. He received a B.A. in psychology from Indiana University and a Master's and Ph.D. from New York University.